Musculoskeletal Pain

Carl Edward Noe
Editor

Musculoskeletal Pain

Evidence-Based Clinical Evaluation and Management

Springer

Editor
Carl Edward Noe
The University of Texas Southwestern Med
Dallas, TX, USA

ISBN 978-3-031-86056-0 ISBN 978-3-031-86057-7 (eBook)
https://doi.org/10.1007/978-3-031-86057-7

This Springer imprint is published by the registered company Springer Nature Switzerland AG
The registered company address is: Gewerbestrasse 11, 6330 Cham, Switzerland

Preface

Musculoskeletal conditions are a major cause of disability and pain worldwide. According to the World Health Organization, approximately 1.7 billion people have musculoskeletal conditions and musculoskeletal conditions are the leading cause of disability in 160 countries.

Evidence-based evaluation and treatment is needed to focus available resources toward optimizing outcomes. Reducing the utilization of ineffective treatments may significantly reduce healthcare costs and treatment complications for patients with musculoskeletal pain. This book will cover a broad range of important musculoskeletal conditions and summarize up-to-date assessment and management options.

Dallas, TX, USA — Carl Edward Noe

Contents

Musculoskeletal Masqueraders of Spine Pain

1

Ankit Patel and Kegan Cunniff

Introduction

Neck and back pain are among the most common pain complaints endorsed by patients. However, identifying the source of a patient's neck or back pain is not always a straightforward task for the clinician as numerous musculoskeletal conditions can mimic spinal pathology. There are a variety of anatomical structures affected by these conditions. Pain experienced in the back or neck can commonly be referred from nearby structures. For example, pain arising from the hip or shoulder joints can radiate into the back and neck. Moreover, pains arising from spinal etiologies often refer to or radiate distally into the extremities, well beyond their spinal origins. Facetogenic pain can refer to the shoulder and hip regions, and radicular symptoms can radiate through the length of the extremities in dermatomal patterns that share similarities with other neuropathies (see Fig. 1.1). The result of this is significant symptom overlap between these musculoskeletal masqueraders and spinal pathologies.

Because of this overlap, clinicians treating spinal pathology will regularly encounter such patients with symptoms arising from non-spinal origins. It is therefore crucial for the clinician to have an understanding of the conditions that can masquerade as spinal pathology and how to pursue their diagnosis and treatment. Evidence-based physical examination techniques can also be helpful in the workup of these patients (*see* Table 1.1). The following chapter will delve into some of the more common conditions that can masquerade as spinal pathologies.

A. Patel (✉)
UT Southwestern Medical Center, Department of Physical Medicine and Rehabilitation, Dallas, TX, USA
e-mail: Ankit.Patel@UTSouthwestern.edu

K. Cunniff
Missoula Bone and Joint, Missoula, MT, USA

C. E. Noe (ed.), *Musculoskeletal Pain*,
https://doi.org/10.1007/978-3-031-86057-7_1

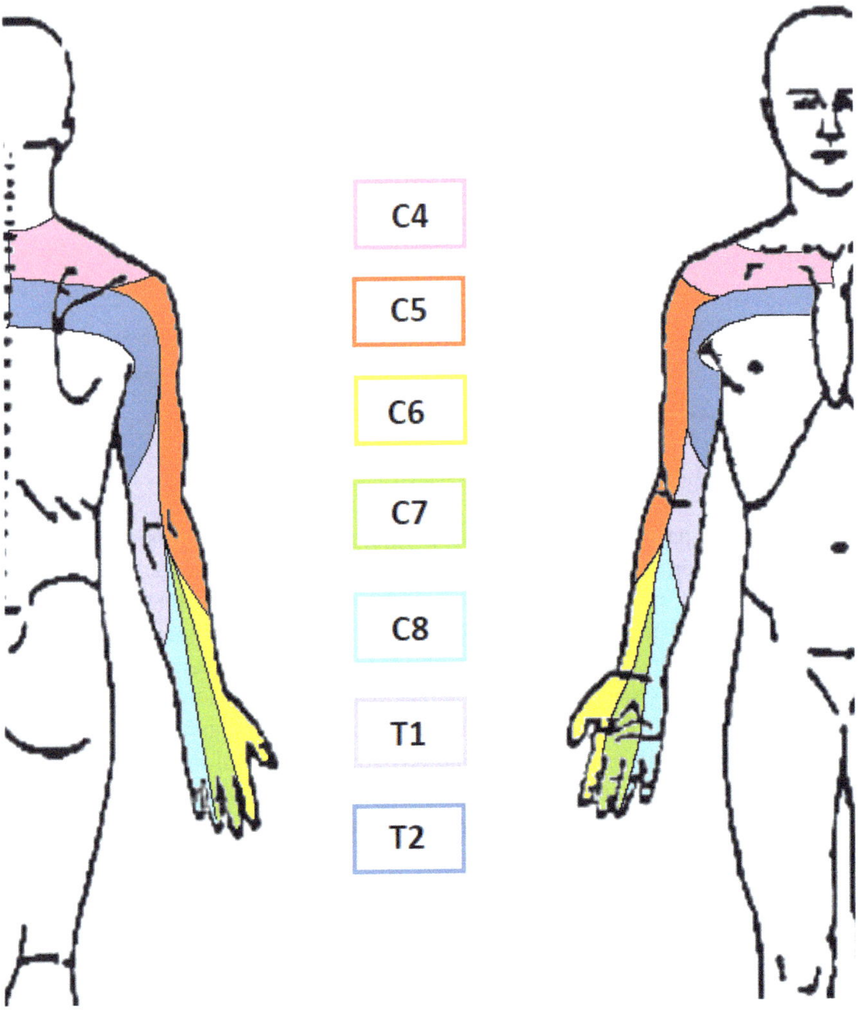

Fig. 1.1 Upper extremity dermatome map

Table 1.1 Evidence-based physical examination maneuvers

Pathology Tested	Maneuver	Sensitivity	Specificity	Source
Cervical Radiculopathy				
	Spurling	0.38–0.97	0.89–1.00	Thoomes et al. 2018
	Lhermitte's	0.09–0.41	0.97	Teoli et al. 2023
Rotator Cuff Tendinitis				
	Hawkins-Kennedy	0.91–0.92	0.25–0.44	Beaudreuil et al. 2009

(continued)

Table 1.1 (continued)

Pathology Tested	Maneuver	Sensitivity	Specificity	Source
	Jobe	0.63–0.95	0.55–0.68	Beaudreuil et al. 2009
	Belly Press	0.34	0.96	Kappe et al. 2018
Biceps Tendinitis				
	Bicipital Groove Tenderness	0.57	0.72	Rosas et al. 2017
	Uppercut	0.73	0.78	Rosas et al. 2017
Lumbar Radiculopathy				
	Straight Leg Raise	0.84	0.78	Tawa et al. 2017
	Femoral Stretch	1	0.83	Tawa et al. 2017
Hip OA/Impingement				
	FABER	0.82	0.25	Maslowski et al. 2010
	FADIR	0.96	0.11	Caliesch et al. 2020
Piriformis Syndrome				
	Active Piriformis	0.78	0.8	Martin et al. 2014
	Seated Stretch	0.52	0.9	Martin et al. 2014
	Straight Leg Raise	0.15	0.95	Martin et al. 2014

Cervical Facet Referral Patterns

While facetogenic pain does arise from the spine, facet-mediated pain is commonly referred to elsewhere in the body and, as such, can masquerade as a non-spinal pathology. Multiple studies have demonstrated cervical zygapophyseal joint referral patterns via stimulation or blocks of these joints or their corresponding medial branches [1–4]. As these referral patterns can extend into the periscapular and shoulder regions, symptomatic cervical facet pain can often be misdiagnosed as pathologies of other structures in those areas. It is therefore helpful for the clinician to be aware of these referral patterns to not only localize symptomatic facets but to limit misdiagnosis of cervical facetogenic pain as a more distal musculoskeletal pain. (*See* Fig. 1.2.)

Atlanto-Occipital Joint

Although not a facet joint, the atlanto-occipital joint is the specialized articulation between the first cervical vertebra and the skull where most of the rotation of the head is performed. This joint has been confirmed as a possible generator of head and neck pain [5]. While not as extensively studied as other cervical joints, the atlanto-occipital joint pain referral territory is more diffuse and vague than its neighbor, the atlantoaxial joint at C1-C2 [5, 6]. Atlanto-occipital joint pain can be experienced in the occipital/suboccipital, periauricular, temporal, periocular, and forehead regions [5, 6]. There may also be a component of radiation to the suprascapular region, as well [6].

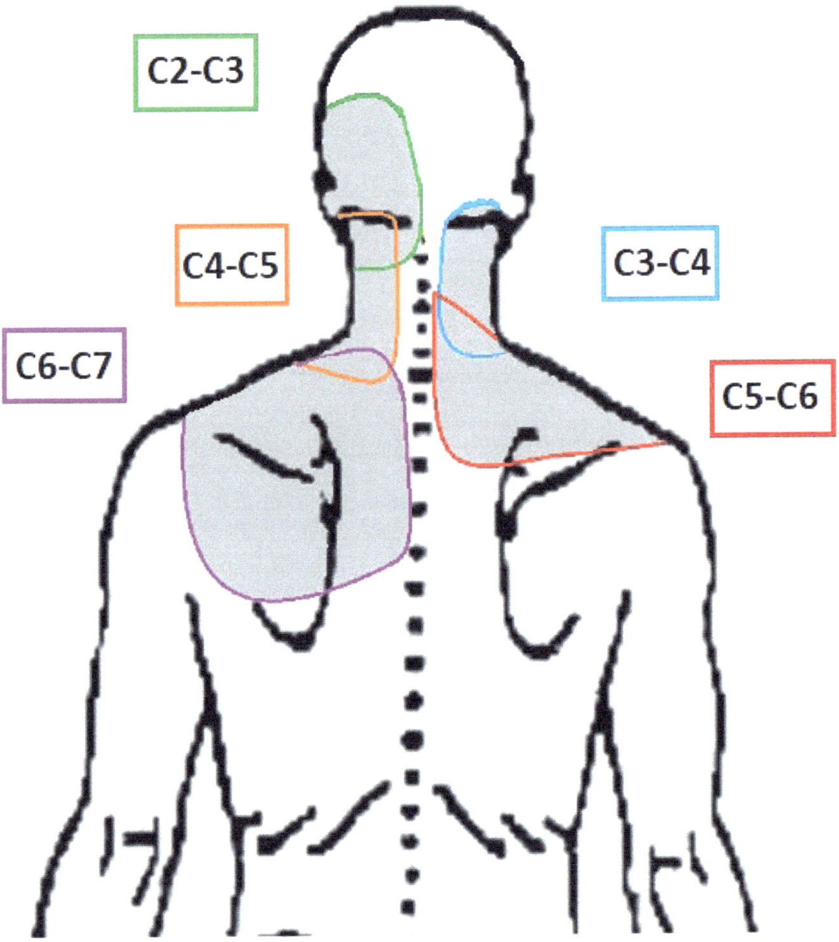

Fig. 1.2 Cervical facet referral patterns

Atlantoaxial (C1-C2) Joint

Pain referral mapping has demonstrated that pain from a symptomatic C1-C2 zygapophyseal joint tends to cluster around the suboccipital region [5]. There can be radiation of this pain into the occipital region, over the vertex of the skull, and as far as the upper forehead and orbital region, but tends to be less diffuse than atlanto-occipital pain [2, 5, 6]. Pain from this joint may also manifest as pain in the ear. This finding can aid in differentiating C1-C2 facet pain from the C2-C3 facet.

C2-C3

The C2-C3 zygapophyseal joint has been found to be one of the most frequently symptomatic joints of the cervical facets, accounting for roughly one-third of symptomatic facet joints in the neck [2]. The distribution of pain referral from the C2-C3 zygapophyseal joint is similar to that of the immediately superior C1-C2 joints but with a more laterally predominant distribution of symptoms. Like the C1-C2 facet joint, pain from the C2-C3 joint can be felt from the occiput to the forehead. However, pain tends to cluster laterally over the occiput, mastoid region, and upper temporoparietal regions [1, 2].

C3-C4

In Cooper et al's 2007 study of zygapophyseal joint pain, pain arising from the C3-C4 joint was rare (<5%) [2]. Pain from these particular joints could arise anywhere throughout the posterolateral aspect of the neck, as well as the occipital region of the head.

C4-C5

Pain from the C4-C5 zygapophyseal joints has been mapped to typically refer to the lower quadrant of the neck with a wide referral pattern extending from the suboccipital region of the neck to the proximal shoulder girdle. Pain extending into the upper extremity or head was not exhibited by symptomatic C4-C5 facets [2].

C5-C6

The C5-C6 zygapophyseal joint is also one of the most commonly symptomatic facet joints in the neck, having been identified in 35% of subjects with axial neck pain [2]. Pain from this joint has been demonstrated to refer from the base of the neck, through the upper trapezius and shoulder girdle, and laterally into the proximal humerus. Pain can occasionally be experienced over the scapular region, but typically does not extend into the head or beyond the elbow [2].

C6-C7

Pain arising from the C6-C7 joint is similar to the C5-C6 but is less commonly symptomatic and tends to refer more to the scapular region. Particularly, C6-C7 pain tends to cluster along the medial and inferior aspects of the scapula and typically does not radiate into the humerus. Moreover, pain from C6-C7 is rarely referred superiorly to the neck and did not demonstrate any referral to the head [2].

Shoulder Pathology Masquerading as Cervical Pathology

The symptoms of axial cervical spine pain can often be mimicked by shoulder pathologies [7]. However, it is also common for pain from the cervical spine to refer to the shoulder and vice versa. Pathologies of the neck or shoulder can arise concurrently with or as a direct result of one another, further complicating the diagnosis of these conditions [7–9]. Given the significant overlap in the presentation of these pathologies, it is critical for the examining provider to be able to identify and differentiate them from one another. Some common intrinsic shoulder pathologies that can masquerade as cervical spine pathologies are reviewed below.

Rotator Cuff Syndrome

Shoulder impingement and rotator cuff syndrome are among the most common causes of pain arising from the shoulder. In fact, it has been estimated that almost one-third of people over age 60 have some degree of rotator cuff tear [10]. The muscles of the rotator cuff work together to facilitate the rotation of the humerus at the glenohumeral joint. The supraspinatus, infraspinatus, teres minor, and subscapularis are the four muscles that comprise the rotator cuff. The most commonly impacted among these are the infraspinatus and supraspinatus, but all muscles in the rotator cuff are prone to degeneration over time due to both mechanical and intrinsic biological factors [11].

Pain from rotator cuff pathology can arise acutely or insidiously. The incidence of rotator cuff tears is positively correlated with age [12]. Pain is typically distributed along the anterolateral shoulder with pain that can radiate down the lateral humerus and proximally into the upper trapezius and neck [12]. This pattern of pain overlaps significantly with myofascial neck pain and the referral pattern from the more inferior cervical facets. Radiating pain can also increase the suspicion of radiculopathy; however, radiating arm pain from shoulder pathology rarely extends below the elbow. Aspects of the history and physical exam can be used to help identify rotator cuff pathology and differentiate it from spinal etiologies. Shoulder pain that worsens with repetitive overhead activities is a hallmark symptom of rotator cuff syndrome. Shoulder pain when lifting heavy objects or while lying on the affected side are also common symptoms suggestive of rotator cuff disease [13]. Weakness and atrophy of the rotator cuff muscles may be present in higher-grade tears which can sometimes mimic the muscle atrophy secondary to denervation seen in cervical radiculopathy [14].

There are numerous described physical examination maneuvers used in the diagnosis of rotator cuff disease. However, the sensitivity and specificity of these maneuvers are variable. Some of the higher-yield of these maneuvers are reviewed briefly below:

First, the Hawkins-Kennedy test is one of the most extensively studied exam findings for rotator cuff disease, specifically impingement of the supraspinatus. This maneuver is highly sensitive (91–92%), but poorly specific (25–44%) [15]. It is performed by abducting the shoulder and flexing the elbows each to 90 degrees. The examiner then internally rotates the shoulder, which produces pain in the shoulder when positive (See Fig. 1.3). The test can be further modified by repeating this maneuver with the tested arm in progressively more cross-body adduction.

Jobe's test, also known as the empty can test, is another maneuver used to detect supraspinatus tendinopathy. In this maneuver, the shoulder is placed in 90 degrees of flexion and abducted slightly from the midline so as to keep the humerus aligned with the scapular plane. The patient's thumb should be pointed at the floor, which places the shoulder in internal rotation. A shoulder is then stabilized by the examiner who concurrently applies a downward directed force on the arm (See Fig. 1.4). Pain or weakness during resistance is a positive test and is 63–95% sensitive and 55–68% specific for supraspinatus injury. Notably, weakness was a much more sensitive finding than pain [15].

The belly press test is used to isolate and test the subscapularis muscle which performs internal rotation of the shoulder joint. The sensitivity of this test for subscapularis lesions is low at 34%, but it was found to be 96% specific [16]. The belly press test is performed with the patient standing or sitting upright. Their elbows should be flexed to 90 degrees with the palm of the tested extremity pressed against the upper abdomen. The examiner fixes the tested elbow with one hand and then tries to pull the patient's hand away from the abdomen while the patient resists. Pain

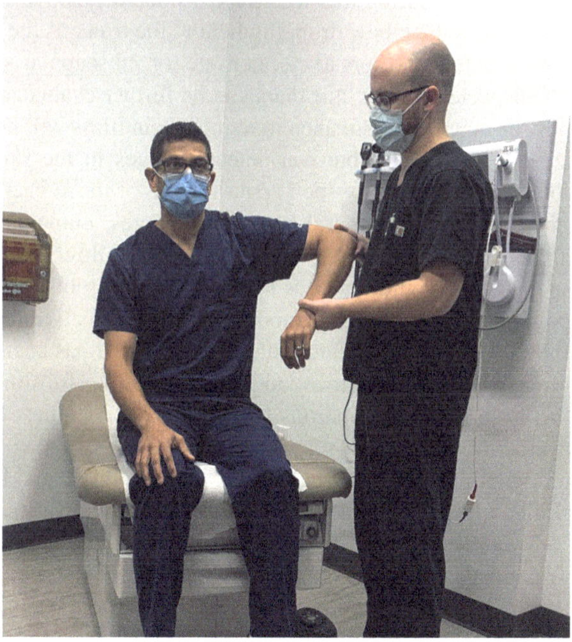

Fig. 1.3 Hawkins-Kennedy test

Fig. 1.4 Jobe's test

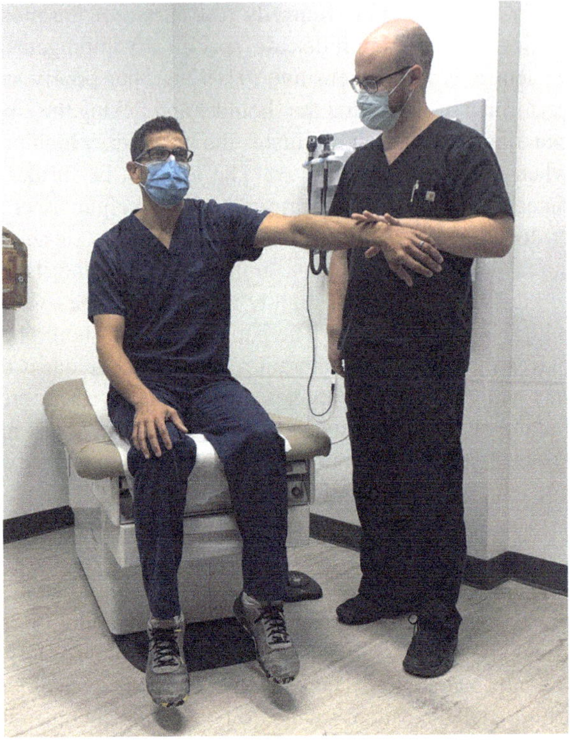

or weakness during this test are considered positive results. Weakness will often manifest as the elbow dropping behind the trunk as the patient resists as this allows the shoulder extensors to compensate for subscapularis weakness.

Suspected rotator cuff tears can be further evaluated with X-rays, ultrasonography, or magnetic resonance imaging. Plain films will not be able to directly visualize the rotator cuff but can detect changes in the skeletal structure that suggest rotator cuff pathology such as narrowing of the subacromial space due to superior migration of the humeral head, osteophytes, humeral subluxation, or rotator cuff arthropathy [13]. Ultrasound and MRI both allow for direct imaging of the soft tissues of the shoulder and as such can be key tools in the diagnosis of rotator cuff pathology. Both imaging modalities boast sensitivities and specificities over 80% for the diagnosis of rotator cuff tears, but MRI has been demonstrated to be slightly more sensitive than ultrasound when detecting full-thickness tears [17]. However, there are unique limitations to each of these studies. MRI may be limited by the availability of an MRI scanner, payor coverage, and cost to the patient. Ultrasound, on the other hand, may be more readily available and less expensive but requires a skilled ultrasonographer and/or radiologist to perform and interpret the scans.

Treatment options for rotator cuff syndrome depend on the nature of the tear. Treatment of mild and/or chronic rotator cuff tendinopathy often includes physical therapy and conservative pain management. For more persistent pain, steroid injection into the subacromial and/or subdeltoid bursa can provide more significant and long-lasting pain relief [18]. For patients with acute large tears, weakness, and/or pain refractory to the aforementioned treatments, surgery may be considered. Arthroscopic repair has become the predominant method of surgical intervention and has similar success rates to open repair with shorter recovery times. However, massive tears are difficult to repair and failure rates of these repairs are high. If there are massive tears not amenable to surgical repair, severe rotator cuff arthropathy, and/or pseudoparalysis, shoulder arthroplasty may be considered [19].

Biceps Tendinitis

Biceps tendinitis is a common mimicker of both axial neck pain and cervical radiculopathy and is often seen in patients with rotator cuff tendinopathy due to their anatomic relationship within the rotator interval. Biceps tendinitis is defined as the inflammation and/or degeneration of the tendon of the long head of the biceps [20]. Patients typically describe a throbbing or aching pain that localizes to the anterior shoulder and often radiates distally along the anterior aspect of the humerus. These radiating pains are frequently radially distributed, which significantly overlaps with the distribution of pain from a C5 radiculopathy [20, 21].

Biceps tendinopathy is most commonly degenerative in origin and associated with repetitive overuse; however, the traumatic rupture of the biceps tendon is also one of the most common tendon tears. Patients will often report exacerbation of symptoms with repetitive pulling, lifting, throwing, or overhead activities. Pain from biceps tendinitis also may worsen at night if the patient sleeps on the affected shoulder.

There are a number of physical examination signs and provocative maneuvers described to identify the pathology of the biceps tendon:

Tenderness of the long head tendon in the bicipital groove is assessed beginning with the patient's elbow flexed to 90 degrees and their humerus in slight internal rotation. The examiner palpates the tendon within the bicipital groove while externally rotating the shoulder. Tenderness to palpation at this location denotes a positive test for biceps tendinitis. This is one of the most powerful single examination maneuvers for detecting proximal biceps tendinitis with a sensitivity of 57% and specificity of 82% [22].

The Yergason test is performed by stabilizing the patient's arm against their side with the elbow in 90 degrees of flexion. The patient then performs wrist supination against resistance applied by the examiner. Pain elicited at or near the bicipital groove denotes a positive Yergason test. The sensitivity of the Yergason test for biceps and/or labral pathology is relatively poor at 41% but has a specificity of 79% [22].

The uppercut test is performed with the patient's tested arm beginning with the shoulder in a neutral position with the elbow flexed to about 90 degrees. The examiner grasps the patient's wrist or fist and asks the patient to thrust their fist across their body towards their contralateral shoulder as if throwing an uppercut punch in boxing. The examiner provides resistance to this motion. Pain or popping during the maneuver denotes a positive test. This exam maneuver has a sensitivity of 73% and a specificity of 78% in the detection of biceps tendinitis [22]. Combining the uppercut test with the tenderness of the biceps tendon within the bicipital groove has been found to be the most accurate exam maneuver for detecting biceps tendinitis and/or labral pathologies, boasting a sensitivity of 88% and specificity of 93% [22].

Imaging studies for the investigation of biceps tendinitis often begin with plain radiographs. Direct evaluation of the biceps tendon is not possible with X-rays but can be utilized to investigate possible areas of impingement and rule out alternate shoulder pathologies. Ultrasonography is typically the best imaging study to assess the extra-articular portions of the biceps tendon and is usually sufficient to establish a diagnosis of biceps tendinopathy. MRI or CT scan of the shoulder is often not necessary unless evaluating the most proximal aspects of the biceps tendon but is frequently obtained in anticipation of surgical intervention. MRI arthrography can be utilized to detect labral tears, which often occur alongside biceps tendon tears due to the long head of the biceps tendon's anatomical attachment to the superior aspect of the labrum. If the aforementioned studies are negative for shoulder pathology, cervical spine imaging and/or electrodiagnostic studies of the affected limb should be considered to rule out cervical radiculopathy [20].

The treatment for nontraumatic biceps tendinitis typically begins with conservative management with rest and avoidance of exacerbating activities, ice, and analgesic medications, such as NSAIDs or acetaminophen. Physical therapy emphasizing shoulder range of motion, rotator cuff strengthening, and scapulothoracic strengthening should also be utilized. Biceps tendon sheath injections with local anesthetic and steroids can be both diagnostic and therapeutic. Biceps tendon rupture or tendinitis that does not respond to at least three months of conservative management may be considered for surgical intervention [20].

Glenohumeral Arthritis

Another common musculoskeletal masquerader of neck and upper back pain is arthritis of the glenohumeral joint. Glenohumeral arthritis is one of the most common shoulder pathologies and is the third most common large joint impacted by osteoarthritis [23]. The majority of cases are degenerative in nature and strongly associated with age, with only about 2% of people in their 40s found to have glenohumeral arthritis and increasing to 27.5% of those in their 80s [23].

Pain from glenohumeral arthritis is typically described as gradual in onset and distributed throughout the shoulder with radiation into the upper trapezius. This does create a significant amount of overlap in pain distribution with pain referring from the axial cervical spine. Diagnosis is further obfuscated by the fact that patients with glenohumeral arthritis frequently have arthritis affecting the cervical spine as well. However, glenohumeral arthritis can be differentiated from that of the spine by pain with the range of motion of the shoulder, including pain during the passive range of motion. This can also differentiate pain due to glenohumeral arthritis from pain due to tendinopathy, which typically is not significantly painful during passive range of motion. Similar to rotator cuff tendonitis, pain from shoulder arthritis is also typically exacerbated by overhead activities [11].

Physical examination should focus on assessing range of motion. As previously stated, pain during both active and passive range of motion should increase suspicion of glenohumeral arthritis. Crepitus and decreased range of motion are also commonly seen in more advanced cases. Plain radiographs of the shoulder are typically all that is required to confirm the diagnosis of glenohumeral arthritis. Advanced imaging is usually only necessary in evaluating shoulder arthritis if surgical intervention is anticipated.

Conservative treatments can reduce symptoms and delay the need for surgical interventions. NSAIDs are a mainstay in the pharmacologic management of symptomatic glenohumeral arthritis. Although acetaminophen has been found to be less effective in reducing these pains when compared to NSAIDs, it has less frequent gastrointestinal and cardiovascular side effects [24]. Physical therapy featuring isometric exercises will allow for strengthening and stabilization of the shoulder girdle while limiting painful motion of the arthritic joint.

Mimickers of Cervical Radiculopathy

Carpal Tunnel Syndrome

Carpal tunnel syndrome is the most common entrapment neuropathy in the upper extremity. Its reported annual incidence is greater than 3% in United States adults but can reach as high as 8% in working adult populations [25, 26]. Carpal tunnel syndrome arises as a result of entrapment of the median nerve as it crosses the wrist through the carpal tunnel. The carpal tunnel is a space contained within the carpal bones dorsally and transverse carpal ligament which lies volarly in the wrist. The median nerve passes through this tunnel along with nine flexor tendons. The narrow aperture of the carpal tunnel combined with the numerous structures that pass through it make the median nerve highly prone to entrapment in this area.

There can be considerable overlap between the symptoms of median mononeuropathy at the wrist (carpal tunnel syndrome) and cervical radiculopathies, particularly those affecting the C6 nerve root [27]. Carpal tunnel syndrome has classically been described as manifesting as pain and/or paresthesia affecting the wrist, radial aspect of the palm, and the first three digits [28].

Due to the C6 innervation of the 1st and 2nd digits and the C7 innervation of the 3rd digit, cervical radiculopathies affecting these levels can be misdiagnosed as carpal tunnel syndrome and vice versa. Both carpal tunnel syndrome and cervical radiculopathies can result in hand weakness. As such, the examiner's knowledge of hand muscle innervation can aid in differentiating the two diagnoses. The thenar eminence is the site of most median innervated muscles in the hand, and it is at this location that atrophy as a result of carpal tunnel syndrome can be seen [28]. Thenar muscle atrophy is not expected in C6 or C7 radiculopathies as these muscles are typically C8 and T1 innervated.

Other findings in the history and physical examination that suggest carpal tunnel syndrome as the etiology of hand pain and paresthesia include: bilateral symptoms, nocturnal exacerbations, relief from shaking the hands, exacerbation by manual activities, and hand weakness [29, 30]. Conversely, findings of neck pain, neck pain, and/or paresthesia exacerbated by neck activity, and lower extremity symptoms argue more strongly for a cervical etiology than carpal tunnel syndrome [29].

Moreover, a thorough physical examination can also help differentiate between carpal tunnel syndrome and cervical radiculopathy. The sensitivities of the exam maneuvers focused on the detection of carpal tunnel syndrome are variable and typically poor in isolation. A Tinel's tap over the median nerve at the wrist, for example, boasts a sensitivity of 36–50% when assessing for carpal tunnel syndrome. Compression of the transverse carpal ligament for 30–60 seconds, also known as Durkan's test, has a reported sensitivity of 64% [30]. The sensitivity of Phalen's test (See Fig. 1.5) is similar at 57–68% sensitivity [30]. However, when the Phalen and Durkan tests are used in combination, sensitivity rises to 80% with a specificity of 92% [30]. Weakness of thumb abductors and thenar atrophy can also help to zero the diagnosis of carpal tunnel syndrome. While the sensitivity of these findings is poor, their reported specificity is higher than most other exam findings at 65–80% and 90–94%, respectively [30].

Electrodiagnostic studies are commonly used for differentiating peripheral nerve entrapments from radiculopathies. When diagnosing carpal tunnel syndrome, EMG/NCS has specificity reported between 94–99% [31]. The sensitivity of this study is lower, ranging from 56–85% [31]. This is in large part due to difficulty detecting mild lesions in nerve conduction studies. Witt et al. reported roughly one-third of these studies will produce normal results in patients with mild CTS [32].

Ultrasonography can also be a useful tool in diagnosing carpal tunnel syndrome. Multiple diagnostic criteria have been investigated in the literature, with the best described being the cross-sectional area of the median nerve at the carpal tunnel [33]. A meta-analysis by Fowler et al. determined the sensitivity and specificity of this measurement on diagnostic ultrasound to be 77.6% and 86.8%, respectively [34].

Fig. 1.5 Phalen's test

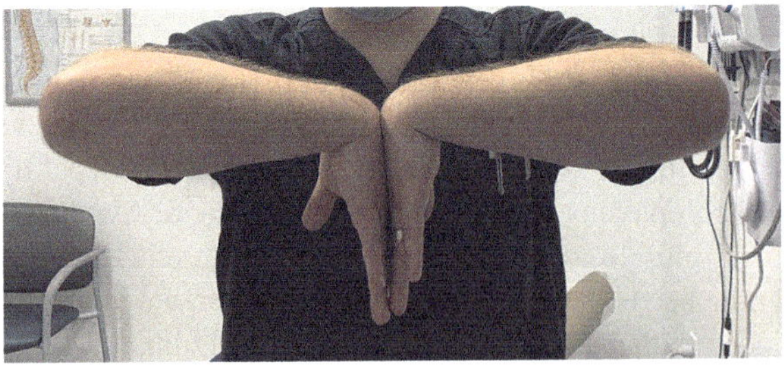

Ulnar Neuropathy

The ulnar nerve can also fall victim to symptomatic entrapment or compression in the upper extremity similar to the median nerve. In fact, ulnar nerve entrapment is the second most common mononeuropathy of the upper extremity behind carpal tunnel syndrome [35]. It is estimated that the incidence of ulnar mononeuropathy in the population is about 3% per year, with a prevalence of around 6% [36]. Compression of the ulnar nerve can classically occur at multiple distinct regions of the upper extremity. This happens most commonly as the ulnar nerve crosses the elbow through the retro-epicondylar groove, although there are three other classically described sites of entrapment of the ulnar nerve about the elbow [37]. Less frequently, the ulnar nerve may also be compressed as it crosses the wrist through Guyon's canal [38].

Similar to carpal tunnel syndrome, the symptoms of ulnar mononeuropathy can be difficult to distinguish from those of cervical radiculopathy, particularly of the C8 and T1 nerve roots [39]. Typically, ulnar nerve mononeuropathy across the elbow manifests as pain and paresthesias affecting the 5th and lateral aspect of the 4th digits. More severe cases of ulnar neuropathy may present with weakness affecting the ulnar innervated hand muscles, (i.e. abductor digiti minimi, interossei, medial lumbricals, adductor pollicis, etc.) while sparing the median innervated muscles (i.e. abductor pollicis brevis, opponens pollicis, flexor pollicis brevis, and lateral lumbricals).

Ulnar patterns of hand weakness can be detected on physical examination through manual motor testing of the aforementioned ulnar-innervated hand muscles, as well as the use of certain exam maneuvers. Similar to carpal tunnel syndrome, the sensitivity of these maneuvers when used in isolation is often poor. The elbow flexion sign, in which the patient's symptoms are reproduced by placing the elbow in full supination and maximal flexion for at least thirty seconds, has a sensitivity of 32% [40]. However, when this maneuver is combined with compression of the ulnar nerve in the retrocondylar groove, the sensitivity for ulnar neuropathy at the elbow rises to 91% with a specificity of 97% [40]. A Tinel's tap of the ulnar nerve at this location is also a useful exam maneuver with a sensitivity of 70% and a specificity of 98% [40].

There is a wide variety of additional physical examination tests to evaluate for ulnar motor weakness; however, there is little data on their sensitivity, specificity, and clinical utility in the literature [41]. Some of the more well-known of these tests include Froment's sign and Wartenberg's sign. To assess for a Froment's sign, the patient is asked to grab a piece of paper using a lateral pinch between the thumb and radial aspect of the second digit (See Fig. 1.6). A positive Froment's sign is characterized by the IP joint of the thumb needing to flex in order to maintain the grasp on the piece of paper. IP flexion at the thumb is maintained in ulnar neuropathy as the median-innervated flexor pollicis brevis is unaffected by the ulnar motor palsy [41]. In the case of cervical radiculopathy, this muscle would not be spared as it is C8-T1 innervated. Similarly, Wartenberg's sign assesses for weakness in the ulnar-innervated hypothenar muscles. A positive Wartenberg sign is described as an

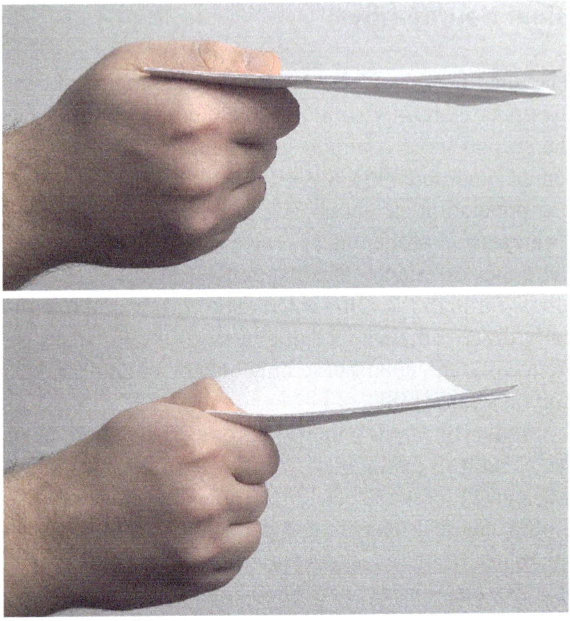

Fig. 1.6 Froment's sign (lower picture)

inability to adduct the 5th digit to touch the medial aspect of the 4th digit [41, 42]. This finding would be more suggestive of an ulnar nerve injury as opposed to cervical radiculopathy, in which hand weakness and atrophy would be more globally distributed throughout the hand and would include the median-innervated hand muscles.

Because of the variety of entrapment locations of the ulnar nerve as it courses the upper extremity, determining the exact site of a lesion can be troublesome. As such, electrodiagnostic studies are an essential tool to localize the site of an ulnar nerve lesion. Electrodiagnosis becomes particularly valuable when used to determine the site of intervention to treat an ulnar nerve lesion due to the multiple possible sites of entrapment. However, the sensitivity of electrodiagnostic testing of ulnar neuropathies is not well established. Electrodiagnosis of ulnar mononeuropathy of the elbow has sensitivities reported between 37% and 86% [43]. The specificity of electrodiagnostic testing for ulnar nerve mononeuropathy at the elbow has been reported as high as 95% [44].

However, when compared to carpal tunnel syndrome, electrodiagnosis of ulnar mononeuropathy is less accurate in the clinical diagnosis of mild pathology. EMG/NCS has been reported to have a sensitivity of 47% for the detection of mild ulnar mononeuropathy at the elbow. For patients with clinically very mild symptoms, the sensitivity of EMG/NCS dropped to 3% [45]. Pelosi and Mulroy reported a sensitivity of 62% and 20% percent for ultrasonographic diagnosis of mild and very mild ulnar mononeuropathy, respectively [45]. As such, ultrasound evaluation can play a crucial complementary role to electrodiagnostic testing in diagnosing ulnar nerve lesions. Moreover, ultrasonography may be of higher utility in the detection of milder ulnar nerve mononeuropathies. Overall, ultrasonographic diagnosis of ulnar neuropathies may boast sensitivity and specificity as high as 84% and 80%, respectively [46].

Thoracic Outlet Syndrome

Brachial plexopathies are another subset of pathologies that can mimic cervical radiculopathy. One such plexopathy commonly described is neurogenic thoracic outlet syndrome (TOS). TOS in general arises as the result of neurovascular structures that travel through the thoracic outlet. Classically, these structures are usually compressed between the anterior scalene muscle and the first rib, but compression can occur at various regions at or near the thoracic outlet [47]. The cause of TOS is the result of compression by a soft tissue structure in 70% of cases, with bony compression comprising the remaining 30% [47]. TOS can arise congenitally but is most commonly the result of trauma to the area. The presence of cervical ribs or large C7 transverse processes likely predisposes to this condition, with roughly 80% of traumatic TOS with these bony abnormalities only developing symptoms after trauma [48].

There are three described forms of TOS: neurogenic, arterial, and venous. Due to its similar symptom profile to cervical radiculopathy, this review will focus on neurogenic TOS in which the brachial plexus is the structure impacted by compression or entrapment. The incidence of thoracic outlet syndrome has been reported between 0.3 and 8.0% per year. Neurogenic TOS accounts for 90% of these cases and affects females at a 3.5 to 1 ratio when compared to males [47].

Neurogenic TOS can present with weakness, paresthesias, and/or pain in the upper extremity, usually in a nonradicular pattern. Neurogenic TOS can affect the upper brachial plexus; however, lower plexus lesions account for up to 90% of cases [49]. Neurogenic TOS affecting the lower plexus usually manifests with weakness of C8-T1 innervated muscles and sensory deficits in the ulnar hand, as well as the ulnar aspect of the forearm [50]. Upper plexus TOS involves the C5-C7 nerve fibers with weakness affecting muscles in these associated myotomes, as well as pain and paresthesia in the supraclavicular region that can radiate into the upper chest, neck, head, and radial aspect of the forearm and hand [50].

Differentiating thoracic outlet syndrome from other similar diagnoses such as cervical spinal pathology, shoulder pathology, and more distal peripheral mononeuropathies can be difficult. The symptoms of TOS as compared to the other aforementioned diagnoses tend to be distributed more diffusely and in a nonradicular pattern. This differs from typical cervical spinal pain which is usually more constant, exacerbated by movement of the neck, and refers to a more dermatomal pattern. Similarly, shoulder pathology also tends to be more constant and worsens with movement of the shoulder. Symptoms from upper extremity mononeuropathies can overlap with neurogenic TOS, particularly ulnar neuropathies. However, these mononeuropathies tend to be distributed along predictable nerve distributions and rarely radiate proximally to the elbow [50].

A number of provocative maneuvers have been described to aid in the detection of thoracic outlet syndrome; however, their utility is limited in isolation and are best used in combination. It is possible to find a positive Tinel's sign when percussing over the supraclavicular and infraclavicular regions; however, the sensitivity of this finding was found to be 46% with a specificity of 56% [51]. The pressure over the scalene muscles and the upper limb tension test (ULTT) were each found to produce positive findings in over 90% percent of patients with neurogenic TOS [52]. The upper limb tension test is performed by abducting the shoulders to just above 90 degrees with the forearm supinated, elbows flexed to 90 degrees, and the wrist and fingers fully extended by the examiner. Next, the elbow is then passively extended by the examiner while the neck is laterally flexed towards the opposite shoulder. A positive test is denoted by pain down the arm, especially around the elbow, in either arm [52].

Roos test, in which the patient holds their arms overhead with elbows in 90 degrees of flexion and repeatedly opens and closes the hands for three minutes, is a commonly described maneuver for the detection of TOS with a relatively high sensitivity of 84%. However, this finding is nonspecific. When combined with the Adson test, which has a similar sensitivity, the positive findings are 82% specific for thoracic outlet syndrome [51]. Adson's test can be performed by placing the patient's shoulder in 30 degrees of abduction and maximal extension. The radial pulse is palpated at the wrist, and the patient is then asked to rotate their head towards the extended shoulder, inhale deeply, and then hold their breath. A decrease or obliteration of the radial pulse is a positive finding for thoracic outlet syndrome. It is important to note, however, that both Roos' and Adson's tests are more useful in identifying vascular TOS.

Imaging and electrodiagnostics tend to be limited in their diagnostic utility when detecting TOS. Plain X-rays of the cervical spine can play a limited role in the diagnosis of thoracic outlet syndrome in that they can quickly and effectively identify cervical ribs or large cervical transverse processes that predispose to TOS [52]. Similarly, electrodiagnostic testing is typically normal in patients suffering from TOS. Moreover, when there are positive findings on EMG/NCS, the findings are often nonspecific [52, 53]. Decreased amplitude of sensory nerve action potentials have been found to be most sensitive in detecting neurogenic TOS but still is normal in approximately half of affected patients [54]. MR neurography may have a role in the diagnosis of neurogenic TOS; however, there is not yet a consensus on imaging protocols or diagnostic criteria [54]. Ultrasonography is an emerging tool for the diagnosis of TOS, via Doppler studies and direct measurement of nerves [53]. Diagnostic blocks with local anesthetic have also been suggested in the literature, but the diagnostic value of these has not been established.

Treatment of neurogenic thoracic outlet syndrome is typically conservative and clinical in nature. Physical therapy centered on strengthening and stretching the neck and shoulder girdle and postural correction is a mainstay of treatment. Anti-inflammatory drugs are useful in decreasing pain. For patients in which the area of compression can be discretely identified, chemodenervation of the scalene muscles with botulinum toxin can reduce symptoms in some patients. Surgery may be indicated in refractory cases to address anatomical sites of plexus compression or entrapment [47].

Lumbar Spine Referred Pain Versus Hip Pain

Musculoskeletal disorders involving the lower back and hip region are common reasons for patients to seek medical attention. Lower back pain has an estimated worldwide point prevalence of 18.3% and is a leading cause of disability [55]. Hip pain is also a common musculoskeletal complaint in adults and the prevalence increases with age. In adults over the age of 45, it is estimated that 6.7–9.7% have osteoarthritis of the hip, and one in four adults will develop symptomatic hip osteoarthritis [56].

For clinicians that manage patients with musculoskeletal and spine conditions, it is important to obtain a thorough history and to perform a comprehensive physical examination. Analysis of the patient's pain referral pattern can also be a very useful tool in formulating a differential diagnosis. It is estimated that 90% of lower back pain is nonspecific, and approximately one-third of cases do not have a triggering event [55]. Patients with mechanical lower back pain may complain of pain that is aggravated with activity and alleviated with rest. Patients with lumbosacral spine conditions such as lumbar facet-mediated pain, discogenic lower back pain, vertebrogenic lower back pain, and sacroiliac joint pain can often present with referred pain in the hip, buttock, and thigh region. (See Fig. 1.7) This type of referred pain can present a diagnostic dilemma for clinicians as it has a significant overlap with other musculoskeletal pain generators including the hip.

While patients with hip pain may describe symptoms in the anterior, lateral, and/or posterior aspect of the hip, intra-articular sources of hip pain present with predominantly anterior hip pain [57]. These patients may present with painful and limited internal rotation of the hip which can interfere with ambulation, donning and doffing shoes, and transferring in and out of a vehicle [11]. Many patients often present for clinical attention with pain from both the lumbar spine and the hip. In these scenarios, treatment of one condition may not necessarily resolve all of the patient's pain.

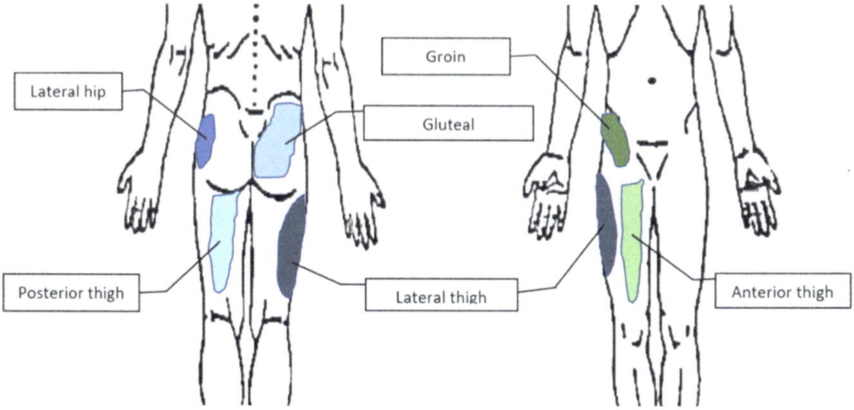

Fig. 1.7 Lumbar pain referral patterns

For patients with lower back pain, physical examination should include a comprehensive neurologic exam and musculoskeletal exam including spinal inspection, palpation, and range-of-motion testing [58]. There is a paucity of strong evidence to support any specific provocation tests on physical examination to diagnose lumbar facet-mediated pain, discogenic pain, and vertebrogenic pain. For patients with suspected lumbar facet-mediated pain, a recent multispecialty-based consensus guideline concluded that there is no pathognomonic history or physical examination findings that predicted response to facet joint blocks in patients with chronic lower back pain [59]. If the sacroiliac joint is suspected as a pain generator, there are some proponents who support the use of sacroiliac joint provocation maneuvers, such as the FABER (Patrick's) test (see Fig. 1.8), Gaenslen test, compression test, distraction test, and Yeoman test. Based upon a recent review of the literature, Buchanan et al. concluded that the sacroiliac joint may be a potential source of pain if the patient has reproduction of pain with at least three of these provocative maneuvers [60].

Physical examination maneuvers such as passive hip flexion, hip adduction, and hip internal rotation may demonstrate restriction in range of motion and can reproduce pain in the hip. This combination of physical exam maneuvers has an estimated sensitivity of 59–100% and specificity of 4–75% for intra-articular hip pathology [57]. For hip osteoarthritis, decreased hip adduction on physical examination was noted to have a sensitivity of 80% and specificity of 81% [61]. In a study by Brown et al., the presence of a limp, groin pain, or limited internal range of motion of the hip significantly predicted a disorder of the hip over the spine. They specifically found that patients with a limp were seven times more likely to have a hip disorder or a combination of a hip and spine disorder, compared to only a spine disorder [62]. While physical examination is an important part of the overall evaluation of patients with hip pain, a systematic review with meta-analysis found limited evidence to support the use of hip physical examination tests as stand-alone diagnostic tools for patients with suspected hip pathology [63].

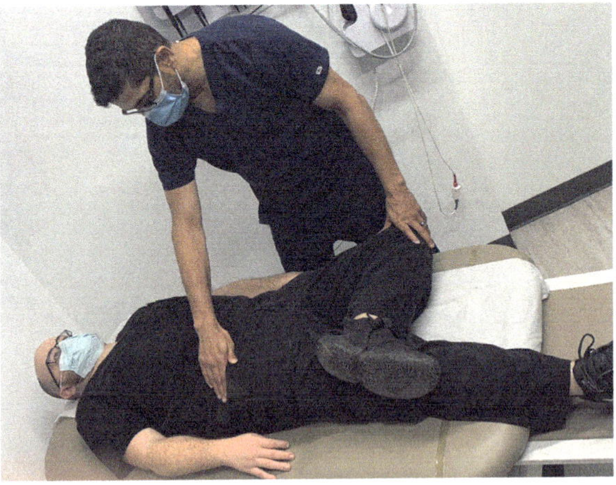

Fig. 1.8 FABER test

For patients who present with nonspecific mechanical low back pain, without red flag symptoms, imaging is generally not indicated early on. There are recommendations from several clinical guidelines that discourage routine imaging in these scenarios [64, 65]. Furthermore, a systematic review of several randomized controlled trials did not show improvement in clinical outcomes with imaging [66].

Radiography is the first-line imaging study for hip pain [67]. An anteroposterior radiograph of the pelvis, to evaluate for joint space narrowing and osteophyte formation, should be considered the starting point [57], however relying solely on hip radiographs is not advisable. In two large studies of patients with osteoarthritis, only 20.7% to 23.8% of patients with radiographic evidence of hip osteoarthritis had hip pain [68]. These studies also revealed that 9.1% to 15.6% of patients with frequent hip pain had radiographic evidence of hip osteoarthritis. A systematic review also noted a poor correlation between intra-articular hip pathology noted on imaging and symptomatic hip pain [69].

In circumstances in which the history, physical exam, radiographic findings, and pain pattern evaluation do not lead to a clear-cut etiology of pain, diagnostic injection therapy can be useful in delineating the primary pain generator and subsequently formulating an appropriate treatment plan. For patients with suspected lumbar facet-mediated pain, diagnostic lumbar facet joint nerve blocks can be given consideration. This intervention has received a moderate to strong strength of recommendation by recent evidence-based guidelines published by the American Society of Interventional Pain Physicians [70]. Similarly, in patients with suspected sacroiliac joint-mediated pain, the diagnostic sacroiliac joint block can be considered a confirmatory tool [71]. Ultrasound-guided hip injections can be a safe and accurate tool for both diagnostic and therapeutic purposes [72]. In a systematic review evaluating surgical outcomes of patients who underwent diagnostic hip injections, Lynch et al. concluded that imaging findings are not reliable predictors of injection response, and that nonresponse to injection was a strong negative predictor of surgical outcome [73].

Lumbar Spinal Stenosis Versus Hip Osteoarthritis

In the US, the prevalence of lumbar spinal stenosis is approximately 11% and it increases with age [74]. Lumbar spinal stenosis can lead to neurogenic claudication and symptoms that masquerade as symptomatic hip osteoarthritis. Some patients may have coexisting hip osteoarthritis and lumbar spinal stenosis, or hip-spine syndrome, making it a challenge clinically to distinguish the primary source of the patients' complaints. Similar to patients with painful hip osteoarthritis, patients with symptomatic lumbar spinal stenosis can experience pain in the lower extremities while standing or walking. These claudication symptoms typically improve with sitting, lying down, or bending forward at the waist. Evaluation of the pain patterns can be useful but should be interpreted with caution. While radiating pain symptoms extending distal to the knee can often be from a lumbar spine etiology, one study noted that 47% of patients with isolated hip arthritis experienced pain radiating below the knee [75]. Physical examination of this patient population is often normal in the seated position [76]. A small percentage may have a reproduction of radicular symptoms with a straight leg test or femoral stretch test [77]. Some authors have suggested that patients with lumbar spinal stenosis may demonstrate an increase in symptoms with lumbar extension, and they may have sensorimotor changes in a specific dermatome if there is chronic nerve root compression [78].

Rainville et al. surveyed musculoskeletal physicians who co-manage hip and spine conditions to gain insight into the potential diagnostic value of several signs and symptoms [79]. The survey found the following items favored symptomatic hip osteoarthritis over lumbar spinal stenosis: groin pain, pain that decreased with continued walking, pain that occurs immediately with walking, pain that occurs immediately with standing, pain getting in/out of a car, pain with dressing the symptomatic leg, and difficulty reaching the foot of the symptomatic leg while dressing. The survey study also found that pain below the knee, leg tingling and/or numbness, and some pain in both legs favored the diagnosis of symptomatic lumbar spinal stenosis over hip osteoarthritis. The physicians in the survey also favored the diagnosis of hip osteoarthritis over lumbar spinal stenosis if the physical examination revealed a limp, limited weight-bearing on a painful leg when standing, and painful and restricted range of motion with hip maneuvers.

There is an absence of strong evidence to support any one stand-alone history or physical examination finding to rule in or rule out symptomatic spinal stenosis. In a systematic review investigating the clinical evaluation for lumbar spinal stenosis, Suri et al. found that the symptoms that most strongly increased the likelihood of having the clinical syndrome of lumbar spinal stenosis were no pain when seated, improvement of symptoms when bending forward, the presence of bilateral buttock or leg pain, and neurogenic claudication. The authors also noted that the absence of neurogenic claudication decreased the likelihood of the diagnosis. The presence of a wide-based gait and abnormal Romberg test also increased the likelihood of having the clinical syndrome of lumbar spinal stenosis [80]. A more recent systematic review noted several factors that may increase the probability of diagnosing lumbar spinal stenosis in patients, including no pain when seated, numbness of the perineal region, or symptoms after a march test [81]. The same study also noted a greater probability of diagnosing lumbar spinal stenosis if there was an abnormal Romberg test on physical examination.

Based on their systematic review, Petersen et al. proposed a set of clinical criteria to help accurately diagnose lumbar spinal stenosis [82]. According to their research, the diagnosis is more likely if there are ≥3 out of 5 of the following history items: age >48 years, bilateral symptoms, leg > back pain, pain while walking/standing, and pain relief with sitting. They also noted a higher likelihood of symptomatic lumbar spinal stenosis if the patient experiences improvement in walking tolerance with the spine in flexion and relief of symptoms by forward bending.

Magnetic resonance imaging has a high sensitivity for evaluating lumbar spinal stenosis and is the preferred imaging modality to evaluate the neural elements and the size of the spinal canal [76]. However, it should be noted that imaging findings of stenosis do not necessarily correspond to symptomatic patients. A systematic review by Jensen et al. revealed that 11% of asymptomatic patients had radiologic evidence of lumbar spinal stenosis [83].

In circumstances in which the history, physical exam, radiographic assessment, and pain pattern evaluation do not lead to a clear-cut etiology of pain, diagnostic injection therapy can be useful in delineating the primary pain generator and subsequently formulating an appropriate treatment plan. There is a lack of strong evidence to support the role of diagnostic injections for lumbar spinal stenosis, however diagnostic hip injection can be given consideration. Ultrasound or fluoroscopy-guided intra-articular hip injections have been utilized with varying degrees of accuracy to isolate intra-articular hip pathology as the primary pain generator [84–86].

Lumbosacral Radiculopathy Mimickers

Sciatica refers to pain radiating down the lower extremity in the sciatic nerve distribution. The most common cause of sciatica symptoms is nerve root compression in the lumbar spine. The annual prevalence of sciatica in the population is estimated to be 9.9–25% [87]. It is also not uncommon for patients with lumbar radiculopathy to have other coexisting musculoskeletal disorders [88]. Less common disorders such as piriformis syndrome and meralgia paresthetica can mimic sciatica symptoms or radiculopathy by causing pain in similar distributions as lumbosacral radiculopathies (See Fig. 1.9) [11].

Piriformis syndrome involves sciatic nerve compression as the nerve passes through or near the piriformis muscle. It is estimated that piriformis syndrome

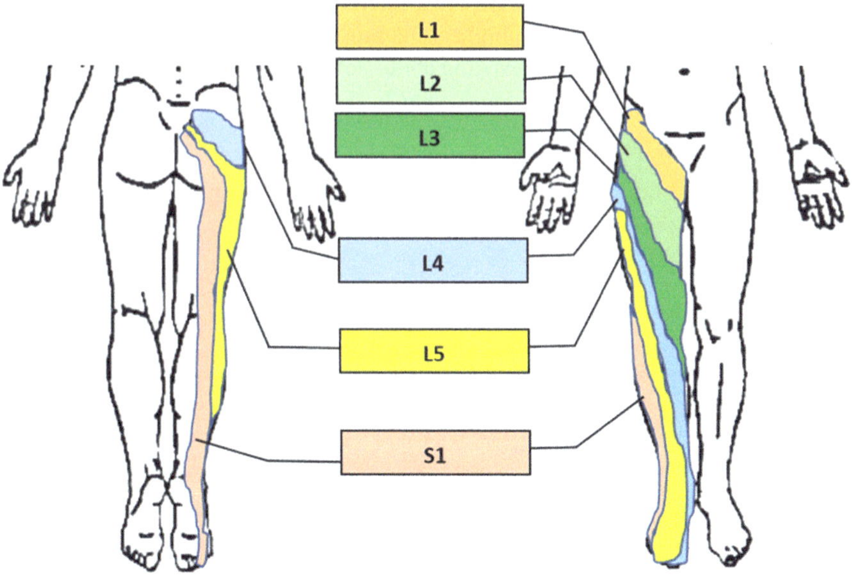

Fig. 1.9 Lumbosacral radicular pain patterns

accounts for 6 to 8% of all sciatica cases [89]. Patients with piriformis syndrome may complain of paresthesias and/or pain radiating from the gluteal region into the posterolateral aspect of the lower leg. This distribution of pain can mimic L5 and S1 radiculitis. In a systematic review of patients with piriformis syndrome, the presence of buttock pain and worsening of sciatica symptoms with sitting were common clinical features [90].

It is recommended that patients with suspected radiculopathy undergo a comprehensive musculoskeletal and neurologic exam. Physical examination using a straight leg raise test (SLR) may help delineate lumbosacral radiculopathy due to a herniated disc (See Fig. 1.10). A systematic review by Nee et al. revealed a fair degree of inter-rater reliability when provocation of lower extremity radicular symptoms was a requirement for a positive SLR [91].

Hopayian et al. found that the most common physical exam features in patients with piriformis syndrome included tenderness over the greater sciatic notch and worsening of pain with exam maneuvers that increased tension in the piriformis muscle [90]. In the physical examination of a patient with suspected piriformis syndrome, the examiner can attempt to reproduce the lower extremity pain symptoms using the FADIR test. This maneuver involves passively flexing, adducting, and internally rotating the hip on the symptomatic side to stretch the piriformis muscle (See Fig. 1.11). The examination is considered positive if it reproduces the patient's sciatica pain symptoms in patients reporting sciatica-like symptoms.

In a study of 33 patients with sciatica nerve entrapment in the gluteal region, the SLR test was positive in 17% [92], suggesting that a positive SLR should not be used to exclude the possibility of the patient having piriformis syndrome. This study also found that a combination of an active piriformis test and a seated piriformis stretch test provided the highest diagnostic accuracy. The active piriformis test involves the examiner resisting abduction and external rotation of the hip

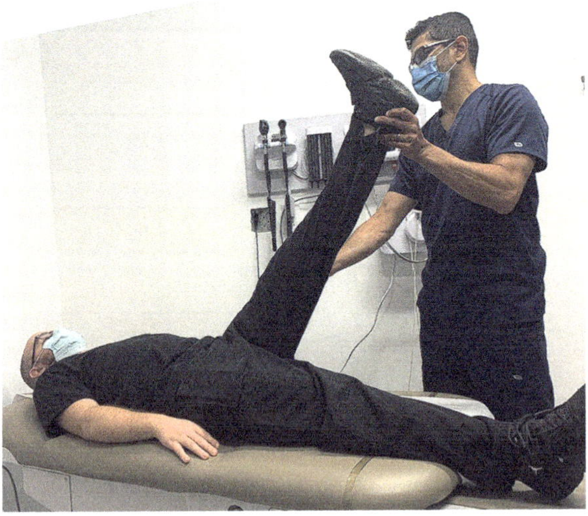

Fig. 1.10 Straight leg raise test

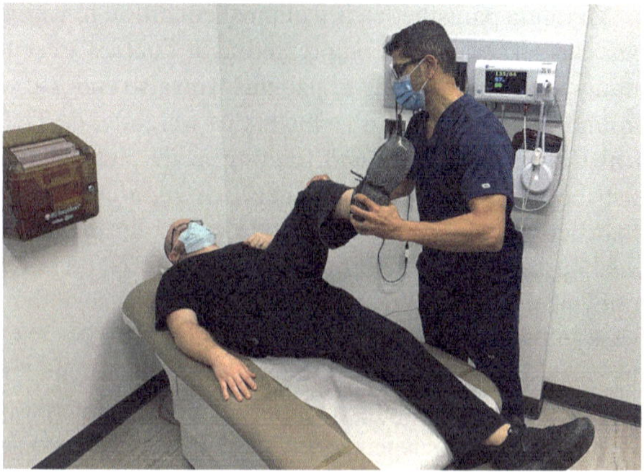

Fig. 1.11 FADIR test

joint. The seated stretch test involves having the patient seated off the edge of the exam with the hip flexed and the knee extended on the symptomatic side. The examiner then palpates the greater sciatic notch while adducting and internally rotating the leg.

Imaging of patients with suspected lumbar radiculopathy typically starts with plain radiographs to assess alignment, spondylosis, instability, fractures, and prior surgical changes. The next step is often magnetic resonance imaging to evaluate for neural compression and to assess soft tissue including disc herniations. Diagnostic imaging can reveal asymptomatic spinal pathology [93]; therefore, it is imperative to correlate the imaging findings with the patient's clinical signs and symptoms. For patients with suspected piriformis syndrome, a recent study of magnetic resonance neurography (or MR Neurography) to assess piriformis muscle bulk asymmetry and sciatic nerve signal changes at the level of the sciatica notch demonstrated high specificity and moderate sensitivity [94].

In some scenarios in which the history, physical exam, and imaging findings are inconclusive, electrodiagnostic testing can be considered to differentiate between radiculopathy versus a peripheral nerve disorder [95]. Electromyography (EMG) can serve a complementary role to diagnostic imaging and has a high specificity and modest sensitivity for radiculopathy [96]. It should be noted; however, that electrodiagnostic testing is operator-dependent and the findings need to be correlated clinically. For patients with piriformis syndrome, the EMG would be expected to be negative, and there is insufficient evidence to support the role of electrodiagnostic testing for this condition. In patients with suspected radiculopathy in which the diagnosis remains unclear, lumbar selective nerve root blocks can be considered however there is limited clinical evidence at this time to support their diagnostic accuracy [97]. Ultrasound-guided piriformis muscle injections and peri-sciatic nerve blocks have been utilized diagnostically; however, there is a paucity of clinical evidence at this time.

Meralgia paresthetica is a clinical condition in which the lateral femoral cutaneous nerve (LFCN) is compressed as it courses over the groin region. It is commonly seen in the setting of patients who also endorse wearing tight-fitting clothing around the waist and with a history of weight gain. The presentation often involves a history of numbness and tingling in the anterolateral aspect of the thigh. The distribution of this condition overlaps significantly with radiculopathy in the L3 distribution. Meralgia paresthetica would not be expected to present with motor weakness or patellar reflex deficit as the LFCN is a purely sensory nerve. Therefore, a physical examination may demonstrate sensory deficits to light touch and pinprick in the dermatomal distribution of the LFCN. The patient with L3 radiculopathy may present with a patellar reflex deficit and in severe cases quadriceps weakness. The femoral stretch test can be considered for the physical examination of a patient with suspected L3 radiculopathy. This exam maneuver is considered positive if passive hip extension produces radicular pain while the patient is in the prone position. Nerve conduction studies (NCS) can be considered for evaluation of lateral femoral cutaneous neuropathy however the examination can be technically limited by several factors including patient body habitus. Ultrasound-guided nerve block of the LFCN can be considered diagnostically if there is a high clinical index of suspicion but the diagnosis remains unconfirmed.

Conclusion

Patients with musculoskeletal disorders and spine pain can present with overlapping symptoms. The evaluation should start with a thorough history and physical examination. Evaluation of the pain referral pattern can be very useful in formulating a differential diagnosis. Imaging studies and electrodiagnostic testing can aid in narrowing down the differential however clinical correlation is highly recommended. Diagnostic injections can also be considered, particularly for patients who have more than one potential pain generator. Overall, there is a growing recognition of the importance of a comprehensive and systematic approach to the evaluation of this patient population, however further research is warranted in this field to provide evidence-based and cost-effective care.

Bullet Points

- Overlapping pain and symptom patterns exist between the spine, shoulder, and hip
- Peripheral nerve disorders can mimic symptoms of radiculopathy or myelopathy
- Patients may have coexisting spine and musculoskeletal conditions that require a comprehensive management approach
- The history, physical examination, and pain pattern are important to help distinguish spine versus musculoskeletal etiology of pain
- Imaging, electrodiagnostic testing, and injections can be helpful when the diagnosis remains unclear

References

1. Dwyer A, Aprill C, Bogduk N. Cervical zygapophyseal joint pain patterns. I: a study in normal volunteers. Spine (Phila Pa 1976). 1990;15(6):453–7. https://doi.org/10.1097/00007632-199006000-00004. PMID: 2402682.
2. Cooper G, Bailey B, Bogduk N. Cervical zygapophysial joint pain maps. Pain Med. 2007;8(4):344–53. https://doi.org/10.1111/j.1526-4637.2006.00201.x. PMID: 17610457.
3. Windsor RE, Nagula D, Storm S, Overton A, Jahnke S. Electrical stimulation induced cervical medial branch referral patterns. Pain Physician. 2003;6(4):411–8. PMID: 16871290.
4. Fukui S, Ohseto K, Shiotani M, Ohno K, Karasawa H, Naganuma Y, Yuda Y. Referred pain distribution of the cervical zygapophyseal joints and cervical dorsal rami. Pain. 1996;68(1):79–83. https://doi.org/10.1016/S0304-3959(96)03173-9. PMID: 9252002.
5. Dreyfuss P, Michaelsen M, Fletcher D. Atlanto-occipital and lateral atlanto-axial joint pain patterns. Spine (Phila Pa 1976). 1994;19(10):1125–31. https://doi.org/10.1097/00007632-199405001-00005. PMID: 8059267.
6. Lee DG, Cho YW, Jang SH, Son SM, Kim GJ, Ahn SH. Effectiveness of intra-articular steroid injection for atlanto-occipital joint pain. Pain Med. 2015;16(6):1077–82. https://doi.org/10.1111/pme.12474. Epub 2014 Aug 8. PMID: 25105892.
7. Katsuura Y, Bruce J, Taylor S, Gullota L, Kim HJ. Overlapping, masquerading, and causative cervical spine and shoulder pathology: a systematic review. Global Spine J. 2020;10(2):195–208. https://doi.org/10.1177/2192568218822536. Epub 2019 Feb 17. PMID: 32206519.
8. Zhang AL, Theologis AA, Tay B, Feeley BT. The association between cervical spine pathology and rotator cuff dysfunction. J Spinal Disord Tech. 2015;28(4):E206–11. https://doi.org/10.1097/BSD.0000000000000223. PMID: 25393668.
9. Gumina S, Carbone S, Arceri V, Rita A, Vestri AR, Postacchini F. The relationship between chronic type III acromioclavicular joint dislocation and cervical spine pain. BMC Musculoskelet Disord. 2009;10:157. https://doi.org/10.1186/1471-2474-10-157. PMID: 2001.
10. Dang A, Davies M. Rotator Cuff disease: treatment options and considerations. Sports Med Arthrosc Rev. 2018;26(3):129–33. https://doi.org/10.1097/JSA.0000000000000207. PMID: 30059447.
11. Pateder DB, Brems J, Lieberman I, Bell GR, McLain RF. Masquerade: nonspinal musculoskeletal disorders that mimic spinal conditions. Cleve Clin J Med. 2008;75(1):50–6. https://doi.org/10.3949/ccjm.75.1.50. PMID: 18236730.
12. Sambandam SN, Khanna V, Gul A, Mounasamy V. Rotator cuff tears: an evidence based approach. World J Orthop. 2015;6(11):902–18. https://doi.org/10.5312/wjo.v6.i11.902. PMID: 26716086; PMCID: PMC4686437.
13. May T, Garmel GM. Rotator Cuff injury. [Updated 2022 Jun 27]. In: StatPearls [Internet]. Treasure Island: StatPearls Publishing; 2022. Available from: https://www.ncbi.nlm.nih.gov/books/NBK547664/.
14. van Kampen DA, van den Berg T, van der Woude HJ, Castelein RM, Scholtes VA, Terwee CB, Willems WJ. The diagnostic value of the combination of patient characteristics, history, and clinical shoulder tests for the diagnosis of rotator cuff tear. J Orthop Surg Res. 2014;9:70.
15. Beaudreuil J, Nizard R, Thomas T, Peyre M, Liotard JP, Boileau P, Marc T, Dromard C, Steyer E, Bardin T, Orcel P, Walch G. Contribution of clinical tests to the diagnosis of rotator cuff disease: a systematic literature review. Joint Bone Spine. 2009;76:15.
16. Kappe T, Sgroi M, Reichel H, Daexle M. Diagnostic performance of clinical tests for subscapularis tendon tears. Knee Surg Sports Traumatol Arthrosc. 2018;26(1):176–81. https://doi.org/10.1007/s00167-017-4617-4. Epub 2017 Jul 4. PMID: 28676889.
17. Liu F, Dong J, Shen WJ, Kang Q, Zhou D, Xiong F. Detecting Rotator Cuff Tears: a network meta-analysis of 144 diagnostic studies. Orthop J Sports Med. 2020;8(2):2325967119900356. https://doi.org/10.1177/2325967119900356. PMID: 32076627; PMCID: PMC7003181.

18. Marder RA, Kim SH, Labson JD, Hunter JC. Injection of the subacromial bursa in patients with rotator cuff syndrome: a prospective, randomized study comparing the effectiveness of different routes. J Bone Joint Surg Am. 2012;94(16):1442–7. https://doi.org/10.2106/JBJS.K.00534.
19. Schmidt CC, Jarrett CD, Brown BT. Management of rotator cuff tears. J Hand Surg Am. 2015;40(2):399–408. https://doi.org/10.1016/j.jhsa.2014.06.122. Epub 2015 Jan 1. PMID: 25557775.
20. Churgay CA. Diagnosis and treatment of biceps tendinitis and tendinosis. Am Fam Physician. 2009;80(5):470–6. PMID: 19725488.
21. Ahrens PM, Boileau P. The long head of biceps and associated tendinopathy. J Bone Joint Surg Br. 2007;89(8):1001–9. https://doi.org/10.1302/0301-620X.89B8.19278. PMID: 17785735.
22. Rosas S, Krill MK, Amoo-Achampong K, Kwon K, Nwachukwu BU, McCormick F. A practical, evidence-based, comprehensive (PEC) physical examination for diagnosing pathology of the long head of the biceps. J Shoulder Elb Surg. 2017;26(8):1484–92. https://doi.org/10.1016/j.jse.2017.03.002.
23. Ibounig T, Simons T, Launonen A, Paavola M. Glenohumeral osteoarthritis: an overview of etiology and diagnostics. Scand J Surg. 2021;110(3):441–51. https://doi.org/10.1177/1457496920935018. Epub 2020 Jul 14. PMID: 32662351.
24. Millett PJ, Gobezie R, Boykin RE. Shoulder osteoarthritis: diagnosis and management. Am Fam Physician. 2008;78(5):605–11. PMID: 18788237.
25. Jackson R, Beckman J, Frederick M, Musolin K, Harrison R. Rates of Carpal Tunnel syndrome in a state workers' compensation information system, by industry and occupation - California, 2007-2014. MMWR Morb Mortal Wkly Rep. 2018;67(39):1094–7. https://doi.org/10.15585/mmwr.mm6739a4.
26. Centers for Disease Control and Prevention. Morbidity and Mortality Weekly Report, 2011. Available at: https://www.cdc.gov/mmwr/preview/mmwrhtml/mm6049a4.htm?s_cid=mm6049a4_w. Accessed 5 January 2023.
27. Caridi JM, Pumberger M, Hughes AP. Cervical radiculopathy: a review. HSS J. 2011;7(3):265–72. https://doi.org/10.1007/s11420-011-9218-z. Epub 2011 Sep 9. PMID: 23024624; PMCID: PMC3192889.
28. Padua L, Coraci D, Erra C, Pazzaglia C, Paolasso I, Loreti C, Caliandro P, Hobson-Webb LD. Carpal tunnel syndrome: clinical features, diagnosis, and management. Lancet Neurol. 2016;15(12):1273–84. https://doi.org/10.1016/S1474-4422(16)30231-9. Epub 2016 Oct 11
29. Chow CS, Hung LK, Chiu CP, Lai KL, Lam LN, Ng ML, Tam KC, Wong KC, Ho PC. Is symptomatology useful in distinguishing between carpal tunnel syndrome and cervical spondylosis? Hand Surg. 2005;10(1):1–5. https://doi.org/10.1142/S0218810405002425. PMID: 16106494.
30. Wipperman J, Goerl K. Carpal Tunnel Syndrome: diagnosis and management. Am Fam Physician. 2016;94(12):993–9. PMID: 28075090.
31. Jablecki CK, Andary MT, Floeter MK, et al. Practice parameter: electrodiagnostic studies in carpal tunnel syndrome. Report of the American Association of Electrodiagnostic Medicine, American Academy of Neurology, and the American Academy of Physical Medic.
32. Witt JC, Hentz JG, Stevens JC. Carpal tunnel syndrome with normal nerve conduction studies. Muscle Nerve. 2004;29(4):515–22.
33. Lin TY, Chang KV, Wu WT, Özçakar L. Ultrasonography for the diagnosis of carpal tunnel syndrome: an umbrella review. J Neurol. 2022;269(9):4663–75. https://doi.org/10.1007/s00415-022-11201-z. Epub 2022 May 31. PMID: 35639198.
34. Fowler JR, Gaughan JP, Ilyas AM. The sensitivity and specificity of ultrasound for the diagnosis of carpal tunnel syndrome: a meta-analysis. Clin Orthop Relat Res. 2011;469(4):1089–94. https://doi.org/10.1007/s11999-010-1637-5. Epub 2010 Oct 21. PMID: 20963527
35. Bains S, Rocha CF. Electrodiagnostic evaluation of ulnar neuropathy. In: StatPearls [Internet]. Treasure Island: StatPearls Publishing; 2022. PMID: 33232078.
36. Shook SJ, Ginsberg M, Narayanaswami P, Beekman R, Dubin AH, Katirji B, Swaminathan B, Werner RA, Cartwright MS. Evidence-based guideline: neuromuscular ultrasound for the

diagnosis of ulnar neuropathy at the elbow. Muscle Nerve. 2022;65(2):147–53. https://doi.org/10.1002/mus.27460.
37. Landau ME, Campbell WW. Clinical features and electrodiagnosis of ulnar neuropathies. Phys Med Rehabil Clin N Am. 2013;24(1):49–66. https://doi.org/10.1016/j.pmr.2012.08.019. Epub 2012 Oct 25. PMID: 23177030.
38. Stewart JD. The variable clinical manifestations of ulnar neuropathies at the elbow. J Neurol Neurosurg Psychiatry. 1987;50(3):252–8.
39. Stoker GE, Kim HJ, Riew KD. Differentiating c8-t1 radiculopathy from ulnar neuropathy: a survey of 24 spine surgeons. Global Spine J. 2014;4(1):1–6. https://doi.org/10.1055/s-0033-1354254. Epub 2013 Aug 28. PMID: 24494175; PMCID: PMC3908974.
40. Novak CB, Lee GW, Mackinnon SE, Lay L. Provocative testing for cubital tunnel syndrome. J Hand Surg Am. 1994;19(5):817–20. https://doi.org/10.1016/0363-5023(94)90193-7. PMID: 7806810.
41. Goldman SB, Brininger TL, Schrader JW, Koceja DM. A review of clinical tests and signs for the assessment of ulnar neuropathy. J Hand Ther. 2009;22(3):209–19; quiz 220. https://doi.org/10.1016/j.jht.2008.10.010. Epub 2009 Feb 1. Erratum in: J Hand Ther. 2010.
42. Wartenberg R. A SIGN OF ULNAR PALSY. JAMA. 1939;112(17):1688. https://doi.org/10.1001/jama.1939.62800170002011a.
43. AAEM Quality Assurance Committee, Campbell WW, Carroll DJ, Greenberg MK, Krendel DA, Pridgeon RM, Sitaram KP, et al. Practice parameter. Electrodiagnostic studies in ulnar neuropathy at the elbow. Neurology. 1999;52:688–90.
44. Robertson C, Saratsiotis J. A review of compressive ulnar neuropathy at the elbow. J Manip Physiol Ther. 2005;28(5):345. https://doi.org/10.1016/j.jmpt.2005.04.005. PMID: 15965409.
45. Pelosi L, Mulroy E. Diagnostic sensitivity of electrophysiology and ultrasonography in ulnar neuropathies of different severity. Clin Neurophysiol. 2019;130(2):297–302. https://doi.org/10.1016/j.clinph.2018.11.018. Epub 2018 Dec 7. PMID: 30552047.
46. Rayegani SM, Raeissadat SA, Kargozar E, Rahimi-Dehgolan S, Loni E. Diagnostic value of ultrasonography versus electrodiagnosis in ulnar neuropathy. Med Dev (Auckl). 2019;12:81–8. https://doi.org/10.2147/MDER.S196106. PMID: 30863191; PMCID: PMC6390865.
47. Masocatto NO, Da-Matta T, Prozzo TG, Couto WJ, Porfirio G. Thoracic outlet syndrome: a narrative review. Rev Col Bras Cir. 2019;46(5):e20192243. Portuguese, English. https://doi.org/10.1590/0100-6991e-20192243. PMID: 31859722.
48. Sanders RJ, Hammond SL. Management of cervical ribs and anomalous first ribs causing neurogenic thoracic outlet syndrome. J Vasc Surg. 2002;36(1):51–6. https://doi.org/10.1067/mva.2002.123750. PMID: 12096257.
49. Atasoy E. A hand surgeon's further experience with thoracic outlet compression syndrome. J Hand Surg Am. 2010;35(9):1528–38. https://doi.org/10.1016/j.jhsa.2010.06.025. PMID: 20807632.
50. Kuhn JE, Lebus VGF, Bible JE. Thoracic outlet syndrome. J Am Acad Orthop Surg. 2015;23(4):222–32.
51. Gillard J, Pérez-Cousin M, Hachulla E, Remy J, Hurtevent JF, Vinckier L, Thévenon A, Duquesnoy B. Diagnosing thoracic outlet syndrome: contribution of provocative tests, ultrasonography, electrophysiology, and helical computed tomography in 48 patients. Joint Bone Spine. 2001;68:416.
52. Sanders RJ, Hammond SL, Rao NM. Diagnosis of thoracic outlet syndrome. J Vasc Surg. 2007;46(3):601–4. https://doi.org/10.1016/j.jvs.2007.04.050. PMID: 17826254.
53. Goedee HS, Seeber AA, van Hattum ES. Value and pitfalls of imaging and electrodiagnosis in neurogenic thoracic outlet syndrome: lessons learned from present and past. Muscle Nerve. 2022;65(1):4–6. https://doi.org/10.1002/mus.27431. Epub 2021 Oct 21. PMID: 346097.
54. Mul K, Pesser N, Vervaart K, Teijink J, van Nuenen B, van Alfen N. Variability in electrodiagnostic findings associated with neurogenic thoracic outlet syndrome. Muscle Nerve. 2022;65(1):34–42. https://doi.org/10.1002/mus.27395. Epub 2021 Aug 21. PMID: 34378193
55. Maher C, Underwood M, Buchbinder R. Non-specific low back pain. Lancet. 2017;389(10070):736–47. https://doi.org/10.1016/S0140-6736(16)30970-9.

56. Murphy L, Helmick CG. The impact of osteoarthritis in the United States: a population-health perspective. Am J Nurs. 2012;112(3 suppl 1):S13–9.
57. Chamberlain R. Hip pain in adults: evaluation and differential diagnosis [published correction appears in Am Fam Physician. 2021;103(5):263]. Am Fam Physician. 2021;103(2):81–9.
58. Urits I, Burshtein A, Sharma M, et al. Low back pain, a comprehensive review: pathophysiology, diagnosis, and treatment. Curr Pain Headache Rep. 2019;23(3):23. Published 2019 Mar 11. https://doi.org/10.1007/s11916-019-0757-1.
59. Cohen SP, Bhaskar A, Bhatia A, et al. Consensus practice guidelines on interventions for lumbar facet joint pain from a multispecialty, international working group. Reg Anesth Pain Med. 2020;45(6):424–67. https://doi.org/10.1136/rapm-2019-101243.
60. Buchanan P, Vodapally S, Lee DW, et al. Successful diagnosis of Sacroiliac joint dysfunction. J Pain Res. 2021;14:3135–3143. Published 2021 Oct 8. https://doi.org/10.2147/JPR.S327351.
61. Katz JN, Arant KR, Loeser RF. Diagnosis and treatment of hip and knee Osteoarthritis: a review. JAMA. 2021;325(6):568–78. https://doi.org/10.1001/jama.2020.22171.
62. Brown MD, Gomez-Marin O, Brookfield KF, Li PS. Differential diagnosis of hip disease versus spine disease. Clin Orthop Relat Res. 2004;419:280–4. https://doi.org/10.1097/00003086-200402000-00044.
63. Reiman MP, Goode AP, Hegedus EJ, Cook CE, Wright AA. Diagnostic accuracy of clinical tests of the hip: a systematic review with meta-analysis. Br J Sports Med. 2013;47(14):893–902. https://doi.org/10.1136/bjsports-2012-091035.
64. Koes BW, van Tulder M, Lin CW, Macedo LG, McAuley J, Maher C. An updated overview of clinical guidelines for the management of non-specific low back pain in primary care. Eur Spine J. 2010;19(12):2075–94. https://doi.org/10.1007/s00586-010-1502-y. Epub 2010 Jul.
65. Oliveira CB, Maher CG, Pinto RZ, et al. Clinical practice guidelines for the management of non-specific low back pain in primary care: an updated overview. Eur Spine J. 2018;27(11):2791–803. https://doi.org/10.1007/s00586-018-5673-2.
66. Chou R, Fu R, Carrino JA, Deyo RA. Imaging strategies for low-back pain: systematic review and meta-analysis. Lancet. 2009;373(9662):463–72. https://doi.org/10.1016/S0140-6736(09)60172-0. PMID: 19200918.
67. Walsh PJ, Walz DM. Imaging of osteoarthritis of the hip. Radiol Clin North Am. 2022;60(4):617–28. https://doi.org/10.1016/j.rcl.2022.03.005.
68. Kim C, Nevitt MC, Niu J, et al. Association of hip pain with radiographic evidence of hip osteoarthritis: diagnostic test study. BMJ. 2015;351:h5983. Published 2015 Dec 2. https://doi.org/10.1136/bmj.h5983.
69. Heerey JJ, Kemp JL, Mosler AB, et al. What is the prevalence of imaging-defined intra-articular hip pathologies in people with and without pain? A systematic review and meta-analysis. Br J Sports Med. 2018;52(9):581–93. https://doi.org/10.1136/bjsports-2017-098264.
70. Manchikanti L, Kaye AD, Soin A, et al. Comprehensive evidence-based guidelines for facet joint interventions in the management of chronic spinal pain: American Society of Interventional Pain Physicians (ASIPP) guidelines facet joint interventions 2020 guidelines. Pain Physician. 2020;23(3S):S1–S127.
71. Jung MW, Schellhas K, Johnson B. Use of diagnostic injections to evaluate Sacroiliac joint pain. Int J Spine Surg. 2020;14(Suppl 1):30–4. Published 2020 Feb 10. https://doi.org/10.14444/6081.
72. Payne JM. Ultrasound-guided hip procedures. Phys Med Rehabil Clin N Am. 2016;27(3):607–29. https://doi.org/10.1016/j.pmr.2016.04.004.
73. Lynch TS, Steinhaus ME, Popkin CA, Ahmad CS, Rosneck J. Outcomes after diagnostic hip injection. Arthroscopy. 2016;32(8):1702–11. https://doi.org/10.1016/j.arthro.2016.02.027.
74. Katz JN, Zimmerman ZE, Mass H, Makhni MC. Diagnosis and management of Lumbar Spinal Stenosis: a review. JAMA. 2022;327(17):1688–99. https://doi.org/10.1001/jama.2022.5921.
75. Khan AM, McLoughlin E, Giannakas K, Hutchinson C, Andrew JG. Hip osteoarthritis: where is the pain? Ann R Coll Surg Engl. 2004;86(2):119–21. https://doi.org/10.1308/003588404322827518. PMID: 15005931; PMCID: PMC1964166.

76. Deer T, Sayed D, Michels J, Josephson Y, Li S, Calodney AK. A review of Lumbar Spinal Stenosis with intermittent neurogenic claudication: disease and diagnosis. Pain Med. 2019;20(Suppl 2):S32–44. https://doi.org/10.1093/pm/pnz161.
77. Devin CJ, McCullough KA, Morris BJ, Yates AJ, Kang JD. Hip-spine syndrome. J Am Acad Orthop Surg. 2012;20(7):434–42. https://doi.org/10.5435/JAAOS-20-07-434.
78. Issack PS, Cunningham ME, Pumberger M, Hughes AP, Cammisa F. Degenerative Lumbar Spinal Stenosis: evaluation and management. J Am Acad Orthop Surg. 2012;20(8):527.
79. Rainville J, Bono JV, Laxer EB, Kim DH, Lavelle JM, Indahl A, Borenstein DG, Haig AJ, Katz JN. Comparison of the history and physical examination for hip osteoarthritis and lumbar spinal stenosis. Spine J. 2019;19(6):1009–18. https://doi.org/10.1016/j.spinee.2.
80. Suri P, Rainville J, Kalichman L, Katz JN. Does this older adult with lower extremity pain have the clinical syndrome of lumbar spinal stenosis? JAMA. 2010;304(23):2628–36. https://doi.org/10.1001/jama.2010.1833.
81. Cook CJ, Cook CE, Reiman MP, Joshi AB, Richardson W, Garcia AN. Systematic review of diagnostic accuracy of patient history, clinical findings, and physical tests in the diagnosis of lumbar spinal stenosis. Eur Spine J. 2020;29(1):93–112. https://doi.org/10.1007/s005.
82. Petersen T, Laslett M, Juhl C. Clinical classification in low back pain: best-evidence diagnostic rules based on systematic reviews. BMC Musculoskelet Disord. 2017;18(1):188. https://doi.org/10.1186/s12891-017-1549-6. PMID: 28499364; PMCID: PMC5429540..
83. Jensen RK, Jensen TS, Koes B, Hartvigsen J. Prevalence of lumbar spinal stenosis in general and clinical populations: a systematic review and meta-analysis. Eur Spine J. 2020;29(9):2143–63. https://doi.org/10.1007/s00586-020-06339-1.
84. Ashberg L, Close MR, Perets I, Walsh JP, Chaharbakhshi EO, Domb BG. The hip-spine connection: how to differentiate hip conditions from spine pathology. Orthopedics. 2021;44(6):e699–706. https://doi.org/10.3928/01477447-20211001-06. Epub 2021 Oct 1. PMID: 34.
85. Yoong P, Guirguis R, Darrah R, Wijeratna M, Porteous MJ. Evaluation of ultrasound-guided diagnostic local anaesthetic hip joint injection for osteoarthritis. Skeletal Radiol. 2012;41(8):981–5. https://doi.org/10.1007/s00256-011-1290-4.
86. Pateder DB, Hungerford MW. Use of fluoroscopically guided intra-articular hip injection in differentiating the pain source in concomitant hip and lumbar spine arthritis. Am J Orthop (Belle Mead NJ). 2007;36(11):591–3.
87. Konstantinou K, Dunn KM. Sciatica: review of epidemiological studies and prevalence estimates. Spine (Phila Pa 1976). 2008;33(22):2464–72.
88. Cannon DE, Dillingham TR, Miao H, Andary MT, Pezzin LE. Musculoskeletal disorders in referrals for suspected lumbosacral radiculopathy. Am J Phys Med Rehabil. 2007;86(12):957–61. https://doi.org/10.1097/PHM.0b013e31815b614a.
89. Probst D, Stout A, Hunt D. Piriformis syndrome: a narrative review of the anatomy, diagnosis, and treatment. PM R. 2019;11(Suppl 1):S54–63. https://doi.org/10.1002/pmrj.12189.
90. Hopayian K, Song F, Riera R, Sambandan S. The clinical features of the piriformis syndrome: a systematic review. Eur Spine J. 2010;19(12):2095–109. https://doi.org/10.1007/s00586-010-1504-9.
91. Nee RJ, Coppieters MW, Boyd BS. Reliability of the straight leg raise test for suspected lumbar radicular pain: a systematic review with meta-analysis. Musculoskelet Sci Pract. 2022;59:102529. https://doi.org/10.1016/j.msksp.2022.102529.
92. Martin HD, Kivlan BR, Palmer IJ, Martin RL. Diagnostic accuracy of clinical tests for sciatic nerve entrapment in the gluteal region. Knee Surg Sports Traumatol Arthrosc. 2014;22(4):882–8. https://doi.org/10.1007/s00167-013-2758-7.
93. DeFroda SF, Daniels AH, Deren ME. Differentiating radiculopathy from lower extremity arthropathy. Am J Med. 2016;129(10):1124.e1–1124.e11247. https://doi.org/10.1016/j.amjmed.2016.06.019.
94. Filler AG, Haynes J, Jordan SE, et al. Sciatica of nondisc origin and piriformis syndrome: diagnosis by magnetic resonance neurography and interventional magnetic resonance imaging with outcome study of resulting treatment. J Neurosurg Spine. 2005;2(2):99.

95. Berry JA, Elia C, Saini HS, Miulli DE. A review of lumbar radiculopathy, diagnosis, and treatment. Cureus. 2019;11(10):e5934. https://doi.org/10.7759/cureus.5934. PMID: 31788391; PMCID: PMC6858271.
96. Dillingham TR, Annaswamy TM, Plastaras CT. Evaluation of persons with suspected lumbosacral and cervical radiculopathy: Electrodiagnostic assessment and implications for treatment and outcomes (Part II). Muscle Nerve. 2020;62(4):474–84. https://doi.org/10.1002/mus.27008.
97. Datta S, Manchikanti L, Falco FJ, et al. Diagnostic utility of selective nerve root blocks in the diagnosis of lumbosacral radicular pain: systematic review and update of current evidence. Pain Physician. 2013;16(2 Suppl):SE97–SE124.

Movement Can Be Pain Medicine

2

Maria Lyuksyutova, Samuel Moshofsky, and Kavita Trivedi

Introduction

The benefits of physical activity and exercise are inarguably numerous, especially in the context of health benefits. Physical activity is defined as any bodily movement produced by the contraction of skeletal muscles that results in an increase in caloric requirements over resting energy expenditure [1]. Exercise, on the other hand, is a type of physical activity consisting of planned, structured, and repetitive bodily movements that are performed to improve or maintain one or more components of physical fitness [2]. The American College of Sports Medicine recommends 30 minutes of moderate-intensity exercise 5 days per week in order to maintain cardiorespiratory, musculoskeletal, and neuromuscular fitness for healthy adults [3].

The specific benefits of exercise are multifold, with advantages in many aspects. For example, aerobic exercise training programs have well-established benefits for decreasing cardiovascular risk factors, including lowering heart rate at rest and submaximal exercise, smaller increases in blood pressure, improved whole-body insulin action, and reduced plasma lipid concentrations [4]. Strengthening exercise programs for the core and hip muscles can enhance the mobility of older adults, reduce kyphotic posturing, and reduce the risk of osteoporotic vertebral fractures [5]. In older patients with osteoarthritis, strengthening exercises also have favorable benefits [6]. A systematic review concluded that exercise improves selected sleep outcomes in adults [7]. Exercise has also been shown to have beneficial effects on cognition and mood. Studies in aging humans show that endurance exercise is protective against cognitive decline, especially executive planning and working memory [8].

M. Lyuksyutova
Texas Tech University, Lubbock, TX, USA

S. Moshofsky · K. Trivedi (✉)
UT Southwestern Medical Center, Dallas, TX, USA
e-mail: kavita.trivedi@utsouthwestern.edu

C. E. Noe (ed.), *Musculoskeletal Pain*,
https://doi.org/10.1007/978-3-031-86057-7_2

Exercise has been considered to be a method for pain management as it has been observed that exercise can influence the perception of pain in both pain-free and chronic pain conditions [9]. Exercise has been found to be effective in relieving pain and benefiting patients' daily physical function in various chronic musculoskeletal pain disorders [10]. This phenomenon is known as exercise-induced hypoalgesia, and it is often defined as a reduction in sensitivity to pain during and/or following an acute bout of aerobic or resistance exercise [11, 12]. The most common proposed mechanism of exercise-induced hypoalgesia is activation of the endogenous opioid system [13]. It has been suggested that exercise intensity and duration may affect the magnitude of the exercise-induced hypoalgesia response [14]. In addition to exercise-induced hypoalgesia, overall pain reduction has been observed following long-term training in individuals with chronic pain [15].

Table 2.1 is a brief list of examples for assessing physical activity levels—it is not meant to be a comprehensive list. These assessments are best used as initial screening tools for which providers can inquire further during their history and physical exam in order to counsel and prescribe appropriate exercise programs for patients.

Table 2.1 Assessment tools for physical activity levels

Evidence Based Assessment			
Assessment Tool	Description	Evidence	Comments
Exercise as a Vital Sign (EVS)	Two item questionnaire in electronic health records inquiring if the individual can walk for 10 minutes at a reasonable pace (~3 mph), and if they can climb 2 flights of stairs without symptoms.	Good face validity and discriminant validity. Patients were more likely to report physician exercise counseling and were more likely to receive exercise related referrals when EVS performed during a visit.	A very brief tool that can give providers a basic understanding of physical activity level in patients.
Duke Activity Status Index (DASI)	12 item self-administered assessment asking questions related to mobility, activities of daily living, and exercise.	DASI survey questions were given to study participants, then underwent exercise testing with Vo2 Max testing performed. DASI correlated significantly to peak oxygen uptake (Spearman correlation coefficient 0.58).	Slightly more detailed tool in which individual questions are assessing more functional status rather than duration of physical activity.
International Physical Activity Questionnaire (IPAQ)	27 item (long form), or 7 item (short form), self-reported questionnaire assessing various types and duration of physical activity.	Short form recommended for monitoring, and long form recommended for research purposes. Validated in at least 12 countries.	Used clinically as well as in research. Focuses on duration of physical activity rather than functional status.

Aerobic Exercise

The American College of Sports Medicine (ACSM) defines cardiovascular exercises as those exercises that are rhythmic, continuous, and performed with large muscles of the body. Under this definition, cardiovascular exercise can include running, jogging, walking, cycling, hiking, stair climbing, skating, rowing, swimming, jumping rope, skiing, and dancing. The ACSM recommends exercising 20–60 minutes, three to five times a week, at a level that raises your heart rate between 60 and 90 percent of your maximum heart rate (MHR) [16]. To calculate your MHR, subtract your age from 220. Then multiply the MHR by 60 and 90 percent to determine your cardiovascular exercise target heart rate. Though wearable technology has made monitoring heart rate during exercise significantly easier, one can also listen to one's body and exercise at a level that leaves you short of breath but still able to maintain a conversation. Low-impact cardiovascular exercise includes but is not limited to walking and water aerobics, while high-impact cardiovascular exercise includes but is not limited to running, dance, and cross-fit style forms of exercise.

In this section, we will focus on discussing how cardiovascular exercise can have an impact on pain, with a special focus on osteoarthritis-related pain, rheumatological pain, fibromyalgia, low back pain, and vascular claudication pain.

Cycling is a popular and outstanding conditioning exercise (Fig. 2.1).

To begin, we can review the different types of pain your patients may be experiencing. Osteoarthritis, the most common cause of arthritis, is a degenerative joint process characterized by cartilage degradation and skeletal changes. Patients experience joint pain, tenderness, stiffness, and range of motion limitations with the disease [17]. Currently, no cure is available for osteoarthritis; thus, focusing on treating symptoms and preventing further disease progression are the mainstays of care. Pain from rheumatological arthritis is caused by an autoimmune inflammatory process that primarily attacks joints in the hands, wrist, and knees. This process causes damage to joint tissue which can result in chronic pain, instability, and deformity of the joints [18]. There is no cure for rheumatoid arthritis, so treatment focuses on symptom management to relieve pain and stiffness and improve joint range of motion. Fibromyalgia is characterized by widespread musculoskeletal pain associated with symptoms of poor sleep, chronic fatigue, mood issues, and memory changes. Symptoms can occur after significant psychological or physical stress and gradually accumulate over time. The mechanism is believed to be due to the brain perceiving painful sensations from painful and nonpainful signals. There is no cure for fibromyalgia, so treatment focuses on symptom management [19]. Chronic lower back pain can stem from a variety of structural causes. This includes degenerative joint and disc disease, radiculopathy, and neurogenic claudication. Treatment includes physical therapy to improve the biomechanical chain, symptom management with pharmaceuticals, and surgery. Vascular claudication pain is experienced through the mechanism of atherosclerotic disease, narrowing blood vessels and thus decreasing oxygen delivery to tissues causing a painful aching sensation to muscles.

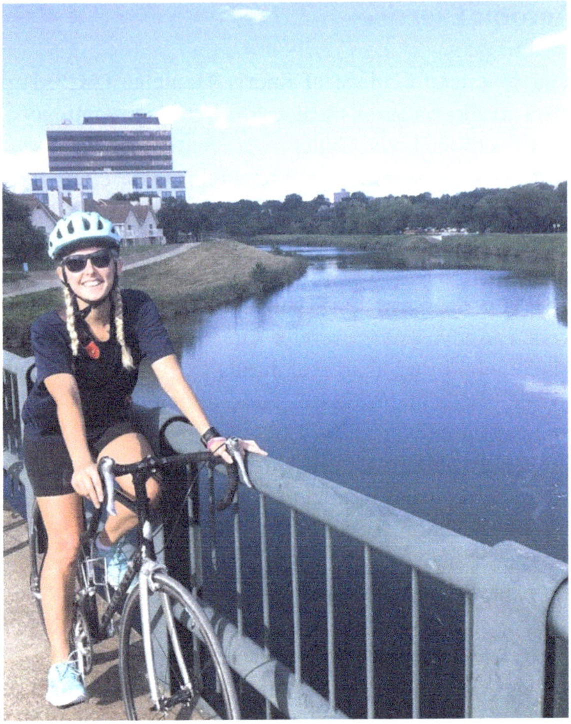

Fig. 2.1 Cyclist with a helmet for safety

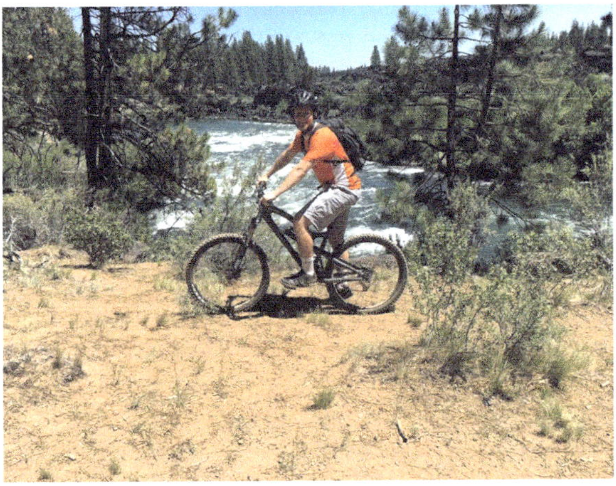

Fig. 2.2 Off-road cyclist

It can be challenging to treat as the underlying mechanism of vascular occlusion prevents prolonged exercise. Thus, many patients lean to pharmacological agents for symptom relief that are not without side effects.

Off-road cycling is a great way to explore nature while exercising (Fig. 2.2).

Walking

Most international clinical guidelines recommend that general aerobic exercise is an effective pain management treatment for patients with knee osteoarthritis. Aerobic walking improves the quality of life, functional status, and short-term pain in patients with knee osteoarthritis [20, 21]. Walking exercises should be performed in multiple bouts instead of one continuous bout due to the risk of undesirable knee joint loading in walking exercise durations of 30 minutes or greater [22] (Fig. 2.3). For patients with rheumatoid arthritis, performing up to 35 minutes of low-intensity aerobic activity, such as walking, improves patient aerobic capacity, exercise time, and painful joint counts. Further, patients report improvements in activities of daily living and reduced joint pain and fatigue. Even as little as 15 minutes of exercise three times a week is sufficient to improve aerobic capacity in rheumatoid arthritis patients [23].

Walking is an ideal, free, and accessible activity for patients with fibromyalgia, it is beneficial in pain relief and anxiety reduction [24]. Most patients with fibromyalgia can manage low to moderate-intensity exercise, and it appears to improve symptoms and overall functioning, high-intensity exercise should be undertaken with care [25].

A systematic review of lower back pain and walking found low evidence for treadmill walking as an effective management strategy for low back pain. However, it should be noted that the studies included in the systematic review had poor

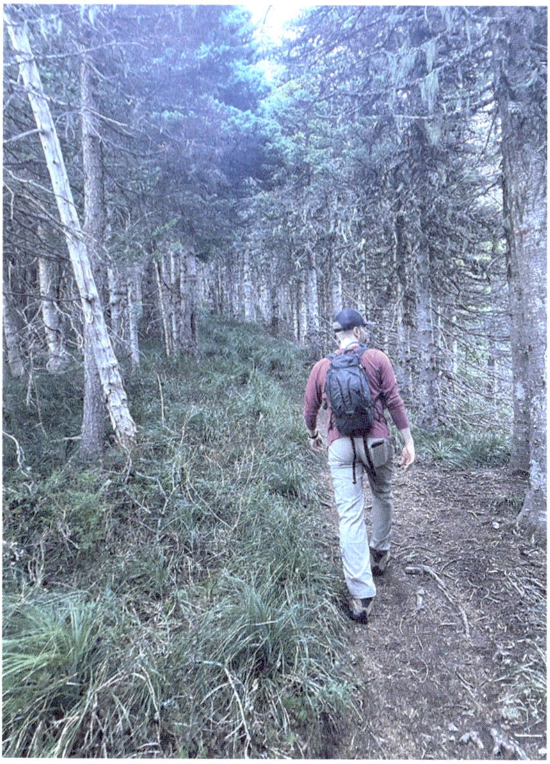

Fig. 2.3 Hiker enjoying exercise in the forest

methodological quality. Though further research is required to characterize the role of walking in lower back pain, clinicians can continue advising patients with low back pain to remain active [26]. Walking is beneficial for those patients experiencing pain secondary to vascular claudication. Walking has been found to be just as effective when compared to alternative exercises such as cycling, strength training, and upper-arm ergometry for improving the maximum and pain-free walking distance of patients with intermittent claudication [27]. Studies comparing walking with usual pharmacological care versus placebo demonstrated that maximum walking distance, maximal walking time, and pain-free walking distance were statistically significantly improved in the walking group compared to the pharmacological-only groups and placebo groups, with improvements noted for up to 2 years [28]. In summary, walking as an aerobic exercise is beneficial for pain relief in short bursts for knee osteoarthritis pain and rheumatoid arthritis pain. It is also an excellent low-intensity exercise for pain reduction in patients with fibromyalgia, indeterminate evidence for low back pain, and beneficial in vascular claudication pain.

Running

Running is recommended for its cardiovascular benefits to many patients. However, in patients with osteoarthritis and rheumatoid arthritis, there is inconclusive evidence regarding the efficacy of pain relief. In theory, the high-impact forces sustained during running exercise may, in fact, be too uncomfortable for patients to continue. Running as a physical activity for people with fibromyalgia improves heart and lung function, lowers cardiovascular risk, and improves psychosocial function. Running is helpful for the benefits. However, the increased impact and intensity of running, when compared to exercises such as swimming or biking, may be detrimental [29] (Fig. 2.4).

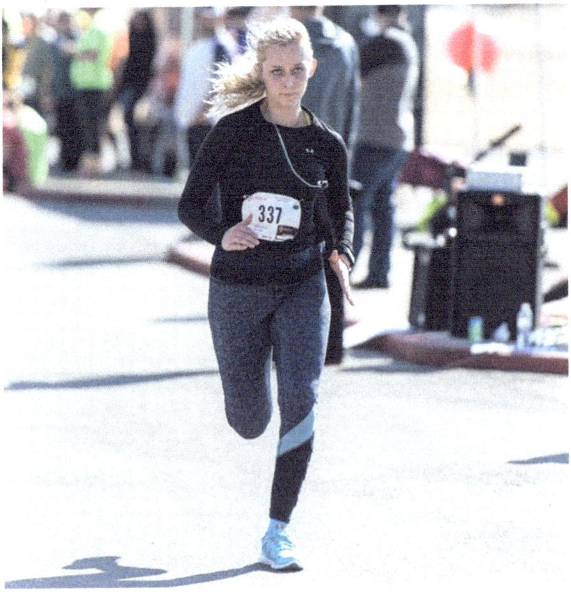

Fig. 2.4 Competitive runner

Aquatic Exercise

Water-based exercise is used in a variety of activity settings, including community exercise, injury rehabilitation, and pain relief. Depending on the activity, aquatic exercise can incorporate components of aerobic exercise, resistance training, stretching, and range of motion exercises and, if accessible, can be a great catalyst for physical improvements in certain populations. One of the main advantages of water-based activities is the buoyancy of water reduces the force that weight-bearing joints, bones, and muscles must bear [30]. Furthermore, the warmth and pressure of the water can promote blood circulation and reduce joint pain and stiffness [31]. It is an ideal introduction to cardiovascular exercise and has the benefits of quad complex and hip adductor strengthening, which will, in turn, benefit patients on dry land by offloading the forces onto the hip and knee joints. Evidence points to aquatic exercise providing short-term pain reduction in patients with hip and knee osteoarthritis but should be considered preferentially in patients as the first part of a more longitudinal exercise regimen as it does not worsen the joint condition and has been found to have a higher level of treatment compliance [32]. Aquatic exercise has been found to be beneficial in patients suffering from joint pain as a result of rheumatoid arthritis. The goal in symptom management of pain associated with rheumatoid arthritis is to increase the range of motion of joints and break up the intra-articular pannus. The literature demonstrates that patients with rheumatoid arthritis find benefits in aquatic exercise in pain reduction, improvements in joint tenderness, improved mood and tension symptoms, and increased grip strength [33]. Once again, it seems that the warmth, pressure, and buoyancy of the water are beneficial for joint pain reduction, be it rheumatological or osteoarthritic in nature. Patients with fibromyalgia-related pain can find benefits in aquatic therapy. Consideration must be made for deep water running/jogging as it has been found to be as effective as land-based exercises with pain experienced in fibromyalgia patients, with equivocal aerobic gains, but with improvements in emotional well-being compared to land-based exercises [34]. Evidence has shown that in as few as 10 treatment sessions of aquatic therapy, in this case, an Ai Chi (Tai Chi in water), patients had significant improvements in pain perceptions, vitality, mental health, and perceived quality of life [35]. Fibromyalgia pain is multifactorial, with widespread musculoskeletal pain accompanied by fatigue, sleep, memory, and mood issues. Aquatic therapy, in theory, targets musculoskeletal pain by gently stretching and warming the affected muscles and trigger point areas and can improve sleep by physically fatiguing the body and, as a result, reducing sleep onset and promoting more restful sleep. Aquatic therapy is additionally beneficial in patients with low back pain as it has been found, when compared to traditional physical therapy, to have a long-term, lasting improvement in disability perception, reported pain anxiety, and sleep quality. Water buoyancy benefits patients with chronic lower back pain by removing the force of gravity and its effect on the posterior chain. This allows patients to relearn the proper biomechanics and strengthen and stretch their muscles to help correct the lower cross syndrome so commonly associated with lower back pain. The benefit of aquatic therapy allows for a gentler reintroduction of movement as many patients suffering from chronic lower back pain develop kinesiophobia and fear avoidance behaviors [36].

Recent work on examining the effects of a 12-week aquatic walking exercise on peripheral arterial disease has found that after an aquatic walking protocol, there was a statistically significant reduction in arterial stiffness, which has been associated with shorter walking distances in patients with PAD. Though these patients did not demonstrate structural changes in their vasculature (analyzed by the arterial brachial index), the change in arterial stiffness may be a result of increased nitric oxide bioavailability, which in turn improves tissue perfusion by enhancing blood flow and alleviating the ischemic claudication symptoms. Aquatic exercise additionally decreases resting heart rate and improves cardiorespiratory capacity, exercise tolerance, muscle strength, and physical function in patients suffering from vascular claudication [37]. Consider aquatic exercise as an option for patients with chronic pain, particularly those who have problems adapting to land-based exercises or have lower limb limitations, but be mindful of the constraints of aquatic therapy, which includes pool availability, access, and patient comfort in shallow water.

Water-based exercise is used in many other populations, especially those associated with chronic pain and or higher risk of falls. There is good evidence to show that stroke water-based therapy is effective in improving balance, walking, muscular strength, and overall quality of life for patients who have suffered a stroke [38], as well as patients with multiple sclerosis [39]. Although not universally accepted, some studies revealed that aquatic exercise for stroke patients may even be superior to land-based therapy [40]. Aquatic gait training has been employed for gait improvement for individuals with Parkinson's, and ai chi (aquatic-based exercise similar in theory to tai chi and other MBE) appears to be valid in treating pain, balance, and functional capacity in the Parkinson's population [41].

Children with spastic cerebral palsy (CP) that participated in aquatic therapy showed greater gross motor function measure, even in patients with more severe CP (Gross Motor Function Classification System Level IV) [42].

Aquatic therapy is also starting to be used more in postoperative care after the initial healing of the surgical incisions. It has been shown to be beneficial after total knee arthroplasty [43] and total hip arthroplasty [44]. However, evidence is mixed on whether aquatic vs. land-based exercise is more beneficial in the post-surgical setting. In addition to post-surgical uses for water-based exercise, researchers are also beginning to look into the benefits of aquatic-based pre-habitation programs prior to total knee arthroplasty, with initial results showing improvement in functional outcomes [45].

Aquatic exercise can be a valuable tool for individuals to initiate exercise and rehabilitation programs safely— it is well tolerated, low cost, and beneficial for diverse patient populations. A key limitation of water-based exercises is accessibility. Not everyone has access to pools or safe bodies of water, and even fewer have access to therapists or providers trained in aquatic exercises.

Resistance Training

Resistance training (interchangeable with strength training) is an overarching term for exercises where muscles work against a force with the goal of increasing muscular strength. There are numerous forms of resistance training, with some of the most common types including weight training (using dumbbells, exercise machines, etc.), resistance bands, and bodyweight exercises such as pushups and pullups (Fig. 2.5). Depending on an individual's functional status, the goals for participating in resistance training can vary from simply improving functional strength to performing activities of daily living, all the way to maximizing dynamic strength and muscle mass for high-performing athletes.

Regardless of an individual's goals, resistance training is comprised of three types of exercises: concentric, eccentric, and isometric. All three modalities are associated with increased muscle strength, but there is some evidence to show that high-intensity eccentric exercises may be more effective at increasing muscle strength and cross-sectional area when compared to concentric exercises [46]. Although muscle strength is directly related to the cross-sectional area of the muscle, in the initial weeks of starting a resistance training program, the majority of the gains in strength are attributed to improved efficiency in motor neuron recruitment and increased neuron output from the spinal cord to the muscle [47], with muscle hypertrophy first seen around 6–7 weeks of resistance training [48].

Numerous resistance exercise routines and theories exist, and individualized plans can optimize outcomes based on individuals' goals. In general, it is thought that lower weight and higher repetition exercise routines lead to more muscular endurance, and higher weight lower repetition routines lead to increased hypertrophy and strength. Evidence shows that muscular strength is increased at all load levels if exercised to the point of muscular fatigue, but that heavier loads do in fact lead to superior gains in dynamic strength compared to lighter loads [49].

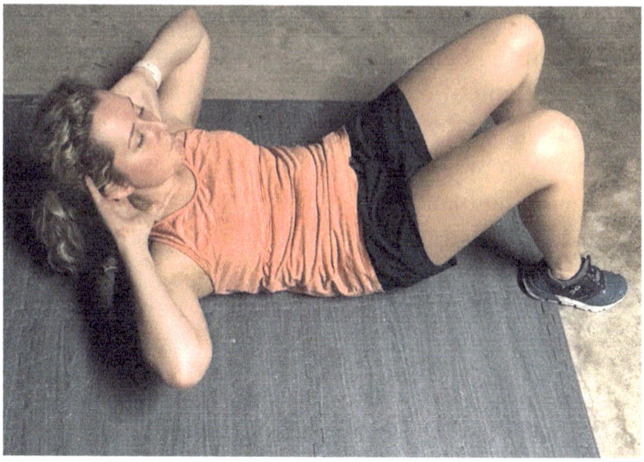

Fig. 2.5 Abdominal exercise

Resistance training, like most forms of exercise, is associated with many positive outcomes. Physical and functional benefits include improved movement control, walking speed, and functional dependence. It is also related to physiologic changes such as increased bone density, lowered resting blood pressure, and decreased LDL cholesterol and triglycerides. Resistance exercise is also associated with higher cognitive abilities and self-esteem [50]. As a commonly prescribed physical modality, strength training has exhibited benefits in all areas of a patient's timeline, including injury and pain prevention, post-injury rehabilitation, and post-surgical recovery.

Preventative Resistance Training

It is common to think of resistance training as a mode of injury prevention with the idea that stronger muscles stabilize joints and prevent injury. Evidence has shown that there is a dose-dependent reduction of injuries with increasing volume of participation in strength training programs [51] (Fig. 2.6). Not only can general strength training reduce injury, but specific programs can be implemented in populations that are at higher risk, given their activity participation. For example, the inclusion of Nordic hamstring exercises into an athlete's resistance training program can reduce the risk of hamstring injury among soccer players [52]. These principles also carry over to the general population, and there is strong evidence to show that implementation of a resistance training program can reduce the risk of workplace-related injury [53].

Strength training has been implemented in populations across the age and ability spectrum. Women with osteoporosis and elderly patients are at higher risk of injury secondary to falls, and resistance training has been shown to increase dynamic balance and strength and decrease fear of falling [54, 55]. Alternatively, high-performing athletes, unsurprisingly, are a common focus amongst resistance training research, and the incorporation of strength training even in endurance-focused triathletes has been shown to prevent overuse injuries [56]. Even for children, under appropriate supervision and guidance, resistance training can be effective at reducing activity-related injuries and promotes the development of physical literacy [57].

Although resistance training cannot eliminate the risk of acute musculoskeletal pathology, it plays a significant role in the prevention of injury for individuals of all ages and functional abilities. It is important to note that strength training is not without risk, and overuse injury is a common area of concern with repetitive forms of exercise.

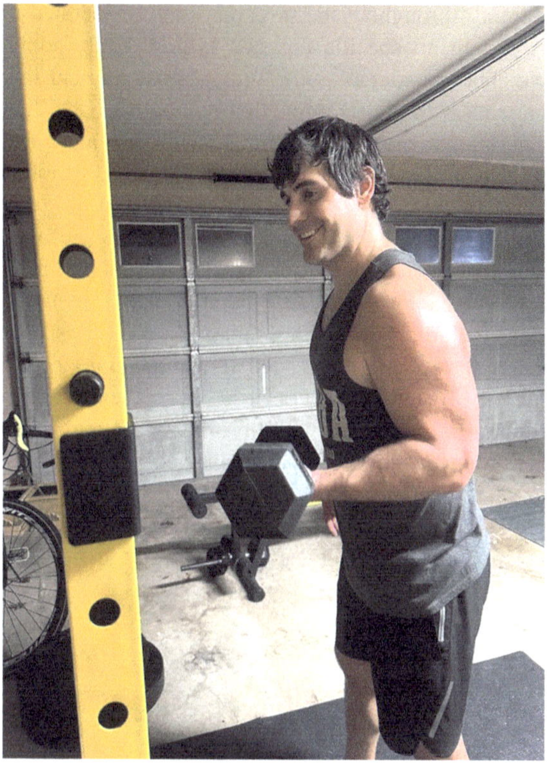

Fig. 2.6 Strength training with dumbbell

Resistance Training as Treatment

Resistance training is often one of the first-line treatments prescribed to individuals with mild to moderate muscular or tendinous injuries. If managed non-operatively and deemed appropriate, progressive resistance exercises are usually initiated early in recovery to begin re-strengthening the tendons and muscles involved in the injury. Ankle injuries are common in athletes and the general population. Various resistance training techniques have been implemented. Regardless of the program, there are benefits seen in strength, balance, and functional measures [58]. Resistance training has also been associated with improved pain, function, strength, and cross-sectional area of affected muscles after muscular strains [59]. For individuals with Achilles tendinopathy, eccentric exercises, and heavy, slow resistance training both show improved patient pain and satisfaction [60].

Orthopedic injuries managed conservatively often benefit significantly from resistance training, as discussed above. Still, post-operative resistance training is exceedingly important for patients to return close to the pre-injury or pre-surgical level of function. ACL reconstruction, one of the most common orthopedic surgeries, is studied extensively in the literature. Resistance training is a staple of recovery for these patients, but there is significant variability in the intensity of resistance training throughout the research, with no defined protocol deemed superior [61]. Although no specific regimen is universally adopted, it is standard of care for patients to undergo some form of post-surgical resistance training. Similarly, for patients with hip fractures that undergo surgical fixation, weekly strength training can improve measured strength, endurance, and gait speed in the immediate follow-up period. However, long-term evidence does not always reveal significant differences [62].

Chronic back and neck pain is extremely prevalent in our society, and there is an abundance of research aimed at interventions to reduce pain, including various forms of exercise. Physical therapy often implements a variety of exercise modalities, including stretching, balance, and resistance training for these patients. Resistance exercise has been shown to improve patient-reported chronic neck and back pain, but not necessarily more than general exercise [63, 64] (Fig. 2.7). Similarly, individuals with fibromyalgia often suffer from chronic pain, which has been shown to improve with resistance training, though aerobic exercise may exhibit greater pain relief in this population [65]. Generally, exercise is encouraged for patients with chronic pain from all causes, including resistance training, although no single form of exercise is superior to others.

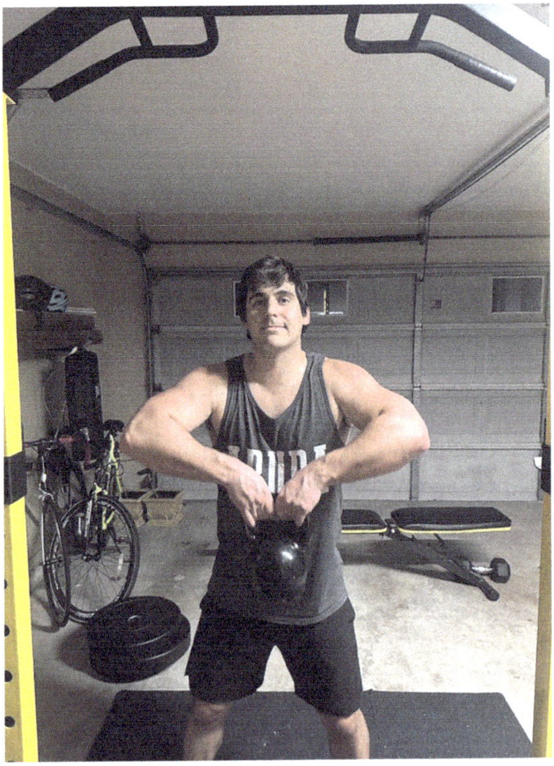

Fig. 2.7 Kettlebell exercises

Summary

Resistance training is rarely used as a treatment in isolation. It is a tool in the toolbox of providers to increase the strength and stability of targeted muscle groups. Much of the evidence for resistance training is influenced by other confounding treatment modalities, variable exercise prescriptions and intensities, patient effort, and pre-morbid level of function. Often there are positive benefits seen acutely, but if resistance training is discontinued some of those benefits may diminish over time. The physical benefits of resistance training are evident, but not necessarily prolonged unless training is sustained. Additionally, resistance training and exercise in general have psychiatric benefits including decreased depression, fatigue, and improved cognition, suggesting a strong connection between mental and emotional health with physical activity.

Mind-Body Exercise

It is well documented that pain is more than just a transmission of signals triggered by noxious stimuli, rather it is a complex perceived sensory experience that is heavily influenced by biopsychosocial factors. There are a variety of interventions aimed to treat some of these factors, including psychotherapy, meditation, biofeedback, as well as mind-body exercises (MBE) such as yoga, tai-chi, pilates, and qigong. When looked at as a group, MBE can significantly decrease chronic pain symptoms, especially in older populations [66].

Tai chi is a historic Chinese practice that combines a continuous flow of slow and gentle movements with stretching, body control, deep breathing, and mindfulness (Fig. 2.8). It is the most studied form of MBE and has numerous health benefits including decreased blood pressure, depression, falls, pain, and increased balance confidence, muscle strength, and cognition [67]. The American College of

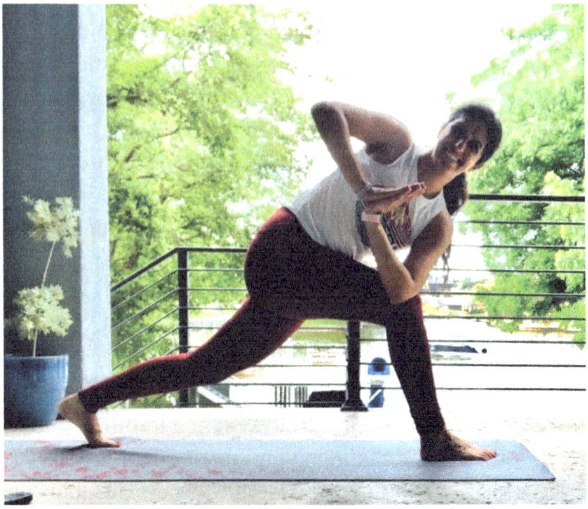

Fig. 2.8 Tai chi position example

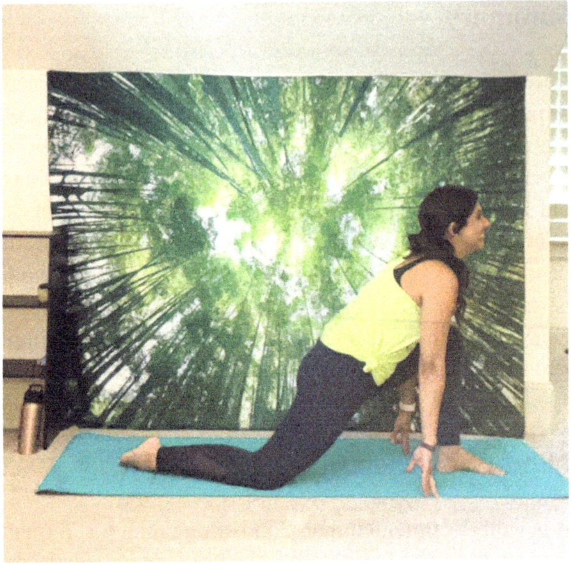

Fig. 2.9 Yoga position example

Rheumatology guidelines for the management of osteoarthritis (OA) strongly recommend tai chi for patients with knee and hip OA, noting improvements in strength, balance, fall prevention, as well as depression and self-efficacy [68]. Tai chi has been implemented in many populations at higher risk of falling and has nearly universally been deemed a useful intervention to prevent further falls and injuries. In regards to pain control, tai chi is most commonly studied in musculoskeletal conditions, shows improved pain in populations with chronic arthritis, and lower back pain, and is even shown to have similar if not greater improvement in pain symptoms for individuals with fibromyalgia when compared to aerobic exercise (the most common exercise prescription for patients with fibromyalgia) [69].

Yoga is another form of MBE that originated as a Hindu practice and incorporates a flow of various postures and poses in combination with meditation and controlled breathing (Fig. 2.9). Although many of the same benefits that are seen in tai chi are documented in yoga research, it is far less studied, and there is an overall lack of evidence to be able to strongly recommend the practice at this time [68]. There is some evidence to show the benefits of yoga for the treatment of lower back pain, but it is unclear if there is any difference between yoga and other forms of exercise or if yoga, in addition to other forms of exercise is more beneficial [70]. Similarly, pilates, qijong and other forms of MBE all have common threads of mindfulness, posture, flexibility, and muscle control. Many may find personal benefits from these practices, although the evidence is scarce for the promotion of these activities.

With emphasis placed on mindfulness, and stress relief in MBE programs, it is no surprise that MBE is associated with decreased depressive symptoms, although there is evidence that MBE, resistance training, and aerobic exercise have comparable efficacy in reducing symptoms of depression [71].

MBE are generally considered to be safe, and have the capability to increase strength, reduce falls and thus secondary injuries, and may reduce pain in certain populations There is a continued need for strong research and evidence to further promote these activities.

Table 2.2 summarizes evidenced based treatments.

Table 2.2 Evidence-based treatment

Evidence Based Treatment		
Diagnosis/ cause of pain	Evidence Based Exercise Recommendation	Comments
Osteoarthritis	Tai chi	Recommended by American College of Rheumatology. Benefits include improved pain control, balance, strength, and fall prevention.
	Aquatic exercise [31]	Benefits include reduced gravitational load, improved pain and walking function in the short term.
	Aerobic exercise	Walking improves pain, quality of life, and functional status [20, 21]
Fibromyalgia	Tai chi [69]	Shown to be similar if not more efficacious than aerobic exercise at improving fibromyalgia related pain.
	Aerobic exercise	The most commonly prescribed form of exercise for treatment/prevention of fibromyalgia pain. Walking is helpful for pain relief and reducing anxiety [24].
	Resistance training [65]	Shown to improve chronic fibromyalgia pain, though may not be as beneficial as aerobic exercise in this population.
Low back pain	Tai Chi [68]	The American College of Physicians in their practice guideline for noninvasive treatment of low back pain recommend tai chi and general exercise among other non-pharmacologic interventions for physicians to prescribe.
	Aquatic Exercise	Shown to be beneficial, though not more efficacious than other forms of exercise.
	Resistance Training [63, 64]	Shown to be beneficial overall though similar to other forms of exercise in terms of low back pain reduction.
	Aerobic exercise.	Low evidence for walking for pain management for low back pain [26].
Orthopedic injuries	Resistance training [51–59]	Prevents injury in most populations. Prevents falls in high risk populations. Improves strength and functional measures after injury. Improved strength, endurance, and gait following lower extremity orthopedic surgeries.
	Aquatic exercise [43–45]	Beneficial for post-operative care as well as prehabilitation for certain surgeries.
Chronic pain	Tai Chi [66]	Mind body exercises as a whole can reduce chronic pain symptoms (especially in elderly populations), with Tai chi having the strongest evidence.
	Aquatic exercise	Reduces force of gravity, and promotes gentle reintroduction of movement to combat kinesiophobic and fear avoidance behaviors [36]
	Resistance training [65]	Shown to decrease chronic pain symptoms, but aerobic exercise and tai chi may be more beneficial.

Conclusions

- Physical activity and exercise have numerous health benefits including cardiovascular benefits, cognitive and mood benefits, improved sleep and mobility and benefits for patients with osteoarthritis.
- Exercise can influence the perception of pain in both pain-free and chronic pain conditions.
- Cardiovascular exercise can have a positive benefit in patients with osteoarthritis-related pain, rheumatological pain, fibromyalgia, lower back pain and vascular claudication pain.
- Walking should be performed in multiple bouts as opposed to one continuous bout for maximum benefit.
- Water-based exercise incorporates components of aerobic exercise, resistance training, stretching, range of motion exercises and can be beneficial in injury rehabilitation and pain relief.
- Resistance training (also known as strength training) includes weight training, resistance bands and bodyweight exercises and can be used to improve functional strength as well as maximize dynamic strength and muscle mass in high performing athletes.
- Resistance training is often the first-line treatment for muscular or tendon injuries and has also been used to manage neck pain, back pain and chronic pain due to different reasons including fibromyalgia.
- The benefits of resistance training is optimized when it is used in conjunction with other forms of treatment and exercise.
- Mind-body exercises include yoga, tai-chi, pilates and qigong and are associated with improved pain in patients with knee and hip osteoarthritis, lower back pain and fibromyalgia.

Bibliography

1. Caspersen CJ, Powell KE, Christenson GM. Physical activity, exercise and physical fitness: definitions and distinctions for health-related research. Public Health Rep. 1985;100(2):126–31.
2. Howley ET. Type of activity: resistance, aerobic and leisure versus occupational physical activity. Med Sci Sport Exer. 2001;33(6):S364–S9.
3. Garber CE, Blissmer B, Deschenes MR, et al. American College of Sports Medicine position stand. Quantity and quality of exercise for developing and maintaining cardiorespiratory, musculoskeletal, and neuromuscular fitness in apparently healthy adults: guidance for prescribing exercise. Med Sci Sports Exerc. 2011;43(7):1334–59.
4. Chodzko-Zajko WJ, Proctor DN, Fiatarone Singh MA, et al. Exercise and physical activity in older adults. Med Sci Sports Exerc. 2009;41(7):1510–30.
5. Sinaki M. Exercise for patients with osteoporosis: management of vertebral compression fractures and trunk strengthening for fall prevention. PM R. 2012;4(11):882–8.
6. Galloza J, Castillo B, Micheo W. Benefits of exercise in the older population. Phys Med Rehabil Clin N Am. 2017;28(4):659–69. https://doi.org/10.1016/j.pmr.2017.06.001.

7. Kelley GA, Kelley KS. Exercise and sleep: a systematic review of previous meta-analyses. J Evid Based Med. 2017;10(1):26–36. https://doi.org/10.1111/jebm.12236.
8. Kramer AF, Hahn S, Cohen NJ, et al. Ageing, fitness and neurocognitive function. Nature. 1999;400:418–9.
9. Rice D, Nijs J, Kosek E, et al. Exercise-induced hypoalgesia in pain-free and chronic pain populations : state of the art and future directions. J Pain. 2019;20(11):1249–66. https://doi.org/10.1016/j.pain.2019.03.005.
10. Polaski AM, Phelps AL, Kostek MC, et al. Exercise-induced hypoalgesia: a meta-analysis of exercise dosing for the treatment of chronic pain. PLoS One. 2019;14(1):e0210418. https://doi.org/10.1371/journal.pone.0210418.
11. Gajsar H, Nahrwold K, Titze C, et al. Exercise does not produce hypoalgesia when performed immediately after a painful stimulus. Scandanav J Pain. 2018;18(2):311–20. https://doi.org/10.1515/sjpain-2018-0024.
12. Drury D, Stuempfle K, Shannon R, et al. An investigation of exercise-induced hypoalgesia after isometric and cardiovascular exercise. J Exer Physiol. 2004;7(4):1–5.
13. Koltyn KF. Analgesia following exercise: a review. Sports Med. 2000;29(2):85–98. https://doi.org/10.2165/00007256-200029020-00002.
14. Misra G, Paris TA, Archer DB, et al. Dose-response effect of isometric force production on the perception of pain. PLoS One. 2014;9(2) https://doi.org/10.1371/journal.pone.0088105.
15. Jan M, Lin J, Liau J, et al. Investigation of clinical effects of high and low resistance training for patients with knee osteoarthritis : a randomized controlled trial. Phys Ther. 2008;88(4):427–36.
16. Alton F, Baldey L, Caplan S, Morrissey MC. A kinematic comparison of overground and treadmill walking. Clin Biomech. 1998;13(6):434–40. https://doi.org/10.1016/S0268-0033(98)00012-6.
17. Felson DT. Developments in the clinical understanding of osteoarthritis. Arthritis Res Ther. 2009;11:203.
18. Centers for Disease Control and Prevention. Rheumatoid Arthritis, 2020. Retrieved from https://www.cdc.gov/arthritis/basics/rheumatoid-arthritis.html.
19. Fibromyalgia. National Institute of Arthritis and Musculoskeletal and Skin Diseases. http://www.niams.nih.gov/Health_Info/Fibromyalgia/default.asp.
20. Zhang W, Nuki G, Moskowitz RW, Abramson S, Altman RD, Arden NK, et al. OARSI recommendations for the management of hip and knee osteoarthritis: part III: changes in evidence following systematic cumulative update of research published through January 2009. Osteoarthr Cartil. 2010;18:476–99.
21. Bautch JC, Malone DG, Vailas AC. Effects of exercise on knee joints with osteoarthritis: a pilot study of biologic markers. Arthritis Care Res. 1997;10:48–55.
22. Farrokhi S, Jayabalan P, Gustafson JA, Klatt BA, Sowa GA, Piva SR. The influence of continuous versus interval walking exercise on knee joint loading and pain in patients with knee osteoarthritis. Gait Posture. 2017;56:129–133. https://doi.org/10.1016/j.gaitpost.2017.05.015. Epub 2017 May 17. PMID: 28544950; PMCID: PMC5669616.
23. Harkcom TM, et al. Therapeutic value of graded aerobic exercise training in rheumatoid arthritis. Arthritis Rheum. 1985;28(1):32.
24. Exercise training for adults with fibromyalgia. Cochrane Database Syst Rev. 6(6):CD012700. https://doi.org/10.1002/14651858.CD012700.
25. Mannerkorpi K. Physical activity and body functions in patients with fibromyalgia syndrome. J Musculoskelet Pain. 2009;17:287–94. https://doi.org/10.1080/10582450903088294.
26. Hendrick P, Te Wake AM, Tikkisetty AS, Wulff L, Yap C, Milosavljevic S. The effectiveness of walking as an intervention for low back pain: a systematic review. Eur Spine J. 2010;19(10):1613–20. https://doi.org/10.1007/s00586-010-1412-z. Epub 2010 Apr 23. PMID: 20414688; PMCID: PMC2989236.
27. Lauret GJ, Fakhry F, Fokkenrood HJ, Hunink MG, Teijink JA, Spronk S. Modes of exercise training for intermittent claudication. Cochrane Database Syst Rev. 2014;(7):CD009638. https://doi.org/10.1002/14651858.CD009638.pub2. Update in: Cochrane Database Syst Rev. 2020 Aug 20;8:CD009638. PMID: 24993079.

28. Lane R, Ellis B, Watson L, Leng GC. Exercise for intermittent claudication. Cochrane Database Syst Rev. 2014;(7):CD000990. https://doi.org/10.1002/14651858.CD000990.pub3. Update in: Cochrane Database Syst Rev. 2017 Dec 26;12 :CD000990. PMID: 25037027.
29. Goldenberg DL. Fibromyalgia: patient education beyond the basics. In: Post TW, editor. UpToDate. Waltham: UpToDate. Accessed September 15, 2022.
30. Biscarini A, Cerulli G. Modeling of the knee joint load in rehabilitative knee extension exercises under water. J Biomech. 2007;40:345–55. https://doi.org/10.1016/j.jbiomech.2005.12.018.
31. Bartels EM, Juhl CB, Christensen R, Hagen KB, Danneskiold-Samsøe B, Dagfinrud H, Lund H. Aquatic exercise for the treatment of knee and hip osteoarthritis. Cochrane Database Syst Rev. 2016;3:CD005523. https://doi.org/10.1002/14651858.CD005523.pub3. PMID: 27007113.
32. Lund H, Weile U, Christensen R, et al. A randomized controlled trial of aquatic and land-based exercise in patients with knee osteoarthritis. J Rehabil Med. 2008;40:137–44. https://doi.org/10.2340/16501977-0134.
33. Al-Qubaeissy KY, Fatoye FA, Goodwin PC, Yohannes AM. The effectiveness of hydrotherapy in the management of rheumatoid arthritis: a systematic review. Musculoskeletal Care. 2013;11(1):3–18. https://doi.org/10.1002/msc.1028. Epub 2012 Jul 16. PMID: 22806987.
34. Assis MR, Silva LE, Alves AM, Pessanha AP, Valim V, Feldman D, Neto TL, Natour J. A randomized controlled trial of deep water running: clinical effectiveness of aquatic exercise to treat fibromyalgia. Arthritis Rheum. 2006;55(1):57–65. https://doi.org/10.1002/art.21693. PMID: 16463414.
35. Pérez de la Cruz S, Lambeck J. A new approach towards improved quality of life in fibromyalgia: a pilot study on the effects of an aquatic Ai Chi program. Int J Rheum Dis. 2018;21(8):1525–32. https://doi.org/10.1111/1756-185X.12930. Epub 2016 Jul 26. PMID: 27457628.
36. Peng M, Wang R, Wang Y, et al. Efficacy of therapeutic aquatic exercise vs physical therapy modalities for patients with chronic low back pain: a randomized clinical trial. JAMA Netw Open. 2022;5(1):e2142069. https://doi.org/10.1001/jamanetworkopen.2021.42069).
37. Park S-Y. Impacts of aquatic walking on arterial stiffness, exercise tolerance, and physical function in patients with peripheral artery disease: a randomized clinical trial. J Appl Physiol. 2019;127:940.
38. Veldema J, Jansen P. Aquatic therapy in stroke rehabilitation: systematic review and meta-analysis. Acta Neurol Scand. 2021;143(3):221–41.
39. Corvillo I, et al. Efficacy of aquatic therapy for multiple sclerosis: a systematic review. Eur J Phys Rehabil Med. 2017;53(6):944–52.
40. Rutz DG, Benninger DH. Physical therapy for freezing of gait and gait impairments in Parkinson disease: a systematic review. PM R. 2020;12(11):1140–56.
41. Pérez de la Cruz S. Effectiveness of aquatic therapy for the control of pain and increased functionality in people with Parkinson's disease: a randomized clinical trial. Eur J Phys Rehabil Med. 2017;53(6):825–32.
42. Lai CJ, et al. Pediatric aquatic therapy on motor function and enjoyment in children diagnosed with cerebral palsy of various motor severities. J Child Neurol. 2015;30(2):200–8.
43. Pozzi F, Snyder-Mackler L, Zeni J. Physical exercise after knee arthroplasty: a systematic review of controlled trials. Eur J Phys Rehabil Med. 2013;49(6):877–92.
44. Papalia R, et al. The role of physical activity and rehabilitation following hip and knee arthroplasty in the elderly. J Clin Med. 2020;9(5):1401.
45. Kim S, et al. A pilot study of aquatic prehabilitation in adults with knee osteoarthritis undergoing total knee arthroplasty - short term outcome. BMC Musculoskelet Disord. 2021;22(1):388.
46. Roig M, et al. The effects of eccentric versus concentric resistance training on muscle strength and mass in healthy adults: a systematic review with meta-analysis. Br J Sports Med. 2009;43(8):556–68.

47. Del Vecchio A, et al. The increase in muscle force after 4 weeks of strength training is mediated by adaptations in motor unit recruitment and rate coding. J Physiol. 2019;597(7):1873–87.
48. Deschenes MR, Kraemer WJ. Performance and physiologic adaptations to resistance training. Am J Phys Med Rehabil. 2002;81(11 Suppl):S3–16.
49. Carvalho L, et al. Muscle hypertrophy and strength gains after resistance training with different volume-matched loads: a systematic review and meta-analysis. Appl Physiol Nutr Metab. 2022;47(4):357–68.
50. Westcott WL. Resistance training is medicine: effects of strength training on health. Curr Sports Med Rep. 2012;11(4):209–16.
51. Lauersen JB, Andersen TE, Andersen LB. Strength training as superior, dose-dependent and safe prevention of acute and overuse sports injuries: a systematic review, qualitative analysis and meta-analysis. Br J Sports Med. 2018;52(24):1557–63.
52. Al Attar WSA, et al. Effect of injury prevention programs that include the Nordic hamstring exercise on hamstring injury rates in Soccer players: a systematic review and meta-analysis. Sports Med. 2017;47(5):907–16.
53. Van Eerd D, et al. Effectiveness of workplace interventions in the prevention of upper extremity musculoskeletal disorders and symptoms: an update of the evidence. Occup Environ Med. 2016;73(1):62–70.
54. Stanghelle B, et al. Effects of a resistance and balance exercise programme on physical fitness, health-related quality of life and fear of falling in older women with osteoporosis and vertebral fracture: a randomized controlled trial. Osteoporos Int. 2020;31(6):1069–78.
55. Lopez P, et al. Benefits of resistance training in physically frail elderly: a systematic review. Aging Clin Exp Res. 2018;30(8):889–99.
56. Etxebarria N, Mujika I, Pyne DB. Training and competition readiness in triathlon. Sports (Basel). 2019;7(5):101.
57. Zwolski C, Quatman-Yates C, Paterno MV. Resistance training in youth: laying the foundation for injury prevention and physical literacy. Sports Health. 2017;9(5):436–43.
58. Cain MS, et al. Four-week ankle-rehabilitation programs in adolescent athletes with chronic ankle instability. J Athl Train. 2020;55(8):801–10.
59. Bayer ML, et al. Chronic sequelae after muscle strain injuries: influence of heavy resistance training on functional and structural characteristics in a randomized controlled trial. Am J Sports Med. 2021;49(10):2783–94.
60. Beyer R, et al. Heavy slow resistance versus eccentric training as treatment for Achilles Tendinopathy: a randomized controlled trial. Am J Sports Med. 2015;43(7):1704–11.
61. Nichols ZW, O'Brien D, White SG. Is resistance training intensity adequately prescribed to meet the demands of returning to sport following anterior cruciate ligament repair? A systematic review. BMJ Open Sport Exerc Med. 2021;7(3):e001144.
62. Ramadi A, et al. Progressive resistance training program characteristics in rehabilitation programs following hip fracture: a meta-analysis and meta-regression. Geriatr Orthop Surg Rehabil. 2022;13:21514593221090799.
63. Iversen VM, et al. Resistance training vs general physical exercise in multidisciplinary rehabilitation of chronic neck pain: a randomized controlled trial. J Rehabil Med. 2018;50(8):743–50.
64. Iversen VM, et al. Resistance band training or general exercise in multidisciplinary rehabilitation of low back pain? A randomized trial. Scand J Med Sci Sports. 2018;28(9):2074–83.
65. Busch AJ, et al. Resistance exercise training for fibromyalgia. Cochrane Database Syst Rev. 2013;2013(12):Cd010884.
66. Wen YR, et al. Are mind-body exercise beneficial for treating pain, function, and quality of life in middle-aged and old people with chronic pain? A systematic review and meta-analysis. Front Aging Neurosci. 2022;14:921069.
67. Solloway MR, et al. An evidence map of the effect of Tai Chi on health outcomes. Syst Rev. 2016;5(1):126.

68. Kolasinski SL, et al. 2019 American College of Rheumatology/Arthritis Foundation guideline for the management of osteoarthritis of the hand, hip, and knee. Arthritis Care Res (Hoboken). 2020;72(2):149–62.
69. Wang C, et al. Effect of tai chi versus aerobic exercise for fibromyalgia: comparative effectiveness randomized controlled trial. BMJ. 2018;360:k851.
70. Wieland LS, et al. Yoga treatment for chronic non-specific low back pain. Cochrane Database Syst Rev. 2017;1(1):Cd010671.
71. Miller KJ, et al. Aerobic, resistance, and mind-body exercise are equivalent to mitigate symptoms of depression in older adults: a systematic review and network meta-analysis of randomised controlled trials. F1000Res. 2020;9:1325.

Nutrition, Obesity, and Musculoskeletal Pain

3

Joseph T. Rinaldi, Biral T. Patel, and Robert S. Ackerman

Introduction

Obesity and pain represent prevailing challenges within contemporary healthcare systems, collectively imposing substantial burdens [2, 3]. Individually, each exerts a significant impact on well-being; however, their confluence escalates the toll on individuals. Numerous cross-sectional investigations have unveiled a pronounced correlation between obesity and pain, with longitudinal studies further establishing obesity as a pivotal risk factor in pain development, accompanied by a consequential diminishment in quality of life [3]. Obesity exhibits a multifaceted and intricate interplay with pain, primarily stemming from factors such as mechanical overloading, the pro-inflammatory milieu induced by obesity, and intricate neurohumoral processes [3, 4]. Conversely, chronic pain can lead to obesity, often due to a sedentary lifestyle or the adoption of eating behaviors for their rewarding or analgesic outcomes [3].

A wealth of compelling evidence underscores the influence of obesity's pathophysiological mechanisms on a range of pain conditions, notably including fibromyalgia, lower back pain, and pediatric pain [3–5]. In combatting obesity, an array of interventions exists, spanning dietary approaches, pharmacotherapy, and surgical

J. T. Rinaldi
Department of Physical Medicine and Rehabilitation, Tufts Medical Center, Boston, MA, USA

B. T. Patel (✉)
Division of Pain Management, Department of Anesthesiology and Pain Management, University of Texas Southwestern Medical Center, Dallas, TX, USA
e-mail: biral.patel@utsouthwestern.edu

R. S. Ackerman
Morsani College of Medicine, University of South Florida, Tampa, FL, USA

Division of Interventional Pain Medicine, Department of Anesthesiology, Moffitt Cancer Center and Research Institute, Tampa, FL, USA

C. E. Noe (ed.), *Musculoskeletal Pain*,
https://doi.org/10.1007/978-3-031-86057-7_3

interventions. Insightful investigations have demonstrated that nutritional strategies wield significant power in ameliorating both pain and overall health, primarily through the attenuation of systemic inflammation [8]. While pain medications stand as an acute symptom-relief avenue, their administration in these contexts becomes notably intricate due to obesity-induced alterations in the pharmacokinetics and pharmacodynamics of diverse medications, potentially resulting in suboptimal dosing [6]. While dietary adjustments and pharmaceutical interventions form the cornerstone of pain management in individuals with obesity, emerging evidence hints at the potential utility of bariatric surgery in enhancing musculoskeletal well-being and functionality [7].

Obesity: General Overview

In 2015, approximately 604 million adults worldwide were affected by obesity [9]. The global prevalence of obesity has witnessed a troubling trend since 1980, with over 70 countries experiencing a doubling of obesity rates, while most other nations also observed a consistent rise in cases [9]. A notable example is the United States, where the age-adjusted overall prevalence of obesity progressively increased from 22.9% to 42.4% between 1988 and 2018, with a balanced distribution between males and females [10]. Within this period, from 2007 to 2018, severe obesity (defined as a body mass index [BMI] $\geq$ 40 kg/m^2) saw an upward trajectory from 5.7% to 9.2% [10]. The National Health Statistics Report highlighted that from 2017 to March 2020, obesity prevalence stood at 19.7% among children and adolescents aged 2 to 19, while adults aged 20 and older faced a prevalence rate of 41.9% [12].

Projections based on current trends paint a concerning picture for the future. If these patterns persist, it is anticipated that nearly half of all adults in the United States will grapple with obesity, and close to one-fourth will battle severe obesity [11, 12]. Alarmingly, almost 60% of today's children are predicted to experience obesity by the age of 35 [13].

The escalating obesity epidemic has profound economic ramifications as well. Among adults, the association between obesity and excess annual medical costs translates to $1861 per person, contributing to a total annual expenditure of $172.74 billion [14]. Severe obesity compounds this burden, with excess costs amounting to $3097 per adult [14]. Among children, obesity-related expenses stand at $116 per person, totaling $1.32 billion in medical spending, while severe obesity incurs $310 in excess costs per child [14]. Notably, interventions targeting obesity at an early stage hold the potential to significantly mitigate healthcare costs. A study by Wang et al. estimates that a mere 1% reduction in overweight or obese individuals aged 16 to 17 could lead to a future reduction of 52,812 adults with obesity, resulting in a decrease of $586 million in lifetime medical costs [15].

Beyond its economic implications, obesity's far-reaching impact on individuals encompasses factors such as school attendance, education levels, earning capacity, and social interactions, thereby exerting a substantial toll throughout their lifetimes [16].

Addressing obesity is a complex challenge due to its intricate pathophysiology, influenced by a myriad of biological, psychosocial, and behavioral factors [17]. Some prominent risk factors include genetics, low socioeconomic status, cultural influences, epigenetics, maternal age, fecundity, sleep deficiency, endocrine disorders, mobility limitations, and pharmaceutical influences [17, 18]. Compounding this complexity is obesity's association with a heightened risk of complications such as hypertension, dyslipidemia, type 2 diabetes, coronary artery disease, stroke, gallbladder disease, obstructive sleep apnea, various cancers, mental health disorders, osteoarthritis, reduced quality of life, bodily pain, and diminished functionality [1]. This underscores the urgency of surmounting effective management strategies.

Despite substantial insights into obesity's pathophysiology, treatment and prevention approaches have predominantly focused on the psychological and social components of the disease. Current noninvasive interventions primarily center on dietary management and behavioral modifications. While pharmacotherapy has shown some efficacy in managing obesity among adults, its effectiveness remains limited, particularly for children. Among the array of available treatments, bariatric surgery stands out for yielding the best outcomes. Genetic testing, though available for select patients, is still evolving in its capacity to guide therapy, necessitating further research to enhance its effectiveness [4, 19, 20].

Fibromyalgia

Introduction and Epidemiology

Fibromyalgia is frequently identified by the presence of persistent, widespread pain that occurs without signs of peripheral musculoskeletal inflammation or structural damage [21]. This pain is often accompanied by fatigue, tenderness, sleep disorders, cognitive impairments, and commonly, mental health disorders such as anxiety and depression [22]. Notably, this condition affects women significantly more frequently than men, with a ratio of approximately six to one [23]. In the United States, the prevalence of fibromyalgia is estimated to be around 2–3%; however, this prevalence tends to rise with age [24, 25].

Diagnostic Criteria

The initial diagnosis of fibromyalgia relied on the 1990 criteria set forth by the American College of Rheumatology (ACR) [26]. These criteria stipulated that individuals needed to experience widespread pain lasting for at least three months [26]. This pain had to be present both above and below the waist, impacting both sides of the body [26]. Additionally, individuals needed to exhibit tenderness when pressure was applied to 11 or more of the 18 designated tender points [26]. While these criteria exhibited a sensitivity and specificity of 85%, it's important to note that they were not designed for practical clinical use [26].

As a result, in 2010, the American College of Rheumatology introduced a preliminary set of clinical criteria, shifting the focus towards a widespread pain index (WPI) and symptom severity (SS) scale. [27] According to these new criteria, fibromyalgia diagnosis would involve a WPI score exceeding 7, along with an SS score surpassing 5 [27]. Alternatively, a WPI score between 3 and 6, coupled with an SS score surpassing 9, could also indicate fibromyalgia [27]. This new approach eliminated the requirement for tender point examinations [27]. The WPI quantifies the number of painful regions on the body from a predefined list of 19 areas, while the SS score incorporates evaluations of fatigue, unrefreshing sleep, cognitive symptoms, and general somatic symptoms [27]. Importantly, these symptoms still needed to persist for a minimum of three months, and no other medical condition could better explain the patient's symptoms [27].

Over the subsequent years, these diagnostic criteria underwent several modifications, culminating in the most recent update in 2016. This revised version shifted the criteria, referring to individuals with pain in four out of five specific regions as having multisite pain (MSP), a departure from the 1990 definition of chronic widespread pain (CWP) [25]. Furthermore, this iteration integrated both physician assessments and questionnaire-based criteria, while discarding the prior recommendation concerning diagnostic exclusions [28].

Pathophysiology

Fibromyalgia is widely believed to be a disorder rooted in central sensitization, resulting in heightened responses to both painful and non-painful stimuli [23]. This altered pain processing within the central nervous system comprises various aspects, such as diminished endogenous pain inhibition, modifications in pain receptors and pain-related neuropeptides, temporal summation of pain, as well as central hypersensitivity [29].

Evidence suggests malfunctioning endogenous analgesic systems, leading to reduced pain inhibition plays a key role in the pathogenesis of fibromyalgia [30]. Notably, fibromyalgia is also associated with changes in the regulation of pain receptors, particularly in the opioid receptor system. In this context, delta-opioid and kappa-opioid receptors are upregulated in peripheral tissues, while mu-opioid receptors are downregulated in the brain [31, 32]. Pain-related neuropeptides, including brain-derived neurotrophic factor (BDNF), have also been found to exhibit elevated levels both in the brain and plasma of individuals with fibromyalgia [33].

Another hallmark of the disorder is the temporal summation of pain, which refers to the phenomenon where individuals experience a more pronounced increase in the perceived intensity of pain when subjected to rapidly repetitive noxious stimuli [34]. Finally, central hypersensitivity, characterized by heightened sensitivity to sensory stimuli encompassing visual, auditory, and olfactory domains is thought to play a key role in the pathogenesis of fibromyalgia [35]. This generalized hypersensitivity is believed to contribute to increased pain sensitivity [35]. This notion is supported by research showing amplified brain responses to both the onset and cessation of pain in individuals with fibromyalgia [35].

Relation to Obesity

Obesity has been proposed as a significant risk factor for the emergence of fibromyalgia [36, 37]. While evidence remains limited, earlier investigations have revealed a striking increase of 37–51% in the prevalence of fibromyalgia among obese individuals, compared to the reported 4% in the general population [38, 39]. While establishing a definitive causal relationship is challenging due to the scarcity of data, several pathophysiological hypotheses have been formulated to elucidate the link between obesity and the prominent clinical aspect of fibromyalgia—pain [5]. Despite its modest impact, multiple studies have identified a noteworthy association between obesity and the severity of pain in fibromyalgia [5]. Obesity's potential connection to fibromyalgia centers around mechanical strain on joints and tissues, possibly compounded by nociceptive input contributing to widespread pain [40]. This interaction with mechanical stimuli and altered neural pain pathways could also give rise to allodynia [41]. Excessive weight might serve as a trigger, potentially amplifying pain responses, particularly in susceptible individuals [42]. Within this context, changes in muscles and tendons due to obesity could create an environment conducive to pain initiation [43]. Another mechanism that has been postulated is that leptin, elevated in obesity, may exacerbate pain sensitivity by enhancing pronociceptive glutamate receptor function [44, 45]. While not the primary cause, inflammation could have a role, as evidenced by elevated pro-inflammatory cytokines and reduced anti-nociceptive mediators in fibromyalgia patients [46]. Findings from animal studies strongly support the role of cytokines and chemokines in promoting central sensitization, enhancing nociception, and contributing to the onset of chronic muscle pain [47–49]. Considering obesity's pro-inflammatory nature, it's plausible that this could intensify the inflammatory context associated with pain signaling, potentially heightening the severity of pain experienced by individuals with fibromyalgia [5]. These inflammatory processes might also extend to influencing other symptoms such as depression, fatigue, and sleep disorders, however, several limitations exist hindering the ability to properly interpret existing data [50–52].

The relationship between fibromyalgia and obesity is marked by a convergence of shared underlying mechanisms, resulting in a complex relationship. In this intricate dynamic, obesity assumes a dual role—not only as a potential exacerbating factor but also as a potential trigger [52, 53]. Concurrently, fibromyalgia's influence on obesity's development is a noteworthy consideration. A compelling supplementary perspective suggests that obesity might function as a "facilitator," intensifying fibromyalgia symptoms due to its impact on the underlying systemic inflammation [5]. Within this framework, weight loss emerges as a promising strategy to enhance the comprehensive treatment of fibromyalgia patients [5, 52]. While further investigations are imperative, clinicians should consider using weight loss as an adjunctive avenue for promoting overall well-being and striving for symptom mitigation among individuals with fibromyalgia.

Low Back Pain

Introduction and Epidemiology

Low back pain is a prevalent and intricate health concern that transcends age and socioeconomic boundaries on a global scale. This pervasive issue imposes a substantial weight on individuals, healthcare infrastructures, and economies due to its far-reaching repercussions encompassing quality of life, work efficiency, and healthcare expenditures [54]. Notably, studies have highlighted that low back pain will affect nearly 84% of adults at some juncture [54].

The prevalence of low back pain exhibits notable variance contingent upon geographical landscapes, age, and a constellation of variables. Extensive investigations reveal that a striking 60–80% of individuals will grapple with at least one episode of low back pain during their lifespan. The point prevalence of low back pain registers at an approximate range of 12–30%, while the scope of one-year prevalence extends from 22% to 65% [55].

Low back pain's prevalence is accentuated with the passage of years, culminating in the highest rates among individuals aged 30 to 60 years. However, it is imperative to acknowledge that low back pain recognizes no age boundaries, permeating through all age brackets from pediatrics to the elderly. Furthermore, intriguing gender dynamics come to the fore, with certain studies suggesting a heightened prevalence among females [56, 57].

The gravity of low back pain's global prevalence naturally precipitates a consequential economic impact, amplifying its significance. It surges to the forefront as a paramount contributor to the burden of disability-adjusted life years (DALYs), a metric that gauges the societal toll of health conditions [58]. In light of these compelling statistics, it becomes evident that low back pain demands attention as a pivotal healthcare concern resonating across a diverse spectrum of individuals and societies [58].

Etiologies

Low back pain often manifests as brief episodes with minimal or no lasting consequences [58]. However, it frequently recurs and is increasingly recognized as a chronic condition characterized by a variable course [58]. This complexity arises from the multifaceted nature of low back pain, with contributions from diverse factors encompassing psychological, social, biophysical, comorbid, and pain-processing mechanisms [59].

Numerous risk factors are associated with complaints of low back pain, including but not limited to smoking, obesity, advancing age, female gender, physically demanding occupations, sedentary work, psychologically strenuous work, lower educational attainment, workers' compensation insurance, job dissatisfaction, and psychosocial factors such as somatization disorder, anxiety, and depression [59–63]. The multitude of contributing factors makes pinpointing a specific nociceptive source exceedingly challenging [58].

The majority of patients presenting with back pain lack an identifiable underlying condition and fall into the category of nonspecific cases. Thankfully, most cases follow a self-limiting trajectory, resolving within a matter of weeks [64, 65]. However, in instances where a specific etiology is discernible, common pathologies encompass fractures, radiculopathies, spinal stenosis, herniated discs, degenerative diseases, osteoporosis, and congenital conditions such as scoliosis and kyphosis [67]. It's crucial to highlight that more serious etiologies should not be overlooked, including metastatic cancer, vertebral osteomyelitis, spinal epidural abscess, and cauda equina syndrome [66]. These conditions typically present with specific risk factors, underscoring the paramount importance of a thorough medical history and physical examination for accurate diagnosis [64–67].

Relation to Obesity

Numerous studies conducted over the years have consistently revealed a compelling link between obesity and low back pain, with a recent comprehensive systematic review in 2021 notably underscoring the role of central adiposity in this relationship [68]. The intricate interplay between these two conditions is primarily expounded through two pivotal mechanisms: the imposition of heightened physical loads and the orchestration of systemic metabolic processes. Within overweight or obese individuals, the surplus adipose tissue precipitates augmented stress upon specific anatomical regions, consequently inducing perturbed posture and aberrant movement patterns that invariably give rise to sensations of pain and debilitation. Concurrently, a mounting body of evidence substantiates the influence of systemic metabolic factors, with research indicating that adiposity exerts a palpable impact on pain even in non-weight-bearing areas, such as the hand [69]. Functioning as a metabolically active entity, adipose tissue actively discharges an array of pro-inflammatory cytokines and adipokines, thereby potentially triggering inflammatory transformations within a given locale that invariably culminate in the manifestation of pain [70]. Furthermore, the cascade of inflammation has been demonstrated to modulate the excitation thresholds and responsivity of peripheral nerves, consequently setting off processes of peripheral and central sensitization [71, 72].

The substantial prevalence of low back pain and obesity highlights the noteworthy health concern stemming from their interrelated nature [54, 68]. This intricacy arises from multifaceted elements encompassing psychological, social, and physiological aspects, with obesity standing out as a prominent risk factor for low back pain. This connection involves heightened physical strain and metabolic mechanisms that elevate systemic inflammation, consequently inducing nerve sensitization and fostering pain [68]. This pathophysiologic framework underscores obesity's pivotal role as a modifiable risk factor for low back pain, prompting healthcare professionals to incorporate weight loss as an adjunctive approach for both preventing and managing low back pain.

Pediatric Pain

Obesity

The Centers for Disease Control and Prevention (CDC) utilizes body mass index (BMI) percentiles to categorize weight in the pediatric population. This classification system includes [73]:

- Underweight: BMI < 5th percentile for age and sex.
- Normal Weight: BMI between 5th and <85th percentile for age and sex.
- Overweight: BMI between >85th percentile and 95th percentile for age and sex.
- Obesity:
  - Class I: BMI ≥95th percentile for age and sex, or BMI ≥30 (whichever is lower).
  - Class II: BMI ≥120 percent of the 95th percentile values or BMI ≥35 kg/m^2 (whichever is lower), roughly equivalent to the 98th percentile.
  - Class III: BMI ≥140 percent of the 95th percentile values or BMI ≥40 kg/m^2.

Approximately one-third of children in the United States grapple with overweight or obesity. Statistics reveal the following prevalences based on age groups [74]:

- Overweight: 12.3% of children aged 2–5 years, 15.4% of those aged 6–11 years, and 19.4% of adolescents aged 12–19 years.
- Class I Obesity: 11.7% of children aged 2–5 years, 12.3% of those aged 6–11 years, and 8.9% of adolescents aged 12–19 years.
- Class II or III Obesity: Prevalent in 2.0% of children aged 2–5 years, 6.4% of those aged 6–11 years, and affecting 10.1% of females and 13.2% of males aged 12–19 years.

Pediatric obesity demonstrates disparities among ethnic groups, with Native American, Black, and Mexican American children exhibiting higher rates in comparison to non-Hispanic White children [75]. Risk factors for childhood obesity encompass parental obesity, lower socioeconomic status, lower educational attainment, and rural residence [76–78].

Studies indicate a significant upsurge in obesity prevalence from the late twentieth century up to 2018. Among children 6 to 11 years, obesity prevalence surged from 6.5% in 1976–1980 to 19.3% in 2015–2018 [75]. For adolescents 12 to 19 years, obesity rates increased from 5% in 1976–1980 to 20.9% in 2015–2018 [75]. In contrast, preschool-aged children evidenced a plateau in prevalence with an upward trajectory through 2018 [75, 79].

Of notable concern is the compelling evidence that many obese children persist into adulthood [80, 81]. The likelihood of this persistence correlates with age, parental obesity, obesity severity, and BMI trajectory during childhood [78, 80–82]. Notably, Ward et al. pooled data to simulate the trajectory of childhood obesity in the United States and demonstrated that almost 60% of children will be obese by the time they are 35 years old, thus highlighting the significance of early intervention in obesity management [13].

Low Back Pain

Research examining the link between musculoskeletal pain and obesity within the pediatric population remains relatively limited [83–86]. Nonetheless, emerging evidence suggests that akin to adults, obesity stands as a modifiable risk factor for low back pain in children. In parallel with adults, children frequently report experiencing back pain in the cervical, thoracic, and lumbar spine, with the lower lumbar spine emerging as the most common site of discomfort. As children grow older, the prevalence of this condition tends to increase, eventually reaching levels comparable to those seen in adults by the age of 18 [87–89].

In a noteworthy study conducted in 2020 by Palmer et al., researchers adjusted for various confounding variables, revealing that overweight or obese children face an elevated risk of developing back pain in the cervical, thoracic, or lumbar spine. Furthermore, this study unveiled a dose-response relationship between back pain and different weight categories. The cumulative incidence of back pain, as diagnosed by community pediatricians, was observed to rise with age, affecting approximately 9% of children with normal weight compared to almost 12% among obese children [90].

While it can be hypothesized that similar pathophysiological mechanisms underlie pediatric back pain as seen in adults, more research is indispensable to delve into the precise etiology within this unique population. Unraveling the intricate relationship between childhood obesity and low back pain is essential for developing effective preventive strategies and targeted interventions, ultimately alleviating the burden of pain among our younger generation.

Management

Children who grapple with excess weight, being either overweight or obese, face a significantly heightened risk of developing back pain [90]. Notably, the incidence of back pain rises with age and appears to be most prevalent among overweight females hailing from socioeconomically disadvantaged backgrounds [91]. It is imperative to recognize that childhood back pain often foreshadows similar issues in adulthood, underscoring the importance of initiating preventive measures from an early age [90].

However, it's worth noting that significant evidence for primary prevention of back pain in children remains limited [83–86]. In the adolescent population, only education and ergonomic school furniture have been analyzed [92]. The available data indicate that educational efforts are generally ineffective, while the quality of evidence supporting the use of ergonomically designed furniture to prevent back pain, as compared to conventional furniture, is of very low quality.

Exercise, particularly when coupled with educational initiatives, has demonstrated potential for preventing back pain in adulthood and thus warrants further exploration in child populations [83]. Such investigations could provide valuable insights into effective preventive and management strategies.

Diet

Introduction

While there is an abundance of evidence demonstrating the efficacy of dietary interventions in managing obesity, the relationship between diet and musculoskeletal pain has not received as much attention in the literature. Nevertheless, extensive studies have shed light on the significant influence of dietary choices on an individual's perception of pain. Recent scientific investigations have revealed a direct link, particularly between a high-fat diet and elevated serum glucose and cytokine levels [93]. Recent research suggests that dietary interventions can offer substantial relief to individuals dealing with chronic pain, operating through various molecular systems believed to support neural function and plasticity [94]. Cutting-edge dietary strategies, including intermittent fasting, time-restricted feeding, caloric restriction, the ketogenic diet, and the Mediterranean diet, have garnered attention in this context [94–96]. It is hypothesized that the effectiveness of these dietary approaches in managing chronic musculoskeletal pain may be linked to their influence on central nervous system sensitization and pain hypersensitivity [94–96].

Intermittent Fasting

Intermittent fasting reduces meal frequency, enhancing cellular efficiency by reducing inflammation and oxidative stress [97]. This approach has shown promise in improving both functional and mechanical outcomes while reducing pain perception and inflammation, although evidence regarding its long-term effectiveness is still evolving [97]. Some studies present conflicting findings, suggesting that intermittent fasting may have little to no significant effect on chronic pain [98]. Nevertheless, intermittent fasting can enhance mitochondrial metabolism, especially when combined with regular exercise, potentially reducing insulin resistance and inflammation, thereby contributing to improved glucose metabolism, cognitive function, and cardiovascular health [97].

Caloric Restriction and Time-Restricted Feeding

Caloric restriction, a widely used dietary strategy for weight loss, involves reducing daily calorie intake without compromising nutrition. It plays a vital role in promoting longevity and overall health, with significant benefits observed in musculoskeletal pain management, especially in cases with a rheumatologic etiology [99, 100]. Similarly, time-restricted feeding has shown promising evidence. This approach regulates food intake within specific time windows, designating certain hours for fasting and others for eating [101]. A variant of intermittent fasting, involves fasting periods lasting 12 to 18 hours [101, 102]. Time-restricted feeding has demonstrated benefits in enhancing various circadian rhythm processes such as blood pressure, sleep cycle, respiration, heart rate, and cognitive functions, and has been shown to be a first step to caloric restriction [102].

Mediterranean and Ketogenic Diet

The Mediterranean diet, characterized by regular consumption of olive oil, fruits, vegetables, fish, unrefined cereals, and moderate meat intake, along with various spices and occasionally wine, is renowned for its rich nutrients and bioactive compounds with anti-inflammatory properties [103]. While promising evidence suggests that a Mediterranean diet may reduce musculoskeletal pain levels, conflicting results are observed when assessing pain frequency and articular stiffness in individuals adhering to this diet [104–107]. In contrast, the ketogenic diet, initially designed for epilepsy management, maintains carbohydrate intake below 50 grams per day or no more than 10% of total energy intake [108, 109]. Although it is hypothesized that ketolytic metabolism can reduce pain and inflammation, current studies do not support its effectiveness in pain management. However, limitations in the existing literature hinder definitive conclusions, and more research is needed to evaluate potential benefits, especially in the context of breast cancer as there is some evidence to suggest it may be there may be some benefit in this population [110].

Other Diets

Beyond these modern diet strategies, current research suggests that several other diets have the potential to alleviate musculoskeletal pain. These include low glutamate diets, vegetarian/vegan diets, diets rich in polyunsaturated fatty acids, supplementation with antioxidant vitamins and minerals, increased fruit and fiber intake, and the elimination of monosodium glutamate in individuals suffering from conditions like fibromyalgia and rheumatoid arthritis [100, 103, 111, 112].

The body of research on dietary strategies for chronic pain management and overall health is promising. Proper nutrition and diet play an essential role in achieving musculoskeletal health and well-being. Therefore, further research is needed to explore the effects of diverse dietary approaches on pain as well as quality of life, circadian rhythm, and sleep quality, not in isolation but through comprehensive analyses as well.

Pharmacology

Drug Absorption

In individuals with obesity, several physiological changes occur, including increased gut permeability, altered gastric emptying, and potential impairments in CYP-mediated gut and liver metabolism [113]. The process of drug absorption from the intestine is influenced by various factors, such as the rate of absorption and bioavailability, which refers to the total amount of a drug absorbed. Bioavailability depends on the fraction of the drug absorbed and the extent of gut and hepatic (first-pass) metabolism [113–116]. These changes in physiology associated with obesity are believed to affect drug absorption and, consequently, bioavailability [113–116].

However, the extent to which obesity impacts drug absorption remains uncertain due to limited available evidence. While there is evidence of increased gut permeability and potential decreases in gut CYP3A4 metabolism in obesity, the only drug that has demonstrated significant changes in bioavailability in severely obese individuals is midazolam [117]. It is important to note that this increase in bioavailability was observed in severely obese patients, suggesting that it may be most pronounced in cases of extreme obesity [117]. Nevertheless, more comprehensive research is needed to draw definitive conclusions.

Volume Distribution

The volume of distribution is a crucial pharmacokinetic parameter determined by the peak concentration of a drug after each dose [118]. Along with drug clearance, it determines a drug's elimination or half-life. This information is vital when dosing medications, as the volume of distribution helps calculate the optimal loading dose, while the drug's half-life is used to determine the dose required to reach and maintain a steady state [118]. Predicting the volume of distribution of a drug is challenging because various drug properties influence it, such as lipophilicity, ionization properties, blood-to-plasma ratio, and protein binding [119, 120].

While it is theoretically expected that lipophilic compounds would easily diffuse into adipose tissue, leading to an increase in volume of distribution with higher body weight, results have been mixed for lipophilic drugs. For instance, diazepam's volume distribution significantly increases with increasing body weight, whereas other lipophilic drugs like propofol and digoxin show no changes in volume distribution with increasing body weight [121–123]. This underscores the importance of considering all drug properties when predicting changes in volume distribution. Serum protein concentrations, which play a crucial role in drug binding, have also been shown to be increased in obesity [124]. While albumin and total protein concentrations seem unaffected, there is evidence that alpha-1 acid glycoprotein (AAG) levels may be elevated in obesity, potentially affecting the pharmacokinetics of basic drugs [124]. However, the role of AAG in altering pharmacokinetics in obese individuals is still theoretical.

Differences in tissue penetration between obese and non-obese individuals can also be significant, as observed in studies involving several antibiotics. For example, cefazolin and ciprofloxacin demonstrated significantly reduced tissue penetration in obese individuals, potentially necessitating higher dosages or increased dosing frequency to maintain adequate plasma concentrations [125–127].

Clearance

Clearance, divided into hepatic and renal components, is a critical factor with the greatest impact on clinical implications. The liver plays a central role in drug metabolism, involving both phase I (modification) and phase II (conjugation) processes, influenced by liver enzyme activity and transport proteins. This, along with hepatic blood flow and protein binding, determines hepatic clearance. Predicting drug clearance for hepatically metabolized drugs is challenging, especially in obese patients, where enzymes for both phase I and phase II metabolism are altered. For instance, CYP1E1 activity increases, while CYP3A4 decreases in phase I metabolism, and phase II metabolism seems to increase overall. Therefore, understanding multiple aspects of a drug, including its metabolic phases, specific enzymes involved, liver size, hepatic blood flow, and the influence of transport proteins, is imperative to determine overall plasma clearance.

Renal clearance also plays a significant role, especially for drugs primarily eliminated through the kidneys. Renal physiology changes with obesity. Initially, glomerular filtration rate (GFR) increases in overweight individuals, but over time, it may decrease, potentially explaining the mixed evidence in the literature. For instance, drugs like gentamicin, tobramycin, and vancomycin, primarily excreted unchanged in urine, showed increased clearance in morbidly obese patients [128–130]. In another study, clearance of lithium was shown to be enhanced in obesity and was hypothesized to be due to impaired tubular reuptake of lithium [131]. Conversely, drugs like cefazolin and fluconazole, also renally excreted, exhibited similar total drug clearances in morbidly obese and nonobese subjects [131, 132]. The influence of obesity on drug clearance may vary depending on factors such as chronicity, comorbidities like diabetes mellitus or sepsis, and the balance between glomerular and tubular processes in renal excretion, thus emphasizing the complexity of determining drug clearance.

Pharmacodynamics

There is limited research on the pharmacodynamics (PD) of drugs in obesity. Some antibiotics have shown decreased efficacy in obese patients, leading to worse outcomes [133]. Also, researchers have hypothesized that hypnosedative drugs such as benzodiazepines can exacerbate prevalent comorbidities in the obese population like obstructive sleep apnea (OSA) by reducing effective breathing, however, no trials have been executed to discern this theory [134, 135]. With few studies exploring pharmacodynamic parameters in obesity, it is difficult to translate pharmacokinetic models into dosing regimens for various pharmacological domains, such as anesthetics, antibiotics, or sedatives. Thus, it is crucial for more research to be conducted in order to elucidate the pharmacodynamics of these drugs in obesity thoroughly.

Bariatric Surgery and Musculoskeletal Pain

Introduction

Bariatric surgery has witnessed remarkable evolution as one of the fastest-evolving operative procedures performed worldwide, with over 579,000 operations conducted in 2014 [136]. The field has transformed from predominantly open surgery to nearly 98% laparoscopic procedures between 1993 and 2016 [137]. In the United States alone, close to two million individuals underwent bariatric surgery during this period [137]. Thanks to advanced developments in these procedures, complication and mortality rates have significantly decreased, from 11.7% and 1% in 1998 to a mere 1.4% and 0.04% in 2016 [137].

The decision to undergo bariatric surgery is typically guided by specific criteria. These criteria include [138]:

1. BMI $\geq$ 40 kg/m^2.
2. BMI between 35–39.9 kg/m^2 along with the presence of obesity-related comorbidities such as diabetes mellitus, hypertension, gastroesophageal reflux disease, osteoarthritis, etc.
3. BMI > 30 kg/m^2 in individuals struggling with difficult-to-control type 2 diabetes mellitus or dysmetabolic syndrome X.

Extensive evidence underscores the sustained and substantial weight loss achieved through bariatric surgery [139]. These procedures are categorized based on their mechanisms for weight loss, whether through restriction, malabsorption, or a combination of both [140]. Restrictive procedures limit caloric intake by reducing stomach size, examples being vertical banded gastroplasty, laparoscopic adjustable gastric banding, and sleeve gastrectomy [141]. Malabsorptive procedures curtail nutrient absorption by shortening the small intestine, either through bypassing the absorptive surface or diverting biliopancreatic secretions that facilitate absorption [141]. In contrast, Roux-en-Y gastric bypass combines restrictive and malabsorptive mechanisms, making it one of the most prevalent bariatric procedures to date [141].

Relationship to Musculoskeletal Pain

To address the health risks and joint complaints associated with obesity, the initial treatment approach typically emphasizes lifestyle changes, particularly diet and exercise. However, achieving a normal weight or maintaining weight loss is often challenging for individuals with obesity [142]. This difficulty can partly be attributed to significant barriers to exercise, as certain activities may exacerbate joint pain [143]. For such individuals, bariatric surgery becomes a viable consideration.

Evidence reveals bariatric surgery as the most effective means to achieve significant weight loss and alleviate comorbid conditions, such as cardiovascular disease and diabetes [144]. Musculoskeletal pain ranks among the common comorbidities in bariatric surgery patients. Even when considering the potential side effects and postoperative risks like nutritional deficiencies, dumping syndrome, gastroesophageal reflux, venous thromboembolism, and anastomotic leakage, bariatric surgery has the potential to be an indirect yet effective treatment for joint pain, and may even delay or eliminate the need for joint replacement surgery [145].

Current literature features several studies that demonstrate improvements in preoperative pain following bariatric surgery. For instance, multiple studies have reported a positive association between weight loss and a reduction in hip and knee joint complaints [146, 147]. Recent research has also shown that bariatric surgery can positively impact lower back pain [148]. Gill et al. conducted a systematic review specifically focused on studies concerning hip and knee osteoarthritis outcomes [149]. Their review, encompassing six studies (five case series and one case control), concluded that there is evidence supporting the effectiveness of weight loss resulting from bariatric surgery in improving osteoarthritis-related hip and knee pain [149]. Heuts et al. conducted a systematic review as well that revealed similar findings. They critically assessed the results of 23 studies involving over 3400 participants who underwent bariatric surgery [150]. While the evidence for hip pain was not robust enough for significant conclusions, weight loss post-bariatric surgery corresponded to reduced knee pain intensity and overall prevalence in these patients [150].

The pathophysiological effects of bariatric surgery on musculoskeletal pain are akin to other weight loss interventions. Research suggests that bariatric surgery not only diminishes mechanical load but also reduces inflammatory mediators, primarily adipokines (adipose tissue-derived cytokines), which have been hypothesized to play a role in alleviating knee pain, particularly in individuals with osteoarthritis [151, 152].

In summary, the existing literature provides substantial evidence supporting the positive influence of bariatric surgery on musculoskeletal pain, reflecting a real biological relationship between weight loss and joint pain. Nonetheless, conclusive evidence remains elusive due to prevalent biases in many studies, the absence of standardized joint pain measures in randomized control trials, and significant gaps in knowledge concerning pain in the bariatric surgery patient population [150]. Furthermore, although evidence suggests that bariatric surgery patients experience improved presurgical pain conditions, the time course, predictors of pain resolution, and its relationship to surgical weight loss remain unknown.

Conclusion

In conclusion, this chapter has provided a comprehensive overview of the multifaceted relationship between obesity and various aspects of health. The global obesity epidemic has reached alarming proportions, impacting not only individuals but also economies worldwide. Obesity's far-reaching consequences extend beyond physical health, affecting psychological well-being, quality of life, and even healthcare costs.

We have explored how obesity intersects with conditions such as fibromyalgia and low back pain, highlighting its dual role as both a potential trigger and an exacerbating factor. Weight loss emerges as a promising strategy for improving the overall well-being of individuals dealing with these conditions.

Furthermore, we delved into dietary interventions and their potential in managing musculoskeletal pain. While diets like intermittent fasting, caloric restriction, and the Mediterranean diet show promise, more research is needed to establish their long-term efficacy and suitability for different populations.

The pharmacokinetic considerations discussed underscore the importance of personalized medicine in obese individuals. Drug absorption, distribution, clearance, and pharmacodynamics may all be affected by obesity, necessitating careful dosing and monitoring.

In summary, addressing the obesity epidemic is an urgent public health imperative. It requires a multifaceted approach that includes lifestyle modifications, healthcare policy changes, and ongoing research to better understand the intricate relationship between obesity and health. As we continue to grapple with this complex challenge, it is essential to prioritize prevention, intervention, and personalized treatment strategies to improve the well-being of individuals and alleviate the societal burden associated with obesity-related conditions.

References

1. Obesity: preventing and managing the global epidemic. Report of a WHO consultation. World Health Organ Tech Rep Ser. 2000;894:i–xii., 1–253. PMID: 11234459
2. Jensen MD, Ryan DH, Apovian CM, Ard JD, Comuzzie AG, American College of Cardiology/American Heart Association Task Force on Practice Guidelines; Obesity Society, et al. 2013 AHA/ACC/TOS guideline for the management of overweight and obesity in adults: a report of the American College of Cardiology/American Heart Association Task Force on Practice Guidelines and The Obesity Society. Circulation. 2014;129(25 Suppl 2):S102–38. https://doi.org/10.1161/01.cir.0000437739.71477.ee. Epub 2013 Nov 12. Erratum in: Circulation. 2014 Jun 24;129(25 Suppl 2):S139–40. PMID: 24222017; PMCID: PMC5819889
3. Taylor R Jr, Pergolizzi JV, Raffa RB, Nalamachu S, Balestrieri PJ. Pain and obesity in the older adult. Curr Pharm Des. 2014;20(38):6037–41. https://doi.org/10.2174/1381612820666140316131431. PMID: 24641223
4. Apovian CM. Obesity: definition, comorbidities, causes, and burden. Am J Manag Care. 2016;22(7 Suppl):S176–85. PMID: 27356115
5. D'Onghia M, Ciaffi J, Lisi L, Mancarella L, Ricci S, Stefanelli N, Meliconi R, Ursini F. Fibromyalgia and obesity: a comprehensive systematic review and meta-analysis. Semin Arthritis Rheum. 2021;51(2):409–24. https://doi.org/10.1016/j.semarthrit.2021.02.007. Epub 2021 Mar 3. PMID: 33676126
6. Pilková A, Hartinger JM. Obesity-associated changes in drug pharmacokinetics. Vnitr Lek. 2020;66(8):465–71. English. PMID: 33740844
7. Speck RM, Bond DS, Sarwer DB, Farrar JT. A systematic review of musculoskeletal pain among bariatric surgery patients: implications for physical activity and exercise. Surg Obes Relat Dis. 2014;10(1):161–70. https://doi.org/10.1016/j.soard.2013.08.001. Epub 2013 Aug 17. PMID: 24182448

8. Cuevas-Cervera M, Perez-Montilla JJ, Gonzalez-Muñoz A, Garcia-Rios MC, Navarro-Ledesma S. The effectiveness of intermittent fasting, time restricted feeding, caloric restriction, a ketogenic diet and the Mediterranean diet as part of the treatment plan to improve health and chronic musculoskeletal pain: a systematic review. Int J Environ Res Public Health. 2022;19(11):6698. https://doi.org/10.3390/ijerph19116698. PMID: 35682282; PMCID: PMC9180920
9. GBD 2015 Obesity Collaborators, Afshin A, Forouzanfar MH, Reitsma MB, et al. Health effects of overweight and obesity in 195 countries over 25 years. N Engl J Med. 2017;377(1):13–27. https://doi.org/10.1056/NEJMoa1614362. Epub 2017 Jun 12. PMID: 28604169; PMCID: PMC5477817
10. Hales CM, Carroll MD, Fryar CD, Ogden CL. Prevalence of obesity and severe obesity among adults: United States, 2017–2018. NCHS Data Brief. 2020;360:1–8. PMID: 32487284
11. Ward ZJ, Bleich SN, Cradock AL, Barrett JL, Giles CM, Flax C, Long MW, Gortmaker SL. Projected U.S. State-level prevalence of adult obesity and severe obesity. N Engl J Med. 2019;381(25):2440–50. https://doi.org/10.1056/NEJMsa1909301. PMID: 31851800
12. Stierman B, et al. National Health and Nutrition Examination Survey 2017–March 2020 Prepandemic Data Files Development of Files and Prevalence Estimates for Selected Health Outcomes. 2021. (158).
13. Ward ZJ, Long MW, Resch SC, Giles CM, Cradock AL, Gortmaker SL. Simulation of growth trajectories of childhood obesity into adulthood. N Engl J Med. 2017;377(22):2145–53. pmid:29171811
14. Ward ZJ, Bleich SN, Long MW, Gortmaker SL. Association of body mass index with health care expenditures in the United States by age and sex. PLoS One. 2021;16(3):e0247307. https://doi.org/10.1371/journal.pone.0247307.
15. Wang LY, Denniston M, Lee S, Galuska D, Lowry R. Long-term health and economic impact of preventing and reducing overweight and obesity in adolescence. J Adolesc Health. 2010;46(5):467–73. https://doi.org/10.1016/j.jadohealth.2009.11.204. Epub 2010 Jan 13. PMID: 20413083
16. Janssen I, Craig WM, Boyce WF, Pickett W. Associations between overweight and obesity with bullying behaviors in school-aged children. Pediatrics. 2004;113(5):1187–94.
17. Skelton JA, Irby MB, Grzywacz JG, Miller G. Etiologies of obesity in children: nature and nurture. Pediatr Clin N Am. 2011;58(6):1333–54., ix. https://doi.org/10.1016/j.pcl.2011.09.006.
18. McAllister EJ, Dhurandhar NV, Keith SW, et al. Ten putative contributors to the obesity epidemic. Crit Rev Food Sci Nutr. 2009;49(10):868–913. https://doi.org/10.1080/10408390903372599.
19. Skelton JA, DeMattia L, Miller L, Olivier M. Obesity and its therapy: from genes to community action. Pediatr Clin N Am. 2006;53(4):777–94.
20. Haywood C, Sumithran P. Treatment of obesity in older persons-a systematic review. Obes Rev. 2019;20(4):588–98. https://doi.org/10.1111/obr.12815. Epub 2019 Jan 15. PMID: 30645010
21. Abeles AM, et al. Narrative review: the pathophysiology of fibromyalgia. Ann Intern Med. 2007;146(10):726–34.
22. Arnold LM, et al. Comorbidity of fibromyalgia and psychiatric disorders. J Clin Psychiatry. 2006;67(8):1219–25.
23. Sluka KA, Clauw DJ. Neurobiology of fibromyalgia and chronic widespread pain. Neuroscience. 2016;338:114–29. https://doi.org/10.1016/j.neuroscience.2016.06.006. Epub 2016 Jun 9. PMID: 27291641; PMCID: PMC5083139
24. Clauw DJ. Fibromyalgia: a clinical review. JAMA. 2014;311(15):1547–55. https://doi.org/10.1001/jama.2014.3266. PMID: 24737367
25. Jones GT, Atzeni F, Beasley M, Flüß E, Sarzi-Puttini P, Macfarlane GJ. The prevalence of fibromyalgia in the general population: a comparison of the American College of Rheumatology 1990, 2010, and modified 2010 classification criteria. Arthritis Rheumatol. 2015;67(2):568–75. https://doi.org/10.1002/art.38905. PMID: 25323744

26. Wolfe F, Smythe HA, Yunus MB, Bennett RM, Bombardier C, Goldenberg DL, Tugwell P, Campbell SM, Abeles M, Clark P, et al. The American College of Rheumatology 1990 criteria for the classification of fibromyalgia. Report of the Multicenter Criteria Committee. Arthritis Rheum. 1990;33(2):160–72. https://doi.org/10.1002/art.1780330203. PMID: 2306288
27. Wolfe F, Clauw DJ, Fitzcharles MA, Goldenberg DL, Katz RS, Mease P, Russell AS, Russell IJ, Winfield JB, Yunus MB. The American College of Rheumatology preliminary diagnostic criteria for fibromyalgia and measurement of symptom severity. Arthritis Care Res (Hoboken). 2010;62(5):600–10. https://doi.org/10.1002/acr.20140. PMID: 20461783
28. Dean LE, Arnold L, Crofford L, Bennett R, Goldenberg D, Fitzcharles MA, Paiva ES, Staud R, Clauw D, Sarzi-Puttini P, Jones GT, Ayorinde A, Flüß E, Beasley M, Macfarlane GJ. Impact of moving from a widespread to multisite pain definition on other fibromyalgia symptoms. Arthritis Care Res (Hoboken). 2017;69(12):1878–86. https://doi.org/10.1002/acr.23214. Epub 2017 Nov 2. PMID: 28182834
29. Staud R. Abnormal pain modulation in patients with spatially distributed chronic pain: fibromyalgia. Rheum Dis Clin N Am. 2009;35(2):263–74. https://doi.org/10.1016/j.rdc.2009.05.006. PMID: 19647141; PMCID: PMC2720882
30. Jensen KB, Kosek E, Petzke F, Carville S, Fransson P, Marcus H, Williams SC, Choy E, Giesecke T, Mainguy Y, Gracely R, Ingvar M. Evidence of dysfunctional pain inhibition in Fibromyalgia reflected in rACC during provoked pain. Pain. 2009;144(1–2):95–100. https://doi.org/10.1016/j.pain.2009.03.018. Epub 2009 May 1. PMID: 19410366
31. Salemi S, Aeschlimann A, Wollina U, Gay RE, Michel BA, Gay S, Sprott H. Up-regulation of delta-opioid receptors and kappa-opioid receptors in the skin of fibromyalgia patients. Arthritis Rheum. 2007;56(7):2464–6. https://doi.org/10.1002/art.22735. PMID: 17599756
32. Harris RE, Clauw DJ, Scott DJ, McLean SA, Gracely RH, Zubieta JK. Decreased central mu-opioid receptor availability in fibromyalgia. J Neurosci. 2007;27(37):10000–6. https://doi.org/10.1523/JNEUROSCI.2849-07.2007. PMID: 17855614; PMCID: PMC6672650
33. Haas L, Portela LV, Böhmer AE, Oses JP, Lara DR. Increased plasma levels of brain derived neurotrophic factor (BDNF) in patients with fibromyalgia. Neurochem Res. 2010;35(5):830–4. https://doi.org/10.1007/s11064-010-0129-z. PMID: 20119637
34. O'Brien AT, Deitos A, Triñanes Pego Y, Fregni F, Carrillo-de-la-Peña MT. Defective endogenous pain modulation in fibromyalgia: a meta-analysis of temporal summation and conditioned pain modulation paradigms. J Pain. 2018;19(8):819–36. https://doi.org/10.1016/j.jpain.2018.01.010. Epub 2018 Feb 15. PMID: 29454976
35. Staud R, Godfrey MM, Robinson ME. Fibromyalgia patients are not only hypersensitive to painful stimuli but also to acoustic stimuli. J Pain. 2021;22(8):914–25. https://doi.org/10.1016/j.jpain.2021.02.009. Epub 2021 Feb 23. PMID: 33636370
36. Arreghini M, et al. Impact of fibromyalgia on functioning in obese patients undergoing comprehensive rehabilitation. PLoS One. 2014;9(3):e91392.
37. Warkentin LM, et al. Predictors of health-related quality of life in 500 severely obese patients. Obesity (Silver Spring). 2014;22(5):1367–72.
38. Mork PJ, Vasseljen O, Nilsen TI. Association between physical exercise, body mass index, and risk of fibromyalgia: longitudinal data from the Norwegian Nord-Trondelag Health Study. Arthritis Care Res (Hoboken). 2010;62(5):611–7.
39. Markkula RA, Kalso EA, Kaprio JA. Predictors of fibromyalgia: a population-based twin cohort study. BMC Musculoskelet Disord. 2016;17:29.
40. Hauser W, et al. Fibromyalgia. Nat Rev Dis Primers. 2015;1:15022.
41. Tomlinson DJ, et al. The impact of obesity on skeletal muscle strength and structure through adolescence to old age. Biogerontology. 2016;17(3):467–83.
42. Scott A, et al. Lipids, adiposity and tendinopathy: is there a mechanistic link? Critical review. Br J Sports Med. 2015;49(15):984–8.
43. McKendall MJ, Haier RJ. Pain sensitivity and obesity. Psychiatry Res. 1983;8(2):119–25.
44. Shanley LJ, Irving AJ, Harvey J. Leptin enhances NMDA receptor function and modulates hippocampal synaptic plasticity. J Neurosci. 2001;21(24):RC186.

45. Kutlu S, et al. Effects of central and peripheral administration of leptin on pain threshold in rats and mice. Neuro Endocrinol Lett. 2003;24(3–4):193–6.
46. Rodriguez-Pinto I, et al. Fibromyalgia and cytokines. Immunol Lett. 2014;161(2):200–3.
47. Zhang JM, An J. Cytokines, inflammation, and pain. Int Anesthesiol Clin. 2007;45(2):27–37.
48. Kawasaki Y, et al. Cytokine mechanisms of central sensitization: distinct and overlapping role of interleukin-1beta, interleukin-6, and tumor necrosis factoralpha in regulating synaptic and neuronal activity in the superficial spinal cord. J Neurosci. 2008;28(20):5189–94.
49. Dina OA, Green PG, Levine JD. Role of interleukin-6 in chronic muscle hyperalgesic priming. Neuroscience. 2008;152(2):521–5.
50. Miller AH, Raison CL. The role of inflammation in depression: from evolutionary imperative to modern treatment target. Nat Rev Immunol. 2016;16(1):22–34.
51. Louati K, Berenbaum F. Fatigue in chronic inflammation – a link to pain pathways. Arthritis Res Ther. 2015;17:254.
52. Irwin MR. Sleep and inflammation: partners in sickness and in health. Nat Rev Immunol. 2019;19(11):702–15. Ursini F, Naty S, Grembiale RD. Fibromyalgia and obesity: the hidden link. Rheumatol Int 2011 Nov;31(11):1403–8. https://doi.org/10.1007/s00296-011-1885-z. Epub 2011 Apr 8. PMID: 21476098
53. Kaltsas G, Tsiveriotis K. Fibromyalgia. In: Feingold KR, Anawalt B, Blackman MR, Boyce A, Chrousos G, Corpas E, de Herder WW, Dhatariya K, Dungan K, Hofland J, Kalra S, Kaltsas G, Kapoor N, Koch C, Kopp P, Korbonits M, Kovacs CS, Kuohung W, Laferrère B, Levy M, McGee EA, McLachlan R, New M, Purnell J, Sahay R, Shah AS, Singer F, Sperling MA, Stratakis CA, Trence DL, Wilson DP, editors. Endotext [Internet]. South Dartmouth: MDText.com, Inc; 2020. 2000–. PMID: 25905317.
54. Deyo RA, Tsui-Wu YJ. Descriptive epidemiology of low-back pain and its related medical care in the United States. Spine (Phila Pa 1976). 1987;12(3):264–8. https://doi.org/10.1097/00007632-198704000-00013. PMID: 2954221
55. Hoy D, Bain C, Williams G, March L, Brooks P, Blyth F, Woolf A, Vos T, Buchbinder R. A systematic review of the global prevalence of low back pain. Arthritis Rheum. 2012;64(6):2028–37. https://doi.org/10.1002/art.34347. Epub 2012 Jan 9. PMID: 22231424
56. Cassidy JD, Carroll LJ, Côté P. The Saskatchewan health and back pain survey. The prevalence of low back pain and related disability in Saskatchewan adults. Spine (Phila Pa 1976). 1998;23(17):1860–6.; discussion 1867. PMID: 9762743. https://doi.org/10.1097/00007632-199809010-00012.
57. Skovron ML, Szpalski M, Nordin M, Melot C, Cukier D, Sociocultural factors and back pain. A population-based study in Belgian adults. Spine (Phila Pa 1976). 1994;19(2):129–37. https://doi.org/10.1097/00007632-199401001-00002. PMID: 8153818
58. Hartvigsen J, Hancock MJ, Kongsted A, Louw Q, Ferreira ML, Genevay S, Hoy D, Karppinen J, Pransky G, Sieper J, Smeets RJ, Underwood M, Lancet Low Back Pain Series Working Group. What low back pain is and why we need to pay attention. Lancet. 2018;391(10137):2356–67. https://doi.org/10.1016/S0140-6736(18)30480-X. Epub 2018 Mar 21. PMID: 29573870
59. Steffens D, Ferreira ML, Latimer J, Ferreira PH, Koes BW, Blyth F, Li Q, Maher CG. What triggers an episode of acute low back pain? A case-crossover study. Arthritis Care Res (Hoboken). 2015;67(3):403–10. https://doi.org/10.1002/acr.22533. PMID: 25665074
60. Katz JN. Lumbar disc disorders and low-back pain: socioeconomic factors and consequences. J Bone Joint Surg Am. 2006;88(Suppl 2):21–4. https://doi.org/10.2106/JBJS.E.01273. PMID: 16595438
61. Macfarlane GJ, Thomas E, Papageorgiou AC, Croft PR, Jayson MI, Silman AJ. Employment and physical work activities as predictors of future low back pain. Spine (Phila Pa 1976). 1997;22(10):1143–9. https://doi.org/10.1097/00007632-199705150-00015. PMID: 9160474

62. Croft PR, Papageorgiou AC, Thomas E, Macfarlane GJ, Silman AJ. Short-term physical risk factors for new episodes of low back pain. Prospective evidence from the South Manchester Back Pain Study. Spine (Phila Pa 1976). 1999;24(15):1556–61. https://doi.org/10.1097/00007632-199908010-00009. PMID: 10457575
63. Croft PR, Papageorgiou AC, Ferry S, Thomas E, Jayson MI, Silman AJ. Psychologic distress and low back pain. Evidence from a prospective study in the general population. Spine (Phila Pa 1976). 1995;20(24):2731–7. https://doi.org/10.1097/00007632-199512150-00015. PMID: 8747252
64. Deyo RA, Weinstein JN. Low back pain. N Engl J Med. 2001;344(5):363–70. https://doi.org/10.1056/NEJM200102013440508. PMID: 11172169
65. Chou R, Qaseem A, Snow V, Casey D, Cross JT Jr, Shekelle P, Owens DK, Clinical Efficacy Assessment Subcommittee of the American College of Physicians, American College of Physicians, American Pain Society Low Back Pain Guidelines Panel. Diagnosis and treatment of low back pain: a joint clinical practice guideline from the American College of Physicians and the American Pain Society. Ann Intern Med. 2007;147(7):478–91. https://doi.org/10.7326/0003-4819-147-7-200710020-00006. Erratum in: Ann Intern Med 2008 Feb 5;148(3):247–8. PMID: 17909209
66. Chou R, Qaseem A, Owens DK, Shekelle P, Clinical Guidelines Committee of the American College of Physicians. Diagnostic imaging for low back pain: advice for high-value health care from the American College of Physicians. Ann Intern Med. 2011;154(3):181–9. https://doi.org/10.7326/0003-4819-154-3-201102010-00008. Erratum in: Ann Intern Med 2012 Jan 3;156(1 Pt 1):71. PMID: 21282698
67. Jarvik JG, Deyo RA. Diagnostic evaluation of low back pain with emphasis on imaging. Ann Intern Med. 2002;137(7):586–97. https://doi.org/10.7326/0003-4819-137-7-200210010-00010. PMID: 12353946
68. Peiris WL, Cicuttini FM, Hussain SM, Estee MM, Romero L, Ranger TA, Fairley JL, McLean EC, Urquhart DM. Is adiposity associated with back and lower limb pain? A systematic review. PLoS One. 2021;16(9):e0256720. https://doi.org/10.1371/journal.pone.0256720. PMID: 34520462; PMCID: PMC8439494
69. Pan F, Laslett L, Blizzard L, Cicuttini F, Winzenberg T, Ding C, et al. Associations between fat mass and multisite pain: a five-year longitudinal study. Arthritis Care Res. 2017;69(4):509–16. https://doi.org/10.1002/acr.22963. PMID: 27390162
70. Cao H. Adipocytokines in obesity and metabolic disease. J Endocrinol. 2014;220(2):T47–59. https://doi.org/10.1530/JOE-13-0339. PMID: 24403378
71. Neogi T. The epidemiology and impact of pain in osteoarthritis. Osteoarthr Cartil. 2013;21(9):1145–53. https://doi.org/10.1016/j.joca.2013.03.018. PMID: 23973124
72. Hartvigsen J, Natvig B, Ferreira M. Is it all about a pain in the back? Best Pract Res Clin Rheumatol. 2013;27(5):613–23.
73. Hampl SE, Hassink SG, Skinner AC, Armstrong SC, Barlow SE, Bolling CF, Avila Edwards KC, Eneli I, Hamre R, Joseph MM, Lunsford D, Mendonca E, Michalsky MP, Mirza N, Ochoa ER, Sharifi M, Staiano AE, Weedn AE, Flinn SK, Lindros J, Okechukwu K. Clinical practice guideline for the evaluation and treatment of children and adolescents with obesity. Pediatrics. 2023;151(2):e2022060640. https://doi.org/10.1542/peds.2022-060640. PMID: 36622115
74. Skinner AC, Ravanbakht SN, Skelton JA, Perrin EM, Armstrong SC. Prevalence of obesity and severe obesity in US children, 1999–2016. Pediatrics. 2018;141(3):e20173459. https://doi.org/10.1542/peds.2017-3459. Erratum in: Pediatrics 2018 Sep;142(3): PMID: 29483202; PMCID: PMC6109602
75. Ogden CL, Fryar CD, Martin CB, Freedman DS, Carroll MD, Gu Q, Hales CM. Trends in obesity prevalence by race and Hispanic Origin-1999-2000 to 2017–2018. JAMA. 2020;324(12):1208–10. https://doi.org/10.1001/jama.2020.14590. PMID: 32857101; PMCID: PMC7455882

76. Ogden CL, Fryar CD, Hales CM, Carroll MD, Aoki Y, Freedman DS. Differences in obesity prevalence by demographics and urbanization in US children and adolescents, 2013–2016. JAMA. 2018;319(23):2410–8. https://doi.org/10.1001/jama.2018.5158. PMID: 29922826; PMCID: PMC6393914
77. Eagle TF, Sheetz A, Gurm R, Woodward AC, Kline-Rogers E, Leibowitz R, Durussel-Weston J, Palma-Davis L, Aaronson S, Fitzgerald CM, Mitchell LR, Rogers B, Bruenger P, Skala KA, Goldberg C, Jackson EA, Erickson SR, Eagle KA. Understanding childhood obesity in America: linkages between household income, community resources, and children's behaviors. Am Heart J. 2012;163(5):836–43. https://doi.org/10.1016/j.ahj.2012.02.025. PMID: 22607862
78. Whitaker RC, Wright JA, Pepe MS, Seidel KD, Dietz WH. Predicting obesity in young adulthood from childhood and parental obesity. N Engl J Med. 1997;337(13):869–73. https://doi.org/10.1056/NEJM199709253371301. PMID: 9302300
79. Ogden CL, Carroll MD, Lawman HG, Fryar CD, Kruszon-Moran D, Kit BK, Flegal KM. Trends in obesity prevalence among children and adolescents in the United States, 1988-1994 through 2013–2014. JAMA. 2016;315(21):2292–9. https://doi.org/10.1001/jama.2016.6361. PMID: 27272581; PMCID: PMC6361521
80. Parsons TJ, Power C, Logan S, Summerbell CD. Childhood predictors of adult obesity: a systematic review. Int J Obes Relat Metab Disord. 1999;23(Suppl 8):S1–107. PMID: 10641588
81. Rundle AG, Factor-Litvak P, Suglia SF, Susser ES, Kezios KL, Lovasi GS, Cirillo PM, Cohn BA, Link BG. Tracking of obesity in childhood into adulthood: effects on body mass index and fat mass index at age 50. Child Obes. 2020;16(3):226–33. https://doi.org/10.1089/chi.2019.0185. PMID: 32191541; PMCID: PMC7099417
82. Mead E, Batterham AM, Atkinson G, Ells LJ. Predicting future weight status from measurements made in early childhood: a novel longitudinal approach applied to Millennium Cohort Study data. Nutr Diabetes. 2016;6(3):e200. https://doi.org/10.1038/nutd.2016.3. PMID: 26950481; PMCID: PMC4817076
83. Foster NE, Anema JR, Cherkin D, et al. Prevention and treatment of low back pain: evidence, challenges, and promising directions. Lancet. 2018;391:2368–83.
84. Krul M, van der Wouden JC, Schellevis FG, et al. Musculoskeletal problems in overweight and obese children. Ann Fam Med. 2009;7:352–6.
85. Paulis WD, Silva S, Koes BW, et al. Overweight and obesity are associated with musculoskeletal complaints as early as childhood: a systematic review. Obes Rev. 2014;15:52–67.
86. Hestbaek L, Leboeuf-Yde C, Kyvik KO. Are lifestyle-factors in adolescence predictors for adult low back pain? A cross-sectional and prospective study of young twins. BMC Musculoskelet Disord. 2006;7:27.
87. Aartun E, Hartvigsen J, Wedderkopp N, et al. Spinal pain in adolescents: prevalence, incidence, and course: a school-based two-year prospective cohort study in 1,300 Danes aged 11–13. BMC Musculoskelet Disord. 2014;15:187.
88. MacDonald J, Stuart E, Rodenberg R. Musculoskeletal low back pain in school-aged children: a review. JAMA Pediatr. 2017;171:280–7.
89. Calvo-Muñoz I, Gómez-Conesa A, Sánchez-Meca J. Prevalence of low back pain in children and adolescents: a meta-analysis. BMC Pediatr. 2013;13:14.
90. Palmer AJ, Poveda JL, Martinez-Laguna D, Reyes C, de Bont J, Silman A, Carr AJ, Duarte-Salles T, Prieto-Alhambra D. Childhood overweight and obesity and back pain risk: a cohort study of 466 997 children. BMJ Open. 2020;10(9):e036023. https://doi.org/10.1136/bmjopen-2019-036023. PMID: 32948552; PMCID: PMC7500301
91. Hartvigsen J, Hancock MJ, Kongsted A, et al. What low back pain is and why we need to pay attention. Lancet. 2018;391:2356–67.
92. Michaleff ZA, Kamper SJ, Maher CG, et al. Low back pain in children and adolescents: a systematic review and meta-analysis evaluating the effectiveness of conservative interventions. Eur Spine J. 2014;23:2046–58.

93. Sjaarda LA, Radin RG, Swanson C, Kuhr DL, Mumford SL, Galai N, Silver RM, Wactawski-Wende J, Perkins NJ, Schisterman EF. Prevalence and contributors to low-grade inflammation in three U.S. populations of reproductive age women. Paediatr Perinat Epidemiol. 2018;32:55–67.
94. Owen L, Corfe B. The role of diet and nutrition on mental health and wellbeing. Proc Nutr Soc. 2017;76:425–6.
95. Totsch SK, Waite ME, Tomkovich A, Quinn TL, Gower BA, Sorge RE. Total Western diet alters mechanical and thermal sensitivity and prolongs hypersensitivity following complete Freund's adjuvant in mice. J Pain. 2016;17:119–25.
96. Nijs J, Elma Ö, Yilmaz ST, Mullie P, Vanderweeën L, Clarys P, Deliens T, Coppieters I, Weltens N, Van Oudenhove L, et al. Nutritional neurobiology and central nervous system sensitisation: missing link in a comprehensive treatment for chronic pain? Br J Anaesth. 2019;123:539–43.
97. Masino SA, Ruskin DN. Ketogenic diets and pain. J Child Neurol. 2013;28:993–1001. https://doi.org/10.1177/0883073813487595.
98. Field R, Pourkazemi F, Turton J, Rooney K. Dietary interventions are beneficial for patients with chronic pain: a systematic review with meta-analysis. Pain Med. 2021;22:694–714. https://doi.org/10.1093/pm/pnaa378.
99. Elma Ö, Yilmaz ST, Deliens T, Clarys P, Nijs J, Coppieters I, Polli A, Malfliet A. Chronic musculoskeletal pain and nutrition: where are we and where are we heading? PMR. 2020;12:1268–78. https://doi.org/10.1002/pmrj.12346.
100. Lowry E, Marley J, McVeigh JG, McSorley E, Allsopp P, Kerr D. Dietary interventions in the management of Fibromyalgia: a systematic review and best-evidence synthesis. Nutrients. 2020;12:2664. https://doi.org/10.3390/nu12092664.
101. Sibille KT, Bartsch F, Reddy D, Fillingim RB, Keil A. Increasing neuroplasticity to bolster chronic pain treatment: a role for intermittent fasting and glucose administration? J Pain. 2016;17:275–81. https://doi.org/10.1016/j.jpain.2015.11.002.
102. Caristia S, De Vito M, Sarro A, Leone A, Pecere A, Zibetti A, Filigheddu N, Zeppegno P, Prodam F, Faggiano F, et al. Is caloric restriction associated with better healthy aging outcomes? A systematic review and meta-analysis of randomized controlled trials. Nutrients. 2020;12:2290. https://doi.org/10.3390/nu12082290.
103. Elma Ö, Yilmaz ST, Deliens T, Coppieters I, Clarys P, Nijs J, Malfliet A. Do nutritional factors interact with chronic musculoskeletal pain? A systematic review. J Clin Med. 2020;9:702. https://doi.org/10.3390/jcm9030702.
104. Che T, Yan C, Tian D, Zhang X, Liu X, Wu Z. Time-restricted feeding improves blood glucose and insulin sensitivity in overweight patients with type 2 diabetes: a randomised controlled trial. Nutr Metab. 2021;18:88. https://doi.org/10.1186/s12986-021-00613-9.
105. Veronese N, Stubbs B, Noale M, Solmi M, Luchini C, Maggi S. Adherence to the Mediterranean diet is associated with better quality of life: data from the osteoarthritis initiative. Am J Clin Nutr. 2016;104:1403–9. https://doi.org/10.3945/ajcn.116.136390.
106. Ingegnoli F, Schioppo T, Scotti I, Ubiali T, De Lucia O, Murgo A, Marano G, Boracchi P, Caporali R. Adherence to Mediterranean diet and patient perception of rheumatoid arthritis. Complement Ther Med. 2020;52:102519. https://doi.org/10.1016/j.ctim.2020.102519.
107. Ortolá R, García-Esquinas E, Sotos-Prieto M, Struijk EA, Caballero FF, Lopez-Garcia E, Rodríguez-Artalejo F. Mediterranean diet and changes in frequency, severity, and localization of pain in older adults: the seniors-ENRICA cohorts. J Gerontol Ser A. 2022;77:122–30. https://doi.org/10.1093/gerona/glab109.
108. Pureza IRDOM, de Lima Macena M, da Silva Junior AE, Praxedes DRS, Vasconcelos LGL, Bueno NB. Effect of early time-restricted feeding on the metabolic profile of adults with excess weight: a systematic review with meta-analysis. Clin Nutr. 2021;40:1788–99. https://doi.org/10.1016/j.clnu.2020.10.031.
109. Adafer R, Messaadi W, Meddahi M, Patey A, Haderbache A, Bayen S, Messaadi N. Food timing, circadian rhythm and Chrononutrition: a systematic review of time-restricted eating's effects on human health. Nutrients. 2020;12:3770. https://doi.org/10.3390/nu12123770.

110. D'Andrea Meira I, Romão TT, Do Prado HJP, Krüger LT, Pires MEP, Da Conceição PO. Ketogenic diet and epilepsy: what we know so far. Front Neurosci. 2019;13:5. https://doi.org/10.3389/fnins.2019.00005.
111. Carter T, D'Cunha NM, Georgousopoulou EN, Isbel S, Davey R, Mellor DD, Kellett J, McKune AJ, Naumovski N. Assessing the diet quality of individuals with rheumatic conditions: a cross-sectional study. Rheumatol Int. 2020;40:1439–48. https://doi.org/10.1007/s00296-020-04527-2.
112. Dragan S, Şerban M-C, Damian G, Buleu F, Valcovici M, Christodorescu R. Dietary patterns and interventions to alleviate chronic pain. Nutrients. 2020;12:2510. https://doi.org/10.3390/nu12092510.
113. Brill MJE, Diepstraten J, Van Rongen A, et al. Impact of obesity on drug metabolism and elimination in adults and children. Clin Pharmacokinet. 2012;51:277–304.
114. Cardoso-Júnior A, Coelho LGV, Savassi-Rocha PR, et al. Gastric emptying of solids and semi-solids in morbidly obese and non-obese subjects: an assessment using the 13C-octanoic acid and 13C-acetic acid breath tests. Obes Surg. 2007;17:236–41.
115. Xing J, Chen JDZ. Alterations of gastrointestinal motility in obesity. Obes Res. 2004;12:1723–32.
116. Ulvestad M, Skottheim IB, Jakobsen GS, et al. Impact of OATP1B1, MDR1, and CYP3A4 expression in liver and intestine on interpatient pharmacokinetic variability of atorvastatin in obese subjects. Clin Pharmacol Ther. 2013;93:275–82.
117. Brill MJE, Van Rongen A, Houwink API, et al. Midazolam pharmacokinetics in morbidly obese patients following semi-simultaneous oral and intravenous administration: a comparison with healthy volunteers. Clin Pharmacokinet. 2014;53:931–41.
118. Smit C, De Hoogd S, Brüggemann RJM, Knibbe CAJ. Obesity and drug pharmacology: a review of the influence of obesity on pharmacokinetic and pharmacodynamic parameters. Expert Opin Drug Metab Toxicol. 2018;14(3):275–85. https://doi.org/10.1080/17425255.2018.1440287. Epub 2018 Feb 15. PMID: 29431542
119. Berezhkovskiy LM. On the accuracy of estimation of basic pharmacokinetic parameters by the traditional noncompartmental equations and the prediction of the steady-state volume of distribution in obese patients based upon data derived from normal subjects. J Pharm Sci. 2011;100:2482–97.
120. Hinderling PH. Red blood cells: a neglected compartment in pharmacokinetics and pharmacodynamics. Pharmacol Rev. 1997;49:279–95.
121. Abernethy DR, Greenblatt DJ, Divoll M, et al. Prolonged accumulation of diazepam in obesity. J Clin Pharmacol. 1983;23:369–76.
122. Van Kralingen S, Diepstraten J, Peeters MYM, et al. Population pharmacokinetics and pharmacodynamics of propofol in morbidly obese patients. Clin Pharmacokinet. 2011;50:739–50.
123. Abernethy DR, Greenblatt DJ, Smith TW. Digoxin disposition in obesity: clinical pharmacokinetic investigation. Am Heart J. 1981;102:740–4.
124. Benedek IH, Fiske WD, Griffen WO, et al. Serum alpha 1-acid glycoprotein and the binding of drugs in obesity. Br J Clin Pharmacol. 1983;16:751–4.
125. Hollenstein UM, Brunner M, Schmid R, et al. Soft tissue concentrations of ciprofloxacin in obese and lean subjects following weight-adjusted dosing. Int J Obes Relat Metab Disord. 2001;25:354–8.
126. Brill MJE, Houwink API, Schmidt S, et al. Reduced subcutaneous tissue distribution of cefazolin in morbidly obese versus non-obese patients determined using clinical microdialysis. J Antimicrob Chemother. 2014;69:715–23.
127. Bauer MP, Van De Garde EMW, Van Kasteren MEE, et al. SWAB guideline: perioperative antibiotic prophylaxis. 2017. Available at: http://www.swab.nl/richtlijnen
128. Adane ED, Herald M, Koura F. Pharmacokinetics of vancomycin in extremely obese patients with suspected or confirmed *Staphylococcus aureus* infections. Pharmacotherapy. 2015;35:127–39.

129. Blouin RA, Bauer LA, Miller DD, et al. Vancomycin pharmacokinetics in normal and morbidly obese subjects. Antimicrob Agents Chemother. 1982;21:575–80.
130. Bauer LA, Edwards WAD, Dellinger EP, et al. Influence of weight on aminoglycoside pharmacokinetics in normal weight and morbidly obese patients. Eur J Clin Pharmacol. 1983;24:643–7.
131. Reiss RA, Haas CE, Karki SD, et al. Lithium pharmacokinetics in the obese. Clin Pharmacol Ther. 2015;71:1501–8. Brill MJE, Houwink API, Schmidt S, et al. Reduced subcutaneous tissue distribution of cefazolin in morbidly obese versus non-obese patients determined using clinical microdialysis. J Antimicrob Chemother. 2014;69:715–23
132. Alobaid AS, Wallis SC, Jarrett P, et al. Effect of obesity on the population pharmacokinetics of fluconazole in critically ill patients. Antimicrob Agents Chemother. 2016;60:6550–7.
133. Huttunen R, Syrjänen J. Obesity and the risk and outcome of infection. Int J Obes. 2013;37:333–40.
134. Jullian-Desayes I, Revol B, Chareyre E, et al. Impact of concomitant medications on obstructive sleep apnoea. Br J Clin Pharmacol. 2017;83:688–708.
135. Mason M, Cates CJ, Smith I. Effects of opioid, hypnotic and sedating medications on sleep-disordered breathing in adults with obstructive sleep apnoea. Cochrane Database Syst Rev. 2015;7:CD011090.
136. Angrisani L, Santonicola A, Iovino P, Vitiello A, Zundel N, Buchwald H, Scopinaro N. Bariatric surgery and Endoluminal procedures: IFSO worldwide survey 2014. Obes Surg. 2017;27(9):2279–89. https://doi.org/10.1007/s11695-017-2666-x. Erratum in: Obes Surg 2017 Jul 5; PMID: 28405878; PMCID: PMC5562777
137. Campos GM, Khoraki J, Browning MG, Pessoa BM, Mazzini GS, Wolfe L. Changes in utilization of bariatric surgery in the United States from 1993 to 2016. Ann Surg. 2020;271(2):201–9. https://doi.org/10.1097/SLA.0000000000003554. PMID: 31425292
138. Eisenberg D, Shikora SA, Aarts E, Aminian A, Angrisani L, Cohen RV, De Luca M, Faria SL, Goodpaster KPS, Haddad A, Himpens JM, Kow L, Kurian M, Loi K, Mahawar K, Nimeri A, O'Kane M, Papasavas PK, Ponce J, Pratt JSA, Rogers AM, Steele KE, Suter M, Kothari SN. 2022 American Society for Metabolic and Bariatric Surgery (ASMBS) and International Federation for the Surgery of Obesity and Metabolic Disorders (IFSO): indications for metabolic and bariatric surgery. Surg Obes Relat Dis. 2022;18(12):1345–56. https://doi.org/10.1016/j.soard.2022.08.013. Epub 2022 Oct 21. PMID: 36280539
139. Buchwald H, Avidor Y, Braunwald E, Jensen MD, Pories W, Fahrbach K, et al. Bariatric surgery: a systematic review and meta-analysis. JAMA. 2004;292:1724–37.
140. Lim RB, Blackburn GL, Jones DB. Benchmarking best practices in weight loss surgery. Curr Probl Surg. 2010;47(2):79–174. https://doi.org/10.1067/j.cpsurg.2009.11.003. PMID: 20103467; PMCID: PMC3134527
141. Karamanakos SN, Vagenas K, Kalfarentzos F, Alexandrides TK. Weight loss, appetite suppression, and changes in fasting and postprandial ghrelin and peptide-YY levels after Roux-en-Y gastric bypass and sleeve gastrectomy: a prospective, double blind study. Ann Surg. 2008;247(3):401–7. https://doi.org/10.1097/SLA.0b013e318156f012. PMID: 18376181
142. Fildes A, Charlton J, Rudisill C, Littlejohns P, Prevost AT, Gulliford MC. Probability of an obese person attaining normal body weight: cohort study using electronic health records. Am J Public Health. 2015;105(9):e54–9.
143. Wilcox S, Der Ananian C, Abbott J, Vrazel J, Ramsey C, Sharpe PA, Brady T. Perceived exercise barriers, enablers, and benefits among exercising and nonexercising adults with arthritis: results from a qualitative study. Arthritis Care Res. 2006;55(4):616–27.
144. Rogers AM. Current state of bariatric surgery: procedures, data, and patient management. Tech Vasc Interv Radiol. 2020;23(1):100654.
145. DeClaire JH, Savich TT, Montgomery BSALG, Warritay OK. Significant weight loss may delay or eliminate the need for total knee replacement. Int J Prev Med. 2014;5(5):648–52.
146. Jafarzadeh SR, Clancy M, Li JS, et al. Changes in the structural features of osteoarthritis in a year of weight loss. Osteoarthr Cartil. 2018;26(6):775–82.

147. Jafarzadeh SR, Neogi T, Stefanik JJ, et al. Mediating role of bone marrow lesion, synovitis, pain sensitization, and depressive symptoms on knee pain improvement following substantial weight loss. Arthritis Rheumatol. 2020;72(3):420–7.
148. Joaquim AF, Helvie P, Patel AA. Bariatric surgery and low back pain: a systematic literature review. Glob Spine J. 2020;10(1):102–10.
149. Groen VA, van de Graaf VA, Scholtes VABB, et al. Effects of bariatric surgery for knee complaints in (morbidly) obese adult patients: a systematic review. Obes Rev. 2015;16(2):161–70.
150. Heuts EAF, de Jong LD, Hazebroek EJ, Wagener M, Somford MP. The influence of bariatric surgery on hip and knee joint pain: a systematic review. Surg Obes Relat Dis. 2021;17(9):1637–53. https://doi.org/10.1016/j.soard.2021.04.019. Epub 2021 Apr 28. PMID: 34116961
151. Tu C, He J, Wu B, Wang W, Li Z. An extensive review regarding the adipokines in the pathogenesis and progression of osteoarthritis. Cytokine. 2019;113(May):1–12.
152. Gandhi R, Takahashi M, Smith H, Rizek R, Mahomed NN. The synovial fluid adiponectin-leptin ratio predicts pain with knee osteoarthritis. Clin Rheumatol. 2010;29(11):1223–8.

Further Reading

Wells JCK, Fewtrell MS. Measuring body composition. Arch Dis Child. 2006;91:612–7.

Pasco JA, Holloway KL, Dobbins AG, Kotowicz MA, Williams LJ, Brennan SL. Body mass index and measures of body fat for defining obesity and underweight: a cross-sectional, population-based study. BMC Obes. 2014;1:9.

Prospective Studies Collaboration, Whitlock G, Lewington S, Sherliker P, Clarke R, Emberson J, Halsey J, Qizilbash N, Collins R, Peto R. Body-mass index and cause-specific mortality in 900 000 adults: collaborative analyses of 57 prospective studies. Lancet. 2009;373(9669):1083–96. https://doi.org/10.1016/S0140-6736(09)60318-4. Epub 2009 Mar 18. PMID: 19299006; PMCID: PMC2662372

Overuse Injuries

4

Konda Chaitanya

Overuse Injuries are a set of common musculoskeletal disorders that span across multiple regions of the body. They can occur across a wide patient population, and the terminology varies, including repetitive motion injury, repetitive strain injury, and cumulative trauma disorder. The basic mechanisms of overuse injuries are typically repetitive actions or movements that create forces that damage tissues, whether it be tendons, ligaments, muscles, or bones. As opposed to acute injuries, these tend to develop over time to exceed the body's ability to heal and adapt. These chronic injuries affect areas such as the neck, shoulders, elbows, wrists, hips, knees, ankles, and feet. Symptoms that are generally associated with overuse injuries include pain, swelling, stiffness, and decreased range of motion. Risk factors that lead to overuse injuries in activities include poor biomechanics, underlying degenerative disease, inadequate rest, and training errors. The basis of most treatments incorporates rest, ice, compression, elevation (RICE), anti-inflammatory medications, and physical therapy. When patients do not improve from these modalities, the next steps in treatment are typically focused interventions or, in severe cases, surgery. Preventative measures and early interventions are key to managing these injuries. In this chapter, we present the various types of overuse syndromes typically associated with each area of the body.

Neck

Neck Muscle Sprain Sprain of the neck muscles is a common overuse injury with prevalence of nonspecific neck pain reported as high as 50% [5] in some studies. Neck sprains can be a result of external factors such as trauma, poor posture, or even a result of arthritis as people age. It typically presents with pain in the active range

K. Chaitanya (✉)
UT Southwestern Medical Center, Dallas, TX, USA
e-mail: chaitanya.konda@utsouthwestern.edu

C. E. Noe (ed.), *Musculoskeletal Pain*,
https://doi.org/10.1007/978-3-031-86057-7_4

of motion of the neck and subsequently decreased range of motion. Management is typically conservative with stretching, ice, and sometimes physical therapy, as this process is typically self-limited and resolves with conservative measures.

Tension Neck Syndrome Tension neck syndrome occurs when relaxation of neck muscles becomes impaired, resulting in neck stiffness and spasms. It occurs as a result of chronic neck strain and poor posture and can be associated with activities such as long-term computer use. Patients will present with tender or spastic regions of their neck muscles on palpation and decreased range of motion. In addition to conservative management, additional treatment options include acupuncture, dry needling, or trigger point injections. Patients typically have improvement in their symptoms once they have received treatment.

Cervical Radiculopathy Cervical radiculopathy can be defined as the compression or irritation of cervical spine nerve roots that results in neuropathic neck pain with radiation down the upper extremities of the affected side. It is more commonly seen in males, with peak incidence at ages 50–54. On examination, patients can have positive Spurlings and neck distraction tests, and diagnosis can be made by combining clinical symptoms with imaging findings on plain radiographs, CTs, MRIs, and even EMG results. First-line treatment includes conservative measures with consideration of epidural steroid injections if appropriate. The symptoms can be self-limited; however, up to 25% of patients may have persistent symptoms requiring surgical nerve decompression.

Shoulder

Biceps Tendinopathy/Tenosynovitis Biceps tendinopathy is typically found in younger or middle-aged patients. More commonly, it is the proximal biceps tendon that gets injured. Overhead activities and involvement in sports such as baseball, tennis, swimming, or volleyball can increase the risk of developing biceps tendinopathy. Diagnosis is based off of physical exam maneuvers (Yergason, speeds, uppercut—Chou-Tan, Mair) as well as MR imaging. First-line treatment includes conservative measures and anti-inflammatory medications. Consideration can also be given to tendon sheath steroid injections for those who fail first-line treatment. Patients with persistent symptoms may be candidates for tenodesis or tenotomies with reported good surgical outcomes with regard to symptom relief.

Rotator Cuff Tendinopathy Rotator cuff tendinopathy, in addition to cases of trauma, is commonly seen in athletes using overhead mechanics or those with occupations that require repetitive motions of the shoulder. Patients will present with shoulder pain and limited active range of motion. Depending on the specific tendons involved, there are a variety of physical exam maneuvers that aid in the diagnosis of rotator cuff tendinopathy. Diagnosis can be confirmed with imaging studies such as ultrasound or MRI. First-line treatment includes conservative measures and physical therapy. Patients with complete tendon rupture can be considered for surgical intervention. However, those with pre-morbid shoulder pain or high baseline pain are more likely to have poor outcomes.

Subacromial-Subdeltoid Bursitis Inflammation of the subacromial-subdeltoid bursa can be a result of underlying shoulder pathology (tendinopathy, arthritis) or repetitive overhead tasks seen in certain athletes or manual laborers. It presents as shoulder pain, and patients will have a limited range of motion on examination. Ultrasound or MR imaging can assist with diagnosis. First-line therapy is conservative with the use of anti-inflammatory medications. Consideration can be given to intrabursal steroid injections for those who fail first-line treatment. Patients with refractory symptoms may be candidates for surgical intervention via subacromial decompression or bursectomy. The disease process is generally self-limiting, and most patients improve with conservative therapy.

SICK Scapula SICK scapula is a syndrome resulting from altered muscle function around the region of the scapula. It is defined by scapular malposition, inferior medial border prominence, coracoid pain and scapular dyskinesis. The prevalence of this syndrome is higher in overhead athletes and can present as pain with throwing activities that is improved with scapular stabilization. On exam, patients will also have tenderness on palpation of the coracoid. The diagnosis is made clinically, and imaging is generally not needed. Treatment includes physical therapy geared towards pectoralis stretching as well as interval throwing programs to assist with scapular symmetry. Adherence to this treatment program generally has good outcomes with regard to reducing pain.

Shoulder Labral Tears (SLAP—Superior Labral Anterior to Posterior) Repetitive trauma and degeneration from activities overhead athletes engage in can lead to impaired labral integrity and eventual tears. In addition to shoulder pain with movement, patients may demonstrate a positive Jobe or O'Brien's test. MR imaging can assist with diagnosis in addition to determining the severity of the tear. The first line of treatment is conservative, with the use of anti-inflammatory medication. Cryotherapy or surgical repair may also be indicated in specific patient populations. Patients who are good surgical candidates generally have favorable outcomes.

Bennett Lesions of the Shoulder Reactive bone formation into Bennett lesions of the shoulder occur due to activities that result in the repetitive impaction of the posterior humeral head onto the glenoid. This can be seen in athletes, especially with throwing, as seen in baseball pitchers. There is an association with patients that have labral tears. Athletes with Bennett lesions typically have pain in the late cocking phase, follow-through or deceleration motions. A variety of imaging modalities can be used to detect the lesion. Initial treatment is nonoperative with an emphasis on stretching exercises focused on the posterior capsule and strengthening of rotator cuff muscles. Patients with persistent symptoms may opt for arthroscopic removal of the lesion, though operative management may have mixed results.

Elbow

Lateral Epicondylitis Lateral epicondylitis is a result of the irritation or degeneration of the forearm extensors as a result of overuse. It is more commonly seen in middle-aged patients, with increased prevalence among females. Forceful and repetitive arm movements such as those seen in tennis are risk factors for developing lateral epicondylitis. On examination, patients will demonstrate pain with resisted wrist or finger extension and grip weakness. The diagnosis is primary clinical. Initial management is conservative, with anti-inflammatory medications and therapy. Steroid injections can also be considered. Patients with persistent symptoms may be candidates for a variety of surgical interventions. Most patients have good pain relief within a year of compliance with conservative measures.

Medial Epicondylitis Medial epicondylitis is a result of the irritation or degeneration of the flexor tendons of the elbow as a result of overuse. It is more commonly seen in females. Forceful and repetitive arm movements such as those seen in golf, bowling, or other racquet sports are risk factors for developing medial epicondylitis. On examination, patients will have aching pain with movement of their forearm flexors as well as grip weakness in chronic cases. There will be pain with resisted pronation of the forearm or wrist flexion (Kiel/Kaiser). The diagnosis is primarily clinical. Initial management is conservative, with anti-inflammatory medications and therapy. Steroid injections, dry needling, splinting, or elbow taping are alternative treatment modality options. Patients with persistent symptoms may be candidates for tendon release or debridement (Kiel/Kaiser). Most patients are able to return to their prior activities with conservative management.

Elbow Ulnar Collateral Ligament Tear Injury to the ulnar collateral ligament of the elbow can be due to acute trauma or chronic microtrauma and degeneration. It has been associated with activities such as baseball or javelin throwing. On examination, patients will have a positive elbow valgus stress test. CT or MR arthrography and ultrasound imaging provide additional diagnostic information. The first-line treatment is conservative with activity modification (limiting throwing and valgus stress motions). Surgical reconstruction may be considered in certain cases. Patients with complete ligament tears are more likely to fail conservative therapy. Baseball players often return to play but may have a decrease in performance in the post-surgical period or require modification of their playing position.

Posterior Elbow Impingement Inflammation of the elbow joint at the site of the olecranon can result in elbow pain from posterior impingement. It is more commonly seen in overhead throwing athletes who commonly engage in repetitive forced extension of the elbow in their throwing motions. Patients will have a limited range of motion on elbow extension. Radiographs or CT imaging can assist with the detection of osteophytes, though MR imaging is more sensitive. The first-line treatment is conservative with activity modification and anti-inflammatory medication. Patients with disabling pain may be candidates for surgical intervention through open vs. arthroscopic approaches. Many patients have symptoms that resolve with conservative management. Arthroscopic management has been shown to be effective in getting patients back to pre-injury levels of activity.

Radial Tunnel Syndrome Radial tunnel syndrome is a compressive neuropathy of the posterior interosseous nerve at the radial tunnel. A risk factor for the development of this syndrome includes repetitive motions that increase the pressures in the radial nerve. Patients have pain that is worse with prono-supination of the forearm, resisted elbow flexion, and tenderness to palpation just distal to the lateral epicondyle of the humerus. The first-line treatment is conservative with activity modification, anti-inflammatory medications, and splinting. Consideration can be given to radial tunnel steroid injections. Patients with severe or refractory pain may be candidates for surgical release of the radial tunnel. Generally, patients have a good resolution of their pain with radial tunnel injections. In surgical cases, the pain relief may be more delayed.

Wrist and Hand

Ganglion Cyst Ganglion cysts are synovial cysts that arise points along synovial sheaths, which communicate with joints. The exact pathophysiology remains unclear, but current theories speculate that chronic inflammation leads to the formation of a one-way valve for fluid formation [36]. Most ganglionic cysts are asymptomatic, but patients may be concerned about cosmetic defects. The fluid consists of a gelatinous mix of hyaluronic acid, glucosamine, globulins, and albumin [37]. These cysts commonly occur at the dorsal aspect of the wrist, with common locations being the radioscaphoid/scapholunate, scaphotrapezial, and metacarpotrapezial joints [37]. Individuals who are younger and female have been shown to be at a higher risk location; some cysts may be associated with a dull, achy pain, restricted range of motion, and may lead to radiating pain and/or weakness if there is compression of the ulnar or median nerves. Physical examination will show a firm, well-circumscribed mass without associated erythema or warmth, which readily transilluminates with light [37]. Imaging is not needed for diagnosis, but an ultrasound or an MRI can be used if an occult dorsal ganglion cyst is suspected. Occult ganglionic cysts are small ganglionic cysts that cannot be observed or palpated on physical exam [36]. There is wide clinical variance in the management of ganglionic cysts, and asymptomatic patients may just need reassurance on the benign nature of these cysts and the likelihood of regression. Aspiration is a common non-surgical strategy but is associated with high rates of recurrence [37]. Surgical excision has lower rates of recurrence but should be reserved for symptomatic patients for whom regression did not occur. Splinting either post-aspiration or post-excision patients has not been shown to reduce recurrence [37].

Trigger Finger Trigger finger is a condition where inflammation and hypertrophy of the annular pulley system results in clicking and catching during finger extension and flexion. More severe cases may result in a reduced range of motion of the affected fingers [38]. The first annular pulley at the metacarpal head is most commonly involved, but any of the annular pulleys can be involved. Patients who are women, over 50 years of age, and have diabetes are at higher risk [38]. Other at-risk populations may include patients who work in occupations requiring frequent hand flexion. A physical exam may reveal catching and locking with passive finger flexion and extension, which may or may not be painful. Oftentimes, an associated painful nodule in the palmer metacarpophalangeal joint may be appreciated. Imaging is usually not indicated, but ultrasound and an MRI may be considered for unusual presentations or if there is concern for other conditions such as a tendon sheath tumor. Conservative treatment may involve splinting, NSAIDs, and corticosteroid injections. Splints at the PIP joint can initially be trialed at night to reduce the impact of daily function. Steroid injections have been shown to have success rates of up to 90%, but their effectiveness wanes with the chronicity of the condition [39]. Surgical releases can be percutaneous or open and should be reserved for patients who have failed multiple corticosteroid injections [38].

De Quervain's Tenosynovitis De Quervain's tenosynovitis is a tenosynovitis involving the abductor pollicis longus (APL) and extensor pollicis brevis (EBL) tendons as they traverse under the tendon sheath [40]. This is the most common type of tenosynovitis and among the most frequent cause of wrist pain in the general population. Similar to all tenosynovitis, the pathophysiology is related to inflammation caused by repetitive stress, resulting in microtraumas of the tenosynovium [41]. At-risk populations include females and patients who engage in activities that involve frequent radial and ulnar deviations of the wrist. These may include patients engaging in sports such as fishing, golfing, or tennis, patients who use wheelchairs, or even parents/caregivers with newborns [41]. Physical examination will show swelling, tenderness, and crepitus near the radial styloid. Classically, patients will have a Finkelstein test, which involves pain associated with the palmar flexion of the thumb and passive ulnar deviation of the wrist. Imaging is rarely required when there is a high clinical suspicion for De Quervain's. If Imaging is obtained, an MRI of the hand and wrist will show inflammation (often visualized through increased tendon thickness, increased signal, or bursitis) within the first extensor compartment. Treatment depends on the severity and chronicity of wrist pain. Patients with minor pain/functional limitations or have had a recent onset of pain for less than three months often respond to rest and splinting. Gentle isometric strengthening can begin after inflammation has improved. Corticosteroid injections in conjunction with rest and splinting can be considered for more subacute or moderately severe cases. Surgical corrections often involve decompression of the first extensor compartment but are only typically reserved for cases that are severe, functionally limiting cases that have not responded to more conservative treatment modalities [41].

Intersection Syndrome Intersection syndrome involves inflammation and/or bursitis at the point where the tendons of adductor pollicis longus, extensor pollicis brevis, and the wrist extensors muscles cross [42]. Populations at risk include patients who engage in racquet sports, rowers, weightlifters, as well as people who use wheelchairs [41]. Clinically, the presentation is similar to De Quervain's tenosynovitis as patients may complain of pain of the dorsoradial aspect of the forearm and exacerbated by resisted extension of the wrist and thumb. However, the pain is often more proximal compared to De Quervain's tenosynovitis, and there may be associated grip weakness. Imaging is rarely indicated as diagnosis can be made with a careful history and clinical findings. An MRI may show inflammation within the first and second extensor compartments and associated bursitis [42]. Treatment options are similar to De Quervain's tenosynovitis with rest, splints, and corticosteroid injection for mild to moderate cases, with most patients responsive to conservative management [43]. Surgical decompression typically only reserved for more severe cases that are resistant to conservative management.

Flexor Carpi Radialis Tendinitis Flexor carpi radialis (FCR) tenosynovitis is inflammation of the FCR unit, which usually presents as pain located at the palmar aspect of the volar radial wrist near the second metacarpal [40]. The underlying inflammation can be due to either overuse injury or secondary to arthritis of the scaphotrapezial-trapezoid joint [40]. At-risk populations include patients who play golf and racket sports [40]. Physical examination involves a positive Lister test, which involves invoking pain from sudden dorsiflexion of the wrist. A careful history assessing for trauma is needed as the differential diagnosis may also include a scaphoid fracture. If a fracture is suspected, radiographic imaging is needed to identify if further acute surgical management is indicated. If a fracture is not suspected, then initial imaging is typically not necessary with initial treatment involving rest, splinting, NSAIDs, and corticosteroid injections into the flexor carpi radialis sheath. Further imaging may show arthritis of the thumb carpometacarpal joint. Positive MR imaging will show an increased signal around the FCR tendon sheath. Surgical decompression should only be reserved for severe cases where conservative management has failed.

Extensor Carpi Ulnaris Tendinitis The tendon for extensor carpi ulnaris (ECU) passes through the sixth extensor compartment at the distal end of the ulna and is covered by an extensor reticulum. Repetitive wrist activities that require supination, palmar flexion, and ulnar deviation can result in local inflammation from microtraumas, leading to pain from tendinopathy and/or tendosynovitis. Further, because the extensor reticulum is not firmly adhered to the tunnel, there may also be associated subluxation of the ECU tendon leading to further micotraumas. At-risk populations include patients who play sports such as basketball, rowing, or racquet sports [42]. Physical examination will show tenderness to palpation over the sixth dorsal compartment [40]. There may also be a painful snap noted with the supination of the wrist, caused by subluxation of the ECU tendon [40]. Diagnosis can be challenging given the proximity of the ECU to the triangular fibrocartilaginous complex, making it challenging to differentiate tenosynovitis from triangular fibrocartilage complex pathology [40]. In cases of suspected ECU subluxation, ultrasound imaging may be useful to assess for dynamic movement. Treatment options are similar to tenosynovitis with rest/splinting/NSAIDs, and possible corticosteroid injections should be considered for minor cases. A lower threshold for surgery may be warranted for patients with ECU subluxation if there is an underlying rupture of the subsheath [40].

Triangular Fibrocartilage Complex (TFCC) Injuries The triangular fibrocartilage complex (TFCC) is an articular disc and serves as a stabilizer and buffer of the distal wrist [44]. It is located at the distal radioulnar joint, between the sigmoid notch of the radius and the ulnar styloid process [45]. Injuries may result from either trauma or degenerative changes. Traumatic presentations are often the result of patients falling with an extended wrist or as a result of a traction injury to the wrist or from a traction injury. Degenerative changes are associated with overuse and present with a slower onset. Patients often complain of pain worsened by activities that involve the supination of the wrist. Physical examination may include positive ulnar variance (discordance in the length of articulations between the ulna and the radius). There may also be a clicking or point tenderness to palpation between the pisiform and ulnar head (fovea sign). Pain may be worsened with ulnar and/or radial deviation of the wrist. Positive radiographic findings are rare, but MR imaging may show TFCC thinning and chondromalacia of the lunate, triquetrum, and distal ulna [44, 46]. Gold standard imaging is arthroscopy but is reserved for patients who fail conservative therapies [44]. Treatment involves conservative management with immobilization, NSAIDs, and corticosteroid injections. Several surgical interventions are available, but approaches differ depending on the location of the tear. Further details on surgical approaches can be found elsewhere. In most cases, a two-week period of immobilization is required, with rehabilitation beginning after this time period.

Flexor Carpi Ulnaris Tendinitis Flexor carpi ulnaris (FCU) tenosynovitis occurs due to repetitive microtraumas of the FCU tendon. Physical examination will reveal point tenderness along the ulnar aspect of the ankle as well as pain with resisted wrist flexion. The FCU tendon inserts on the pisiform, which may result in concurrent pisotriquetral arthritis. The pisotriquetral grind test can be utilized to screen for pisotriquetral arthritis. This test involves pain when an examiner pinches the pisiform and applies force to attempt to translate the pisiform in both ulnar and radial directions with a pain indicating a positive test. Radiographic imaging is not required but can further evaluate for associated arthritic changes at the Pisotriquetral joint, and calcifications along the FCU tendon may be identified [47]. Treatment remains consistent with other tendinitis with rest/splinting/NSAIDs, and possible corticosteroid injections should be considered for minor cases, and surgical intervention should be reserved for patients who are nonresponsive to conservative management.

Hip

Acetabular Labral Tears Typically present as anterior hip or groin pain and can be accompanied by an audible or palpable snap during hip movement. The anterior acetabular area is a watershed area that is at risk for damage due to wear and tear and poor vascularity for healing capacity. It typically develops in 10% of the population after high-velocity trauma: MVCs, falls, or repetitive trauma. However, this can develop idiopathically in athletes (typically 74% of the time). Patients are at higher risk for developing acetabular labral tears if they have a history of Legg-Calve-Perthes disease, congenital hip dysplasia, or history of FAI. On examination, the patient will be positive on anterior hip impingement tests such as FABER and FADIR. Radiographic imaging should be ordered to assess for alternative pathology. MR arthrography is 90% sensitive for labral tears. Initial treatment is conservative with rest, ice, and NSAIDs. Patients should limit pivoting motions. Image-guided injections can be considered for both diagnostic and therapeutic use. However, caution is advised in a young patient population due to the risk of chondral damage. Surgical intervention can be considered after the failure of conservative treatment or functional limitations are unsatisfactory. Of those who complete arthroscopic repair, 89% of patients report improvement in symptoms at 16.5 months.

Athletic Pubalgia Aka Sports Hernia Injury to the muscular and/or fascial attachments to the anterior pubis from repetitive shearing forces at the pubic symphysis between the external oblique and rectus abdominis against the stronger hip adductor muscles. The imbalance in strength causes injury to the rectus tendon, external oblique aponeurosis, posterior inguinal wall, and transversalis fascia. Rectus tendon tears occur in isolation only 6–8% of the time. Commonly occurs in athletes involved in cutting, kicking, or explosive changes in direction such as hockey, football, or soccer players. On examination, the pain is reproducible with a resisted sit-up. Three out of five criteria is required for diagnosis: tender to palpation at pubic tubercle at the point of tendon insertion (1), tender to palpation of deep inguinal ring, pain and/or dilation of external ring without obvious hernia present (2), pain at the origin of the adductor longus tendon (3), dull diffuse groin pain often radiating to the perineum and inner thigh near the rectus insertion, lateral edge of the rectus, pubic tubercle, adductor longus origin (4), and no true detectable hernia (5). Plain radiographs of the pelvis in the AP and lateral view can be obtained to rule out alternative pathologies. MR imaging would show a tear in the rectus abdominis muscle or alternative adductor strains. Conservative management is initially trialed as most athletes are able to return to play after 6–8 weeks of rest, NSAIDs, and a progressive

PT program. After the failure of conservative treatment, patients can consider surgical repair, with >95% of athletes returning to play within 1 year after surgery.

Bursitis of the Greater Trochanter Presents as chronic intermittent lateral hip or thigh pain that is worse with activity and lying on the side. It is often seen with gluteal tendinopathies. Women are more at risk for the development of bursitis due to a larger pelvic width relative to whole body width and lower femoral shaft angle. Additional risk factors include obesity and arthritis. Can consider radiographic imaging to assess for alternative pathology. Initial treatment includes activity modification, NSAIDs, steroids, or PRP injection. If pain is refractory to conservative treatment, one can consider bursectomy or IT band lengthening. However, 90% of cases improve with conservative measures.

Femoroacetabular Impingement (FAI) An abnormality of the femoral head and/or neck that causes an impingement of the labrum against the femoral neck during hip flexion. This anatomic variance is more commonly seen in women. On examination, there is a decreased range of hip flexion that is painful, limited internal rotation, and adduction of the hip. Anterior hip impingement tests are positive in FAI. Radiography of the hip will show anatomic abnormalities of the femoral head and the head/neck junction. The normal head-neck offset is >7 mm and an alpha angle of <55 degrees. MRI is helpful for evaluating the labrum for lesions and articular damage. In patients with FAI, 88% of patients show a triad of abnormal head-neck anatomy, anterosuperior cartilage abnormality, and labral disorders at the anterosuperior aspect. Initial treatment includes restriction of ROM of the hip, NSAIDs, and physical therapy;. 89% of those who undergo conservative treatment report an improvement in pain six months out, and 79% report continued pain relief at 2 years. However, athletes and those who fail conservative treatment may want to consider surgical correction.

Myofascial Pain Syndrome Hard, palpable, and painful nodules within the band of skeletal muscle. Typically involves the muscle and its surrounding connective tissue. Occurs in low to moderate muscular exertion. Smaller type 1 musculature is recruited first and de-recruited last during static muscle exertion. This leads to the continuous activation of these muscle fibers, placing them at risk for muscle damage and calcium dysregulation. Latent when pain is only present during palpation and active when pain is spontaneous at rest. Both latent and active nodules can cause muscle dysfunction, weakness, and limited range of motion. Pain characterization is dependent on the patient's perception of its characteristics. Affects more than three-fourths of the world's population. Associated with both sleep and mood disruptions. Commonly affects office workers, musicians, dentists, and one with chronic low or moderate physical exertion. Associated with rheumatic diseases, fibromyalgia, and other diseases or syndromes associated with pain such as radiculopathies, tendonitis, etc. Myofascial pain syndrome is a clinical diagnosis. Requires palpation of a hard nodule within a taut muscle band. Pain is elicited on palpation or worsened/recreated during palpation. No current criteria for diagnosis currently. Ultrasound can be considered to show areas of nodular regions of hypo echogenicity, but this is not required for diagnosis. Initial treatment includes physical therapy, targeting normal muscle laxity and improving range of motion. Adjunct therapies that can be considered include botulinum injections and dry needling. Of those who receive dry needling, 31% have permanent relief, 20% have several months of relief, and 22% have weeks of relief.

Osteoarthritis of the Hip Repetitive shear stress at the articular surface. The repetitive stress causes pro-inflammatory mediators in the articular cartilage. As a result of the damage to the articular cartilage, the subchondral bone reactively changes and remodels too, leading to the development of osteoarthritis. Overall, it occurs in 4–10% of the population, and the risk increases with age. Risk factors include age, sex, weight, genetics, ethnicity, occupation, muscular function, joint morphology, joint shape, and femoroacetabular impingement. On examination, there is hip pain with internal hip rotation, internal rotation <15 degrees, stiffness of the hip for less than 69 minutes in the morning, and positive FABER & FADIR. Radiography can be helpful for confirmation, ruling out alternative pathologies, and monitoring disease progression. There is high discord between patient symptoms and radiographic findings. Initial treatment includes weight loss, strength training, and NSAIDs (most efficacious with diclofenac or etoricoxib); however, society guidelines recommend the lowest possible dose and duration of NSAIDs. Recommend oral over topical NSAIDs due to the depth of the hip joint. Steroid, hyaluronic acid, or PRP injection. Surgical management after failure of conservative treatment.

Osteitis Pubis A reaction of the pelvis due to high-stress forces during physical activity that causes injury to the pubic symphysis and surrounding muscles, typically adductor muscles. The repetition of overloading the pubic symphysis causes a stress reaction and lytic response to the bone. Typically seen in athletes that participate in rapid direction changes such as soccer, rugby, or football players. This can present as an anterior or medial groin pain that begins insidiously. Patients often have concomitant pathologies in the abdomen, scrotum, or adductor involvement. On physical examination, there is a restricted range of motion with both internal and external rotation. Will have positive adduction squeeze test, hop test, and FABER. In the acute phase, radiography places the patient in "flamingo view" to demonstrate the instability of the pubic symphysis, characterized by >2 mm superior/inferior or >7 mm widening. Chronic osteitis pubis will show on radiography with bony sclerosis of the pubic symphysis. Treated conservatively with rest, NSAIDs, heat or cold packs. Patients should avoid kicking or running as they undergo an aggressive rehabilitation program that focuses on the ROM of the hips and then strengthening. Surgical management is offered for the treatment of concomitant pathologies.

Piriformis Syndrome Compression of the sciatic nerve by the piriformis muscle at the ischial tuberosity that results in a shooting or burning pain from the glute down the posterior leg. It may also occur if the piriformis is inflamed; then, the sciatic nerve may have associated irritation as well. The piriformis may be injured because of acute internal rotation injuries, muscle hypertrophy, or poor posture during prolonged sitting. Typically occurs in middle-aged patients with female predominance. A diagnosis of exclusion and clinically diagnosed. Patients frequently present for chronic pain in the glute and hip. On examination, there is tenderness at the sciatic notch, pain is reproducible with FADIR and forceful internal and external rotation of the thigh and side lying with the knee flexed off the edge of the table. Additional imaging should be completed to rule out alternative pathologies. Managed conservatively with NSAIDS, muscle relaxants, steroid injection, and therapy targeted at the piriformis muscle. Surgical release or debridement can be considered after the failure of conservative measures. The amount of time required for rehabilitation prior to return to full activity is variable and dependent on the severity of symptoms and interventions taken in treatment. Most patients are symptom-free after 1–3 weeks of conservative management, but relapse is high due to exercise noncompliance.

Snapping Hip Syndrome Internal or external slapping from either the IT band or iliopsoas tendon sliding over bony prominences. Additional intra-articular pathology is found in 50% of patients. Typically affects repetitive extreme hip motions, such as ballet dancers, weight lifts, soccer players, and runners. A clinical diagnosis is made by an audible or palpable snapping sensation during hip movement. Imaging is completed to rule out alternative pathologies. Radiography for anatomic variance, ultrasonography can allow visualization of tendon snapping, MRI for thickened IT band or gluteus maximus. If pain is present, conservative measures are recommended with daily stretching, NSAIDs, steroid injection, and physical therapy. For those with pain refractory to conservative measures, surgical intervention can be considered.

Stress Fractures Fracture to the pubic rami and/or femoral neck after a sudden change in training regimen. Commonly seen in long-distance runners. Pain is described as a slow and progressive onset that is only with activity. On physical exam, tenderness to deep palpation over the pubic ramus, will be unable to stand or put full weight on the affected side. Radiography is negative in the early phase. CT or MRI can confirm the diagnosis if radiography is negative in the early phase. Stress fractures of the pubic ramus are treated with 4–6 weeks of rest and avoidance of activities that exacerbate pain symptoms. Patients with a stress fracture of the superior femoral neck are treated with rest and recommended to be non-weight bearing through the affected limb during this time. Stress fractures to the inferior femoral neck have a higher likelihood of progressing to a complete fracture. Treatment for an inferior femoral neck fracture is prophylactic and requires surgical repair.

Adductor Tendinopathy Medial or anterior hip pain that occurs at the musculotendinous junction or the bone-tendon junction. Accounts for 10% of all injuries in soccer players. Other athletes that are at risk include hockey players and football players. Patients are at higher risk for the development of tendinopathy if there is poor adductor strength or range of motion. Adductor tendinopathy is a clinical diagnosis. On physical exam, the patient will be tender to deep palpation of the involved muscle and will have reproducible pain on resisted adduction. Ultrasound or MRI can be considered in chronic injuries that do not respond to conservative management. Typically treated with NSAIDs and rest, physical therapy is delayed until the pain resolves if the strain is near a bone-tendon junction. Poor evidence for the role of steroid injection for adductor tendinopathy. After failure of conservative management or if imaging reveals a complete tear, one can consider surgical intervention. Athletes are typically able to return to play once strength has returned (approximately 4–8 weeks) with conservative management.

Leg/Ankle/Foot

Patellofemoral Pain Syndrome Common cause of knee pain caused by abnormal patellar tracking and weightbearing on a flexed knee causing peripatellar synovitis. Physical activity adolescents and young adults are most at risk of this condition. Females are two times more likely than males to develop this syndrome. Risk factors for patellofemoral pain syndrome include decreased knee extension strength, increased knee internal rotation, and decreased hip abduction. There is usually a positive patellar grind test on physical exam. There may be crepitus with knee range of motion as well. Imaging is not usually indicated. Treatment is conservative and includes ice, NSAIDS, quadriceps strengthening, activity modifications, patellar taping, and bracing. This condition carries a high likelihood of chronic pain for the patient.

Iliotibial Band Syndrome Characterized by repetitive flexion and extension of the knee that causes friction between the distal iliotibial band and the lateral femoral condyle. It is commonly seen in runners and athletes in endurance sports. Hip abductor weakness and increased knee internal rotation and adduction put individuals at risk of this syndrome. The classic physical exam finding is a positive Ober test. Iliotibial band syndrome is diagnosed clinically. Treatment differs by phase. In the acute phase, ice, anti-inflammatory medications, and ultrasound are the recommended treatments. In the subacute phase, physical therapy with hip abductor strengthening is indicated. Patients typically have resolution of symptoms in 4–8 weeks with conservative treatment.

Osgood-Schlatter Disease Chronic avulsion of the immature tibial tuberosity cartilage from repetitive quadriceps contractions. Preadolescent athletes are at high risk of this condition, especially if involved in activities with repetitive jumping or running. Rapid growth in preadolescents is another significant risk factor. On physical exam, patients usually have swelling and tenderness over the tibial tuberosity and pain with resisted knee extension. While the diagnosis is clinical, X-rays are normally indicated to rule out other causes of pain and swelling. Rest, ice, and physical therapy are the mainstays for treatment. Patients may also trial infrapatellar straps. Most patients have resolution of symptoms with conservative management, however, there is new data to suggest that a significant group of individuals with Osgood-Schlatter disease will have chronic pain.

Sinding-Larsen-Johansson Syndrome Inflammation and avulsion at the insertion of the patellar tendon into the inferior pole of the patella from traction on the patellar ligament. Populations most at risk of this condition include active adolescents aged 10–14, those with rapid skeletal growth, and overweight individuals. Physical exam typically reveals point tenderness and swelling at the inferior pole of the patella. MRI is required to rule out patellar sleeve avulsion. If an ultrasound is performed, the patella will appear hypoechoic and fragmented. Treatment is similar to that of Osgood-Schlatter disease—ice, NSAIDs, rest, and patellar band. However, Sinding-Larsen-Johansson syndrome may require a period of immobilization or surgery.

Pes Anserine Bursitis Common cause of medial knee pain. It is characterized by inflammation of the pes anserine bursa due to friction from excess valgus or rotational stress. There is a higher incidence in women, overweight individuals, and long-distance runners. Risk factors include knee osteoarthritis, valgus deformity, and pes planus. Swelling and tenderness to palpation of medial tibia just distal to the knee are typically seen on physical exam. On ultrasound, there will be increased fluid in the pes anserine bursa and a thickened bursa wall. Rest, NSAIDs, and physical therapy are the initial treatments. Steroid injections can be considered as well. It typically responds to these conservative interventions.

Medial Tibial Stress Syndrome Also known as shin splints, is caused by chronic traction on the tibial periosteum at the periosteal-fascial junction. It is classically seen in runners and individuals who suddenly increase exercise volume. It is more commonly seen in females. A larger navicular drop and excessive pronation while running puts individuals at risk of this syndrome. There is usually tenderness to palpation along the medial tibial border on physical exam. MRI helps to rule out stress fractures. Medial tibial stress syndrome can take up to six months to heal. Treatment is conservative, with modalities of ice, rest, activity modification, stretching, and orthotics.

Chronic Exertional Compartment Syndrome Nerve impingement or tissue ischemia from increased compartment pressure in any of the compartments of the lower leg. Young endurance athletes, especially runners, and individuals with a prior history of lower limb pathology are at risk of developing this. Physical exam classically reveals weakness and numbness of the associated muscles and a firm compartment. Diagnosis is made with compartment pressure studies using a manometer. Initial treatment includes activity modification, though most patients need surgical fasciotomy. The majority of patients have good outcomes after fasciotomy.

Retrocalcaneal Bursitis Inflamed and thickened bursa between the posterior calcaneus and Achilles tendon from repetitive pressure. Most frequently seen in females. Risk factors include wearing high heels or poorly fitting shoes. The physical exam finding most commonly seen his swelling and tenderness to palpation of the distal Achilles tendon. No imaging is needed. Symptoms usually resolve with conservative treatment, including changing footwear.

Calcaneal Apophysitis (Sever's disease) One of the most common causes of heel pain in children. It occurs when the calcaneal growth plate becomes inflamed from receptive gastrocnemius activation. This is seen most often in growing children involved in gymnastics, soccer, ballet, or track. Pes planus, hyperpronation of the foot, tight plantar fascia, inappropriate footwear, and running on hard surfaces are all known to put patients at higher risk of this disease. Physical exam is usually notable for tenderness to palpation at the insertion of the Achilles into the calcaneus. Patients may also have a positive squeeze test of the calcaneus. Imaging is not needed for diagnosis. Rest, ice, NSAIDs, stretching, and heel lifts usually provide resolution of symptoms within a few weeks to months.

Plantar Fasciitis Inflammation and microtears of the plantar fascia from increased tension. There is a higher incidence in females and overweight individuals, particularly those that participate in running, jumping, or dancing sports. Risk factors include pes cavus or pes planus, tight Achilles tendon, and bone spurs. Common physical exam findings are tenderness to palpation of the medial heel and plantar fascia and pain with passive dorsiflexion of the toes. X-rays can be obtained to look for bone spurs. Ultrasound typically reveals a thickened and hypoechoic plantar fascia. Conservative treatments are highly effective. These include heel pads, Achilles and plantar fascia stretching, night splints to hold the foot in slight dorsiflexion, NSAIDs, and physical therapy.

Anterior Impingement Syndrome of the Ankle Impingement and inflammation of the synovial tissues from recurrent dorsiflexion. It is frequently seen in athletes of sports that require forced dorsiflexion, such as running, dancing, and high jumping. Recurrent inversion injuries and tibiotalar osteophytes are risk factors. There is usually tenderness to palpation of the anteromedial or anterolateral ankle joint line. Ankle X-rays are needed to look for osteophytes. Initial management options are ice, rest, heel lifts, and injections. A large subgroup of these patients will ultimately require surgery.

Posterior Impingement Syndrome of the Ankle Impingement of the synovial tissue from compression of the talus and the soft tissue between the calcaneus and the tibia. As opposed to anterior impingement syndrome, this is commonly seen in athletes of sports that require forced plantarflexion, such as dancing, football, soccer, and martial arts. Flexor hallucis longus tendinopathy, os trigonum, and Stieda process put patients at risk of developing this syndrome. Physical exam classically reveals tenderness to palpation deep to the Achilles tendon medially or laterally and pain with forced hyperplantarflexion. X-rays of the ankle may reveal bony abnormalities like the os trigonum Stieda process. Most cases resolve with conservative treatment of ice, rest, NSAIDs, and heel lifts.

Bullet Points

- Overuse injuries are due to repetitive actions or movements that create forces that damage tissues, whether it be tendons, ligaments, muscles, or bones.
- These injuries usually occur over time.
- Conservative measures such as rest, ice/heat, compression, elevation(RICE), and physical therapy are the mainstay initial treatments.
- When these injuries do not respond to conservative measures, interventions such as injections can help alleviate symptoms.
- Surgery is rare but indicated for failed previous interventions.
- Key to management is prevention and early treatment.

Table 4.1 summarizes important clinical information about musculoskeletal overuse syndromes of the hip.

Table 4.2 summarizes important clinical information about musculoskeletal overuse syndromes of the wrist and hand.

Table 4.3 summarizes important clinical information about musculoskeletal overuse syndromes of the leg.

Table 4.4 summarizes important clinical information about musculoskeletal overuse syndromes of the neck shoulder and elbow.

Table 4.1 Hip musculoskeletal overuse injuries

Condition	Pathophysiology	Epidemiology	Risk factors	Physical exam	Imaging	Treatment	Outcomes
Hip and Pelvis							
Acetabular labral Tears (Groh, Hickman, Hunt, Kelly, Lewis)	Audible or palpable snapping that occurs during hip movement. Additionally, presents with anterior hip or groin pain (seen in 90% of patients). Most occur anteriorly (86–94%), a watershed region, making it more at risk for damage from wear and tear with poor healing capability	10% of the population. Motor vehicle accidents, falls, femoracetabular impingement, capsular laxity, dysplasia, and degeneration When occurring in isolation, typically due to high velocity trauma, idiopathic (74% of the time in athletes)	Legg-calve-Perthes disease, FAI, hip dysplasia (72%)	Anterior hip impingement test, FADIR, Faber test	Lateral & frog X-ray: Assess for alternative etiologies, 49% of patient with symptomatic labral tears had at least 1 radiographic abnormality	Rest, NSAID, PT. limit pivoting motions Injection: Diagnostic image guided intraarticular hip injection Surgical repair after failure of conservative treatment or if functional limitations are unsatisfactory	89% of patients after arthroscopy report improvement in symptoms at approximately 16.5 months after Mixed literature on whether PT works in conservative therapy

(continued)

Table 4.1 (continued)

Condition	Pathophysiology	Epidemiology	Risk factors	Physical exam	Imaging	Treatment	Outcomes
Athletic Pubalgia (Caudill, Elattar, Paajanen)	Injury to muscular and or fascial attachments to the anterior pubis. Occurs due to repetitive shearing of the pelvis by the stronger adductor muscles against the pubic symphysis. Additional structures at risk for injury includes the external oblique aponeurosis, posterior inguinal wall, and transversalis fascia	Athletes involved in cutting, kicking, and explosive turns or changes in direction Most often seen in soccer, ice hockey, football, or rugby athletes	Weak lower abdominal muscles	Reproducible pain with a resisted sit up 3/5 of the below needed: Tender to palpation at pubic tubercle at the point of tendon insertion Tender to palpation of deep inguinal ring Pain and/or dilation of external ring without obvious hernia present Pain at the origin of the adductor longus tendon Dull diffuse groin pain often radiating to the perineum and inner thigh near the rectus insertion, lateral edge of the rectus, pubic tubercle, adductor longus origin No true detectable hernia	Radiography: To rule out other potential conditions MRI: Demonstrate partial or complete tear of rectus muscle or adductor strains	Rest 6–8 weeks. NSAIDs or heat or ice. Progressive PT plan Not enough evidence to support US guided steroid injection After failure of conservative treatment can consider surgery	Conservative treatment: 50% return to play After surgery >95% return to play within 1 year

Bursitis of greater Trochanter (Reid)	Chronic intermittent lateral hip/thigh/buttock pain	Often coincides with gluteal tendinopathies and bursitis	Female Obesity and arthritis	Localized lateral hip pain with focal tenderness over the trochanter on palpation	Radiographic evidence is seen 4–46% A clinical diagnosis	Activity modification, NSAIDs, local steroid injection, PRP injection. Bursectomy or IT band lengthening for refractory cases	90% of people improve with conservative measures
Femoroacetabular impingement (Byrd, Ejnisman, Emara, Ganz, Gerhardt, Matsuda, Notzli)	Most commonly due to anatomic abnormalities of the femoral head/neck that cause impingement of the labrum against the femoral neck during hip flexion		Anatomic variance Seen more commonly in women	Anterior impingement test, decreased range of motion & painful limitation with flexion, internal rotation, and adduction of the hip Sensitivity of 75% and specificity of 43%	X-ray of the hip with both AP and lateral view, show abnormalities of the femoral head and head/neck junction MRI: best to show lesions of the labrum and articular cartilage	First-line treatment: Restriction of ROM of the hip, PT, and NSAIDs Athletes and those who fail conservative treatment may consider surgical correction	Those who undergo conservative treatment >89% saw significant improvement in pain at 6 months and 72% still saw improvement after 2 years
Myofascial pain Syndrome (Shah, Weller)	Hard, palpable, and painful nodules within the band of skeletal muscle. Occurs in low to moderate muscular exertion. A result of continuous muscle activation, that increases the risk for muscle damage and calcium dysregulation	Affects >3/4 of the world's population. Associated with sleep and mood disruptions Commonly affects office workers, musicians, dentists, any one with chronic low or moderate physical exertion	Associated with rheumatic diseases, fibromyalgia, and other diseases or syndromes associated with pain such as radiculopathies, tendonitis etc.	A clinical diagnosis. Requires, palpation of a hard nodule within a taut muscle band. Pain is elicited on palpation or worsened/recreated during palpation. No current criteria for diagnosis currently	US to show areas of nodular regions of hypo echogenicity	Conservative treatment is physical therapy, targeting normal muscle laxity and range of motion Adjunct therapies that can be considered include botulinum injections and dry needling	31% of those who receive dry needling, studies show permanent relief, 20% at several months, and 22% have several weeks of relief

(continued)

Table 4.1 (continued)

Condition	Pathophysiology	Epidemiology	Risk factors	Physical exam	Imaging	Treatment	Outcomes
Osteoarthritis of the Hip (Katz, Murphy)	Repetitive shear stress at the articular surface. As a result of the damage to the articular cartilage, the subchondral bone reactively changes and remodels too	Approximately 4–10% population prevalence. A 25% lifetime risk of symptomatic hip osteoarthritis who live to the age of 85 and 10% lifetime risk of undergoing total hip replacement for end stage osteoarthritis	Age, sex, weight, genetics, ethnicity, occupation, muscular function, joint morphology, joint shape, and femeoracetabular impingement syndrome	Hip pain, internal rotation <15 degrees, pain with internal hip rotation, stiffness of the hip for less than 69 minutes in the morning. Faber and Fadir	XR of the hip for diagnosis confirmation, ruling out alternative pathology High discord between radiographic features and patient symptomatology	Weight management, strength training, NSAIDs. Steroid, hyaluronic acid, or PRP injection. Surgical management after failure of conservative treatment	SMD = standard mean difference in pain score compared to placebo HA: 0.18 Steroid 1.65 Opioids 0.21 Oral NSAID 0.24–0.43 Exercise program 0.19–0.49 THR 90% reports little to no pain after surgical recovery
Osteitis Pubis (Beatty)	HIgh acceleration, deceleration, and directional forces causing injury to the pubic symphysis and surrounding muscle	Typically, an athlete participating in soccer, rugby, football, or ice hockey	Rapid direction changes	Anterior or medial groin pain with insidious onset. Often has concomitant pathologies Positive adduction squeeze test, hop test, and FABER Restricted ROM with internal and external rotation	XR: If chronic, bony sclerosis of the symphysis In "flamingo view", AP view with the patient standing on one leg may reveal pubic symphysis instability, characterized by >2 mm superior/inferior shear or > 7 mm widening. MRI to assess for labral tear	Rest, NSAIDs, heat or cold packs. Physical therapy program that focuses on ROM of the hips and strengthening	

Piriformis Syndrome (Hicks)	Compression of the sciatic nerve by the piriformis muscle at the ischial tuberosity. If the piriformis is irritated or inflamed, then the sciatic nerve can also be irritated as well. Piriformis can be injured due to trauma or muscle hypertrophy or prolonged sitting	Typically occurs in middle-aged patients with a ratio of male to female patient being affected 1:6	Chronic poor posture or acute internal hip rotation injuries	A clinical diagnosis and diagnosis of exclusion Palpation may reveal mild to moderate tenderness around the sciatic notch Reproducible symptoms with FADIR, forceful internal rotation of extended thigh, resisted abduction and external rotation of the thigh	US, CT, and MRI are helpful in ruling out alternative diagnosis	NSAIDs, muscle relaxants, and physical therapy targeted at stretching the piriformis muscle Steroid injections can help decrease inflammation. Botulinum toxin may provide temporary relief Surgical management can be considered after failed conservative treatment	Most are symptom free within 1–3 weeks after conservative treatment. Relapse is high due to exercise non-compliance
Snapping hip syndrome (Musick, Nolton)	Extra-articular causes: Internal snapping hip: Iliopsoas tendon snapping on bony prominences External snapping hip: Commonly from the IT band moving over the greater trochanter of the femoral head. Typically, an overuse injury but can be caused by trauma, such as total hip arthroplasty	In 50% of internal snapping hip cases, an additional intra-articular hip pathology is found Seen in sports with extreme hip motions: Ballet dancers, weight lifts, soccer player, or runners In ballet dancers were found to have bilateral involvement in 80%	External hip rotation and abduction over 90 degrees	Clinically diagnosed: Characterized by audible or palpable snapping sensation during hip movement	Imaging can be used to rule out other hip pathology MRI: Thickened iliotibial band or thickened edge of gluteus maximus US: Visualize snapping IT band over the greater trochanter MRA: For concomitant intra-articular hip pathology	Without pain: No intervention needed Pain is present: Stretching, steroid injections, NSAIDs, and PT Surgery: After failure of conservative treatment	

(continued)

Table 4.1 (continued)

Condition	Pathophysiology	Epidemiology	Risk factors	Physical exam	Imaging	Treatment	Outcomes
Stress Fractures (Barry, LeBlanc, noakes Pavlov)	Fracture to the pubic rami and/or femoral neck. Commonly in long distance runners. Describe the pain as slow gradual onset of activity related pain to the groin and hip that improves with rest	Athletes with a sudden change in their training regimen	Long distance running	Tenderness to deep palpation over the pubic ramus and unable to stand and put full weight on affected side	XR: Negative in the early phase. CT/MRI can confirm diagnosis if XR is initially negative	Pubic ramus: 4–6 weeks of rest and avoidance of activities that worsen pain symptoms Superior femoral neck fracture: Rest and non weight bearing for 4–6 weeks Inferior femoral neck stress fractures: Surgical repair	
Adductor tendinopathy (O'Connell, Schilders, Verrall, Werner)	Occurs at the musculotendinous junction or sometimes the bone-tendon junction	10% of all injuries in soccer players	Decreased range of adduction and adductor weakness players, hockey players, football players	Clinical diagnosis. Tender on deep palpation of the involved muscle. Resister adduction	US or MRI can be considered in chronic injuries that are unresponsive to conservative treatment	Rest and NSAIDs If strain is near bony—Tendon junction, delay PT until pain has improved Surgery if: Complete tear or failed conservative treatment after at least 6 months	Return to sports: In acute strains/tears it is recommended to return when strength has returned to >70%, typically after 4–8 weeks In chronic strains return to play can be as long as 6 months.

Table 4.2 Wrist and hand overuse syndromes

Condition	Pathophysiology	Symptoms	Risk factors	Physical exam	Additional tests or imaging	Treatment	Outcomes
Non-focal conditions							
Ganglionic cyst	Repetitive microtrauma results in the development of a synovial cyst that arises along the synovial sheath of the joint space	May be an asymptomatic cystic mass which may or may not be associated with pain, tenderness, and weakness	Younger age Female sex	Firm, well circumscribed 1-2 cm mass that transilluminates with light	*US*: Well defined area of hypogenicity	Immobilization Aspiration Surgical excision	Aspiration improves cosmetic appearance but associated with high rates of recurrence (90%)
Trigger finger	Degenerative changes of the flexor tendons and the annular pulley system	Locking or catching of finger with extension and flexion. May have associated painful nodule at the palmer metacarpophalangeal joint	Diabetes RA Gout >50 years old	Tenderness to palpation and/or presence of a nodule at the level of the annular pulley Fixed flexion of the PIP joint may reproduce symptoms	Not required for diagnosis *US*: Thickened annular pulley with effusions around the synovial sheath	Splints NSAIDs corticosteroid injections Surgical release	Up to 90% of patients may respond positively to corticosteroid injections

(continued)

Table 4.2 (continued)

Condition	Pathophysiology	Symptoms	Risk factors	Physical exam	Additional tests or imaging	Treatment	Outcomes
Radial-sided wrist pain							
De Quervain's tenosynovitis	Inflammation caused by repetitive stress from wrist motion results in inflammation of the abductor pollicis longus and extensor pollicis brevis tendons as they pass through a fibro-osseous tunnel at the first dorsal compartment	Pain over the first dorsal compartment	Female sex Newborn care givers Golf Fishing Racquet sports Wheelchair use	Finkelstein test	Increased thickness or bursitis within the first extensor compartment	Rest and thumb spica splint NSAIDs Corticosteroid injections Surgical decompression	60–80% report improvement with corticosteroid injections Chronic cases can result in development of a ganglion cyst
Intersection syndrome	Inflammation at the point where the APL, EPB, and wrist tensor muscles cross may lead to bursitis and/or tendon hypertrophy	Pain over the dorsal forearm with possible associated grip weakness	Racquet sports Rowers Weightlifters Wheelchair use	Pain over the dorsal forearm and wrist that is worsened with existed extension of the thumb and wrist	*MRI*: Inflammation and/or abnormal signal of the first and second extensor compartments	Rest, splinting, injections, NAIDs	Over 60% of patients respond positively to conservative treatment

Flexor carpi radialis tendinitis	Inflammation of the flexor carpi radialis tendon unit	Pain located over the palmer aspect of the volar radial wrist	Golfers Racquet sports Baseball players	Tenderness at the palmer aspect of the second metacarpal -positive Lister test (pain from rapid dorsiflexion)	*XR*: May be needed to rule out scaphoid fracture *MRI*: Inflammation or abnormal fluid signal from the FCR tendon sheath	Rest, splinting, injections, NAIDs	Frequently resolves with conservative management
Ulnar-sided wrist pain							
Extensor carpi Ulnaris tendinitis	Tenosynovitis of the extensor capari ulnaris from repetitive twisting and/or dorsiflexion	Tenderness to palpation over the sixth dorsal wrist compartment -ulnar wrist pain	Rowers Basketball players Racquet sports	Tenderness to palpation over the sixth dorsal compartment and worsened with wrist extension	*MRI*: Inflammation or abnormal signal intensity of the tendon sheath *Ultrasound*: Subluxation of the ECU tendon during dynamic maneuvers	Rest, splinting, corticosteroid injections, NAIDs. Surgical	Usually responds to conservative management. Lower threshold for surgical intervention is positive subluxation of the ECU

(continued)

Table 4.2 (continued)

Condition	Pathophysiology	Symptoms	Risk factors	Physical exam	Additional tests or imaging	Treatment	Outcomes
Triangular fibrocartilage complex	Damage to the triangular fibrocartilage complex can be due to trauma or degenerative changes from repetitive microtraumas	Pain worsened by activities which involve supination of the wrist	Older age	Positive ulnar variance may be seen with inspection of the wrist with increased variation seen with pronation. There may also be tenderness to palpation between the pisiform and ulnar head (fovea sign)	*MRI*: TFCC thinning and chondromalacia of the lunate, triquetrum, and distal ulna Arthroscopy is the gold standard	Rest, splinting, and corticosteroid injections	
Flexor carpi Ulnaris	Repetitive microtraumas of the FCU tendon	Pain with activities involving wrist flexion. May have associated arthritic pain of the pisotriquentral jont	Racquet sports Rowers Wheelchair users	Pain with resisted wrist flexion Pisotriquentral grind test to screen for concurrent pisotriquentral arthrits	*XR*: Calcified tendinitis and associated pisotriquentral arthrtis *MRI*: Increased signal and calcification along the FCU tendon	Rest, splinting, and corticosteroid injections	Frequently resolves with conservative management

Table 4.3 Leg overuse syndromes

Condition	Pathophysiology	Epidemiology	Risk Factors	Physical Exam	Imaging	Treatment	Outcomes
Knee/shin/calf/foot/ankle							
Patellofemoral pain syndrome	Abnormal patellar tracking [81] Weight bearing on a flexed knee [82] Peripatellar synovitis	Physically active adolescents and young adults Females 2 times more likely than males	Decreased knee extension strength [83] Females: Increased knee internal rotation and decreased hip abduction	Positive patellar grind test Possible crepitus with knee ROM	No abnormal findings on imaging	Ice, NSAIDS, quadriceps strengthening, activity modifications, patellar taping or bracing	Highly likelihood of chronic pain
Iliotibial band syndrome	Repetitive flexion/extension of the knee causes friction between the IT band distally and the lateral femoral condyle [84]	Runners Athletes in endurance sports	Hip abductor weakness Increased knee internal rotation and adduction	Positive Ober test	Diagnosed clinically, no imaging needed	Acute phase: Rest, ice, anti-inflammatory medications, ultrasound Subacute phase: PT with hip abductor strengthening	Typically heal in 4–8 weeks with conservative treatment

(continued)

Table 4.3 (continued)

Condition	Pathophysiology	Epidemiology	Risk Factors	Physical Exam	Imaging	Treatment	Outcomes
Patellar tendonitis	Forceful eccentric quadriceps contractions [85] (jumping and squatting) Microtears of the patellar tendon	Usually skeletally mature athletes	Decreased flexibility of quadriceps and hamstrings [86]	Tenderness to palpation at inferior (more common) or superior pole of the patella	None needed	Ice, NSAIDS, quadriceps strengthening, activity modifications, patellar taping or bracing	Usually resolves after 6 weeks of conservative treatment
Osgood-Schlatter disease	Chronic avulsion of the immature tibial tuberosity cartilage from repetitive quadriceps contraction [87]	Preadolescent athletes	Repetitive running or jumping Fast growth	Tenderness or swelling over tibial tuberosity Pain with resisted knee extension	Usually only needed to rule out other causes Diagnosis is clinical	Rest Ice Infrapatellar strap PT	Most patients have resolution of symptoms, but new data shows there may be a significant subgroup of patient with chronic pain [88]
Sinding-Larsen-Johansson syndrome	Inflammation and avulsion at the insertion of the patellar tendon into the inferior pole of the patella from traction on the patellar ligament [89]	Active adolescents aged 10–14	Rapid skeletal growth Overweight	Point tenderness and swelling at inferior pole of patella	MRI is needed to rule out patellar sleeve avulsion Patella appears hypoechoic and fragmented on ultrasound	Ice, NSAIDs, rest, activity modification, patellar band	May require immobilization or surgery

Pes anserine bursitis	Inflammation of pes anserine bursa due to friction from excess valgus or rotational stress	Higher incidence in women, overweight individuals, and long-distance runners	Obesity Knee OA Valgus deformity Pes planus	Swelling of bursa Tenderness to palpation of medial tibia just distal to the knee [90]	Increased fluid in the pes anserine bursa with thickened bursa wall	Rest, NSAIDs, physical therapy, steroid injections	Typically resolves with conservative treatment
Medial tibial stress syndrome	Chronic traction on tibial periosteum at the periosteal-fascial junction [91]	Runners, more commonly in females	Larger navicular drop Excessive pronation while running [92]	Tenderness to palpation along medial tibial border	MRI helps to rule out stress fractures	Rest, activity modification, stretching, ice, orthotics	Can take up to 6 months to heal
Chronic exertional compartment syndrome	Nerve impingement or tissue ischemia from increased compartment pressure	Young endurance athletes, especially runners	Previous lower limb pathology	Weakness and numbness of associated muscles Firm compartment	Compartment pressure studies using manometer	Fasciotomy	Good to excellent outcomes in 60–96% of patients [93]
Retrocalcaneal bursitis	Inflamed and thickened bursa between the posterior calcaneus and Achilles tendon from receptive pressure	Females	Wearing high heels or poor fitting shoes	Swelling and tenderness to palpation of distal Achilles tendon insertion	None needed	Change footwear	Typically resolves with conservative treatment

(continued)

Table 4.3 (continued)

Condition	Pathophysiology	Epidemiology	Risk Factors	Physical Exam	Imaging	Treatment	Outcomes
Achilles tendonitis	Forceful eccentric gastrocnemius and soleus contractions cause micro-tears and inflammation	Runners and jumpers	Training errors Increased pronation Tight hamstrings Pes cavus Genu varum	Tenderness to palpation of tendon insertion on calcaneus	None needed	Rest, ice, NSAIDs, stretching and strengthening, heel lifts	Most resolve with conservative treatment. Can lead to tendon rupture
Calcaneal apophysitis (Sever's disease)	Caused by receptive gastrocnemius activation	Young female gymnasts	Pes planus Hyper pronation of the foot Tight plantar fascia or Achilles tendon Inappropriate footwear Running on hard surfaces [94]	Tenderness to palpation at the insertion of Achilles into calcaneus	None needed	Rest, ice, NSAIDs, stretching, heel lifts	Usually resolves within a few weeks to months with conservative treatment
Plantar fasciitis	Inflammation of plantar fascia from increased tension	Higher incidence in females	Pes cavus or pes planus Tight Achilles tendon Obesity Bone spurs	Tenderness to palpation of medial heel and plantar fascia	XR to look for bone spur	Heel pads, Achilles and plantar fascia stretching, night splints to hold in slight dorsiflexion, NSAIDS, PT	Conservative 90–95% effective

Flexor hallucis longus tendonitis (Dancer's tendonitis)	Inflammation of the tendon as it passes behind the lateral malleolus from repetitive push-off maneuvers	Commonly seen in dancers and soccer players	Motor imbalance Decreased dorsiflexion of hallux with ankle dorsiflexed [95]	Tenderness to palpation at posteromedial aspect of hallux Decreased toe flexion Pain with active plantarflexion and passive dorsiflexion	None needed	Ice, rest, stretching	Most cases improve in a few weeks with conservative treatment
Anterior impingement syndrome of ankle	Recurrent dorsiflexion causes impingement and inflammation of synovial tissue usually due to talotibial osteophytes [96]	Athletes that require forced dorsiflexion (runners, dancers, high jumpers)	Recurrent inversion injuries Tibiotalar osteophytes	Tenderness to palpation of anteromedial or anterolateral ankle joint line	XR to evaluate for osteophytes	Ice, rest, heel lifts, injections, surgery	Surgery frequently required
Posterior impingement syndrome of ankle	Compression of the talus and nearby soft tissue between the calcaneus and the tibia causing impingement of synovial tissue [97]	Athletes that require forced plantarflexion (dancing, football, soccer, martial arts)	Bony lesions such as os trigonum or Stieda process Flexor hallucis longus tendinopathy	Tenderness to palpation deep to the Achilles tendon medially or laterally Positive posterior ankle impingement test (pain with forced hyperplantarfelxion)	XR may reveal bony abnormalities such as os trigonum or Stieda process [98]	Ice, rest, NSAIDs, heel lifts	Usually resolves with conservative treatment

Table 4.4 Neck, shoulder, and elbow overuse syndromes

Condition	Pathophysiology	Epidemiology	Risk factors	Physical exam	Imaging	Treatment	Outcomes
Neck							
Neck muscle sprain	Injury/tearing of the muscle fibers of the neck	Non-specific neck pain has annual prevalence between 15 and50%, and is more common in females than males [5]	Poor posture, trauma, arthritis, lifting heavy objects	Limited ROM, pain with active ranging	Not generally needed	Physical therapy, stretching, ice,	Typically self-limited
Cervical radiculopathy	Compression or irritation of cervical spine nerve roots	Peak incidence 50–54 years of age, more commonly in males with incidence of about 100 pr 100,000	Prior lumbar radiculopathy, tobacco use, Caucasian	+Spurlings, +Neck traction +Neck distraction	Plain radiograph, CT, MRI, EMG	Conservative treatment w/ NSAIDs, physical therapy, Consideration of epidural steroid injections, Persistent: Surgical decompression	Can be self-limited, 75–90% patients w/ symptom improvement w/ conservative management, Up to 25% patients will have persistent symptoms requiring surgical management

Tension neck syndrome	Impaired relaxation of neck muscles with resulting pain, stiffness, spasms	*	Computer mouse use, long-term use of computers, poor posture, chronic neck strain, stress	Palpable tense, tender, spasmodic regions of trapezius, sternocleidomastoid muscles; decreased ROM of neck; pain on resistance	Not generally needed	Physical therapy, stretching exercises of neck muscle groups; acupuncture; trigger point injections; dry needling	Generally, with improvements in pain, muscle tension with treatment
Shoulder							
Biceps tendinopathy/tenosynovitis	Injury, traction, or degeneration of the long head of the biceps tendon	Typically seen in young or middle aged patients, proximal biceps injuries more common	Baseball pitching, tennis players, swimming, volleyball players; overhead manual labor	+Yergason, +speeds +Uppercut (Mair)	Increased signal on MR, fluid in biceps tendon sheath; IUS w/ fluid/debris in tendon sheath, tendon thickening	1st line: Physical therapy, activity modification, NSAIDs Persistent: Tendon sheath steroid injection Increased tendon fraying: Debridement Other: tenodesis, tenotomy	For those w/ pdebilitating symptoms: Improvement in patient-reported pain, good long-term outcomes in surgical patients

(continued)

Table 4.4 (continued)

Condition	Pathophysiology	Epidemiology	Risk factors	Physical exam	Imaging	Treatment	Outcomes
Subacromial-subdeltoid bursitis	Inflammation of the subacromial-subdeltoid bursa as a result of injury, infection, overuse leading to fluid collection in the bursa	Equal gender prevalence, elder people more prone; comprises about 0.4% of all primary care visits—subacromial bursitis in general	Rotator cuff tendinopathy, osteoarthritis, infection, rheumatoid arthritis. More often seen in people participating in repetitive overhead activities	Shoulder pain and limited ROM	US/MR imaging w/ fluid/debris in bursa	1st line: Rest + NSAIDs Persistent: Intrabursal steroid injection Surgical: If not fixed by the above, subacromial decompression, bursectomy	Generally good outcomes as process is self-limiting; most patients improve with conservative therapy.
Rotator cuff tendinopathy	Injury to or degeneration of supraspinatus, infraspinatus, teres minor or subscapularis muscle tendons	Incidence 0.3–5%, annual prevalence 0.5–7.4%. Associated with increasing age	Overhead athletes, occupations w/ repetitive shoulder use, shoulder trauma	Limited active ROM, +Jobes, +drop-arm test, lift-off tests Variety of tests in combination assist with diagnosis of tendinopathy of specific tendons in rotator cuff group	Tendon thickening, increased T2 signal on MR; hypoechogeneity on US	1st line: Physical therapy Persistent: Tendon debridement vs. primary repair for full tendon tears	Prior shoulder pain and high baseline pain/disability associated with poorer outcomes

SICK scapula (scapular malposition—Inferior medial border prominence, coracoid pain/ malposition and scapla dyskinesis)	Altered muscle function around the region of scapula	Increased prevalence of scapular dyskinesis specifically in overhead athletes	Overhead athletes	Tenderness on coracoid palpation, pain w/ throwing that is improved with scapular stabilization maneuvers	Generally, not needed	Physical therapy with attention to stretching of pectoralis minor, activity modification; interval throwing program to improve scapular symmetry	Good resolution of pain symptoms achieved with achieving scapular symmetry and treatment compliance
Shoulder labral tears (SLAP—Superior labral anterior to posterior (same as general labral tear?)	Impaired labral integrity due to trauma/ degeneration resulting in tear	Highest incidence in 20–29 and 40–49-year-olds	Overhead athletes	+Jobe relocation and O'Brien for labral pathology	MRI can be useful in diagnosis of anterior labral tears	Physical therapy, activity modification, NSAIDS, cryotherapy. Surgical repair may be indicated	Generally favorable outcomes in following arthroscopic repairs if patients were good surgical candidates

(continued)

Table 4.4 (continued)

Condition	Pathophysiology	Epidemiology	Risk factors	Physical exam	Imaging	Treatment	Outcomes
Bennett lesion of shoulder	Reactive bone formation due to impaction of posterior humeral head on glenoid	Overhead athletes	Overhead throwing athletes (ie baseball pitchers); associated with labral tears	Pain in late cocking phase, follow-through or deceleration	Radiographs may show lesion in certain views CT, MRI, arthrography	Initial: Nonoperative management w/ posterior capsule stretching, strengthening rotator cuff Persistent symptoms: Arthroscopic intervention to remove lesion Operative management w/ mixed results	Limited outcome data*
Elbow							
Lateral epicondylitis	Degenerative changes or irritation of forearm extensor tendons, most commonly extensor carpi radialis brevis as result of overuse	Effecting 1–3% adults yearly, higher incidence in males in their 40 s and females in their 50 s 0.3–12.2% prevalence in adults, higher prevalence in females	forceful and repetitive arm movements, tennis playing; ipsilateral rotator cuff tear	+pain w/ resisted wrist/finger extension, grip weakness	Diagnosis primarily clinical, radiograph/US/ MRI can be used to evaluate for other etiologies of pain	Initial: Conservative management w/ NSAIDs, orthotics, physical therapy, injections Persistent: Surgical management with multiple approaches	Most patients have pain relief within a year of conservative treatment, noncompliant patients will often have symptom recurrence

Medial epicondylitis	Denerative changes/irritation of wrist flexor tendons of elbow as result of overuse	Prevalence of 0.4 percent, more common in female, tend to be more present in dominant arm	Forceful or repetitive movements, golf playing Bowling, tennus, or racquet sports, overhead athletes	+aching pain with movement and weakness in forearm flexors; chronic cases will have weakened grip strength, tenderness distal and anterior to medial epicondyle, paint w/ resisted pronation or wrist flexion	Diagnosis primarily clinical, US can help distinguish from other etiologies of pain, chronic degeneration seen as hyoechoic tissue, MRI can be used to rule out other causes	Nonsurgically mostly with activity modification, NSAIDS/APAP, ice, topical nitroglycern, physical therapy, Other modalities: Dry needling, night splinting/ elbow taping, US-guided steroid injection Persistent/ REfractory: surgical management with tendon release and debridement	Favorable prognosis, most patients can return to work or their sports activity with conservative management

(continued)

Table 4.4 (continued)

Condition	Pathophysiology	Epidemiology	Risk factors	Physical exam	Imaging	Treatment	Outcomes
Elbow ulnar collateral ligament tear	Rupture of ulnar collateral ligament due to acute trauma or chronic microtrauma and degeneration	* only found data among specific athletic groups	Often associated with baseball players, javelin throwers	+elbow valgus stress test	Static radiograph, valgus stress radiograph, CT or MR arthrography and US provide most diagnostic information	Non-surgical treatment: Physical therapy, activity modification (no throwing, no valgus stress), Certain populations can be good candidates for surgical reconstruction	Complete tears distally more likely to fail non-surgical treatment; Baseball players often return to play but may have decreased performance post-reconstruction, may require position change

Posterior elbow impingement	Inflammation of the elbow joint at the olecranon	Uncommon in general population, seen in overhead throwing athletes/tennis players	Repetitive forced extension of elbow such as overhead throwing motions; associated w/ UCL insufficiency	Limited ROM on elbow extension activities	Radiographs can detect olecranon or posterior fossa osteophytes, CT for posterior osteophytes, MRI w/ intraarticular contrast more sensitive	Most can be treated conservatively with NSAIDS and activity modification Surgical intervention for disabling pain or continued loss of function despite conservative treatment. Open surgery vs. arthroscopic debridement are options	Many patients treated conservatively with good outcomes, Arthroscopic management is effective as well and can result in return to pre-injury levels of activity

(continued)

Table 4.4 (continued)

Condition	Pathophysiology	Epidemiology	Risk factors	Physical exam	Imaging	Treatment	Outcomes
radial tunnel syndrome (entire section Shamrock and Das)	Compressive neuropathy of posterior interosseous nerve (PIN) at the radial tunnel resulting in pain	Rare, annual incidence estimated 0.003%, often misdiagnosed as PIN compression syndeome which is a separate entity	Repetitive prono-supination with elbow fleed at 0–45 degrees (increases pressure in radial tunnel)	Pain worse with prono-supination of forearm, resisted elbow flexion, tenderness to palpation few centimeteres distl to lateral epicondyle of humerus;	Limited role of MRI in diagnosis, but can evaluate for other causes	Initial: Non-operative treatment w/ activity modification, NSAIDS, splinting, Other options: Radial tunnel steroid injections, Severe, refractory case: Surgical radial tunnel release	Good resolution of pain w/ radial tunnel injections, post-op pain relief in surgical cases can be delayed with 60–70% success rate

*47% of frequent computer users have some degree of tension neck syndrome
Source: Kashmeera et al. [16]

Bibliography

Neck/Shoulder/Elbow

1. Barry NN, McGuire JL. Acute injuries and specific problems in adult athletes. Rheum Dis Clin N Am. 1996;22:531–49.
2. Beatty T. Osteitis pubis in athletes. Curr Sports Med Rep. 2012;11(2):96–8. https://doi.org/10.1249/JSR.0b013e318249c32b. PMID: 22410702
3. Byrd JW, Jones KS. Arthroscopic femoroplasty in the management of cam-type femoroacetabular impingement. Clin Orthop Relat Res. 2009;467:739–46.
4. Caudill P, Nyland J, Smith C, Yerasimides J, Lach J. Sports hernias: a systematic literature review. Br J Sports Med. 2008;42(12):954–64. https://doi.org/10.1136/bjsm.2008.047373. Epub 2008 Jul 4. PMID: 18603584
5. Cohen SP. Epidemiology, diagnosis, and treatment of neck pain. Mayo Clin Proc. 2015;90(2):284–99. https://doi.org/10.1016/j.mayocp.2014.09.008. PMID: 25659245
6. Ejnisman L, Philippon M, Lertwanich P. Femoroacetabular impingement: the femoral side. Clin Sports Med. 2011;30:369–77.
7. Elattar O, Choi HR, Dills VD, Busconi B. Groin injuries (athletic Pubalgia) and return to play. Sports Health. 2016;8(4):313–23. https://doi.org/10.1177/1941738116653711. Epub 2016 Jun 14. PMID: 27302153; PMCID: PMC4922526
8. Emara K, Samir W, Motasem el H, Ghafar KA. Conservative treatment for mild femoroacetabular impingement. J Orthop Surg (Hong Kong). 2011;19:41–5.
9. Ganz R, Parvizi J, Beck M, Leunig M, Nötzli H, Siebenrock KA. Femoroacetabular impingement: a cause for osteoarthritis of the hip. Clin Orthop Relat Res. 2003;417:112–20.
10. Gerhardt MB, Romero AA, Silvers HJ, Harris DJ, Watanabe D, Mandelbaum BR. The prevalence of radiographic hip abnormalities in elite soccer players. Am J Sports Med. 2012;40:584–8.
11. Groh MM, Herrera J. A comprehensive review of hip labral tears. Curr Rev Musculoskelet Med. 2009;2(2):105–17. https://doi.org/10.1007/s12178-009-9052-9. Epub 2009 Apr 7. PMID: 19468871; PMCID: PMC2697339
12. Hickman JM, Peters CL. Hip pain in the young adult: diagnosis and treatment of disorders of the acetabular labrum and acetabular dysplasia. Am J Orthop. 2001;30:459–67.
13. Hicks BL, Lam JC, Varacallo M. Piriformis syndrome. 2022 Sep 4. In: StatPearls [Internet]. Treasure Island: StatPearls Publishing; 2022 Jan–. PMID: 28846222.
14. Hunt D, Clohisy J, Prather H. Acetabular tears of the hip in women. Phys Med Rehabil Clin N Am. 2007;18(3):497–520.
15. J Rehabil Res Dev. Author manuscript; available in PMC 2015 Sep 28. Published in final edited form as: J Rehabil Res Dev. 2014;51(10):1515–24. https://doi.org/10.1682/JRRD.2013.09.0211.
16. Kashmeera PK, Vijay Selvan N, Megha A. Prevalence of tension neck syndrome in frequent computer users. Medical & Clinical Case Reports Journal. 2023;1:67–71. https://doi.org/10.51219/MCCRJ/Vijay-Selvan-N/20.
17. Katz JN, Arant KR, Loeser RF. Diagnosis and treatment of hip and knee osteoarthritis: a review. JAMA. 2021;325(6):568–78. https://doi.org/10.1001/jama.2020.22171. PMID: 33560326; PMCID: PMC8225295
18. Kelly BT, Weiland DE, Schenker ML, Philippon MJ. Arthroscopic labral repair in the hip: surgical technique and review of the literature. Arthroscopy. 2005;21:1496–504.
19. LeBlanc KE, LeBlanc KA. Groin pain in athletes. Hernia. 2003;7:68–71.
20. Lewis CL, Sahrmann SA. Acetabular labral tears. Phys Ther. 2006;86:110–21. [PubMed] [Google Scholar] [Ref list]
21. Matsuda DK, Carlisle JC, Arthurs SC, Wierks CH, Philippon MJ. Comparative systematic review of the open dislocation, mini-open, and arthroscopic surgeries for femoroacetabular impingement. Arthroscopy. 2011;27:252–69.

22. Murphy NJ, Eyles JP, Hunter DJ. Hip osteoarthritis: etiopathogenesis and implications for management. Adv Ther. 2016;33(11):1921–46. https://doi.org/10.1007/s12325-016-0409-3. Epub 2016 Sep 26. PMID: 27671326; PMCID: PMC5083776
23. Musick SR, Varacallo M. Snapping hip syndrome. [Updated 2022 Sep 4]. In: StatPearls [Internet]. Treasure Island: StatPearls Publishing; 2022 Jan-. Available from: https://www.ncbi.nlm.nih.gov/books/NBK448200/
24. Noakes TD, Smith JA, Lindberg G, Wills CE. Pelvic stress fractures in long distance runners. Am J Sports Med. 1985;13:120–3.
25. Nolton EC, Ambegaonkar JP. Recognizing and managing snapping hip syndrome in dancers. Med Probl Perform Art. 2018;33(4):286–91.
26. Nötzli HP, Wyss TF, Stoecklin CH, Schmid MR, Treiber K, Hodler J. The contour of the femoral head-neck junction as a predictor for the risk of anterior impingement. J Bone Joint Surg Br. 2002;84:556–60.
27. O'Connell MJ, Powell T, McCaffrey NM, O'Connell D, Eustace SJ. Symphyseal cleft injection in the diagnosis and treatment of osteitis pubis in athletes. AJR Am J Roentgenol. 2002;179:955–9.
28. Paajanen H, Brinck T, Hermunen H, Airo I. Laparoscopic surgery for chronic groin pain in athletes is more effective than nonoperative treatment: a randomized clinical trial with magnetic resonance imaging of 60 patients with sportsman's hernia (athletic pubalgia). Surgery. 2011;150(1):99–107. https://doi.org/10.1016/j.surg.2011.02.016. Epub 2011 May 5
29. Pavlov M, Nelson TL, Warren RF, Torg JS, Burnstein AH. Stress fractures of the pubic ramus. A report of twelve cases. J Bone Joint Surg Am. 1982;64:1020–5.
30. Reid D. The management of greater trochanteric pain syndrome: a systematic literature review. J Orthop. 2016;13(1):15–28.
31. Shah JP, Thaker N, Heimur J, Aredo JV, Sikdar S, Gerber L. Myofascial trigger points then and now: a historical and scientific perspective. PM R. 2015;7(7):746–61. https://doi.org/10.1016/j.pmrj.2015.01.024. Epub 2015 Feb 24. PMID: 25724849; PMCID: PMC4508225
32. Schilders E, Bismil Q, Robinson P, O'Connor PJ, Gibbon WW, Talbot JC. Adductor-related groin pain in competitive athletes. Role of adductor enthesis, magnetic resonance imaging, and entheseal pubic cleft injections. J Bone Joint Surg Am. 2007;89:2173–8.
33. Verrall GM, Slavotinek JP, Fon GT. Incidence of pubic bone marrow oedema in Australian rules football players: relation to groin pain. Br J Sports Med. 2001;35:28–33.
34. Weller JL, Comeau D, Otis JAD. Myofascial pain. Semin Neurol. 2018;38(6):640–3. https://doi.org/10.1055/s-0038-1673674. Epub 2018 Dec 6
35. Werner J, Hägglund M, Waldén M, Ekstrand J. UEFA injury study: a prospective study of hip and groin injuries in professional football over seven consecutive seasons. Br J Sports Med. 2009;43:1036–40.

Wrist/Hand

36. Versteeg G, Goyal K. Radiologist identification of occult dorsal wrist ganglion cysts on MRI. J Wrist Surg. 2019;08(04):276–9. https://doi.org/10.1055/s-0039-1683847.
37. Gude W, Morelli V. Ganglion cysts of the wrist: pathophysiology, clinical picture, and management. Curr Rev Musculoskelet Med. 2008;1(3–4):205–11. https://doi.org/10.1007/s12178-008-9033-4.
38. Makkouk AH, Oetgen ME, Swigart CR, Dodds SD. Trigger finger: etiology, evaluation, and treatment. Curr Rev Musculoskelet Med. 2008;1(2):92–6. https://doi.org/10.1007/s12178-007-9012-1.
39. Freiberg A, Mulholland RS, Levine R. Nonoperative treatment of trigger fingers and thumbs. J Hand Surg Am. 1989;14(3):553–8. https://doi.org/10.1016/S0363-5023(89)80024-3.
40. Rettig AC. Wrist and hand overuse syndromes. Clin Sports Med. 2001;20(3):591–611. https://doi.org/10.1016/S0278-5919(05)70271-4. PMID: 11494843.

41. Apple DF, Cody R, Allen A. Chapter five overuse syndrome of the upper limb in people with spinal cord injury in rehabilitation research and development service. Phys Fit A Guid Individ with Spinal Cord Inj. 2004;13:97–107.
42. Banks KP, Ly JQ, Beall DP, Grayson DE, Bancroft LW, Tall MA. Overuse injuries of the upper extremity in the competitive athlete: magnetic resonance imaging findings associated with repetitive trauma. Curr Probl Diagn Radiol. 2005;34(4):127–42. https://doi.org/10.1067/j.cpradiol.2005.04.001.
43. Balakatounis K, Angoules AG, Angoules NA, Panagiotopoulou K. Synthesis of evidence for the treatment of intersection syndrome. World J Orthop. 2017;8(8):619–23. https://doi.org/10.5312/wjo.v8.i8.619.
44. Löw S, Erne H, Pillukat T, Mühldorfer-Fodor M, Unglaub F, Spies CK. Diagnosing central lesions of the triangular fibrocartilage as traumatic or degenerative: a review of clinical accuracy. J Hand Surg Eur. 2017;42(4):357–62. https://doi.org/10.1177/1753193416684658.
45. Rein S, Krenn V, Hagert E, et al. Degeneration of the articular disc in the human triangular fibrocartilage complex. Arch Orthop Trauma Surg. 2021;141(4):699–708. https://doi.org/10.1007/s00402-021-03795-2.
46. Oneson SR, Scales LM, Timins ME, Erickson SJ, Chamoy L. MR imaging interpretation of the palmer classification of triangular fibrocartilage complex lesions. Radiographics. 1996;16(1):97–106. https://doi.org/10.1148/radiographics.16.1.97.
47. Vezeridis PS, Yoshioka H, Han R, Blazar P. Ulnar-sided wrist pain. Part I: anatomy and physical examination. Skeletal Radiol. 2010;39(8):733–45. https://doi.org/10.1007/s00256-009-0775-x.

Hip

48. Barry NN, McGuire JL. Acute injuries and specific problems in adult athletes. Rheum Dis Clin N Am. 1996;22:531–49.
49. Beatty T. Osteitis pubis in athletes. Curr Sports Med Rep. 2012;11(2):96–8. https://doi.org/10.1249/JSR.0b013e318249c32b. PMID: 22410702
50. Byrd JW, Jones KS. Arthroscopic femoroplasty in the management of cam-type femoroacetabular impingement. Clin Orthop Relat Res. 2009;467:739–46.
51. Caudill P, Nyland J, Smith C, Yerasimides J, Lach J. Sports hernias: a systematic literature review. Br J Sports Med. 2008;42(12):954–64. https://doi.org/10.1136/bjsm.2008.047373. Epub 2008 Jul 4
52. Ejnisman L, Philippon M, Lertwanich P. Femoroacetabular impingement: the femoral side. Clin Sports Med. 2011;30:369–77.
53. Elattar O, Choi HR, Dills VD, Busconi B. Groin injuries (athletic Pubalgia) and return to play. Sports Health. 2016;8(4):313–23. https://doi.org/10.1177/1941738116653711. Epub 2016 Jun 14. PMID: 27302153; PMCID: PMC4922526
54. Emara K, Samir W, Motasem el H, Ghafar KA. Conservative treatment for mild femoroacetabular impingement. J Orthop Surg (Hong Kong). 2011;19:41–5.
55. Ganz R, Parvizi J, Beck M, Leunig M, Nötzli H, Siebenrock KA. Femoroacetabular impingement: a cause for osteoarthritis of the hip. Clin Orthop Relat Res. 2003;417:112–20.
56. Gerhardt MB, Romero AA, Silvers HJ, Harris DJ, Watanabe D, Mandelbaum BR. The prevalence of radiographic hip abnormalities in elite soccer players. Am J Sports Med. 2012;40:584–8.
57. Groh MM, Herrera J. A comprehensive review of hip labral tears. Curr Rev Musculoskelet Med. 2009;2(2):105–17. https://doi.org/10.1007/s12178-009-9052-9. Epub 2009 Apr 7. PMID: 19468871; PMCID: PMC2697339
58. Hickman JM, Peters CL. Hip pain in the young adult: diagnosis and treatment of disorders of the acetabular labrum and acetabular dysplasia. Am J Orthop. 2001;30:459–67.

59. Hicks BL, Lam JC, Varacallo M. Piriformis syndrome. 2022 Sep 4. In: StatPearls [Internet]. Treasure Island: StatPearls Publishing; 2022 Jan–. PMID: 28846222.
60. Hunt D, Clohisy J, Prather H. Acetabular tears of the hip in women. Phys Med Rehabil Clin N Am. 2007;18(3):497–520.
61. J Rehabil Res Dev. Author manuscript; available in PMC 2015 Sep 28. Published in final edited form as: J Rehabil Res Dev. 2014;51(10):1515–24. https://doi.org/10.1682/JRRD.2013.09.0211.
62. Katz JN, Arant KR, Loeser RF. Diagnosis and treatment of hip and knee osteoarthritis: a review. JAMA. 2021;325(6):568–78. https://doi.org/10.1001/jama.2020.22171. PMID: 33560326; PMCID: PMC8225295
63. Kelly BT, Weiland DE, Schenker ML, Philippon MJ. Arthroscopic labral repair in the hip: surgical technique and review of the literature. Arthroscopy. 2005;21:1496–504.
64. LeBlanc KE, LeBlanc KA. Groin pain in athletes. Hernia. 2003;7:68–71.
65. Lewis CL, Sahrmann SA. Acetabular labral tears. Phys Ther. 2006;86:110–21. [PubMed] [Google Scholar] [Ref list]
66. Matsuda DK, Carlisle JC, Arthurs SC, Wierks CH, Philippon MJ. Comparative systematic review of the open dislocation, mini-open, and arthroscopic surgeries for femoroacetabular impingement. Arthroscopy. 2011;27:252–69.
67. Murphy NJ, Eyles JP, Hunter DJ. Hip osteoarthritis: etiopathogenesis and implications for management. Adv Ther. 2016;33(11):1921–46. https://doi.org/10.1007/s12325-016-0409-3. Epub 2016 Sep 26. PMID: 27671326; PMCID: PMC5083776
68. Musick SR, Varacallo M. Snapping Hip syndrome. [Updated 2022 Sep 4]. In: StatPearls [Internet]. Treasure Island: StatPearls Publishing; 2022 Jan-. Available from: https://www.ncbi.nlm.nih.gov/books/NBK448200/
69. Noakes TD, Smith JA, Lindberg G, Wills CE. Pelvic stress fractures in long distance runners. Am J Sports Med. 1985;13:120–3.
70. Nolton EC, Ambegaonkar JP. Recognizing and managing snapping hip syndrome in dancers. Med Probl Perform Art. 2018;33(4):286–91.
71. Nötzli HP, Wyss TF, Stoecklin CH, Schmid MR, Treiber K, Hodler J. The contour of the femoral head-neck junction as a predictor for the risk of anterior impingement. J Bone Joint Surg Br. 2002;84:556–60.
72. O'Connell MJ, Powell T, McCaffrey NM, O'Connell D, Eustace SJ. Symphyseal cleft injection in the diagnosis and treatment of osteitis pubis in athletes. AJR Am J Roentgenol. 2002;179:955–9.
73. Paajanen H, Brinck T, Hermunen H, Airo I. Laparoscopic surgery for chronic groin pain in athletes is more effective than nonoperative treatment: a randomized clinical trial with magnetic resonance imaging of 60 patients with sportsman's hernia (athletic pubalgia). Surgery. 2011;150(1):99–107. https://doi.org/10.1016/j.surg.2011.02.016. Epub 2011 May 5. PMID: 21549403
74. Pavlov M, Nelson TL, Warren RF, Torg JS, Burnstein AH. Stress fractures of the pubic ramus. A report of twelve cases. J Bone Joint Surg Am. 1982;64:1020–5.
75. Reid D. The management of greater trochanteric pain syndrome: a systematic literature review. J Orthop. 2016;13(1):15–28.
76. Shah JP, Thaker N, Heimur J, Aredo JV, Sikdar S, Gerber L. Myofascial trigger points then and now: a historical and scientific perspective. PM R. 2015;7(7):746–61. https://doi.org/10.1016/j.pmrj.2015.01.024. Epub 2015 Feb 24. PMID: 25724849; PMCID: PMC4508225
77. Schilders E, Bismil Q, Robinson P, O'Connor PJ, Gibbon WW, Talbot JC. Adductor-related groin pain in competitive athletes. Role of adductor enthesis, magnetic resonance imaging, and entheseal pubic cleft injections. J Bone Joint Surg Am. 2007;89:2173–8.
78. Verrall GM, Slavotinek JP, Fon GT. Incidence of pubic bone marrow oedema in Australian Rules football players: relation to groin pain. Br J Sports Med. 2001;35:28–33.
79. Weller JL, Comeau D, Otis JAD. Myofascial pain. Semin Neurol. 2018;38(6):640–3. https://doi.org/10.1055/s-0038-1673674. Epub 2018 Dec 6. PMID: 30522139
80. Werner J, Hägglund M, Waldén M, Ekstrand J. UEFA injury study: a prospective study of hip and groin injuries in professional football over seven consecutive seasons. Br J Sports Med. 2009;43:1036–40.

Leg/Ankle/Foot

81. Sillanpää P, Dirisamer F, Arendt EA, Dejour D, Zaffagnini S. Patellofemoral pain, instability, and arthritis : clinical presentation, imaging, and treatment. 2nd ed. Springer; 2020.
82. Pazzinatto MF, de Oliveira SD, Pappas E, Magalhães FH, de Azevedo FM. Is quadriceps H-reflex excitability a risk factor for patellofemoral pain? Med Hypotheses. 2017;108:124–7. https://doi.org/10.1016/j.mehy.2017.08.019.
83. Boling MC, Nguyen A-D, Padua DA, Cameron KL, Beutler A, Marshall SW. Gender-specific risk factor profiles for patellofemoral pain. Clin J Sport Med. 2021;31(1):49–56. https://doi.org/10.1097/JSM.0000000000000719.
84. Miccio S, Berardi A, Tofani M, Galeoto G. Conservative rehabilitation treatments of iliotibial band syndrome: a systematic review. Muscles Ligaments Tendons J. 2021;11(1):29–40. https://doi.org/10.32098/mltj.01.2021.04.
85. Pezzullo DJ, Whitney SL, Irrgang JJ. Patellar tendonitis: Jumper's knee. J Sport Rehabil. 2016;1:56–68.
86. Witvrouw E, Bellemans J, Lysens R, Danneels L, Cambier D. Intrinsic risk factors for the development of patellar tendinitis in an athletic population. A two-year prospective study. Am J Sports Med. 2001;29(2):190–5. https://doi.org/10.1177/03635465010290021201.
87. Cooper G (Physiatrist). Essential physical medicine and rehabilitation. Humana Press; 2006.
88. Holden S, Olesen JL, Winiarski LM, Krommes K, Thorborg K, Hölmich P, Rathleff MS. Is the prognosis of Osgood-Schlatter poorer than anticipated? A prospective cohort study with 24-month follow-up. Orthop J Sports Med. 2021;9(8):1–9.
89. Kuehnast M, Mahomed N, Mistry B. Sinding-Larsen-Johansson syndrome. South African J Child Health. 2012;6(3):90–2. https://doi.org/10.7196/SAJCH.423.
90. Choudhary M, Richa SG, Gaur AK. Effect of ultrasound-guided pes anserine bursa injection on knee scores: a comparative study. J Orthop Spine. 2022;10(1):24–9. https://doi.org/10.4103/JOASP.JOASP_19_21.
91. Cuccurullo S. Physical medicine and rehabilitation board review. Springer Publishing Company, Inc; 2004.
92. Saeki J, Nakamura M, Nakao S, et al. Ankle and toe muscle strength characteristics in runners with a history of medial tibial stress syndrome. J Foot Ankle Res. 2017;10:1–6. https://doi.org/10.1186/s13047-017-0197-2.
93. Trew CAJ, Kocialkowski C, Parsons T, Barton T. Predictors of positive outcomes and a scoring system to guide management after fasciotomy for chronic exertional compartment syndrome. Orthop J Sports Med. 2022;10(6):1–6. https://doi.org/10.1177/23259671221101328.
94. Belikan P, Färber L-C, Abel F, Nowak TE, Drees P, Mattyasovszky SG. Incidence of calcaneal apophysitis (Sever's disease) and return-to-play in adolescent athletes of a German youth soccer academy: a retrospective study of 10 years. J Orthop Surg Res. 2022;17(1):83. https://doi.org/10.1186/s13018-022-02979-9.
95. Michelson JD, Bernknopf JW, Charlson MD, Merena SJ, Stone LM. What is the efficacy of a nonoperative program including a specific stretching protocol for flexor hallucis longus tendonitis? Clin Orthop Relat Res. 2021;479(12):2667–76. https://doi.org/10.1097/CORR.0000000000001867.
96. Niek van Dijk C. Anterior and posterior ankle impingement. Foot Ankle Clin. 2006;11(3):663–83. https://doi.org/10.1016/j.fcl.2006.06.003.
97. Kudaş S, Dönmez G, Işık Ç, Çelebi M, Çay N, Bozkurt M. Posterior ankle impingement syndrome in football players: case series of 26 elite athletes. Acta Orthop Traumatol Turc. 2016;50(6):649–54. https://doi.org/10.1016/j.aott.2016.03.008.
98. Maffulli N, Aicale R, Migliorini F, et al. The double posteromedial portals endoscopy for posterior ankle impingement syndrome in athletes. J Orthop Traumatol. 2022;23:28. https://doi.org/10.1186/s10195-022-00651-w.

Rheumatoid Arthritis

5

Nilofar Syed and Fatemeh Ezzati

Introduction

Rheumatoid arthritis (RA) is a chronic autoimmune disorder that predominantly causes inflammation of the joints. The joint involvement is typically symmetrical, and usually leads, if uncontrolled, to destruction of the joints due to erosion of the bone and cartilage and development of joint deformities.

Epidemiology

The prevalence of RA is approximately 1% of the population in the USA [1]. The average age of onset is 40–60 years old, and it occurs 2–3 times more frequently in women compared to men. The specific etiology of RA is unknown, but it is felt to be multifactorial due to genetic and environmental associations. HLA-DRB1 is a genetic risk factor associated with the development of RA [2]. There are also environmental factors associated with RA, which include smoking, obesity, and silicosis.

Clinical Manifestations

Rheumatoid arthritis frequently presents as a gradual onset of symmetric polyarticular involvement; however, some patients can present with an acute onset, palindromic symptoms, and even monoarticular disease. RA is classically associated with pain and swelling of the small joints in the hands and feet. The

N. Syed (✉) · F. Ezzati
Division of Rheumatology, University of Texas Southwestern Medical Center, Dallas, TX, USA
e-mail: nilofar.syed@utsouthwestern.edu

C. E. Noe (ed.), *Musculoskeletal Pain*,
https://doi.org/10.1007/978-3-031-86057-7_5

metacarpophalangeal (MCP), proximal interphalangeal (PIP), and metatarsophalangeal (MTP) joints are typically involved early in the disease with joint swelling, erythema, and warmth. Other joints, such as the wrists, elbows, shoulders, knees, and ankles, can also be affected. Patients can also have myalgias, fatigue, and generalized weakness associated with their joint disease.

Patients with palindromic rheumatism have recurrent attacks of monoarticular, polyarticular arthritis, or tendonitis, which may last hours to days, with symptom-free periods that may last from days to months. About 28–67% of these patients will eventually develop a well-defined rheumatic disease, mainly RA, but some of the remaining patients develop systemic lupus erythematosus (SLE) and other systemic disorders.

Chronic joint inflammation can lead to reduced range of motion and deformities of the joints such as ulnar deviation of the fingers. Swan neck deformity is caused by hyperextension of the proximal interphalangeal joints (PIP) with flexion of the distal interphalangeal joints (DIP). Boutonniere deformity occurs due to flexion contracture of the PIP and extension of the DIP joints. Patients can also develop soft tissue rheumatoid nodules on the extensor surfaces.

Diagnostic Evaluation

A combination of clinical findings, laboratory data, and imaging is important to diagnose early cases of RA. Auto-antibodies have been used to guide the diagnosis of various autoimmune diseases. Rheumatoid factor (RF) is present in 70–80% of patients with RA with a sensitivity of 69% and a specificity of 85%. RF is usually measured as an IgM antibody that binds to the Fc part of IgG [3].

RF may also be found in patients with chronic infections, and healthy individuals, albeit in low titers. It is seen in 5% of the general population and up to 15% of elderly people. It may also be present in other connective tissue diseases such as systemic lupus erythematosus, Sjogren syndrome, scleroderma, and granulomatosis with polyangiitis.

Higher RF titers (>100 IU/mL) are more likely to be RA; however, RF levels do not correlate with disease activity. High titers are associated with more severe RA and risk for extra-articular manifestations [4].

Antibodies against CCP (also called ACPA) have also proven to be a useful diagnostic tool, especially in early patients with RA [4]. ACPA is present in 70-80% of patients with a sensitivity of 67% and a specificity of 95%. The specificity is greater in patients with higher titers of ACPAs. Another test, anti-mutated citrullinated vimentin, gives similar results to ACPA and is used as an alternative in some laboratories [5].

If both RF and ACPA are positive, the sensitivity and specificity of the diagnosis increase substantially. RF and ACPA are present for months to years before the onset of clinical arthritis [6].

Acute Phase Reactants

Elevations of the erythrocyte sedimentation rate (ESR) and/or C-reactive protein (CRP) level are consistent with the presence of an inflammatory state, such as RA. However, these markers may be elevated in other inflammatory and infectious processes, other rheumatologic disorders, pregnancy, and malignancy. Moreover, in active RA, the ESR or CRP may be elevated only in 60% of patients. Thus, when elevated, these biomarkers may support an RA diagnosis, but their positive and negative predictive values are limited [7].

Classification Criteria

According to the *2010 ACR/EULAR classification criteria for RA* [8], the definite RA is based upon the presence of synovitis in at least one joint, the absence of an alternative diagnosis that better explains the synovitis and the achievement of a total score of at least 6 (of a possible 10) from the individual scores in four domains.

The highest score achieved in each domain is used for this calculation. These domains and their values are:

- *Number and site of involved joints*
  - 2–10 large joints (from among shoulders, elbows, hips, knees, and ankles) = 1 point
  - 1–3 small joints (from among the metacarpophalangeal joints, proximal interphalangeal joints, second through fifth metatarsophalangeal joints, thumb interphalangeal joints, and wrists) = 2 points
  - 4–10 small joints = 3 points
  - Greater than 10 joints (including at least 1 small joint) = 5 points.
- *Serological abnormality* (rheumatoid factor or anti-citrullinated peptide/protein antibody)
  - Low positive (above the upper limit of normal [ULN]) = 2 points.
  - High positive (greater than three times the ULN) = 3 points.
- *Elevated acute phase response* (erythrocyte sedimentation rate [ESR] or C-reactive protein [CRP]) above the ULN = 1 point
- *Symptom duration at least six weeks* = 1 point

Note that these are classification criteria, so their primary purpose is used in clinical studies of patients with RA, including clinical trials.

The new criteria were noted to better predict the probability of RA, have the same sensitivity as the previous criteria for the diagnosis of RA, and have a higher specificity as well as a higher negative predictive value [9].

Imaging in RA

Conventional Imaging

Progressive radiographic changes occur in the affected joints of patients with active disease, including periarticular osteopenia, joint space narrowing, and bone erosion.

Conventional radiographs of the hands and feet have traditionally been used in the diagnosis, management, and monitoring of patients with rheumatoid arthritis (RA); however, it is not sensitive enough to detect changes such as bone erosions in early disease. Erosion of cortical bone is known to be the main characteristic of erosive RA [10]. Radiographs still represent a useful technique despite its limitations, because of easy availability, reliability, and low cost.

Ultrasound

Ultrasonography is another sensitive tool to evaluate soft tissues and can distinguish synovial thickening, the presence of fluid in joints, bursae, and tendon sheaths, and basic abnormalities of tendons, ligaments, entheses, and small erosions. Synovial hypertrophy is a characteristic of chronic synovitis and is regarded as a very reliable biomarker of aggressive RA [10]. The combination of higher spatial resolution and multi-planar exploration makes the US superior when compared to conventional radiography. Ultrasound-guided joint and soft tissue aspirations allow for increased accuracy of the RA diagnosis. Ultrasound has the following disadvantages: it requires additional training, is examiner-dependent, and is not suited for the assessment of deep joints.

Magnetic Resonance Imaging

Magnetic resonance imaging can assess all the structures affected by RA. These include soft tissue, cartilage, and bones. This imaging method is highly sensitive and can detect early erosions up to 3 years before they may be seen with conventional radiography. The decreased signal from the bone marrow on T1-weighted images and enhancement of the marrow after administration of gadolinium-based contrast is interpreted as bone inflammation. The presence of marrow edema on MRI is predictive of the later development of erosive disease [11]. The presence of MRI-detected synovial proliferation also correlates with the later development of bone erosions [12]. Disadvantages of MRI include the high cost and being less available. Further research is needed to optimize the roles of these advanced imaging modalities in RA to provide cost-effective management for patients.

Differential Diagnosis

Joint pain involving the hands is a common clinical presentation for a variety of conditions. When patients fail to meet criteria or have atypical features for RA, other etiologies should be considered.

Viral Polyarthritis

Several viral infections may cause acute viral polyarthritis. Viral infections such as rubella, parvovirus B19, hepatitis B virus (HBV), hepatitis C virus (HCV), chikungunya virus, or Zika virus can cause an acute polyarthritis syndrome that may be mistaken for the inflammatory polyarthritis of RA. Serologic testing can help identify patients with HBV, HCV, or human parvovirus B19 in some individuals with early disease.

Other Systemic Rheumatic Diseases

Systemic lupus erythematosus (SLE), Sjögren's syndrome, dermatomyositis (DM) and antisynthetase syndrome, and overlap syndromes such as mixed connective tissue disease can cause inflammatory arthritis. In contrast to RA, these disorders are generally characterized by the presence of other systemic features, such as rashes, dry mouth and dry eyes, oral ulcers, Raynauds, and by various autoantibodies not often seen in RA.

Inflammatory Osteoarthritis

A minority of osteoarthritis manifests inflammatory osteoarthritis, distinguished by having inflammatory synovitis and erosive changes in multiple PIP and DIP joints of the hands. Such patients are usually seronegative, and the radiograph erosions of inflammatory OA are distinctly different ("gullwing" central erosions) from those seen in RA.

Crystal Arthritis

Calcium pyrophosphate deposition disease can cause inflammatory symmetric polyarthritis that resembles RA. CPPD is confirmed by arthrocentesis, identification of calcium pyrophosphate crystals, radiographic chondrocalcinosis, and negative serologic tests for RF or ACPA. Chronic untreated gout can also present with polyarticular arthritis resembling RA. Synovial fluid revealing monosodium urate crystals would differentiate these two conditions. The presence of tophi on physical examination, the lack of detection of serologic markers of RA, and the characteristic appearance of gouty erosions are also useful in distinguishing RA from polyarticular gout.

Spondyloarthritis

Reactive arthritis, inflammatory bowel disease, and psoriatic arthritis can be associated with inflammatory arthritis. Reactive arthritis often presents as monoarthritis or oligoarthritis in large joints, such as the knees, and RA may occasionally present like this as well. History of recent urethritis or enteric infection, asymmetric involvement of joints, symptoms or signs of enthesopathy, and the presence of human leukocyte antigen (HLA)-B27 are more suggestive of reactive arthritis. While IBD-related arthritis is more commonly large-joint oligoarticular arthritis or spondyloarthritis with sacroiliitis, patients with IBD may infrequently develop peripheral polyarthritis with prominent involvement of smaller joints that can be mistaken for RA. Psoriatic arthritis can be difficult to distinguish from RA because symmetric polyarthritis can be observed in both disorders. We generally make the diagnosis of psoriatic arthritis in such patients who also have psoriasis; however, in some patients, the joint symptoms of psoriatic arthritis may precede the onset of skin disease by a few years. Such patients should be evaluated for other signs more characteristic of psoriatic arthritis, such as nail changes, sausage fingers, enthesitis, or a family history of psoriasis.

Polymyalgia Rheumatica

Polymyalgia rheumatica (PMR) can sometimes be mistaken for RA in patients presenting with more limited arthritis over the age of 50. Unlike RA, PMR is usually associated with marked myalgias in the shoulders and hips, and joint involvement tends to be milder, more limited, and more often asymmetric. Although both conditions are associated with prolonged morning stiffness, high acute phase reactants, and joint pain, PMR is distinguished from RA with prominence of limb girdle (shoulders, hips) involvement, muscle pain, and lack of RF or ACPA antibodies.

Myelodysplasia

Patients with myelodysplastic syndrome sometimes develop inflammatory polyarthritis that mimics RA [13]. The arthritis may precede the diagnosis of myelodysplasia in at least half of the patients. Symptoms associated with this condition include anemia, other cytopenias, or elevated acute phase reactants despite control of the arthritis.

Hypermobility Syndrome and Fibromyalgia

Patients with hypermobility and fibromyalgia mainly have pain in their joints rather than stiffness or swelling. The hypermobility syndromes are associated with hyperextensible joints. Fibromyalgia is associated with tender points at multiple sites including articular and non-articular sites and chronic widespread pain. Both conditions lack synovitis in the exam.

Neither of them is associated with significant titers of RF or ACPAs or with elevated levels of acute phase reactants.

Treatment of Rheumatoid Arthritis in Adults

The goals of treatment for RA are to control active synovitis and to prevent the progression of the disease which can lead to joint damage. Treatment regimens consist of combinations of pharmaceuticals, weight-bearing exercise, and educating patients about the disease. Treatments are generally customized to a patient's needs. This includes factors such as disease progression, the joints involved, age, overall health, occupation, compliance, and education about the disease.

Nonpharmacologic and Preventive Therapies

This needs a multidisciplinary team approach. Patients may continue to experience problems with physical function, as well as emotional and social function that are not adequately addressed by providing drug therapy alone.The major elements of nonpharmacologic therapy include:

- Patient education and psychosocial interventions.
- Physical and occupational therapy.
- Proper nutrition and diet.

Patient Education and Counseling

Education and counseling are important in the management of RA. Multidisciplinary pain and disease management programs can be beneficial. They may provide general information about the disease, teaching skills for the management of chronic illness, strategies for preserving joint function, and enhanced social support. Various psychosocial interventions can benefit patients with RA. Research has shown that psychosocial interventions and cognitive–behavioral therapy can reduce symptoms of fatigue and brain cognitive dysfunction.

Physical and Occupational Therapy

Patients should be evaluated and receive education and instruction from an expert in physical therapy to optimize strength and joint function. Different modalities of physical therapy depend on the severity of inflammation and include resistance exercise programs or progressive high-intensity strength training (for mild arthritis) versus isometric exercises for moderate arthritis. Patients with severe inflammation may need resting splints, rather than resistance or aerobic exercise, for joint immobilization until the disease is better controlled with medication.

Nutrition and Dietary Therapy

Many patients with active RA suffer from reduced appetite and poor dietary intake. Attempts to overcome these difficulties should, therefore, be a part of the management of the disease [14]. Patients should be encouraged to eat a healthy diet that is high in vegetables and fruits and associated with a reduced risk of cardiovascular disease in observational studies.

Approach to Drug Therapy

All patients diagnosed with active rheumatoid arthritis should receive disease-modifying antirheumatic drugs (DMARDs) to prevent or arrest disease-related injury.

The treatment of rheumatoid arthritis is directed toward the control of synovitis and the prevention of joint injury. In patients whose condition is resistant to an initial course of treatment with a nonbiologic DMARD, timely adjustments in the treatment regimen are required to achieve effective disease control and prevent damage to the joints [15].

Early treatment of RA is important to prevent permanent damage to the joints. The 2015 ACR guidelines on the management of RA recommend a treat-to-target approach to achieve control of the disease. Treatment of early RA, which is defined as a disease duration <6 months, involves starting with traditional disease-modifying antirheumatic drugs (DMARDs). Methotrexate is recommended for initial monotherapy and a typical starting dose of 15mg weekly is used. The dose can be titrated up to a maximum of 25mg weekly if the disease is not controlled. Common adverse effects of methotrexate include hepatotoxicity, bone marrow suppression, GI toxicity such as nausea, vomiting, oral ulcers, and hair loss. Folic acid supplementation is recommended while taking methotrexate to help with side effects.

If there is continued moderate to high disease activity despite monotherapy, then more aggressive therapy is warranted. This can include a combination of DMARD therapy or the use of biological agents. Other DMARD therapies include leflunomide, hydroxychloroquine, and sulfasalazine. Leflunomide is an alternative to methotrexate with a similar side effect profile and can be used in patients with chronic kidney disease. Hydroxychloroquine and sulfasalazine are less effective as monotherapy and are typically only used in combination with other DMARDs. Hydroxychloroquine and sulfasalazine when combined with methotrexate are referred to as triple therapy. There is evidence that triple therapy has similar effectiveness as methotrexate in combination with a TNF inhibitor [16]. Given the side effect profile of DMARDs such as methotrexate, frequent lab monitoring is recommended including complete blood count, liver transaminase levels, and serum creatinine levels often every 3 months.

Biologics, also known as biological DMARDs, are rapidly effective in retarding the progression of the joint damage caused by RA. They are considered to be a more "direct, defined, and targeted" method of treatment [17]; however, they are associated with more side effects including increased risk of infection. Some of the commonly used medications are as follows:

1. Tumor necrosis factor (TNF) is a messenger protein that promotes inflammation in joints. Etanercept, infliximab, adalimumab, golimumab, and certolizumab are all TNF inhibitors that prevent the recruitment of the cells that cause inflammation, bringing rapid symptom relief. They are often used in combination with other DMARDs, especially MTX. TNF inhibitors are contraindicated in patients with congestive heart failure or demyelinating diseases.
2. IL-6 blockers like tocilizumab and sarilumab block IL-6, a chemical messenger of inflammation. They are administered via intravenous infusion given monthly or via weekly subcutaneous injections.
3. Abatacept is a biological medication that works by blocking T cell activation. This is given as an intravenous infusion once a month or subcutaneously once a week.
4. JAK inhibitors have a different mechanism of action and work by blocking Janus kinases within cells, which are enzymes of inflammation. For this reason, it is known as a JAK inhibitor. These medications are used for patients who have not been effectively treated with MTX. Tofacitinib, which was the first medication approved in this group in 2012 is taken orally twice daily, alone or in combination with MTX.

   Other medications in this group are baricitinib and upadacitinib.
5. Rituximab is useful in RA because it depletes the B cells responsible for inflammation and the production of abnormal antibodies.

References

1. Almutairi KB, Nossent JC, Preen DB, Keen HI, Inderjeeth CA. The prevalence of rheumatoid arthritis: a systematic review of population-based studies. J Rheumatol. 2021;48(5):669–76.
2. van Drongelen V, Holoshitz J. Human leukocyte antigen-disease associations in rheumatoid arthritis. Rheum Dis Clin North Am. 2017;43(3):363–76.
3. Nishimura K, Sugiyama D, Kogata Y, Tsuji G, Nakazawa T, Kawano S, Saigo K, Morinobu A, Koshiba M, Kuntz KM, Kamae I, Kumagai S. Meta-analysis: diagnostic accuracy of anti-cyclic citrullinated peptide antibody and rheumatoid factor for rheumatoid arthritis. Ann Intern Med. 2007;146(11):797–808.
4. Nielsen SF, Bojesen SE, Schnohr P, et al. Elevated rheumatoid factor and long-term risk of rheumatoid arthritis: a prospective cohort study. BMJ. 2012;345:e5244.
5. Kroot EJ, de Jong BA, van Leeuwen MA, et al. The prognostic value of anti-cyclic citrullinated peptide antibody in patients with recent-onset rheumatoid arthritis. Arthritis Rheum. 2000;43(8):1831–5.
6. Luime JJ, Colin EM, Hazes JM, Lubberts E. Does anti-mutated citrullinated vimentin have additional value as a serological marker in the diagnostic and prognostic investigation of patients with rheumatoid arthritis? A systematic review. Ann Rheum Dis. 2010;69(2):337. Epub 2009 Mar 15

7. Nielen MM, van Schaardenburg D, Reesink HW, van de Stadt RJ, van der Horst-Bruinsma IE, de Koning MH, Habibuw MR, Vandenbroucke JP, Dijkmans BA. Specific autoantibodies precede the symptoms of rheumatoid arthritis: a study of serial measurements in blood donors. Arthritis Rheum. 2004;50(2):380–6.
8. Cush JJ. Rheumatoid arthritis: early diagnosis and treatment. Rheum Dis Clin North Am. 2022;48(2):537–47.
9. Aletaha D, Neogi T, Silman AJ, et al. 2010 Rheumatoid arthritis classification criteria: an American College of Rheumatology/European League Against Rheumatism collaborative initiative. Arthritis Rheum. 2010;62:2569.
10. Mota HLM, Laurindo IMM, dos Santos Neto LL, et al. Imaging diagnosis of early rheumatoid arthritis. Rev Bras Rheumatol. 2012;52(5):757–66.
11. McQueen FM. Bone marrow edema and osteitis in rheumatoid arthritis: the imaging perspective. Arthritis Res Ther. 2012;14:224–36.
12. McQueen FM, Stewart N, Crabbe J, Robinson E, Yeoman S, Tan PL, McLean L. Magnetic resonance imaging of the wrist in early rheumatoid arthritis reveals progression of erosions despite clinical improvement. Ann Rheum Dis. 1999;58(3):156.
13. Mekinian A, Braun T, Decaux O, Falgarone G, et al. Inflammatory arthritis in patients with myelodysplastic syndromes: a multicenter retrospective study and literature review of 68 cases. Medicine (Baltimore). 2014;93(1):1.
14. Cleland LG, Hill CL, James MJ. Diet and arthritis. Baillieres Clin Rheumatol. 1995;9(4):771–85.
15. Anderson JJ, Wells G, Verhoeven AC, Felson DT. Factors predicting response to treatment in rheumatoid arthritis: the importance of disease duration. Arthritis Rheum. 2000;43(1):22–9.
16. O'Dell JR, Mikuls TR, Taylor TH, et al. Therapies for active rheumatoid arthritis after methotrexate failure. N Engl J Med. 2013;369(4):307.
17. Bullock J, Rizvi SAA, Saleh AM, Ahmed SS, Do DP, Ansari RA, Ahmed J. Rheumatoid arthritis: a brief overview of the treatment. Med Princ Pract. 2018;27(6):501–7.

Soft Tissue Pain

6

Alejandro J. Carruyo, Peter Y. Yi, Biral T. Patel, and Robert S. Ackerman

Introduction and Diagnostic Evaluation of Soft Tissue Pain

The following conditions are amongst the most difficult to diagnose and treat, given their lack of specificity within the history-taking process and physical examination. Despite this, knowledge of the following disease processes can aid physicians in establishing diagnosis and place the patient on a path of relief. When dealing with soft tissue pain, it is essential to retain a broad differential diagnosis that includes nervous, degenerative, traumatic, inflammatory, iatrogenic, and idiopathic causes. Below is a concise summary of the initial presentations of the discussed conditions.

- Myofascial pain syndrome (MPS) is characterized by deep, aching, or throbbing hyperirritable spots within muscles and fascia, known as trigger points. These trigger points are often accompanied by muscle stiffness, reduced range of motion, and referred pain in various areas. MPS can result from chronic micro-stressors due to repetitive activities, leading to discomfort and functional limitations.

A. J. Carruyo
School of Medicine, Duke University, Durham, NC, USA

P. Y. Yi
Division of Pain Medicine, Department of Anesthesiology, Duke University Medical Center, Durham, NC, USA

B. T. Patel (✉)
Division of Pain Management, Department of Anesthesiology and Pain Management, University of Texas Southwestern Medical Center, Dallas, TX, USA
e-mail: biral.patel@utsouthwestern.edu

R. S. Ackerman
Morsani College of Medicine, University of South Florida, Tampa, FL, USA

Division of Interventional Pain Medicine, Department of Anesthesiology, Moffitt Cancer Center and Research Institute, Tampa, FL, USA

C. E. Noe (ed.), *Musculoskeletal Pain*,
https://doi.org/10.1007/978-3-031-86057-7_6

- Fibromyalgia is a complex and challenging-to-treat condition, characterized by tender points, chronic soft tissue pain, and mood and sleep disturbances. The pathophysiology of FM involves a combination of genetic, neurobiological, immune, and environmental factors, with central sensitization playing a key role in the perception of pain.
- Cervical whiplash is a common injury resulting from rapid acceleration-deceleration forces applied to the neck. It can lead to a spectrum of clinical presentations, ranging from mild discomfort to chronic pain and disability.
- Chronic cervical dystonia, or spasmodic torticollis, is a movement disorder characterized by involuntary contractions of neck muscles, resulting in abnormal posturing and repetitive twisting or writhing movements of the head. Its etiology involves various neurobiological, neurochemical, and neuroanatomical factors, including genetic mutations and medication-induced effects.
- Notalgia paresthetica is a rare and poorly understood condition causing recurrent pruritus, thought to be of neurological origin. Its precise cause remains unclear, but cutaneous nerve entrapment is a possible contributing factor.
- Greater trochanteric pain syndrome is a disabling condition involving lateral hip pain and tenderness over the greater trochanter of the femur. The pathophysiology includes mechanical, inflammatory, and degenerative processes, affecting tendons, bursae, and muscles around the hip.
- Gluteal bursitis, and other forms is characterized by inflammation of the greater trochanter bursae of the femur. Repetitive activities, viral prodromes, or trauma can lead to inflammation and pain in the lateral hip region.
- Piriformis syndrome involves compression or irritation of the sciatic nerve by the piriformis muscle, leading to posterior hip pain and radiating symptoms down the posterior thigh. Proper recognition of this syndrome is essential due to its overlapping features with other gluteal and hip conditions.

Myofascial Pain Syndrome

Introduction

Myofascial pain syndrome (MPS) is a regional pain disorder that leads to pain in select locations within muscles and their fascia.

Initial Presentation

Hallmark pain from MPS is often described as deep, aching, or throbbing hyperirritable spots, or trigger points, within select locations of the body, including the trapezius muscles, erector capitis, rhomboids, sternocleidomastoid, and scalene muscles within the neck. Trigger points also commonly occur in the lower body, where the erector spinae, quadratus lumborum, gluteus minimus, and medius, as well as the tensor fasciae latae are frequently involved. These spots are often accompanied by taught bands of muscle. Radiation of pain along the band of muscle can occur, along with burning or tingling that may arise from local nervous tissue entrapment. Sensory stimulation from trigger points can contribute to headaches, autonomic phenomena, and referred pain specific to the musculature involved. For example, trigger points palpation in the trapezius muscles can refer to pain in the upper neck, periauricular area, and ipsilateral forehead. MPS can be a result of chronic micro-stressors that incur on the affected musculature due to repeated exercise and occupational or habitual activities. Patients may experience muscle stiffness and a reduced range of motion in the affected area, making it challenging to perform activities of daily living (ADLs). In some cases, muscle weakness may also be present [1–3].

Anatomical Considerations and Pathophysiology

In MPS, prolonged or repetitive muscle contractions lead to the accumulation of metabolic waste products, reduced blood flow, and oxygen deprivation in the affected muscles. These conditions create a local environment conducive to the formation of trigger points. Taut bands within trigger points contain sarcomeres that remain in a state of sustained contraction, resulting in a palpable nodule or tight band. Psychosocial factors, such as stress, anxiety, and depression, can influence the pathophysiology of MPS. Psychological distress can contribute to muscle tension and altered pain processing, exacerbating the development and persistence of trigger points. In turn, the presence of chronic pain from MPS can impact an individual's emotional well-being and quality of life, creating a complex interplay between physical and psychological factors [4, 5].

Physical Examination

Physical exam findings consistent with MPS include reproduction or exacerbation of pain when applying pressure to the affected muscles or trigger points. When trigger points are stimulated or compressed, patients may experience pain that radiates to distant areas of the body, consistent with the referred pain pattern for the palpated muscle. Increased muscle tension and nodules may be noted, as well as weakness in affected musculature. Changes in posture may be noted in patients to compensate for muscular discomfort, decreased range of motion, or weakness [2–4, 6, 7].

Differential Diagnosis

Physicians should note that although referred pain due to converging sensory innervation with the muscles and other parts of the body occurs in MPS, radicular pain that is selective to one or more dermatomes or muscular weakness that is selective to myotomes or the bilateral proximal musculature is not commonly seen. Patients suspected of MPS should be evaluated based on their clinical presentation and physical examination against fibromyalgia, cervical neuropathies, cervical radiculopathy, cervical trauma/whiplash-associated disorders (WAD), myopathies, or other rheumatological conditions. If clinical presentation is ambiguous, the physician should note that MPS does not often present with any secondary metabolic or anatomic abnormalities like that of radiologic evidence of cervical nerve entrapment, increased ESR and CRP, rashes or cutaneous eruptions, correction of symptoms with corticosteroids, or chronic pain outside of trigger points [1].

Treatment

Like many chronic pain conditions, pain management specialists should look to multimodal approaches to pain relief and treatment, especially in the setting of MPS. Trigger point injections with saline or botulinum toxin can provide patients with short-term relief. Primary and longitudinal treatment of MPS should involve physical therapy and rehabilitation correcting postural compensation/poor posture, exercise of muscles involved, passive stretching, and manual trigger point release. Psychotherapy for the management of stress and emotional contributions to trigger points should be explored when physical management is insufficient. Finally, pharmacological therapy is available and aims to reduce muscle tension and the creation of trigger points. Medications used to treat pain include the use of NSAIDs or acetaminophen, whether oral or topical, muscle relaxers like that of tizanidine or Flexeril, and gabapentanoids. Heating or cooling pads can also be utilized by patients [1, 6–8].

Fibromyalgia

Introduction

Fibromyalgia (FM) is a complex and often difficult-to-treat condition, broadly characterized by tender spots or points, mood and sleep disturbances, chronic and diffuse soft tissue pain, and little evidence of organically driven disease. Due to this presentation, clinicians often have trouble in recognizing and treating the condition, while a select few regard the condition as functional, psychogenic, or psychosomatically driven [9].

Epidemiology

FS is more prevalent in women than men, with a female-to-male ratio of approximately 3:1 to 9:1, while affecting about 2–4% of the general population in developed countries. The prevalence of FS increases with age, peaking in middle-aged individuals, but the condition can affect patients of any age group, including adolescents and, less frequently, children. Prevalence of the condition is thought to be increased within certain subgroups, including individuals with rheumatological or psychiatric disease. Interestingly, familial and twin studies have suggested a hereditary component in FM [9–11].

Pathophysiology

The pathophysiology of fibromyalgia is complex and not fully understood. It involves a combination of genetic, neurobiological, immune, and environmental factors that contribute to the development and maintenance of the condition. While the discussion of the mechanistic contributions to the condition is rich and expansive within the current body of literature, the literature highlights central sensitization, aberrations in normal neurotransmission, autonomic dysfunction, and genetic/environmental factors as the likely culprits. Finally, gender discrepancy in the prevalence of the condition raises questions about potential hormonal and genetic contributing factors [1, 11, 12].

Initial Presentation

The onset of FM pain can be gradual or sudden, while patients may recall a trigger, such as physical trauma (e.g., car accident, fall), an infection, or significant psychological stress, which appears to precede the development of symptoms. For others, symptoms slowly built up over time, becoming increasingly widespread and persistent. Pain is typically generalized and commonly affects the neck, shoulders, upper and lower back, hips, thighs, and knees. Patients often describe a "body-wide" pain, which may include aching, burning, stabbing, or shooting sensations. Allodynia or hyperalgesia may be noted in patients. The pain may be described as "deep" or "diffuse," and patients often have difficulty pinpointing specific areas of pain. Physical overexertion, repetitive movements, and prolonged standing or sitting may worsen symptoms. Changes in weather, sleep disturbances, and high levels of stress can also trigger pain flares. Alleviating factors include rest, gentle stretching, and engaging in low-impact exercises, such as swimming. Heat application may also be noted to help symptoms in history. Finally, other affective and psychosocial symptoms are common, including fatigue, sleep disturbances, cognitive difficulties (often referred to as "fibro fog"), and headaches. Presentation of FM symptoms for 3 months or longer without any other likely cause(s), along with concordant physical examination, is a diagnostic requirement for the condition [9–11].

Physical Examination

FM is most notable for widespread tender points or spots. The American College of Rheumatology (ACR) has outlined diagnostic criteria for tender points in FM. The ACR notes the following points, bilateral and without relatively significant joint pain:

1. Occiput: At the suboccipital muscle insertions (2 points).
2. Low cervical: At the anterior aspect of the intertransverse spaces of C5-C7 (2 points).
3. Trapezius: At the midpoint of the upper border (2 points).
4. Supraspinatus: At the origins, just above the scapular spine (2 points).
5. Second rib: At the second costochondral junctions (2 points).
6. Lateral epicondyle: 2 cm distal to the epicondyles (2 points).
7. Gluteal: In the upper outer quadrants of the buttocks (2 points).
8. Greater trochanter: Posterior to the trochanteric prominence (2 points).
9. Knee: At the medial fat pad proximal to the joint line (2 points).

Patients should have at least 11 of the 18 tender points bilaterally for the diagnosis of FM. Of note, tender points may be experienced in other locations not outlined by the ACR metrics, along with affective or psychiatric disturbances as mentioned above [9–11, 13, 14].

Differential Diagnosis

FM does not present with any aberrations in metabolic, endocrine, or kidney function tests and often highlights normal CBC, CMP, TSH, ESR, CRP, CK, etc. Adequate ruling out of other conditions is a necessity for the diagnosis of FM. Myofascial pain syndrome (MPS), as discussed in this chapter, should be ruled out. In short, MPS presents with trigger points as opposed to tender points, while the former is less frequently bilateral. Referred pain from trigger points is often encountered, and the condition scantly presents with psychosocial symptoms, as in FM. Patients with psychiatric disease should have the condition adequately evaluated and treated if deemed appropriate by specialists. Furthermore, consideration of rheumatological conditions like that of proximal or thyroid-related myopathies, polymyalgia rheumatica, systemic lupus erythematosus. Note that coexisting conditions may be present in FM patients, such as osteoarthritis, axial back pain or lumbar radiculopathy, and migranous headaches. Lastly, FM patients should be evaluated for somatic or functional disorders like somatic symptoms disorder, inflammatory bowel syndrome, and sleep disorders [1].

Treatment

After the diagnosis of FM has been rendered, multimodal treatment should be initiated. This includes patient education about the condition and coping strategies. Evaluation with a psychotherapist for the establishment of care and intervention with cognitive behavioral therapy is beneficial. Adequate treatment of comorbidities should be done, as conditions such as obesity, osteoarthritis, and poor sleep can either impair treatment with low-impact exercise or exacerbate the condition. Low-impact cardiovascular exercise should be initiated, while FM patients can have the most difficulty in initiating the program. Initial pharmacologic therapy should include the use of low-dose tricyclic antidepressants (TCA) or other serotonin-norepinephrine reuptake inhibitors (SNRIs) as monotherapy. Poor response to monotherapy, as commonly experienced in FM patients seeing pain management specialists, requires assessment of therapy adherence or escalation of dosing or the use of joint pharmacotherapy. Additional targets include the musculature, while low-dose (1–4 mg) cyclobenzaprine nightly has been noted to aid in pain, sleep, and fatigue. In patients with prominent sleep issues, the use of gabapentinoids or other alpha-delta fiber ligands, such as pregabalin, may aid in sleep and contribute to pain relief. Little evidence supports the use of NSAIDs or opiates, which may be associated with increased harm. Other therapies with emerging evidence include the use of naltrexone, vitamin D supplementation, and lidocaine infusions [1, 10, 15, 16].

Cervical Whiplash

Introduction

Cervical whiplash is a relatively common injury resulting from rapid acceleration-deceleration forces applied to the neck, occurring due to motor vehicle trauma, sports-related collisions, falls, or other traumatic events. Whiplash-associated disorders (WAD) encompass a spectrum of clinical presentations ranging from mild discomfort to debilitating chronic pain and disability [17–19].

Pathophysiology

During a whiplash event, the head is rapidly forced into hyperextension and, subsequently, flexion, leading to tissue injury due to the sudden stretching and compression forces. The primary structures affected include the cervical muscles and ligaments, leading to traumatic myositis, enthesitis, and cervical tendinopathy. Fracture of zygapophyseal (facet) joints of the cervical vertebrae, which can contribute to short- or long-term axial neck pain from micro- or macro-fractures; intervertebral disc herniation or injury from axial, rostral-dorsal, or lateral shearing forces; spinal cord, mixed spinal nerve, or peripheral cervical nerve injury or entrapment, secondary to disc herniation, bony injury with protrusion, or muscle/tendinous strain. Collectively, injury to one or more structures outlined can lead to painful sequalae characterized as chronic cervical whiplash pain or WAD [17–20].

Initial Presentation

Patients with acute cervical whiplash present with a variety of symptomology that typically develops within 24 hours of the traumatic event. Common initial presentations include neck pain, stiffness, and reduced range of motion, while headaches, dizziness, tinnitus, and cognitive difficulties can be concomitant. Detailed history of the traumatic event is crucial for diagnosis, as well as any preexisting history that can predispose or exacerbate neck injury. Furthermore, key history involving any motor or sensory deficits should be elicited, as prompt recognition of spinal cord compression or spinal nerve injury is favorable for treatment and prognosis. Physicians should gather plain and computed tomography images in the acute setting and establish the degree of stability of the neck prior to the removal of the cervical spine collar [6, 17–21].

Chronic pain secondary to whiplash injury can present similarly to acute pain, while secondary symptoms like cervicogenic headaches, dizziness, tinnitus, or cognitive difficulties are less common in the chronic phase; although, these findings may be present with concomitant post-concussion syndrome along with mood and sleep disturbances. The presence of pain and associated symptoms for more than 3 months is diagnostic for chronic cervical whiplash pain or WAD. Injury severity in the acute setting can directly correlate with the prevalence of chronic symptoms, while chronic states can contribute to loss of productivity and emotional distress [19, 21, 22].

Physical Examination

Patients with chronic cervical whiplash may continue to experience reduced neck mobility. The range of motion (ROM) in all directions (flexion, extension, rotation, lateral bending) may be limited or painful to perform. The loss of flexibility is often more pronounced in the direction that initially caused the injury. Chronic whiplash can lead to myofascial pain syndrome (MPS), characterized by the presence of trigger points in the neck and shoulder muscles amongst other locations. These tender points may refer pain to other areas of the body and can be identified during palpation. See the MPS section for a detailed discussion of the condition and diagnostic considerations. Prolonged muscle disuse or compensatory patterns due to pain can lead to weakness in the cervical and lower neck regions. Muscle spasms may persist in the chronic phase while exacerbating pain and contributing to further limitation of motion. Chronic whiplash can result in altered joint mechanics and dysfunctional movement patterns in the cervical spine, while chronic inflammation and poor healing of soft tissues can lead to the formation of adhesions within the muscles and fascia of the neck. The practitioner should elicit Spurling's sign to test for cervical radiculopathy and test digital strength, including finger abduction, opposition, and digital flexion, to potentially localize an affected myotome. Sensory deficits should be noted as well, with reference to the digital and upper limb dermatomal patterns. Finally, a manual neck distraction test can also be used to evaluate for cervical neuroforaminal stenosis [6, 18].

Differential Diagnosis

Cervical whiplash and cervical strain are often similarly described, although the former is caused by shearing forces secondary to rapid acceleration and deceleration, while the latter is due to habitual or occupational demands on the neck (most commonly because of recurrent or prolonged neck extension) or milder trauma. As discussed in the physical examination section, MPS may be a concomitant condition, while distinction may arise with the presence of taut bands, referred pain, and alleviation with massage and trigger point release. Radiculopathy, discogenic pain, herniated cervical disc, or vertebral dislocation should be ruled out. Red flag symptoms that signal acute process and need for urgent workup include fever or chills, worsening or abnormal intensity headache, history of immunosuppression, chronic glucocorticoid use, history of intravenous drug use, progressive changes in neurologic physical exam including weakness, gait instability, ataxia, perianal anesthesia, bladder, or bowel incontinence. For patients who have persistent pain for more than 6–12 weeks, imaging is encouraged [6, 18, 23].

Treatment

While treatment in the acute phase may differ from the chronic, here we will discuss in detail the stepwise and multimodal treatment reasoning for the treatment of chronic whiplash-related pain. Firstly, patients should be educated on the condition and its course while being taught or referred to a specialist who can assist in pain coping strategies or psychiatry for concomitant depression, anxiety, or post-traumatic stress disorder (PTSD). After imaging has been gathered, physical therapy should be implemented, allowing for direct muscle manipulation and an exercise regimen. Medication history, response to prior treatment, adherence to treatments, and treatment lapses should be elicited. Patients arriving for care in the realm of chronic pain management have frequently tried pharmacologic therapies; however, this may not signify adequate or optimal dosing, scheduling, and adherence. First-line pharmacologic therapies include the use of NSAIDs or analgesics like ibuprofen, naproxen, or acetaminophen. The combination of oral and topical therapies can provide greater relief while maintaining patients on the minimum effective dose.

Escalation in pharmacologic care can be done with muscle relaxers like cyclobenzaprine, tizanidine, or baclofen. Additional treatments for concomitant neuropathic pain include the use of gabapentin, duloxetine, or TCAs. Finally, pain refractory to multiple measures can be treated with weak and low-dose opiates like that of tramadol. Interventional options include dry needling or trigger point injections, while chronic disc or facet joint dysfunction or injury can be treated surgically [17, 21, 24].

Chronic Cervical Dystonia

Introduction

Chronic cervical dystonia, also known as spasmodic torticollis, is a movement disorder categorized by involuntary contractions of neck muscles, leading to abnormal posturing and repetitive twisting or writhing movements of the head. It is a relatively rare condition that can have a profound impact on the quality of life of affected individuals [25, 26].

Pathophysiology

While the exact etiology of cervical dystonia is poorly understood, extensive research showcases various neurobiological, neurochemical, and neuroanatomical factors contributing to its development while broadly categorized into genetic, medication-induced, environmental, and idiopathic causes. Certain gene variants are implicated with an increased risk of dystonia, including TOR1A (DYT1), THAP1 (DYT6), and CIZ1, among others. These genes are involved in diverse cellular functions, such as protein folding, gene regulation, and synaptic transmission. The mutations in these genes likely disrupt the normal functioning of basal ganglia circuits, leading to abnormal motor control and dystonic movements. High-potency first-generation neuroleptics, particularly haloperidol, and fluphenazine, have a greater propensity to cause extrapyramidal symptoms, including acute dystonia or tardive dyskinesias. Chronic use of neuroleptics can change dopaminergic receptor sensitivity in the basal ganglia. Neuroleptics primarily block dopamine D2 receptors, reducing dopaminergic activity. In the chronic state of decreased dopaminergic neurotransmission, compensatory upregulation of D2 receptors occurs to restore neurotransmitter balance. Upregulation of D2 receptors, particularly in the striatum, contributes to the development of tardive dyskinesia [26–29].

Epidemiology

The estimated prevalence of cervical dystonia ranges from 5 to 15 cases per 100,000 individuals in the general population, while the incidence is challenging to accurately determine and is estimated to range from 0.5 to 2 per 100,000 individuals per year [30].

Initial Presentation and Physical Examination

The presentation of cervical dystonia can vary among individuals and is characterized by the onset of involuntary and sustained contractions of neck musculature, leading to abnormal head postures and movements. The symptoms may start gradually, often insidiously, and progress over time. Of note, concomitant abnormal contractures can be noticed in other locations, especially in the setting of medication-induced dystonia or movement disorders. History of the present illness is crucial for accurate diagnosis and management [25, 26].

The hallmark feature of the condition is the abnormal posturing of the head while exhibiting head rotation (torticollis), head tilt (laterocollis), or forward head flexion (anterocollis). The head movements are usually involuntary, repetitive, or sustained, leading to the characteristic dystonic postures mentioned. Neck pain due to sustained muscle contractions and abnormal postures is often experienced while significantly impacting daily activities and quality of life. As mentioned above, certain conditions can contribute to dystonia, including long-term use of neuroleptics, movement disorders like Parkinson's or Huntington's disease, or recent trauma to the affected area. Lastly, dystonia can be secondary to various neurological conditions, such as stroke, brain tumors, or brain infections. These underlying neurological pathologies can affect the basal ganglia-thalamo-cortical motor circuitry, leading to dystonic movements [27–29, 31].

Differential Diagnosis

Other conditions can be mistaken for cervical dystonia, and specific conditions should be kept in mind and ruled out by the practitioner to adequately diagnose the cervical dystonia.

Essential tremor (ET) is a common movement disorder characterized by bilateral, symmetric, and postural tremors that occur during voluntary movements. It can involve the head and neck region, leading to head tremor, which may be mistaken for cervical dystonia. Observation of the tremor pattern during posture and action can help differentiate essential tremors from cervical dystonia. Tremors are typically rhythmic and oscillatory, while dystonic movements are sustained and often have a directional component. ET may temporarily improve with small doses of alcohol, while cervical dystonia usually does not show this response.

Parkinson's disease is a progressive neurodegenerative disorder characterized by bradykinesia, resting tremor, rigidity, and postural instability. Some patients with Parkinson's disease may develop "antecollis," which is an abnormal forward flexion of the neck. Differentiating the sustained, twisting movements of cervical dystonia from the characteristic resting tremor and bradykinesia of Parkinson's disease is crucial. Parkinson's disease usually responds to levodopa, leading to improvements in motor symptoms. Cervical dystonia does not typically show a robust response to levodopa. Cervical radiculopathy or structural spinal pathologies can cause neck pain and abnormal head postures. X-rays or MRIs of the cervical spine can identify any anatomical abnormalities, such as herniated discs or spinal stenosis which can contribute to abnormal posturing. Lastly, some medications, such as neuroleptic drugs and other dopaminergic antagonists or serotonergic agonists, can induce acute dystonic reactions that mimic cervical dystonia. A detailed history of medication use, including neuroleptic drugs, can help identify any drug-induced dystonic reactions [25, 26, 28, 29, 32, 33].

Treatment

The treatment of cervical dystonia aims to improve symptoms, enhance functional abilities, and enhance the quality of life of affected individuals. The approach varies based on the underlying cause of dystonia, with different treatment strategies tailored to primary (idiopathic) dystonia and secondary causes.

Botulinum toxin injections are first-line measures for primary cervical dystonia. These injections are administered directly into the affected neck muscles to block nerve signals and reduce muscle contractions. Repeated treatments are typically required for sustained benefit. Although not as effective as botulinum toxin injections, some oral medications may provide symptomatic relief for primary cervical dystonia. These include anticholinergic drugs (e.g., trihexyphenidyl), muscle relaxants (e.g., baclofen), benzodiazepines, and dopaminergic agents (e.g., levodopa or dopamine receptor agonists) in the setting of neurodegenerative disease or chronic neuroleptic use. However, response to these medications can vary, and their use is often limited due to side effects. Lastly, for individuals with severe and refractory primary cervical dystonia, deep brain stimulation may be considered and has shown promising results in alleviating dystonic symptoms [29, 32, 33].

Notalgia Paresthetica

Notalgia paresthetica is a rare and poorly understood condition, thought to be of neurological origin, that leads to recurrent pruritus. Causes of the condition are not completely elucidated, although prevailing ideas include cutaneous nerve entrapment of posterior rami of T2 or levels below. Presentation of the condition includes pruritus adjacent to the medial border of the scapula and skin overlying lower trapezius muscles. Discoloration of the involved skin may be seen, attributed to recurrent scratching and lichenification as a result; however, cutaneous discoloration is not a diagnostic requirement. Past history of trauma to the spine or back may be noted, although the condition may alternatively occur idiopathically. Differential diagnosis is broad due to the relative rarity of this condition as compared to other chronic causes of pruritus. Consider dermatologic conditions like xerosis, psoriasis, eczematous eruptions, contact dermatitis, urticaria, lichen planus, infection folliculitis, or scarring. Treatment for this condition is appropriate after ruling out more likely dermatological conditions, and patients should seek dermatological consultation. The current body of literature scantly expands on evidence-based tactics; however, initial studies highlight the use of topical agents as preferred methods compared to oral medications. The use of topical capsaicin, pramoxime, lidocaine, ketamine, and amitriptyline; however, symptoms resurface with treatment cessation. Other therapies include the use of oral anticonvulsants or alpha-delta ligands like that of gabapentin or pregabalin. Lastly, nerve block or cutaneous injection with local anesthetic or botulinum toxin can be therapeutic in the short term [34–37].

Greater Trochanteric Pain Syndrome

Introduction

Greater trochanteric pain syndrome (GTPS) is a common and disabling condition characterized by lateral hip pain and tenderness over the greater trochanter of the femur. It encompasses a group of disorders affecting the tendons, bursae, and muscles around the hip, leading to pain and functional limitations [38].

Pathophysiology

The pathophysiology of GTPS involves multiple factors, including mechanical, inflammatory, and degenerative processes. It often involves gluteal tendinopathy, where the gluteus medius and gluteus minimus tendons become degenerated or inflamed. Additionally, trochanteric bursitis, which is inflammation of the bursa overlying the greater trochanter, can contribute to pain and tenderness in the lateral hip region. Other factors include muscle imbalances, iliotibial band tightness, and hip instability, all of which can contribute to abnormal biomechanics and increased stress on the greater trochanter, gluteal ligaments, greater trochanteric bursa, and iliotibial band [38–40].

Epidemiology

GTPS is a prevalent condition, particularly in middle-aged and elderly individuals. It affects both men and women, although it is more common in women. The incidence and prevalence of GTPS increase with age, with degenerative changes in tendons and bursae becoming more common as individuals age. It is also frequently associated with other musculoskeletal conditions, such as hip osteoarthritis, low back pain, and iliotibial band syndrome [41].

Clinical Presentation

Patients with GTPS typically present with lateral hip pain, which may radiate to the thigh or buttock. The pain is often described as aching or burning and is exacerbated by activities involving hip movement, such as walking, climbing stairs, or lying on the affected side. Patients may also experience tenderness over the greater trochanter upon palpation, and they may have difficulty lying on the affected side due to pain [38–40].

Physical Examination

The Ober test evaluates the tightness of the iliotibial band (ITB). The patient lies on their unaffected side with the affected knee flexed, and the examiner attempts to passively abduct the affected leg. A positive test suggests ITB tightness contributing to GTPS [38–40].

Diagnostic Considerations and Differential Diagnosis

Diagnosing GTPS involves ruling out other conditions that may present with similar hip pain. The differential diagnosis includes hip osteoarthritis, which can cause pain in a similar location, especially during weight-bearing activities. Limited range of motion, joint stiffness, and crepitus on palpation, with radiographs showcasing joint space narrowing, osteophyte formation, and subchondral sclerosis, are diagnostic for the condition. Lumbar spine pathologies, such as foraminal stenosis, facet joint arthritis, and herniated discs, can refer to pain in the hip region. A thorough physical examination and imaging studies can help differentiate between lumbar spine-related pain and GTPS. Tears in the hip labrum may present with similar symptoms to GTPS. Diagnostic imaging, such as MRI or hip arthroscopy, can aid in the diagnosis. Piriformis syndrome can cause buttock, hip, hamstring, and calf pain due to compression of the sciatic nerve. Clinical examination, including stretching maneuvers and imaging, can help distinguish between GTPS and piriformis syndrome. Pain from other sources, such as the sacroiliac joint or knee, may refer to the hip area. Isolated greater trochanteric bursa inflammation is most consistent with gluteal bursitis, as described below [38–40].

Diagnostic Evaluation

The diagnosis of GTPS is primarily clinical and based on the patient's history and physical examination. Imaging studies like X-rays and magnetic resonance imaging (MRI) may be ordered to rule out other hip pathologies or to evaluate for gluteal tendon tears. Diagnostic ultrasound can also be valuable in assessing the tendons and bursae around the greater trochanter.

Treatment

The treatment of GTPS aims to alleviate pain, improve function, and address underlying contributing factors. Initial treatment often involves rest, activity modification, and physical therapy to strengthen hip abductor muscles and correct muscle imbalances.

NSAIDs, such as ibuprofen or naproxen, can be used to reduce pain and inflammation associated with GTPS. These medications are often prescribed in the acute phase or during flare-ups, while they may play a lesser role in the chronic state. Local corticosteroid injections can provide short-term pain relief for patients with GTPS. The injection is typically administered into the greater trochanteric bursa or at the point of maximal tenderness. Targeted physical therapy is a cornerstone of conservative management for GTPS. Therapeutic exercises aim to strengthen hip abductor and external rotator muscles, improve hip biomechanics, and correct muscle imbalances. Specific exercises may include side-lying leg lifts, clamshells, hip bridges, and functional training to address functional limitations. Applying ice packs or warm compresses to the affected hip can help reduce pain and inflammation. Other minimally invasive therapies (including ultrasound or transcutaneous electrical nerve stimulation (TENS), extracorporeal shock wave therapy (ESWT), platelet-rich plasma (PRP) injections, gluteal fascial plane blocks, and orthodontics) are options for patients whose pain is refractory to initial therapies. Lastly, surgical intervention, including bursectomy or tendon repair, in situations in which structural abnormalities are present or as a last resort measure [38, 42–45].

Gluteal Bursitis

Introduction

Gluteal bursitis (GB), also referred to as trochanteric bursitis, is a common condition characterized by inflammation of the greater trochanter bursae of the femur. While these bursae act as cushions between tendons, muscles, and bone, reducing friction during hip movements, repetitive activities, viral prodromes, or trauma can contribute to inflammation and pain. GB can lead to lateral hip pain and tenderness, often aggravated by activities involving hip movements, such as walking, running, or climbing stairs. While many intersections exist between the condition and other pain disorders that include bursitis, like that of greater trochanteric pain syndrome (GTPS), these sections will assist in the differentiation and alternative treatment therapies for these conditions [40, 46, 47].

Initial Presentation

Patients with GB typically present with lateral hip pain and tenderness over the greater trochanteric region. The pain may be described as aching or sharp and is commonly aggravated by activities that involve hip movements, such as rising from a chair, walking up or down stairs, or lying on the affected side. Patients may report a history of repetitive activities or direct trauma to the hip as a potential trigger, as well as physical exertion or prolonged pressure on the hip, such as from sleeping on the affected side. GB is a subset condition of greater trochanteric pain syndrome, but other conditions that present similarly include gluteus medius/minimus tendinopathy, iliotibial band syndrome, and hip labral tears. Both GB and GTPS may present with tenderness over the greater trochanter; however, in GB, tenderness is localized to the inflamed bursae, whereas in GTPS, the tenderness may be more widespread, involving other structures like the gluteal tendons or iliotibial band [38, 40, 46–48].

Physical Examination

On physical examination, tenderness is typically elicited over the greater trochanter of the femur. Palpation of this area may reproduce the patient's pain, helping to confirm the diagnosis. Additionally, range of motion testing of the hip joint and looking for other signs of hip pathology or muscle tightness that may be more consistent with GTPS or iliotibial band syndrome [38, 40, 46–48].

Differential Diagnosis

When evaluating a patient with lateral hip pain, it is essential to consider other potential causes to rule out conditions that may mimic gluteal bursitis. As mentioned before, GB exists within a continuum of conditions that affect the hip and underpinnings, including inflammation, ligamentous strain or tightness, muscular discomfort, bursitis, and pain with motion. Conditions that can be mistaken include GTPS, iliotibial band syndrome, gluteal tendonitis, lumbar radiculopathy, sacroiliitis, hip labral tears, and hip osteoarthritis [38, 40, 46–48].

Diagnostic Considerations

The diagnosis of GB is mainly clinical, based on the patient's history and physical examination findings. Diagnostic imaging, such as X-rays or MRI, may be ordered to rule out other hip pathologies or assess for structural abnormalities. In some cases, a diagnostic bursal injection with a local anesthetic may be used to confirm the diagnosis. If the patient experiences significant pain relief after the injection, it supports the diagnosis of gluteal bursitis [38, 46, 48].

Treatment

The treatment of GB focuses on reducing inflammation, alleviating pain, and improving function. Initial management is similar to that of GTPS or other syndromes characterized by bursitis. These treatments are typically conservative and may include avoiding activities that exacerbate symptoms, such as excessive running or prolonged sitting, and the use of heat or ice on the affected area can help reduce pain. NSAIDs may be prescribed to lessen pain and inflammation in the setting of acute flares, while in cases of persistent or severe bursitis, a corticosteroid injection may be administered directly into the inflamed bursa to reduce inflammation and alleviate pain. Like GTPS, ultrasound or shock wave therapy may prove beneficial. Using a cane or crutches may be helpful in reducing pressure on the affected hip during the acute phase of GB. In rare cases where conservative measures are ineffective, surgical options, such as bursectomy (removal of the inflamed bursa) or tendon repair, may be considered [38, 49–51].

Ischial Bursitis

Introduction

Ischial bursitis is a condition characterized by inflammation of the ischial bursa, a small, fluid-filled sac located between the ischial tuberosity and the gluteus maximus tendon. It functions to reduce friction and cushion the area during hip movement. When inflamed, the bursa can cause pain and discomfort in the buttock region [47, 52].

Initial Presentation

Patients with ischial bursitis commonly present with a chief complaint of insidious-onset, posterior hip pain, predominantly concentrated within the ischiogluteal region. The pain is frequently described as an aching or sharp sensation, exacerbated by prolonged periods of sitting or direct pressure on the ischial tuberosity. Etiologically, patients may attribute the pain to overuse or injury of the hip region, although the majority often report a gradual development of symptoms without any specific event. Notably, discomfort may also be reported during sleep or while attempting to transition from a seated to a standing position, highlighting the potential role in the use or position of hip extensor musculature in the aggravation of the ischial bursa. Similarly, activities necessitating engagement of the hip extensors, such as climbing stairs or walking uphill, tend to exacerbate the symptoms [47, 52].

Physical Examination and Differential Diagnosis

Patients with ischial bursitis often report discomfort or pain during hip flexion and extension maneuvers. Gentle palpation of the ischiogluteal region and the ischial bursa, while the patient is in the lateral decubitus or prone position, should reproduce symptoms. Note that symptoms should not be reproduced with isolated flexion or extension of the knee joint. Such a reproduction of pain with stretching of the hamstrings could highlight other conditions like that of hamstring tendinopathy or iliotibial band syndrome. Sacroiliac joint testing should be performed with the FABER maneuver and distraction test, while positive testing can highlight sacroiliitis as a potential diagnosis. Lastly, ischial bursitis should not present with any radicular symptoms primary to the condition. Therefore, the presence of such radiculopathy should que physicians to look for other potential diagnoses or concomitant presentations [47, 52].

Treatment

Patient education constitutes the foundational step in the management of ischial bursitis, with emphasis on the relation between the motions of the hip and the potential exacerbation of symptoms. Physical therapy may prove beneficial to patients, as inflammation of the bursa may stem from chronically tight and flexed musculature that exerts increasing pressure and shearing forces on the bursa. Exercises to both strengthen and increase flexibility may prove beneficial. Like other inflammatory conditions discussed in this chapter, NSAIDs may prove beneficial in the short term and with acute flares of pain. Local corticosteroid injections prove both diagnostic and therapeutic. Lastly, as with other topics mentioned relating to the bursa, ultrasound or shockwave therapy, platelet-rich plasma injections, and surgery are provided to patients who are refractory to conservative and intermediate treatment options [38, 40, 42, 44].

Nerve Entrapment

Introduction

Nerve entrapment is an umbrella term for many conditions that involve injury, inflammation, or mechanical stress to one or more spinal or peripheral nerves. While the term is inclusive of the spinal nerves, its main clinical use is within the context of peripheral nerves and explains abnormal pain presentations due to peripheral nerve aberrations [53–55].

Pathophysiology

Peripheral nerves carry sensory, autonomic, and somatic impulses to and from the CNS. Aberrations in proper signaling, whether increased signaling, decreased signaling, or disorganized signaling, can lead to the sensation of painful or unpleasant stimuli. Nervous tissue damage can occur for a multitude of reasons, whether from trauma, burn, ischemia, radiative necrosis, mechanical compression, or chronic traction from the musculature. Thus, injury or irritation of nerves results in the perception of painful stimuli, allodynia, and hyperalgesia in the areas distal to the approximate area of "entrapment." Hence, all pain from nervous entrapment is a radiculopathy with potential dysesthesia [56–59].

Initial Presentation

There is no one presentation for patients with nervous entrapment. Anterior cutaneous nerve entrapment syndrome, as discussed in the abdominal wall chapter, is one such example where peripheral nerves innervating the abdominal wall musculature and cutaneous tissue are entrapped, contributing to pain, autonomic dysregulation, allodynia, or hyperalgesia. Lumbar and cervical radiculopathies, piriformis syndrome, slipping rib syndrome, peroneal neuropathy, and meralgia paresthetica are all commonly known diseases that involve nervous entrapment of some kind. It is worth mentioning that nervous entrapment can occur anywhere and is not selective towards peripheral nerves but also within the CNS, as in spinal stenosis or cranial nerve palsies due to trauma or mass effect [56, 60].

Physical Examination

Hallmark findings include distal unpleasant stimuli, whether pain, tingling, burning, etc., with potential motor and autonomic dysfunction. As in the case of peroneal neuropathy to the chronic and habitual crossing of the legs, burning and numbness may be replicated when asking the patient to keep legs crossed. Furthermore, neuropathy may be so severe that it could lead to some level of foot drop or tibialis anterior weakness [53, 57, 58].

Treatment

Local anesthetic injections targeting the suspected entrapment sites can be used to both confirm the diagnosis and treatment. However, the diagnostic accuracy of nerve blocks is variable, and false-positive or false-negative results can occur. Factors such as technical expertise, patient variability in response to injections, and the potential for transient symptom relief can impact the interpretation of diagnostic injections. Conservative medical treatments include the use of NSAIDs, gabapentinoids, or tricyclic antidepressants, while interventional treatment options include radiofrequency ablation, peripheral nerve stimulation, and surgical release of entrapped nerves as a last resort [61–64].

Piriformis Syndrome

Introduction

Piriformis syndrome is characterized by compression or irritation of the sciatic nerve by the piriformis muscle, leading to posterior hip pain and radiating symptoms down the thigh. Despite its prevalence, piriformis syndrome is often underdiagnosed, as it shares overlapping features with several other conditions affecting the gluteal and hip region, as discussed in this chapter [65–67].

Pathophysiology

The piriformis muscle is a deep, linearly shaped muscle located in the gluteal region, originating from the anterior surface of the sacrum and inserting onto the greater trochanter of the femur. The sciatic nerve typically courses through or beneath the piriformis muscle, and its proximity makes it vulnerable to compression or irritation. Muscle hypertonicity, spasm, or myofascial trigger points within the piriformis can lead to increased pressure on the sciatic nerve. Prolonged muscle tension can create a state of chronic compression. Activities that involve repetitive hip flexions, such as prolonged sitting or running, can increase tension in the piriformis muscle and worsen the symptoms. Additionally, improper or excessive exercise techniques, poor posture, or hip muscle imbalances can also contribute to the biomechanical stress on the sciatic nerve [65–67].

Initial Presentation

Patients with piriformis syndrome commonly present with posterior hip pain, frequently accompanied by radicular symptoms along the posterior thigh and potentially in the calf in the distribution of the greater peroneal nerve and posterior tibial nerve. The pain is often described as deep, dull, and achy, with episodic exacerbations. Patients frequently report difficulty in sitting or walking for prolonged periods, while the onset of presentation is often insidious. Patients may struggle to recall any specific inciting event or injury and may report a sense of muscle tightness or deep achiness in the gluteal region. Some individuals experience a subjective feeling of muscle spasms or knots within the piriformis muscle, which may be exacerbated by certain positions or activities. Lastly, this condition may present with a peripheral nerve propensity, meaning primary irritation of one component of the nerve, whether the peroneal or tibial component. This signifies that radiative symptoms may have a propensity to travel to the lateral or anterior calf (peroneal propensity) or down the posterior calf and into the ventral foot (posterior tibial propensity) [67–71].

Physical Examination and Differential Diagnosis

For this condition, the hip flexion and internal rotation should reproduce symptoms, as the piriformis muscle aids in the extension and external rotation of the hip. Therefore, flexion and internal rotation, individually or collectively, place the piriformis muscle in a stretched position that intensifies tension on the sciatic nerve. Radicular pain should be more generalized as compared to lumbar radicular pain, which is often limited to specific dermatomal patterns based on the location of foraminal stenosis or impingement. This is because the sciatic nerve contains nervous tissue from several levels; thus, the presence of more generalized or poorly localized radicular pain can assist in discerning from single-level radiculopathy when present. Additionally, ultrasound and MRI techniques may be utilized for visual confirmation of sciatic nerve compression by the piriformis [67–71].

Treatment

Physicians should educate patients about the underlying pathophysiology of the condition, emphasizing the compression or irritation of the sciatic nerve by the piriformis muscle. Physical therapy is a cornerstone in conservative management, with evidence supporting the use of specific exercises targeting the piriformis muscle and associated hip muscles to improve flexibility, reduce muscle tension, and alleviate pressure on the sciatic nerve. Piriformis muscle stretches, myofascial release techniques, and hip range of motion exercises are integral components of physical therapy interventions. NSAIDs are frequently prescribed as the first-line pharmacologic treatment for piriformis syndrome. Muscle relaxants may be considered in cases where there are significant muscle spasms or a recent history of trauma. Gabapentinoids may be considered in the short to intermediate term, although therapy is the most crucial component of treatment. While very seldom used, interventional techniques can be utilized only after ruling out other conditions and assuring adequate patient adherence to physical therapy regimens. Although injections into the piriformis are performed with anecdotal patient relief, there is scant evidence in the form of clinical trials available to evaluate their effectiveness. As such, activity modification and physical therapy remain the mainstays of treatment [68, 69, 71–73].

Treatment Summary

A

References

1. Borg-Stein J. Treatment of fibromyalgia, myofascial pain, and related disorders. Phys Med Rehabil Clin N Am. 2006;17(2):491–510, viii
2. Couppe C, Torelli P, Fuglsang-Frederiksen A, Andersen KV, Jensen R. Myofascial trigger points are very prevalent in patients with chronic tension-type headache – a double-blinded controlled study. Clin J Pain. 2007;23(1):23–7.
3. Skootsky SA, Jaeger B, Oye RK. Prevalence of myofascial pain in general internal medicine practice. West J Med. 1989;151(2):157–60.
4. Duarte FCK, West DWD, Linde LD, Hassan S, Kumbhare DA. Re-examining myofascial pain syndrome: toward biomarker development and mechanism-based diagnostic criteria. Curr Rheumatol Rep. 2021;23(8):69.

5. El-Essawy H. An investigation into the mechanism of "locking" in the myofascial pain dysfunction syndrome (MPD). Int J Oral Surg. 1975;4(2):69–72.
6. Ettlin T, Schuster C, Stoffel R, Bruderlin A, Kischka U. A distinct pattern of myofascial findings in patients after whiplash injury. Arch Phys Med Rehabil. 2008;89(7):1290–3.
7. Fernandez-De-Las-Penas C, Alonso-Blanco C, Cuadrado ML, Gerwin RD, Pareja JA. Myofascial trigger points and their relationship to headache clinical parameters in chronic tension-type headache. Headache. 2006;46(8):1264–72.
8. Hsieh LF, Hong CZ, Chern SH, Chen CC. Efficacy and side effects of diclofenac patch in treatment of patients with myofascial pain syndrome of the upper trapezius. J Pain Symptom Manag. 2010;39(1):116–25.
9. Goldenberg DL. Fibromyalgia syndrome. An emerging but controversial condition. JAMA. 1987;257(20):2782–7.
10. Winslow BT, Vandal C, Dang L. Fibromyalgia: diagnosis and management. Am Fam Physician. 2023;107(2):137–44.
11. Cole JA, Rothman KJ, Cabral HJ, Zhang Y, Farraye FA. Migraine, fibromyalgia, and depression among people with IBS: a prevalence study. BMC Gastroenterol. 2006;6:26.
12. Bennett RM. Emerging concepts in the neurobiology of chronic pain: evidence of abnormal sensory processing in fibromyalgia. Mayo Clin Proc. 1999;74(4):385–98.
13. Cassisi G, Sarzi-Puttini P. Consistency between the 2016 ACR criteria and a previous diagnosis or hypothesis of fibromyalgia in a specialised referral clinic. Clin Exp Rheumatol. 2023;41(6):1283–91.
14. Wolfe F, Smythe HA, Yunus MB, Bennett RM, Bombardier C, Goldenberg DL, et al. The American College of Rheumatology 1990 criteria for the classification of fibromyalgia. Report of the Multicenter Criteria Committee. Arthritis Rheum. 1990;33(2):160–72.
15. Tzadok R, Ablin JN. Current and emerging pharmacotherapy for fibromyalgia. Pain Res Manag. 2020;2020:6541798.
16. Atzeni F, Gerardi MC, Masala IF, Alciati A, Batticciotto A, Sarzi-Puttini P. An update on emerging drugs for fibromyalgia treatment. Expert Opin Emerg Drugs. 2017;22(4):357–67.
17. Carroll LJ, Holm LW, Hogg-Johnson S, Cote P, Cassidy JD, Haldeman S, et al. Course and prognostic factors for neck pain in whiplash-associated disorders (WAD): results of the bone and joint decade 2000–2010 task force on neck pain and its associated disorders. J Manip Physiol Ther. 2009;32(2 Suppl):S97–S107.
18. Kasch H, Bach FW, Stengaard-Pedersen K, Jensen TS. Development in pain and neurologic complaints after whiplash: a 1-year prospective study. Neurology. 2003;60(5):743–9.
19. Spitzer WO, Skovron ML, Salmi LR, Cassidy JD, Duranceau J, Suissa S, et al. Scientific monograph of the Quebec Task Force on Whiplash-Associated Disorders: redefining "whiplash" and its management. Spine (Phila Pa 1976). 1995;20(8 Suppl):1S–73S.
20. Kasch H, Bach FW, Jensen TS. Handicap after acute whiplash injury: a 1-year prospective study of risk factors. Neurology. 2001;56(12):1637–43.
21. Lord SM, Barnsley L, Wallis BJ, Bogduk N. Chronic cervical zygapophysial joint pain after whiplash. A placebo-controlled prevalence study. Spine (Phila Pa 1976). 1996;21(15):1737–44; discussion 44–5
22. Malfliet A, De Kooning M, Inghelbrecht E, Hachimi-Idrissi S, Willems B, Bernheim J, et al. Sex differences in patients with chronic pain following whiplash injury: the role of depression, fear, somatization, social support, and personality traits. Pain Pract. 2015;15(8):757–64.
23. Mehta RS, Arnold R. Evaluation of spinal cord compression #237. J Palliat Med. 2011;14(3):361–2.
24. Cote P, Wong JJ, Sutton D, Shearer HM, Mior S, Randhawa K, et al. Management of neck pain and associated disorders: a clinical practice guideline from the Ontario Protocol for Traffic Injury Management (OPTIMa) Collaboration. Eur Spine J. 2016;25(7):2000–22.
25. Stacy M. Epidemiology, clinical presentation, and diagnosis of cervical dystonia. Neurol Clin. 2008;26(Suppl 1):23–42.
26. Singer C, Velickovic M. Cervical dystonia: etiology and pathophysiology. Neurol Clin. 2008;26(Suppl 1):9–22.

27. Widschwendter CG, Hofer A. Antipsychotic-induced tardive dyskinesia: update on epidemiology and management. Curr Opin Psychiatry. 2019;32(3):179–84.
28. Dilks S, Xavier RM, Kelly C, Johnson J. Implications of antipsychotic use: antipsychotic-induced movement disorders, with a focus on tardive dyskinesia. Nurs Clin North Am. 2019;54(4):595–608.
29. Patel S, Martino D. Cervical dystonia: from pathophysiology to pharmacotherapy. Behav Neurol. 2013;26(4):275–82.
30. Defazio G, Jankovic J, Giel JL, Papapetropoulos S. Descriptive epidemiology of cervical dystonia. Tremor Other Hyperkinet Mov (N Y). 2013;3:tre-03-193-4374-2.
31. Agostino R, Berardelli A, Formica A, Accornero N, Manfredi M. Sequential arm movements in patients with Parkinson's disease, Huntington's disease and dystonia. Brain. 1992;115(Pt 5):1481–95.
32. Christie J. Cholinergic medication for antipsychotic-induced tardive dyskinesia. Issues Ment Health Nurs. 2019;40(12):1049–50.
33. Lu CS, Chen RS, Tsai CH. Double-blind, placebo-controlled study of botulinum toxin injections in the treatment of cervical dystonia. J Formos Med Assoc. 1995;94(4):189–92.
34. Robinson C, Downs E, De la Caridad GY, Nduaguba C, Woolley P, Varrassi G, et al. Notalgia paresthetica review: update on presentation, pathophysiology, and treatment. Clin Pract. 2023;13(1):315–25.
35. Haney B. Notalgia paresthetica: an underdiagnosed condition in primary care. Nurse Pract. 2021;46(9):40–6.
36. Akram A. Notalgia paresthetica: cervical spine disease and neuropathic pruritus. Cureus. 2021;13(1):e12975.
37. Mulkoglu C, Nacir B. Notalgia paresthetica: clinical features, radiological evaluation, and a novel therapeutic option. BMC Neurol. 2020;20(1):191.
38. Mallow M, Nazarian LN. Greater trochanteric pain syndrome diagnosis and treatment. Phys Med Rehabil Clin N Am. 2014;25(2):279–89.
39. Pumarejo Gomez L, Childress JM. Greater trochanteric pain syndrome. StatPearls. Treasure Island (FL) with ineligible companies. Disclosure: John Childress declares no relevant financial relationships with ineligible companies. 2023.
40. Pianka MA, Serino J, DeFroda SF, Bodendorfer BM. Greater trochanteric pain syndrome: evaluation and management of a wide spectrum of pathology. SAGE Open Med. 2021;9:20503121211022582.
41. Segal NA, Felson DT, Torner JC, Zhu Y, Curtis JR, Niu J, et al. Greater trochanteric pain syndrome: epidemiology and associated factors. Arch Phys Med Rehabil. 2007;88(8):988–92.
42. Brennan KL, Allen BC, Maldonado YM. Dry needling versus cortisone injection in the treatment of greater trochanteric pain syndrome: a noninferiority randomized clinical trial. J Orthop Sports Phys Ther. 2017;47(4):232–9.
43. Govaert LH, van Dijk CN, Zeegers AV, Albers GH. Endoscopic bursectomy and iliotibial tract release as a treatment for refractory greater trochanteric pain syndrome: a new endoscopic approach with early results. Arthrosc Tech. 2012;1(2):e161–4.
44. Furia JP, Rompe JD, Maffulli N. Low-energy extracorporeal shock wave therapy as a treatment for greater trochanteric pain syndrome. Am J Sports Med. 2009;37(9):1806–13.
45. Ferreira-Dos-Santos G, Hurdle MFB, Tran J, Eldrige JS, Clendenen SR, Agur AMR. Ultrasound-guided gluteal fascial plane block for the treatment of chronic refractory greater trochanteric pain syndrome – technique description and anatomical correlation study. Pain Med. 2022;23(11):1875–81.
46. Jones DL, Erhard RE. Diagnosis of trochanteric bursitis versus femoral neck stress fracture. Phys Ther. 1997;77(1):58–67.
47. Mears C, Rudra R, John A, Shi W. Inferior gluteal pain with sitting, unrelated to ischial bursitis. BMJ Case Rep. 2021;14(11):e246294.
48. Murphy J, Yusta-Zato J, Patel A, Davies AM, James SL, McBryde C, et al. The use of pelvic radiographs as a predictor for gluteal tendinopathy and bursitis. Hip Int. 2020;30(6):775–8.

49. Lustenberger DP, Ng VY, Best TM, Ellis TJ. Efficacy of treatment of trochanteric bursitis: a systematic review. Clin J Sport Med. 2011;21(5):447–53.
50. Fox JL. The role of arthroscopic bursectomy in the treatment of trochanteric bursitis. Arthroscopy. 2002;18(7):E34.
51. Ege Rasmussen KJ, Fano N. Trochanteric bursitis. Treatment by corticosteroid injection. Scand J Rheumatol. 1985;14(4):417–20.
52. Johnson DB, Varacallo M. Ischial Bursitis. StatPearls. Treasure Island (FL) ineligible companies. Disclosure: Matthew Varacallo declares no relevant financial relationships with ineligible companies. 2023.
53. Applegate WV. Abdominal cutaneous nerve entrapment syndrome. Am Fam Physician. 1973;8(3):132–3.
54. Srinivasan R, Greenbaum DS. Chronic abdominal wall pain: a frequently overlooked problem – practical approach to diagnosis and management. Am J Gastroenterol. 2002;97(4):824–30.
55. van Assen T, Brouns JAGM, Scheltinga MR, Roumen RM. Incidence of abdominal pain due to the anterior cutaneous nerve entrapment syndrome in an emergency department. Scand J Trauma Resusc Emerg Med. 2015;23:19.
56. Franz CK, Murthy NK, Malik GR, Kwak JW, D'Andrea D, Wolfe AR, et al. The distribution of acquired peripheral nerve injuries associated with severe COVID-19 implicate a mechanism of entrapment neuropathy: a multicenter case series and clinical feasibility study of a wearable, wireless pressure sensor. J Neuroeng Rehabil. 2022;19(1):108.
57. Aland RC, Sharp AC. Anomalous plantar intrinsic foot muscle attaching to the medial longitudinal arch: possible mechanism for medial nerve entrapment: a case report. J Med Case Rep. 2021;15(1):58.
58. Hibino N, Hamada Y. Bilateral proximal radial shaft fracture dislocations resulting from 2 separate injuries with the same mechanism, each associated with median nerve entrapment: a case report in a gymnast performing back hand springs: bony entrapment of median nerve at proximal radius. J Hand Microsurg. 2015;7(1):123–6.
59. Johansson AS, Isberg A, Isacsson G. A radiographic and histologic study of the topographic relations in the temporomandibular joint region: implications for a nerve entrapment mechanism. J Oral Maxillofac Surg. 1990;48(9):953–61; discussion 62
60. Hershfield NB. The abdominal wall. A frequently overlooked source of abdominal pain. J Clin Gastroenterol. 1992;14(3):199–202.
61. Minamikawa S, Ueshima E, Yokoi A, Ishida Y, Nakagishi Y. Conservative treatment for an anterior cutaneous nerve entrapment syndrome case. Pediatr Int. 2022;64(1):e14715.
62. Oosterbos C, Rasulic L, Rummens S, Kiekens C, van Loon J, Lemmens R, et al. Controversies in treatment strategies in patients with foot drop due to peroneal nerve entrapment: results of a survey among specialists. Brain Spine. 2022;2:100887.
63. Boelens OB, van Assen T, Houterman S, Scheltinga MR, Roumen RM. A double-blind, randomized, controlled trial on surgery for chronic abdominal pain due to anterior cutaneous nerve entrapment syndrome. Ann Surg. 2013;257(5):845–9.
64. Leider JD, Derise OC, Bourdreaux KA, Dierks GJ, Lee C, Varrassi G, et al. Treatment of suprascapular nerve entrapment syndrome. Orthop Rev (Pavia). 2021;13(2):25554.
65. Natsis K, Totlis T, Konstantinidis GA, Paraskevas G, Piagkou M, Koebke J. Anatomical variations between the sciatic nerve and the piriformis muscle: a contribution to surgical anatomy in piriformis syndrome. Surg Radiol Anat. 2014;36(3):273–80.
66. Windisch G, Braun EM, Anderhuber F. Piriformis muscle: clinical anatomy and consideration of the piriformis syndrome. Surg Radiol Anat. 2007;29(1):37–45.
67. Probst D, Stout A, Hunt D. Piriformis syndrome: a narrative review of the anatomy, diagnosis, and treatment. PM R. 2019;11(Suppl 1):S54–63.
68. Ro TH, Edmonds L. Diagnosis and management of piriformis syndrome: a rare anatomic variant analyzed by magnetic resonance imaging. J Clin Imaging Sci. 2018;8:6.
69. Rodrigue T, Hardy RW. Diagnosis and treatment of piriformis syndrome. Neurosurg Clin N Am. 2001;12(2):311–9.

70. Benson ER, Schutzer SF. Posttraumatic piriformis syndrome: diagnosis and results of operative treatment. J Bone Joint Surg Am. 1999;81(7):941–9.
71. Zhang W, Luo F, Sun H, Ding H. Ultrasound appears to be a reliable technique for the diagnosis of piriformis syndrome. Muscle Nerve. 2019;59(4):411–6.
72. Fishman LM, Konnoth C, Rozner B. Botulinum neurotoxin type B and physical therapy in the treatment of piriformis syndrome: a dose-finding study. Am J Phys Med Rehabil. 2004;83(1):42–50; quiz 1–3
73. Mullin V, de Rosayro M, Quint D. Mechanism of action caudal steroids for piriformis syndrome. Anesth Analg. 1998;86(3):680.

Geriatric Orthopedic Trauma

7

Heba Zakaria, Sahiti Patibandla, and Megan Sorich

Geriatric Trauma

Causes of Geriatric Trauma

Falls are the most common mechanism of trauma in older patients. Ground-level falls result in approximately 2.1 million emergency department (ED) visits every year. The mortality rate for geriatric patients is 7–11% after falls. Furthermore, compared to younger patients, geriatric patients have a higher incidence of hospital and intensive care unit (ICU) admission. Although ground-level falls are much more prevalent in geriatric patients, other mechanisms of trauma like motor vehicle accidents, pedestrians struck by a vehicle, injuries related to other forms of transport, firearm injuries, and lacerations/penetrating injuries are typically seen (Tables 7.1, 7.2, and 7.3) [1].

Table 7.1 Evidence-based points for evaluation of geriatric trauma

Although challenging at times, obtain a detailed history that includes an accurate list of patients' medications and when they last took each to avoid being falsely reassured by the absence of tachycardia or the presence of normal blood pressure (BP).
Consider comorbidities, medications, and baseline functional status.
Older adults have a physiologic decline in respiratory function (decreased functional residual capacity) and a higher incidence of pulmonary comorbidities (chronic obstructive pulmonary disease) that result in decreased lung compliance
Patients were 34% less likely to die if treated at a higher-volume trauma center.
Improved outcomes and decreased hospital length of stay were associated with having a geriatrician available to consult on trauma patients.
Evaluation by physical therapy after a fall is critical for the prevention of further injury.

H. Zakaria · S. Patibandla · M. Sorich (✉)
University of Texas Southwestern Medical Center, Dallas, TX, USA
e-mail: megan.sorich@utsouthwestern.edu

C. E. Noe (ed.), *Musculoskeletal Pain*,
https://doi.org/10.1007/978-3-031-86057-7_7

Table 7.2 Evidence-based points for management of geriatric trauma

Promoting and improving bone health through osteoporosis screening and treatment can significantly improve long-term geriatric patient outcomes.
Polypharmacy may be a risk when administering acute opioid pain medications for patients that are on multiple home medications while underdosing pain medications may cause delirium.
Acetaminophen has few side effects and contraindications compared to nonsteroidal anti-inflammatory drugs (NSAIDs).
Low-dose, short-duration ketamine infusion, regional anesthesia, and peripheral nerve blocks are preferred over opioid analgesia.

Table 7.3 Section highlights of geriatric trauma

Evaluation and management of geriatric trauma can present differently compared to general trauma patients that are seen.
It is important to acknowledge the physiologic changes that are seen in geriatric patients to avoid complications.

Age-Related Changes in Older Adults

Vital Signs

Compared to the younger populations, the geriatric population has more comorbidities. Therefore, the evaluation of normal vital signs in the setting of trauma is important. Given the physiologic changes and increased comorbidities, many geriatric patients are on medications for cardiac conditions. For example, B-blockers may artificially slow their heart rate or blunt a physiologic tachycardic response to the stress or hemorrhage they may potentially be experiencing. In addition, many patients have chronic hypertension that may or may not be controlled with medications. It's critical to obtain a detailed history that includes an accurate list of medications they take and when they last took each. Otherwise, physicians may be falsely reassured by the absence of tachycardia or the presence of normal blood pressure (BP). For example, a geriatric trauma patient with a baseline systolic BP of 160 mm Hg may present with a seemingly normal systolic BP of 110 mm Hg which is, in reality, hypotensive [1].

Frailty

Frailty is defined as the age-associated decline in physiologic function across multiple organ systems. Frail patients are more likely to experience trauma (especially falls) and poor post-trauma outcomes. Geriatric patients with preexisting conditions generally have higher morbidity and are more likely to die within 5 years of traumatic injury. When evaluating geriatric patients, emergency physicians (EPs) should consider comorbidities, medications, and baseline functional status. For example, what are the patient's ambulatory abilities and baseline cognitive deficits (if any) [1]?

Neurologic Considerations

Because geriatric patients are more likely to have neurocognitive impairments like dementia, obtaining an accurate medical history may be challenging at times.

Additionally, prior cerebrovascular accidents that resulted in neurologic deficits can make it difficult to identify new deficits caused by traumatic injury. The use of anticoagulants or antiplatelets along with decreased brain volume make intracranial bleeds more prevalent and difficult to treat [1].

Cardiopulmonary Considerations

Older adults have a physiologic decline in respiratory function (decreased functional residual capacity) and a higher incidence of pulmonary comorbidity (chronic obstructive pulmonary disease) that results in decreased lung compliance. Therefore, rib fractures and pulmonary contusions have significant implications in older patients compared to younger patients. Pneumonia is the most common post-traumatic hospital complication. In patients with poor baseline pulmonary function, infection clearance may be prolonged [1].

Musculoskeletal Considerations

Although osteoporosis causes substantial morbidity and mortality, it remains an undertreated disease entity. Proximal humerus fractures (PFHs) provide an opportunity to intervene with antiresorptive therapy to prevent the occurrence of subsequent fractures. Medications like alendronate, risedronate, zoledronic acid, and denosumab have been shown to reduce the risk of future nonvertebral fractures by about 50%. Because a significant proportion of the US population is vitamin D deficient, vitamin D and calcium supplementation for the management of osteoporosis has been shown to reduce the risk of vertebral and nonvertebral fractures. Nationally, less than 30% of patients that present with fragility fractures are diagnosed or treated for osteoporosis. Promoting and improving bone health through osteoporosis screening and treatment can significantly improve long-term geriatric patient outcomes [2]. Optimizing medical care in other aspects like hearing, vision, and strength in coordination with primary care and geriatricians is important to preventing fractures and decreasing the severity of injury if falls are experienced [1]. Programs like Returning Seniors to Orthopedic Excellence (RESTORE), led by Dr. Megan Sorich, provide new hope for older adults who suffer fractures and subsequent complications. This program consolidates clinical specialties like Geriatric Medicine, Internal Medicine, Emergency Medicine, Anesthesiology and Pain Management, Clinical Nutrition, and Physical Therapy at UT Southwestern [3].

Management

Trauma Activation and Consulting Services

Some studies have shown that geriatric trauma patients who present to a trauma center have better outcomes. One study found that patients were 34% less likely to die if treated at a higher-volume trauma center. In addition to the importance of having access to an equipped trauma team for trauma evaluations, it is also important to have the resources to comprehensively assess geriatric patients. Improved outcomes and decreased hospital length of stay were associated with having a geriatrician available to consult on trauma patients. Lastly, evaluation by physical therapy after a fall, whether in the ED or on follow-up, is critical for the prevention of further injury [1].

Pain Management

Physiologic changes associated with aging can alter the effects and metabolism of pain medication. Having a lower overall plasma volume, decreased muscle mass, and increased body fat can cause lipid-soluble medications a longer duration of action. Medications with lower lipid solubility can also have a more potent effect. Polypharmacy may be a risk when administering acute opioid pain medications for patients that are on multiple home medications. Many physicians are aware of the risk of underdosing pain medications which frequently causes delirium. Overmedication can also cause delirium in addition to exacerbation of dementia and sedation [1].

There are several ways to manage acute pain in geriatric patients. Acetaminophen has few side effects and contraindications compared to nonsteroidal anti-inflammatory drugs (NSAIDs). NSAIDS have a higher risk profile and the potential to cause renal dysfunction and GI bleeds. Topical NSAIDs, however, have similar effects to oral ones but with almost no systemic effects. Low-dose, short-duration ketamine infusion is recommended if other pain management methods fail. Regional anesthesia such as epidural blocks is preferred over opioid analgesia. Peripheral nerve blocks act faster, last longer in geriatric patients, and cause fewer systemic side effects compared to oral or parenteral pain management. Ultrasound-guided nerve blocks are becoming more commonly performed in the ED [1].

Evidence-based points for evaluation and management of hip fracture care are summarized in Tables 7.4 and 7.5.

Table 7.4 Evidence-based points for evaluation and management of hip fracture care

Determining fracture type is a key component of hip fracture evaluation, as it dictates the intervention strategy. Patient demographics, such as age and activity status, must also be considered.	
Both surgical and non-surgical treatment regimens are utilized in hip fracture care. It is important to understand the fracture classification systems, as each classification category typically has a corresponding, well-described care plan.	
Classification Systems and Treatment Range	
Femoral Head	*Pipkin*: conservative treatment, closed reduction, ORIF Osteochondral impaction: total hip arthroplasty
Femoral Neck	*Garden*: internal fixation, percutaneous pinning, hemiarthroplasty, total hip arthroplasty
Intertrochanteric	*Evans:* lateral plate and screw fixation vs. intramedullary nail fixation, proximal femoral nail fixation, gamma nail fixation, total hip arthroplasty
Subtrochanteric	*Russell & Taylor:* conservative management, intramedullary nailing, extramedullary plating

Table 7.5 Section highlights of hip fracture care

Section Highlights
Hip fractures can be anatomically divided into intracapsular and extracapsular fractures based on bony location. More common hip fracture patterns include femoral head, femoral neck, intertrochanteric, and subtrochanteric fractures.
Each hip fracture pattern has a specific treatment regimen dictated by both fracture classification and patient-specific characteristics.
Fracture liaison services are multidisciplinary organizations that help identify patients at risk for hip fractures in order to increase rates of osteoporosis treatment compliance, while decreasing rates of secondary fractures and post-fracture mortality.

Hip Fractures

A significant proportion of geriatric trauma involves providing hip fracture care, as the incidence of this fracture type has been increasing in recent years. Over 300,000 individuals, at or above 65 years old, are hospitalized each year [4]. The most common etiology by far of this injury type is falls. Geriatric hip fractures pose a challenge to healthcare providers as they are associated with high rates of morbidity and mortality. As a response to this, there has been a rise in research addressing appropriate treatment for traumatic hip fractures in geriatric populations. When determining the optimal treatment regimen, patient-specific risk factors, fracture type, stability of the fracture, fixation type, and postoperative outcomes are only a few of the many important prognostic factors that must be considered. Furthermore, there has been growing evidence showing that centers specialized in providing orthogeriatric care may enable patients to have better postoperative outcomes than care received from standard, unspecialized trauma centers.

In general, hip fractures can be categorized based on bony location, with the most common types consisting of femoral head, femoral neck, intertrochanteric, and subtrochanteric fractures. Hip fractures may also be classified as intracapsular or extracapsular depending on the involvement of the hip joint [5].

Intracapsular

Femoral Head

Femoral head fractures may be complete or impaction-related. Complete femoral head fractures are typically the result of high-energy injuries and often occur in conjunction with posterior hip dislocations. Femoral head fractures are typically classified by the Pipkin system into one of four types. Type 1 fractures occur below the fovea centralis, while type 2 fractures occur above the fovea centralis. Pipkin I fractures are typically treated with conservative treatment, a closed reduction, or

ORIF. In contrast, the more serious Pipkin 2 fractures are treated with closed reduction or ORIF. Type 3 fractures can be above or below the fovea centralis but contain an associated femoral neck fracture as well. This fracture type requires an urgent open reduction with internal fixation. Type 4 fractures are type 1 or type 2 fractures that possess a related acetabular rim fracture. Type 4 fractures can be treated with closed reduction and traction or with surgical fracture fixation. Recent studies have proposed utilizing other, more comprehensive classification systems in place of the Pipkin system, however, the Pipkin categories remain the most frequently used in orthopedics [6].

Osteochondral impaction femoral head fractures are typically associated with anterior hip dislocations, though they may be seen with posterior dislocations as well. In geriatric patients, femoral head impaction is typically treated with a total hip arthroplasty to reconstruct the joint and replace the damaged bone. In older patients, high-energy Pipkin fractures are less common, and fractures associated with osteoporosis and medical comorbidities are more typical. Such injuries may result from low-impact trauma and may present occultly with only unspecified hip pain. It is important for providers to remain wary of this presentation to enable timely detection and appropriate intervention for occult femoral head fractures in the geriatric population [5].

Femoral Neck

Femoral neck fractures are often described as basicervical, subcapital, or transcervical based on location. They can be further classified as displaced or nondisplaced depending on where the bone fragments lie in relation to the original femoral anatomical structure. The reason why this classification schema is important is because the blood supply to the femoral head is tenuous and may be impacted by femoral neck injury, posing a risk of avascular necrosis. It is important to note that femoral neck fractures are more common in older populations due to worse bone quality and density in comparison to younger counterparts. Transverse subcapital femoral neck fractures of low-energy traumatic etiology are most common in the geriatric population. The Garden classification system is typically used in this patient population to classify subcapital femoral neck fractures. Stage 1 fractures are incomplete or valgus impacted. Stage 2 fractures are complete and nondisplaced, while stage 3 fractures are complete and partially displaced. Finally, Garden stage 4 subcapital fractures are complete and fully displaced. In elderly patients, internal fixation is the treatment of choice for nondisplaced or impacted femoral neck fractures. The type of fixation is typically dependent on the fracture type as well as the surgeon's preference. Percutaneous pinning is the treatment of choice for nondisplaced femoral neck fractures, including Garden stage 1 and stage 2 [7]. For displaced Garden stage 3 and 4 fractures, a more complex process is required. The fracture must first be manually reduced and evaluated via fluoroscopic imaging. Then, percutaneous pinning is attempted. The benefits of this method are short operative time, high union rates, minimal blood loss, and immediate weight-bearing [8]. Another surgical option to consider, specifically for displaced femoral neck fractures, is hip joint reconstruction via a hemiarthroplasty or total hip arthroplasty procedure. Though arthroplasty eliminates the risks of avascular necrosis and nonunion, it involves the risks of longer operative time, higher blood loss, infection, and hardware failure [9]. Generally, total hip arthroplasty is recommended for active adults or adults with preexisting hip arthritis. The optimal treatment for femoral neck fractures is determined based on fracture classification, patient characteristics, and operative risk stratification [5].

Extracapsular

Intertrochanteric

Intertrochanteric fractures are more commonly seen in older populations than in younger counterparts, so this fracture pattern is of particular interest when discussing geriatric trauma. Specifically, in women older than 60, this fracture pattern has been increasing in prevalence and severity. There are multiple explanations for this phenomenon to consider, including osteoporotic complications and decreased mobility seen in this subpopulation. More generally, this fracture type is highly associated with lateral falls in which the patient lands on the greater trochanter of the femur.

Unlike the femoral head and neck fractures discussed previously, intertrochanteric fractures are categorized as extracapsular. This is a key distinction because the blood supply is more robust in this fracture pattern, so there is a lower risk of complications such as nonunion. However, it is important for the practitioner to realize that intertrochanteric fractures do pose a distinct set of complications, including instability, malunion, and deformity. There is not an agreed-upon classification system for intertrochanteric fractures, however, the Evans system is often utilized. Type 1 fractures have two bony fragments that are not displaced, while type 2 fractures have two bony fragments with displacement. Type 3 fractures contain three bony fragments with posterolateral cortex comminution. Similarly, type 4 fractures contain three bony fragments with posteromedial cortex comminution. Type 5 fractures consist of more than four bony fragments with both medial and lateral cortex comminution. Generally, increased fragment number and medial cortical involvement indicate increased severity of fracture pattern. Another important intertrochanteric fracture variant includes the reverse obliquity pattern. Since this fracture pattern is quite unstable, appropriate fixation is key [5].

Generally, treatment of intertrochanteric fractures in the elderly is aimed at restoring mobility and achieving weight-bearing status. Early surgical intervention is key to achieving these goals and reducing rates of mortality. There are two fixation methods that can be utilized to address intertrochanteric fractures, lateral plate and screw fixation vs. intramedullary nail fixation. Either fixation type can be utilized for simple fracture patterns, though treatment decision-making can become complicated as the fracture pattern gets more complex. The load-bearing axis of a lateral plate and screw fixation results in an increased likelihood of hardware loosening or failure, when compared to intramedullary nail fixation. Additionally, if the fracture is severely comminuted or if internal fixation fails, total hip arthroplasty is indicated [10]. As mentioned previously, the reverse obliquity intertrochanteric fracture pattern may present with extreme instability. Either proximal femoral nail fixation (PFN) or gamma nail fixation (GN) can be used to address this fracture type, though PFN has been shown to have better biomechanical results than GN [11].

Subtrochanteric

Subtrochanteric femoral fractures are a category of proximal femur fractures that are within 5 cm of the lesser trochanter. Over two-thirds of subtrochanteric fractures occur in individuals over the age of 50, and the majority of these fractures occur in women [12]. Again, this is likely due to decreased bone mineral density due to the higher incidence of osteoporosis in the subpopulation [13]. Elderly patients with underlying osteoporosis typically get this fracture type from low-energy falls, which results in spiral fractures with little comminution.

Like intertrochanteric fractures, there is not a universally accepted classification system for this fracture pattern. However, the Russell and Taylor system is commonly utilized as it provides clear guidelines on surgical intervention. This classification schema categorizes subtrochanteric fractures into two major groups. Type 1 fractures have no extension into the piriformis fossa, while type 2 fractures have piriformis fossa extension. Each major group is further classified based on whether a lesser trochanter-posteromedial femoral cortical fracture fragment is present. The reason why assessing piriformis fossa and posteromedial cortex involvement is important is because it determines surgical intervention and fixation choice. Surgical management options include intramedullary nailing and extramedullary plating [14]. Intramedullary nailing is associated with better postoperative functional outcomes and lower rates of complications, so it is considered to be the gold standard of treatment [15, 16]. Furthermore, IMN provides biomechanical advantages that make it an inherently stronger construct.

It is also important to consider the more complicated atypical and reverse obliquity fracture patterns, as these fracture types have a more complex treatment regimen. Reverse fractures have a high rate of failure with internal fixation via sliding hip screws, so intramedullary nailing is the treatment of choice. Atypical fractures are specifically associated with long-term bisphosphonate use [13]. For atypical fractures that are incomplete and not painful, conservative management can be attempted. However, for atypical fractures that are incomplete and painful or complete, intramedullary nailing is the standard of care [17, 18].

To summarize, geriatric hip fractures are typically the result of low-energy falls or injury mechanisms. These fractures can be categorized into intracapsular or extracapsular depending on anatomical location and joint involvement. Intracapsular hip fractures include femoral head and femoral neck fractures. These fracture patterns are of particular interest since there is limited blood supply, increasing the risk of avascular necrosis and nonunion. Extracapsular fractures, in contrast, do not involve the hip joint and consist of subtrochanteric and intertrochanteric fracture patterns. Though the blood supply is more robust with extracapsular, reducing the risk of AVN, these fractures present with their own risks of instability and hardware failure. Treatment is specific to the fracture pattern and determined by the surgeon based on anatomical, as well as patient-specific factors.

Fracture Liaison Services

In attempts to reduce re-fracture risk in patients with recent osteoporosis-related and other fragility fractures, Fracture Liaison Service (FLS) programs have been established. These multidisciplinary programs are effective, monetarily beneficial, and patient-centric and have the goal of closing the gap between patients who need preventative fracture care and those patients that actually receive this care [19]. FLS work to identify, treat, and monitor individuals that have had prior fragility fractures or are at high risk of fragility fractures to prevent secondary fractures [20]. It is a multidisciplinary approach that requires cooperation between different patient settings, including in-patient hospitals, outpatient treatment centers, and clinic visits. It also requires coordination between multiple care providers, including medical physicians, surgeons, nurses, physical therapists, and registered dieticians. Fracture Liaison Services have been shown to increase rates of osteoporosis treatment compliance, decrease the risk of secondary fracture, and significantly decrease the risk of post-fracture mortality [21, 22].

Evidence-based points for evaluation and management of distal radial fracture are summarized in Tables 7.6 and 7.7.

Table 7.6 Evidence-based points for evaluation and management for distal radial fracture

Deciding between a surgical and non-surgical approach to the treatment of DRFs is complex, and factors like the amount of acceptable deformity or displacement, patient demographics and medical comorbidities, desired recovery time, and functional assessment of the patient should be considered.
Short arm casting with fiberglass material and splinting with plaster material using either volar dorsal slab or sugar tong techniques are nonoperative treatment modalities that may be used.
Combining the benefits of a minimally invasive surgical method with the biochemical advantages of intramedullary nailing and locking screw technology, intramedullary nailing is the most recent technique used to treat DRFs.

Table 7.7 Section highlights for distal radial fracture

Wrist fractures are the most common upper extremity fractures in older adults.
The American Academy of Orthopedic Surgeon's recommendation is inconclusive since operative treatment may not lead to improved long-term outcomes.
Upper limb surgery under ultrasound-guided brachial plexus block is becoming increasingly popular because of its safety, effectiveness, and convenience.
Studies have found that an 8-week-long daily rehabilitation program yielded a continuous improvement of wrist ROM.

Distal Radius Fracture

Epidemiology and Risk Factors

In older adults, wrist fractures are the most common upper extremity fractures. The annual incidence of wrist fractures is 8–10 per 1000 person-years. To put things into perspective, the incidence rate for hip fractures is 7 per 1000 person-years. While hip fractures become more common in women over the age of 75, wrist fractures are more common in women under the age of 75. Because wrist fractures are most commonly the result of falls sustained while walking, they occur in those that are healthy, active, and functionally independent. Low bone mineral density, no history of previous estrogen use, a history of two or more falls in the preceding year, and a previous fracture sustained after the age of 50 are all risk factors for wrist fracture. For women over the age of 75, poor cognitive status increases the risk of wrist fracture [23].

Sarcopenia and Frailty

Although osteoporosis is a leading cause of distal radius fractures (DRFs), sarcopenia has been implicated in fragility fractures. Sarcopenia is a condition characterized by decreased muscle mass and function that affects older people. As mentioned before in this chapter, frailty is a status characterized by a decrease in reserve and resistance to stress that results from multiple physiologic changes like a decline in lean body mass, strength, physical performance, balance, and endurance causing vulnerability. Studies show that screening people of older age for frailty is a predictor for DRF [24].

Wrist fractures have been associated with a 48% increased risk of developing clinically important functional decline in older women. Opening and closing jars, carrying heavy objects, cutting food, lifting pots and pans, turning keys, rising from a chair, and opening and closing taps are all tasks affected by wrist fractures. However, the functional decline associated with wrist fracture was found to be like that associated with falls, arthritis, and diabetes mellitus. The development of disability in older people may be partially caused by wrist fractures. However, menopausal women who sustain a wrist fracture usually experience full functional recovery [23].

Operative Versus Nonoperative Treatment

Although DRFs, also known as wrist fractures, are common injuries, there is no gold standard for their treatment. The American Academy of Orthopedic Surgeon's recommendation is inconclusive since operative treatment may not lead to improved long-term outcomes [25]. Like treatments for other fractures, the aims of wrist fracture treatment include restoration of a full pain-free functional capacity of the wrist and lower arm and prevention of post-treatment complications. Accurate anatomical reconstruction and timely rehabilitation result in a good functional post-treatment outcome [26]. Deciding between a surgical and non-surgical approach to the treatment of DRFs is complex. Factors like the amount of acceptable deformity or displacement, patient demographics and medical comorbidities, desired recovery time, and functional assessment of the patient should be used when treating a patient [27].

Nonoperative Treatment

Medical providers should prioritize a patient-centered approach and shared decision-making when creating a treatment plan, especially when a nonoperative route is chosen. Short arm casting with fiberglass material and splinting with plaster material using either volar dorsal slab or sugar tong techniques nonoperative treatment modalities that may be used [27].

Operative Treatment

Surgical methods used to treat unstable DRFs include percutaneous pinning, external fixation, dorsal plating, and volar and dorsal angular stable plating. Although external fixation might be better at maintaining reduction compared to percutaneous pinning, percutaneous pinning yields a better functional outcome. Angular stable locking plates are widely used as the standard of modern treatment for all types of DRFs. Volar and dorsal locking plate fixation have been associated with high rates of tendon irritations or ruptures. Complications like breakage of the plate, screw loosening, carpal tunnel syndrome (CTS), or complex regional pain syndrome (CRPS) are all associated with the implantation of a locking plate. Loss of radial inclination of the distal radius is a less common but serious complication associated with volar angular stable plating fixation [26].

Recent studies have shown that operative fixation can potentially lead to a quicker recovery time and may be beneficial in radiocarpal fracture dislocation patterns. Furthermore, operative intervention should be considered in active geriatric patients or patients with bilateral upper extremity injuries that limit their activities of daily living [25]. Reduction and fixation with a proximal volar locking plate (PVLP) for dorsal displaced DRFs with volar lunate facet fragments is possible. Applying a dorsal volar locking plate (DVLP) to the distal ulnar for volar displaced DRFs may result in favorable postoperative outcomes [28]. The influence of age on 30-day postoperative outcomes has been studied. Data shows that patients 65 years or older that do not have high-risk comorbidities may be offered ORIF since complication risk is low [29].

Combining the benefits of a minimally invasive surgical method with the biochemical advantages of intramedullary nailing and locking screw technology, intramedullary nailing is the most recent technique used to treat DRFs. There are only a few intramedullary implant types that are clinically used for the treatment of wrist fractures. Studies have shown that intramedullary fixation yielded fast functional recovery due to the limited surgical approach at the radial styloid. In terms of fracture reduction, maintenance of reduction, and functional outcomes, internal fixation with the Targon DR is equivalent to open reduction and volar plating. Intramedullary fixation along with placement of a novel hybrid implant like Targon DR between a plate and a nail results in excellent function and low pain levels even during the earlier stages of the post-surgical period [26].

Because of its safety, effectiveness, and convenience, upper limb surgery under ultrasound-guided brachial plexus block is becoming increasingly popular. Due to the uneven distribution of anesthesiologists, surgeons, especially hand surgeons, have been performing ultrasound-guided brachial plexus blocks. Studies have shown that brachial plexus block alone and additional local infiltration anesthesia or intravenous anesthesia is successful in 94.1%. 5.9% of cases, however, were shifted to general anesthesia. Cooperation and coordination with anesthesiologists are necessary for the administration of anesthesia by surgeons [28].

Rehabilitation

Immobilization of the wrist in casts for a prolonged period makes early rehabilitation difficult in geriatric DRFs. Permanent stiffness and residual disability may occur in geriatric patients if controlled mobilization is not initiated in the early stages of fracture healing. Studies have found that an 8-week-long daily rehabilitation program yielded a continuous improvement in wrist ROM. A greater change in ROM was observed in patients with short-term stiffness that underwent rehabilitation. Based on these findings, an 8-week daily rehabilitation program for geriatric patients with limited ROM is recommended [30].

Evidence-based points for evaluation and management of proximal humeral fractures are summarized in Tables 7.8 and 7.9.

Table 7.8 Evidence-based points for evaluation and management of proximal humeral fractures

Patient comorbidities and perioperative risk are important factors to consider when deciding between surgical and nonsurgical treatment.
Proximal humerus fractures (PHFs) have been commonly classified by the Neer classification system which is based on the description of the humeral shaft, the articular part of the humeral head, the greater tuberosity, and the lesser tuberosity on plain AP radiographs.
Patients who received nonoperative treatment had more comorbid conditions, a longer length of stay, and higher mortality at 7 days, 30 days, and 1 year.
Indications for surgery in elderly patients include fracture dislocations, displaced surgical neck fractures without bone contact, those with a head split or head impaction, excessive tuberosity displacement greater than 1 cm, and excessive angulation in the coronal or sagittal planes greater than 45 degrees.

Table 7.9 Section highlights for proximal humeral fractures

PHFs are the third most common fracture in patients 65 years and older.
Most PHFs are caused by ground-level falls, traffic injuries, and ladder-related falls.
Due to the economic burden on healthcare systems, there has been a recent attempt to reduce costs by performing orthopedic procedures in the outpatient setting.

Proximal Humerus Fractures

Running third behind the hip and distal radius fractures, proximal humerus fractures (PHFs) are the third most common fracture in patients 65 years and older. Sixteen percent of all adult fractures and approximately 200,000 ED visits in the US are due to PHFs. The incidence rate is expected to triple in the next few decades due to the demographic change in society. Therefore, the clinical and economic importance of PHFs is on the rise [31].

Classification

PHFs have been commonly classified by the Neer classification system since 1970. It is based on the description of the following four anatomical segments of the PH as they appear on plain AP radiographs: the humeral shaft, the articular part of the humeral head, the greater tuberosity, and the lesser tuberosity. The fracture is considered displaced if any of these segments are displaced more than 1 cm or angulated more than 45°. All other fractures are categorized as minimally displaced fractures regardless of the number of fracture lines. The fractures are termed 2-part, 3-part, or 4-part depending on the number of displaced segments. Fractures can be further classified depending on the involved segments. For example, 86% of all PH fractures are either minimally displaced (49%), 2-part surgical neck fractures (28%), or 3-part greater tuberosity fractures (9%). The AO classification system is, in comparison to the Neer classification system, less commonly used for PH fractures [32].

Get to Know Your Patient and Their Fracture

Deciding on how to treat PHF is complex and requires consideration of multiple factors. So how do you go about making the best decision for your patient? Getting to know your patient and their fracture will help you make a plan that will yield the best possible results for your patient [33].

Start by discussing with the patient their activity level, anticipated demands, and range of motion (ROM). When deciding between surgical and nonsurgical treatment, patient comorbidities and perioperative risk are important factors to consider. For patients that perform most of their activities below shoulder level, a malunion will not be as limiting as for a young patient who may prefer a wider ROM [33].

Defining the specific PHF pattern may be understood through a series of shoulder radiographs. To better appreciate the level of bone impaction, comminution, and bone quality, a CT scan may be obtained. The deltoid tuberosity index (DTI) is strongly correlated with local bone mineral density. Values that are less than 1.4 indicate an increased risk for hardware failure following ORIF [33].

PHFs that are treated conservatively will have a ROM that is generally worse with more displaced fractures. Cohort studies of PHF treated nonoperatively showed that 3-part fractures can expect flexion to 120 ± 22 degrees and 4-part fractures can expect flexion to 90 ± 25 degrees. 80% of elderly patients treated nonoperatively reported good to excellent satisfaction rates with 70% normal flexion. Although many elderly patients tolerate their decreased ROM, it is important to educate them on the limitations they should expect. RTSA may be considered for patients initially treated nonoperatively who experience symptomatic sequelae like malunion. Studies suggest that there is little difference in outcome between acute or delayed reverse total shoulder arthroplasty (RTSA) [33].

Operative Versus Nonoperative Treatment

Nonoperative Treatment

A cohort study of elderly patients with PH fractures was conducted to evaluate mortality, length of stay, discharge data, readmission, and differences based on management. Out of the 42,511 PH fractures, 76.2% received nonoperative treatment. It was found that patients who received nonoperative treatment had more comorbid conditions, a longer length of stay, and higher mortality at 7 days, 30 days, and 1 year [34].

Other studies showed that non-surgical management should be used to treat minimally displaced fractures as well as displaced 2-, 3- and 4-part fractures in older patients. Since articular surface fractures, fracture-dislocations, and isolated tuberosity fractures are not thoroughly studied, they may benefit from surgery. Most PHFs heal with nonunion only seen in 1.1% of all fractures. However, when displaced fractures are treated nonoperatively in adults, malunion is inevitable. This does not necessarily result in poor function or pain. Restoring anatomy or replacing a joint with a prosthesis is not required to obtain satisfactory patient-reported outcomes [32].

Operative Treatment

In deciding between fixation and arthroplasty, DTI and fracture pattern are considered. Indications for surgery in elderly patients include fracture dislocations, displaced surgical neck fractures without bone contact, those with a head split or head impaction, excessive tuberosity displacement greater than 1 cm, and excessive angulation in the coronal or sagittal planes greater than 45 degrees. Surgical neck fractures with 33%–100% displacement are associated with a ten-fold increase in nonunion risk. Greater or lesser tuberosity fractures with greater than 1 cm displacement can result in weakness and impingement. Valgus fractures with greater tuberosity above the articular surface are surgically managed because they can result in impingement, malunion, or nonunion [33].

There are several randomized trials that compared early and late mobilization in non-surgical treatment of PH fractures. Less pain and better function were reported when training was initiated within the first week for most patients except those with unstable 3- and 4-part fractures and tuberosity fractures. Patients should be monitored for secondary displacement by outpatient visits, radiographs, and controlled loading. Most patients experience pain relief after 2–3 weeks of non-surgical treatment while improvement in function and pain relief can be expected 3–6 months after surgery [32].

Although previously believed that most PH fractures were minimally displaced, recent epidemiological studies have reported that most are displaced. Furthermore, the complexity of the fractures increases with advanced age [32]. Unstable surgical neck fractures, varus posteromedial fracture patterns, and isolated displaced tuberosity injuries are usually treated with open reduction and internal fixation (ORIF) [33]. ORIF is contraindicated in patients with preexisting arthritis or rotator cuff pathology [34]. Arthroplasty is considered for patients with fracture dislocation, head-split patterns, articular impaction injuries, or complex 4-part fractures, especially those with irreparable tuberosity injuries [33].

Due to the economic burden on healthcare systems, there has been a recent attempt to reduce costs by performing orthopedic procedures in the outpatient setting. This has been done with surgical fixation of ankle fractures and has resulted in significant cost savings. A study was done to assess the perioperative outcomes of performing ORIF for PHFs in the outpatient setting. In comparison to inpatient procedures, outpatient procedures did not result in increased rates of 30-day perioperative complications or readmissions [31].

Surgical repair of PHFs, when bone quality is impaired, increases the risk of screw penetration, delayed union, or instability despite the use of locked plating [35]. Furthermore, the use of locking plates in displaced 2-part fractures is not recommended since current studies do not demonstrate any benefits in comparison to non-surgical management [32]. Treatment of complex fracture patterns and poor bone quality using head-preserving osteosynthesis with locking plates has yielded high complication and reoperation rates [32]. One special entity of locked plating, the Proximal Humeral Internal Locking System (PHILOS), has been successfully used for the treatment of PHFs. However, recent studies have shown the need for secondary interventions or complications like loss of reduction, screw perforation, and nonunion [32].

Cement-augmented fixation, like biologic or synthetic bone substitutes, has shown biochemical advantages. The demineralized bone matrix has been an effective treatment used in several orthopedic trauma conditions like critical-size defects. Although allografts have been used in several studies, their use in the treatment of PHFs in the elderly has not been fully studied [35]. Osteosynthesis with a lock plate or intramedullary nail is the surgery used if humeral head preservation and tuberosity fixation are possible. A joint prosthesis can be considered if head preservation is not possible. RTSA has become more popular than shoulder hemiarthroplasty in the past 20 years since it is less dependent on tuberosity fixation [32].

Shoulder stiffness, nonunion, malunion, avascular necrosis of the humeral head, and persistent pain are all reported complications that can occur following surgical interventions. Mal-positioning of the implant at the time of surgery or due to subsequent fracture collapse and/or avascular necrosis of the humeral head is also possible. RTSA serves as a salvage option for failed non-surgical treatments and osteosynthesis [32].

Low Energy vs. High Energy Mechanisms

The impact of the mechanism of injury on the outcome of operative fixation of geriatric PHFs was studied. PHFs can be the result of low velocity/energy (LV) or high velocity/energy (HV) mechanisms. Although most HV mechanisms are seen in younger patients, there are some middle-aged and geriatric patients that sustain HV PHFs. Most PHFs are caused by ground-level falls, traffic injuries, and ladder-related falls. It was found that the energy and mechanism had similar outcomes in operatively treated PHFs which implies that these factors shouldn't affect surgical decision-making [36].

References

1. Clare D, Zink KL. Geriatric trauma. Emerg Med Clin North Am. 2021;39(2):257–71.
2. Piple A, Smith CT, Barton DW, Carmouche JJ. Proximal humerus fractures in the geriatric population present an opportunity to improve recognition and treatment of osteoporosis. Geriatr Orthop Surg Rehabil. 2020;11:2151459320935103.
3. Wascovich P. Restore program provides special care for seniors with fractures – CT plus – UT Southwestern. Center Times – UT Southwestern. February 24, 2021.
4. Agency for Healthcare Research and Quality. HCUPnet, healthcare cost and utilization project. Published online 2002.
5. Sheehan SE, Shyu JY, Weaver MJ, Sodickson AD, Khurana B. Proximal femoral fractures: what the orthopedic surgeon wants to know-erratum. Radiographics. 2015;35(5):1624.
6. Romeo NM, Firoozabadi R. Classifications in brief: the pipkin classification of femoral head fractures. Clin Orthop Relat Res. 2018;476(5):1114–9.
7. Bray TJ, Chapman MW. Percutaneous pinning of intracapsular hip fractures. Instr Course Lect. 1984;33:168–79.
8. Kofoed H, Alberts A. Femoral neck fractures. 165 cases treated by multiple percutaneous pinning. Acta Orthop Scand. 1980;51(1):127–36.
9. Lutnick E, Kang J, Freccero DM. Surgical treatment of femoral neck fractures: a brief review. Geriatrics. 2020;5(2) https://doi.org/10.3390/geriatrics5020022.
10. Shih Y, Bartschat NI, Cheng EY. Sliding hip screw and side plate for intertrochanteric hip fractures. JBJS Essent Surg Tech. 2022;12(1) https://doi.org/10.2106/JBJS.ST.19.00038.
11. Min WK, Kim SY, Kim TK, et al. Proximal femoral nail for the treatment of reverse obliquity intertrochanteric fractures compared with gamma nail. J Trauma. 2007;63(5):1054–60.
12. Ng AC, Drake MT, Clarke BL, et al. Trends in subtrochanteric, diaphyseal, and distal femur fractures, 1984–2007. Osteoporos Int. 2012;23(6):1721–6.
13. Napoli N, Schwartz AV, Palermo L, et al. Risk factors for subtrochanteric and diaphyseal fractures: the study of osteoporotic fractures. J Clin Endocrinol Metab. 2013;98(2):659–67.
14. Garrison I, Domingue G, Honeycutt MW. Subtrochanteric femur fractures: current review of management. EFORT Open Rev. 2021;6(2):145–51.
15. Robertson R, Tucker M, Jones T. Provisional plating of subtrochanteric femur fractures before intramedullary nailing in the lateral decubitus position. J Orthop Trauma. 2018;32(4):e151–6.

16. Brumback RJ, Toal TR Jr, Murphy-Zane MS, Novak VP, Belkoff SM. Immediate weight-bearing after treatment of a comminuted fracture of the femoral shaft with a statically locked intramedullary nail. J Bone Joint Surg Am. 1999;81(11):1538–44.
17. Al-Ashqar M, Panteli M, Chakrabarty G, Giannoudis PV. Atypical fractures: an issue of concern or a myth? Injury. 2018;49(3):649–55.
18. Lee KJ, Min BW. Surgical treatment of the atypical femoral fracture: overcoming femoral bowing. Hip Pelvis. 2018;30(4):202–9.
19. Curtis JR, Silverman SL. Commentary: the five Ws of a Fracture Liaison Service: why, who, what, where, and how? In osteoporosis, we reap what we sow. Curr Osteoporos Rep. 2013;11(4):365–8.
20. Fuggle NR, Kassim Javaid M, Fujita M, et al. Fracture risk assessment and how to implement a fracture liaison service. In: Falaschi P, Marsh D, editors. Orthogeriatrics: the management of older patients with fragility fractures. Springer; 2020.
21. Briot K. Fracture liaison services. Curr Opin Rheumatol. 2017;29(4):416–21.
22. Or O, Fisher Negev T, Hadad V, et al. Fracture liaison service for hip fractures: is it a game changer? Isr Med Assoc J. 2021;23(8):490–3.
23. Edwards BJ, Song J, Dunlop DD, Fink HA, Cauley JA. Functional decline after incident wrist fractures—study of osteoporotic fractures: prospective cohort study. BMJ. 2010;341:c3324.
24. Caliskan H, Igdir V, Ozsurekci C, Caliskan E, Halil M. Frailty and sarcopenia in patients with distal radius fracture: a geriatric perspective. Geriatr Orthop Surg Rehabil. 2020;11:2151459320906361.
25. Medda S, Aneja A, Carroll EA. Distal radius fractures: setting yourself up for success in the active geriatric patient. J Orthop Trauma. 2021;35(Suppl 5):S16–20.
26. Falk SSI, Mittlmeier T, Gradl G. Results of geriatric distal radius fractures treated by intramedullary fixation. Injury. 2016;47(Suppl 7):S31–5.
27. Cooper AM, Wood TR, Scholten Ii DJ, Carroll EA. Nonsurgical management of distal radius fractures in the elderly: approaches, risks and limitations. Orthop Res Rev. 2022;14:287–92.
28. Obata H, Naito K, Kaneko A, et al. Clinical outcomes in distal radius fractures accompanied by volar lunate facet fragments: a comparison between dorsal and volar displaced fractures. J Hand Surg Asian Pac. 2020;25(4):417–22.
29. Skochdopole A, Tarabishy S, Hermiz S, Mailey B, Herrera FA. Open reduction internal fixation of distal radius fractures: retrospective cohort analysis of the geriatric population using the NSQIP database. Hand. 2022;17(2):319–25.
30. Zhang W, Wang L, Zhang X, Zhang Q, Liang B. Manual passive rehabilitation program for geriatric distal radius fractures. Medicine. Published online 2021. https://www.ncbi.nlm.nih.gov/pmc/articles/PMC7837967/.
31. Bovonratwet P, Suhardi VJ, Andarawis-Puri N, Ricci WM, Fu MC. Outpatient surgical fixation of proximal humerus fractures can be performed without increased rates of short-term complications or readmissions. J Orthop Trauma. 2021;35(10):e356–63.
32. Brorson S, Palm H. Proximal humeral fractures: the choice of treatment. In: Falaschi P, Marsh D, editors. Orthogeriatrics: the management of older patients with fragility fractures. Springer; 2020.
33. O'Donnell JA, Gage MJ. Proximal humerus geriatric fracture care: fix, replace, or nonoperative treatment? J Orthop Trauma. 2021;35(Suppl 5):S6–S10.
34. Lander ST, Mahmood B, Maceroli MA, et al. Mortality rates of humerus fractures in the elderly: does surgical treatment matter? J Orthop Trauma. 2019;33(7):361–5.
35. Halvachizadeh S, Berk T, Rauer T, et al. Treatment of proximal humerus fractures in geriatric patients – can pathological DEXA results help to guide the indication for allograft augmentation? PLoS One. 2020;15(4):e0230789.
36. Ganta A, Solasz S, Drake J, Littlefield C, Konda S, Egol K. Does mechanism of injury impact the outcome of operative fixation of geriatric proximal humerus fractures. Arch Orthop Trauma Surg. Published online September 13. 2022; https://doi.org/10.1007/s00402-022-04616-w.

Complex Regional Pain Syndrome

8

Albert Huh

Introduction

One of the initial descriptions of complex regional pain syndrome (CRPS) dates to the American Civil War. In 1864, Dr. Silas Weir Mitchell, a neurologist, coined the term "causalgia" after observing burning pain, shining red skin, and muscle atrophy that appeared out of proportion to the extent of injuries suffered by soldiers at the time [1]. Later, in 1946, Dr. James A. Evans noted similar findings in patients' limbs and attributed the sympathetic nervous system to the maintenance of pain and muscle wasting in those areas. He used the term "reflex sympathetic dystrophy" (RSD) to reflect this hypothesis [2]. These terms would continue to be utilized until 1994 when the International Association for the Study of Pain (IASP) developed a set of diagnostic criteria to reference these signs and symptoms (Table 8.1). Subsequently, the name complex regional pain syndrome was established. This was further categorized into two types, with CRPS type I and II describing RSD and causalgia, respectively [3]. The primary distinguishing feature between the two types is the absence (type I) or presence (type II) of "major nerve damage," or a known nerve injury that precedes symptoms. Though the IASP criteria have high sensitivity, it was limited due to low specificity and overdiagnosis of CRPS. In response, the Budapest criteria was developed in 2007 (Table 8.2). The addition of more objective diagnostic requirements (i.e., motor and trophic features) exhibited higher specificity than the original IASP criteria while maintaining high sensitivity [4].

A. Huh (✉)
Department of Anesthesiology and Pain Management, University of Texas Southwestern Medical Center, Dallas, TX, USA
e-mail: ALBERT.HUH@UTSOUTHWESTERN.EDU

C. E. Noe (ed.), *Musculoskeletal Pain*,
https://doi.org/10.1007/978-3-031-86057-7_8

Table 8.1 IASP CRPS Diagnostic Criteria (1994)*

1. The presence of an initiating noxious event, or a cause of immobilization[a]
2. Continuing pain, allodynia, or hyperalgesia in which the pain is disproportionate to any known inciting event
3. Evidence at some time of edema, changes in skin blood flow, or abnormal sudomotor activity in the region of pain (can be a sign of symptom)
4. This diagnosis is excluded by the existence of other conditions that would otherwise account for the degree of pain and dysfunction

*If seen without "major nerve damage" diagnose CRPS I; if seen in the presence of "major nerve damage" diagnose CRPS II

[a]Not required for diagnosis; 5–10% of patients will not have this. Must meet criteria 2, 3, and 4 for diagnosis

Table 8.2 Budapest Diagnostic Criteria for CRPS (2007)*

1. Continuing pain, which is disproportionate to any inciting event
2. Must report ≥ one symptom in three of the four following categories:
   Sensory: hyperesthesia and/or allodynia
   Vasomotor: temperature asymmetry and/or skin color changes and/or skin color asymmetry
   Sudomotor/Edema: edema and/or sweating changes and/or sweating asymmetry
   Motor/Trophic: decreased range of motion and/or motor dysfunction (weakness, tremor, dystonia) and/or trophic changes (hair, nail, skin)
3. Must display ≥ one sign at time of evaluation in two or more of the following categories:
   Sensory: hyperalgesia (to pinprick) and/or allodynia (to light touch and/or temperature sensation and/or deep somatic pressure and/or joint movement)
   Vasomotor: evidence of temperature asymmetry (>1 °C) and/or skin color changes and/or asymmetry
   Sudomotor/Edema: edema and/or sweating changes and/or sweating asymmetry
   Motor/Trophic: decreased range of motion and/or motor dysfunction (weakness, tremor, dystonia) and/or trophic changes (hair, nail, skin)
4. There is no other diagnosis that better explains the signs and symptoms

*If seen without "major nerve damage" diagnose CRPS I; if seen in the presence of "major nerve damage" diagnose CRPS II

While further developments in diagnostic tools have assisted in the continued recognition of this disorder, CRPS remains incompletely understood. The disorder has a wide spectrum of presenting features and lacks a well-defined pathophysiology, making management unrelentingly difficult to achieve. Not only a condition causing physiological chronic pain, CRPS also has implications on cognitive, psychological, and social factors.

Pathophysiology

Several theories on the pathophysiology of CRPS have been proposed based on clinical and scientific studies, suggesting a multifactorial contribution to its etiology. Some of the more comprehensive and well-studied mechanisms include disruptions of the sympathetic nervous system, sensory pathways, and immune system.

Sympathetic Nervous System Dysregulation

Disruptions of the sympathetic nervous system are thought to be involved in certain manifestations of CRPS. One study exhibited increased nociceptive behaviors and hypersensitivity in rats with chronic post-ischemic pain (CRPS type I model) after intradermal injections of norepinephrine, vasopressin, and endothelial NO synthase inhibitor. These results suggested abnormal nociceptive responses to sympathetic nervous system driving agents, which were further reduced by alpha-adrenergic antagonists [5]. In human subjects, limbs that become cool, blue, and painful have been linked with vasoconstriction due to excessive sympathetic efflux. Increased pain duration and hyperalgesia in CRPS-affected limbs were seen in patients after local sympathetic stimulation with intradermal injection of phenylephrine [6].

The coupling of sympathetic neurons with various afferent neurons has been implicated in the pain associated with CRPS, a state referred to as "sympathetically maintained" CRPS. In cutaneous and deep somatic tissues, sympathetic autonomic receptors are upregulated on nociceptive neurons [7]. Consequently, sympathetic stimulation, such as through breath holding, skin cooling, or sensory startle, results in a heightened pain response [8]. Other non-nociceptive neurons also couple with the sympathetic nervous system, leading to changes in temperature, mechano- and thermosensitivity [9]. Some cases of CRPS have been deemed "sympathetically independent" due to the persistence of pain even after the effective sympathetic blockade, indicating a separate mechanism contributing to the pain state [10].

Sensory Pathway Sensitization

Following peripheral nerve injury, several multiple pro-inflammatory factors are released including TNF-α, substance P, bradykinin, and glutamate. If sustained, the threshold for nociceptive stimulation decreases, resulting in peripheral neural sensitization [3]. Persistent nociceptive firing to the central nervous system causes dorsal horn excitability and a "wind up" phenomenon [11]. NMDA receptor activation further contributes to central sensitization, as evidenced by a positive response to NMDA antagonist agents, such as ketamine [12].

Impairments in somatosensory perception also promote central neuroplastic changes. A study investigating skin biopsy samples of affected limbs in CRPS type I patients revealed a reduced density of C and A-fibers compared to unaffected limbs. Consequently, these patients displayed decreased activity in the somatosensory cortex of the affected side with a body midline shift towards the unaffected side, comparable to unilateral neglect from stroke[9]. Functional brain imaging studies performed in CRPS patients revealed significant reorganization in central sensory and motor cortices, with the amount of reorganization positively correlating with the extent of pain intensity. Regions of reorganization were found to be reversible upon adequate reduction of pain, suggesting pain as the primary culprit of these changes [13]. Altogether, the processes of peripheral and central nervous system sensitization result in the symptoms of hyperalgesia and allodynia.

Immune System Disturbances

Both the innate and adaptive immune systems are activated in CRPS. Mast cell accumulation and proliferation occur in CRPS-affected limbs, demonstrated by elevated levels of tryptase in skin biopsy samples. Degranulation of these cells leads to a release of mediators contributing to nociceptive sensitization and neurogenic inflammation [14]. In the chronic stage of CRPS, increased numbers of central memory $CD8^+$ and $CD4^+$ T lymphocytes with pro-inflammatory pathways have also been attributed to continual inflammation and cell damage [15]. Immunoglobulin autoantibodies with agonist properties activating β_2, α_1, and muscarinic-2 receptors have been detected in CRPS [16, 17]. The ensuing release of various cytokines, including TNFα, IL-1β, and IL-6, augments nociceptive signaling [18]. These observations are further upheld by the symptomatic improvement reflected in trials after administration of intravenous immunoglobulin in CRPS patients [19].

Epidemiology

A retrospective study assessing the Nationwide Inpatient Sample database in the United States from 2007 to 2011 revealed that 22,533 out of 33,406,123 admitted patients, or 0.07%, were discharged with a diagnosis of CRPS type I. Demographic analysis showed a higher incidence of CRPS type I for persons between the ages of 45 and 55, the female gender, Caucasian race, a higher median household income, preexisting depression, headache, drug abuse, and patients under private insurance (vs. Medicaid). In contrast, comorbidities of diabetes, obesity, hypothyroidism, and anemia were found to have a lower incidence [20]. A survey performed on 1359 subjects through the Reflex Sympathetic Dystrophy Syndrome Association of America website indicated that CRPS was most triggered by trauma and usually presented in the lower (56%) and upper (38%) extremities. Symptoms also often progressed to involve other regions of the body [21]. Fracture has been noted as the injury most associated with inciting CRPS in multiple studies [22, 23]. Long-term outcomes were worse with non-fracture injuries and upper extremity compared to lower extremity injuries [24]. Studies also suggest a genetic susceptibility, as patients with a familial history of CRPS had a higher incidence and diagnosis at a younger age [25]. Moreover, siblings of patients that developed CRPS before age 50 had a significantly increased risk of acquiring the syndrome themselves [26]. While conditions such as depression, anxiety, and personality disorders have often been linked with CRPS, multiple studies have shown no significant correlation to coexisting psychiatric comorbidities [22].

Clinical Presentation

Based on IASP criteria, CRPS typically follows a noxious event or injury, presents with pain disproportionate to the initiating event, and displays evidence of edema, skin changes, blood flow, or abnormal sudomotor activity in the affected region (Table 8.1). The Budapest criteria for CRPS differs with the requirements of at least one symptom in three of four categories (sensory, vasomotor, sudomotor, motor), at least one sign in at least two of four categories (sensory, vasomotor, sudomotor, motor), and differentiating between CRPS type I and II, or the absence or presence of major nerve damage, respectively (Table 8.2). There must be no other condition that could possibly explain the signs and symptoms.

In the acute, or "warm," phase of CRPS, the affected limb is generally associated with intense pain, erythema, edema, and warmth. Characteristics of allodynia, hyperalgesia, altered sweating, hair and nail growth, and muscle atrophy may also surface [9]. Although acute CRPS occasionally resolves with early, aggressive treatment, cases that last more than 1 year rarely recover [27]. The transition to the chronic, or "cold," phase occurs when pain is sustained despite resolution of vascular alterations and is thought to be related to modifications in central neuroplasticity [28]. The longer that symptoms persist, the more likely that features may spread, oftentimes proximally up the ipsilateral limb, but also even to involve the limb on the opposite side [29]. While the noxious, or "positive," signs of hyperpathia, hyperalgesia, and allodynia are the predominantly described characteristics of CRPS, the development of "negative" sensory deficits (hypoesthesia, hypoalgesia, hypothermesthesia) has also been described [30]. Additionally, there have been reports of associated systemic complications, including neurologic (fatigue, syncope, dystonia, cognitive difficulties), gastrointestinal (gastroparesis, irritable bowel syndrome), and urologic (urinary frequency, incontinence) [31].

Treatment

Treatment for CRPS encompasses the combination of pharmacologic and nonpharmacologic therapies to mitigate pain and improve functionality. Multiple treatment modalities have been utilized, though evidence for each shows varying levels of support.

Pharmacologic Treatment

Anticonvulsants

As CRPS is primarily considered a neuropathic pain condition, anticonvulsants such as gabapentin and pregabalin are typically first-line medications prescribed for treatment. In a double-blind, randomized clinical trial observing multiple neuropathic pain syndromes, including CRPS, gabapentin decreased pain scores and improved quality of life measures over an 8-week period when compared to placebo [32]. One crossover study focusing solely on CRPS through two 3-week periods revealed only mild pain relief from gabapentin when compared to placebo. Subjects achieved significant relief in the first period but noted minimal effect in the second period after a 2-week washout without the medication [33]. A more recent randomized, controlled trial compared gabapentin with amitriptyline in the treatment of CRPS I in pediatric patients, finding that both significantly decreased pain scores and improved sleep. No significant differences were found between the two medications [34]. To date, there have been no clinical trials on the efficacy of pregabalin for CRPS. A case report on a pediatric CRPS patient observed decreased pain and edema within 24–48 hours after transitioning from gabapentin to pregabalin. Upon cessation of the pregabalin, symptoms recurred and subsequently resolved with reinitiation of the medication [35]. A study inducing CRPS-type pain in rats through extremity ischemia found pregabalin alleviated mechanical allodynia for the longest duration compared to other medications (dexamethasone, morphine, ibuprofen, acetaminophen, and amitriptyline) [36].

Anti-inflammatories

A significant component of the pain associated with CRPS has been attributed to inflammation, making nonsteroidal anti-inflammatory drugs (NSAIDs) and corticosteroids potential therapeutic options [14]. One study found a correlation between increased spinal cyclooxygenase-2 levels and the presence of allodynia following nerve injury in rats. Cyclooxygenase-1 levels were not detectable in the same damaged nerve samples, and subsequent intrathecal injection of indomethacin showed no effect on allodynia symptoms 2 weeks after injury. This highlighted the importance of cyclooxygenase-2 as a potential target for therapy in CRPS [37]. Studies in humans have more variable results, with many showing no benefit from NSAIDs [38].

Conversely, there have been several clinical trials utilizing corticosteroids in human subjects with CRPS. One prospective, randomized clinical trial found that 30 mg of prednisone daily resulted in improved pain, edema, and finger dexterity when compared to placebo in early CRPS [39]. Another study comparing prednisolone with piroxicam in post-stroke patients that developed CRPS exhibited significantly lower shoulder-hand syndrome scores (pain, distal edema, passive humeral abduction, and external rotation) in the prednisolone group [40].

Antidepressants

Like anticonvulsant usage for neuropathic pain, antidepressants have also been frequently utilized in the management of CRPS. Serotonin-norepinephrine reuptake inhibitors (SNRIs) and tricyclic antidepressants (TCAs) have successfully treated various neuropathic pain conditions, though no studies directed towards treating CRPS with these medications alone have been performed. SNRIs have been FDA-approved for fibromyalgia, diabetic peripheral neuropathic pain, and chronic musculoskeletal pain, in addition to major depressive disorder [41]. These have yet to be trialed for CRPS. One randomized, controlled trial compared amitriptyline with gabapentin and found both to significantly improve pain and sleep disturbances in

CRPS patients at 6 weeks [34]. Another study revealed the combination of gabapentin and nortriptyline to be effective in treating neuropathic pain, with CRPS included, compared to either medication alone [42].

Opioids

Opioids are potent medications that are effective for several pain conditions, including CRPS. However, these are generally best applied for short durations, given the numerous adverse effects associated with long-term usage (nausea, constipation, sleep disorders, cognitive impairment, addiction, dependence, tolerance, hyperalgesia, and potential overdose) [43]. Even considering short-term use, one study using sustained-release morphine in CRPS patients concluded there was no significant benefit over the course of 8 days, though this study was limited by multiple confounding variables [44]. Opioids with neuropathic therapeutic properties, such as methadone (NMDA antagonism), tramadol, and tapentadol (SNRI), have theoretical benefits for CRPS, though there are no focused studies looking at this. Long-term high-dose opioid usage may progress to a hyperalgesic state and potentially exacerbate allodynia and hyperpathia commonly associated with CRPS [45].

NMDA Antagonists

Sub-anesthetic doses of intravenous ketamine have been utilized in multiple clinical trials and have shown good outcomes in both outpatient and inpatient settings. CRPS patients given intravenous ketamine infusions in ten consecutive outpatient sessions were found to have significant reductions in multiple pain parameters when compared to normal saline placebo 3 months after treatment [46]. Another study administered intravenous ketamine in CRPS patients over a 4.2-day course during inpatient admission and found significantly lower pain scores compared to placebo up to 12 weeks after, but did not result in functional improvement [12]. Adverse effects of hallucinations, psychomotor impairment, dysphoria, cardiovascular stimulation, and potential hepatoxicity have precluded its use at higher doses [47]. Other NMDA receptor antagonists, such as memantine and dextromethorphan, have also been trialed for CRPS with mixed results [48–50].

Topicals

Due to the relative lack of systemic effects, topical analgesics have been an attractive therapeutic modality for CRPS. Of these medications, lidocaine and capsaicin are the more commonly utilized analgesics due to their observed benefits in mitigating neuropathic pain. A prospective observational study completed in Spain over a 6-month period showed ≥50% reduction in pain scores in six out of ten CRPS patients with a 5% lidocaine-medicated plaster applied to the area of pain [51]. Studies on 5% lidocaine patches used for post-herpetic neuralgia have shown a reduction in symptoms that are also present in CRPS, such as allodynia [52]. Topical capsaicin has also shown efficacy for neuropathic pain, which is achieved through the temporary denervation of nociceptive nerve endings. In one trial, large-dose capsaicin was topically administered to CRPS patients, preceded by regional anesthesia to reduce intense burning from the initial application. Nine out of 10 patients achieved pain relief for up to 18 weeks [53]. Topical capsaicin in isolation is generally avoided in CRPS due to the early nociceptive stimulation that occurs and the potential to cause intractable exacerbation of pain [54].

Interventional Management

Sympathetic Blocks

Consideration for the involvement of the sympathetic nervous system in CRPS can be traced back to the 1940s when Dr. James Evans referred to the syndrome as "reflex sympathetic dystrophy." He associated excess sympathetic stimulation with arterial spasms and ischemia leading to edema and temperature changes and noted an improvement of symptoms with blockade of the sympathetic ganglion [2]. Recent evidence suggests this state represents "sympathetically maintained" CRPS, while cases that do not respond to sympathetic block are referred to as "sympathetically independent [10]." The most common targets for sympathetic blocks are the stellate ganglion for upper extremity CRPS and the lumbar sympathetic ganglia at L2/L3 for lower extremity CRPS. In a double-blinded, crossover study, local anesthetic and saline injections of sympathetic ganglia both resulted in similar reductions in pain intensity and mechanical allodynia, but the mean duration of pain relief was significantly longer (3 days vs. 19.9 hours) in the local anesthetic group [55]. Another prospective trial comparing local anesthetic sympathetic block with systemic IV phentolamine in 20 patients with sympathetically maintained CRPS found significant improvement in both groups but no difference between the two. They concluded that either technique could be utilized to differentiate sympathetically maintained versus sympathetically independent CPRS pain [56]. Botulinum toxin has also been used as an injectate, showing an increased duration of analgesia when combined with bupivacaine versus bupivacaine alone for lumbar sympathetic blockade [57]. Despite displaying some efficacy in pain relief, sympathetic blocks have largely fallen out of favor solely as a therapeutic intervention due to their ability to only achieve short-term relief. However, sympathetic blocks have found clinical utility in alleviating pain to provide a short window to gain improved tolerance during rehabilitation sessions and ultimate functional recovery [58].

Neuromodulation

When conservative and pharmacologic management is ineffective for pain control, neuromodulation techniques such as spinal cord stimulation (SCS), dorsal root ganglion (DRG) stimulation, intrathecal drug delivery systems (IDDS), and transcranial stimulation have been shown to reduce pain, improve functionality, and decrease medication requirements in several cases. One of the first trials investigating the utility of spinal cord stimulation for CRPS-related pain was done by Kemler et al., where the group receiving SCS and physical therapy had a significant reduction of pain intensity at 6 months compared to the group receiving physical therapy alone. However, there was no clinically significant improvement in functional status [59]. Follow-up studies at 2 years revealed partially sustained improvements in pain scores and quality of life in the SCS groups [60], but at 5 years, noted a diminished effect with time and was no longer statistically significant after 3 years [61]. A systematic review of 19 studies focusing on spinal cord stimulation for CRPS was done by Visnjevac et al. Outcomes of perceived pain relief, pain score improvement, quality of life, and satisfaction with SCS therapy had high-level evidence (1B+) favoring SCS use. Effects on functional status, sleep hygiene, psychology, and CRPS sign resolution were inconclusive [62].

Further advances in neuromodulation include dorsal root ganglion (DRG) therapy, which has also shown promise in CRPS management. The "ACCURATE" study compared DRG stimulation to SCS for lower extremity pain secondary to CRPS. After 12 months, successful treatment ($\geq$ 50% pain relief in visual analog scale score from baseline) was higher in the DRG (81.2%) compared to the SCS group (56.7%), which was statistically significant. They also found that DRG stimulation exhibited greater improvements in quality of life and psychological measures, less variation in paresthesia with position changes, and reduced stimulation in nonpainful areas, suggesting a more targeted treatment for lower extremity pain [63].

Intrathecal drug delivery systems using various analgesics have been examined in patients with CRPS. A study investigating long-term outcome measures of pain intensity and oral opioid intake was done on patients that underwent IDDS implantation between 2000 and 2013, twenty-six of which were for CRPS-related pain and had at least 4 years of consistent follow-up. The different intrathecal medications used in these devices included opioids, ziconotide, bupivacaine, and clonidine. Upon completion of the study, intrathecal opioids did not result in long-term decreases in oral opioid intake, ziconotide was associated with significantly reduced oral opioid intake at 4-year follow-up, and bupivacaine had an increase in oral opioid intake. Pain intensity scores did not show significant long-term decreases regardless of which medication or dose was used [64]. Baclofen has been utilized intrathecally to assist with severe spasticity. This was trialed in a dose-escalation study of CPRS patients with dystonia, which concluded that dystonia, pain, disability, and quality of life all showed improvement with intrathecal baclofen over the course of 1 year. However, this study was hindered by numerous side effects, including medication-related effects and device system defects, with some even requiring pump explant [65].

Transcranial stimulation techniques have also been utilized, specifically cortical and peripheral repetitive magnetic stimulation (rTMS, rPMS), transcranial direct current stimulation (tDCS), and transcutaneous electrical nerve stimulation (TENS). Pain intensity in CRPS patients was decreased after a single rTMS session when compared to sham, but the pain level would revert to baseline after approximately 45 minutes [66]. Another study concluded that rTMS reduced pain scores and improved emotional scores but did not sustain at 1-week and 3-month follow-ups [67]. tDCS has been studied in case reports for CRPS, most of which showed reduced pain intensity with tDCS used as an add-on to another modality (sensorimotor training, TENS) versus tDCS alone [68, 69]. While studies on TENS application for CRPS are limited, it is generally accepted as a potential treatment option given minimal complications from usage. One randomized clinical trial showed that TENS, along with physical therapy, effectively reduced pain scores and edema and increased finger range of motion in CRPS compared to placebo [70].

Surgery and Ablation

Surgical sympathectomy is another modality used for sympathetically maintained CPRS and is usually reserved for instances where less invasive interventions have failed. These procedures were initially done through an open technique, but modern technology has allowed for minimally invasive methods, including endoscopic and percutaneous routes. A study utilizing thoracoscopic sympathectomy for sympathetically mediated pain disorders, which included ten patients with RDS/CRPS, showed a high rate of symptom relief immediately following the procedure (92%) but diminished at 6 months postoperative follow-up (72%). When compared to historical groups of patients that underwent open sympathectomies for similar resection targets, the thoracoscopic technique had reduced morbidity rates, hospital stay, and time to return to normal activity [71]. Radiofrequency ablation (RFA) through the percutaneous route has also been described, which has the advantage of not requiring general anesthesia, intubation, or lung isolation as required by the thoracoscopic approach. In a series of 148 sympathectomies using RFA, Wilkinson found that 96% of the patients had sustained pain relief after 2 years and 91% after 3 years [72]. RFA usage has largely fallen out of favor due to a lack of high-quality studies and its association with significant complications, including pneumothorax, exacerbation of symptoms, deafferentation syndromes, and post-ablative neuralgia. These problems also occur in cases of neurolytic sympathectomies using alcohol or phenol and are generally reserved for palliative measures in the terminally ill [73].

Key Points

- Previously referred to as "causalgia" and "reflex sympathetic dystrophy," the International Association for the Study of Pain (IASP) established the name complex regional pain syndrome (CRPS) to describe pain, allodynia, or hyperalgesia associated with edema, vasomotor, and sudomotor activity that has been noted by various physicians since the 1800s (Table 8.1).
- CRPS is categorized into two types, type I, and II, based on the presence or absence of known nerve injury preceding symptoms, respectively.
- Due to limited specificity and overdiagnosis of CRPS with the IASP criteria, the addition of more objective diagnostic requirements (sensory, vasomotor, sudomotor, motor symptoms and signs) was established with the Budapest criteria in 2007 (Table 8.2).

- The pathophysiology of CRPS has been attributed to disruptions in the sympathetic nervous system, sensory pathways, and immune system.
- Some of the more common demographic factors associated with a higher incidence of CRPS include age 45–55, female gender, Caucasian race, higher median household income, preexisting depression, headache, drug abuse, and patients under private insurance.
- Pharmacologic treatment consists of anticonvulsants, anti-inflammatories, antidepressants, opioids, NMDA antagonists, and topical medications.
- Interventional techniques have been utilized when conservative measures fail to control symptoms. These include sympathetic blocks, neuromodulation (spinal cord stimulation, dorsal root ganglion stimulation, intrathecal drug delivery systems, and transcranial stimulation), radiofrequency and chemical ablation, and open or endoscopic surgical resection.

References

1. Lau FH, Chung KC. Silas Weir Mitchell, MD: the physician who discovered causalgia. J Hand Surg Am. 2004 Mar;29(2):181–7.
2. Coderre TJ. Complex regional pain syndrome: What's in a name? J Pain. 2011;12(1):2–12.
3. Shim H, Rose J, Halle S, Shekane P. Complex regional pain syndrome: a narrative review for the practising clinician. Br J Anaesth. 2019 Aug;123(2):e424–33.
4. Harden NR, Bruehl S, Perez RSGM, Birklein F, Marinus J, Maihofner C, Lubenow T, Buvanendran A, Mackey S, Graciosa J, Mogilevski M, Ramsden C, Chont M, Vatine JJ. Validation of proposed diagnostic criteria (the "Budapest criteria") for complex regional pain syndrome. Pain. 2010;150(2):268–74.
5. Xanthos DN, Bennett GJ, Coderre TJ. Norepinephrine-induced nociception and vasoconstrictor hypersensitivity in rats with chronic post-ischemia pain. Pain. 2008;137(3):640–51.
6. Drummond PD, Morellini N, Finch PM, Birklein F, Knudsen LF. Complex regional pain syndrome: intradermal injection of phenylephrine evokes pain and hyperalgesia in a subgroup of patients with upregulated α1-adrenoceptors on dermal nerves. Pain. 2018;159(11):2296–305.
7. Schattschneider J, Binder A, Siebrecht D, Wasner G, Baron R. Complex regional pain syndromes: the influence of cutaneous and deep somatic sympathetic innervation on pain. Clin J Pain. 2006;22(3):240–4.
8. Drummond PD, Finch PM, Skipworth S, Blockey P. Pain increases during sympathetic arousal in patients with complex regional pain syndrome. Neurology. 2001;57(7):1296–303.
9. Marinus J, Moseley GL, Birklein F, Baron R, Maihöfner C, Kingery WS, van Hilten JJ. Clinical features and pathophysiology of complex regional pain syndrome. Lancet Neurol. 2011;10(7):637–48.
10. Drummond PD, Finch PM. Persistence of pain induced by startle and forehead cooling after sympathetic blockade in patients with complex regional pain syndrome. J Neurol Neurosurg Psychiatry. 2004;75(1):98–102.
11. Goh EL, Chidambaram S, Ma D. Complex regional pain syndrome: a recent update. Burns Trauma. 2017;5:2.
12. Sigtermans MJ, van Hilten JJ, Bauer MCR, Arbous SM, Marinus J, Sarton EY, Dahan A. Ketamine produces effective and long-term pain relief in patients with complex regional pain syndrome type 1. Pain. 2009;145(3):304–11.
13. Maihöfner C, Seifert F, Markovic K. Complex regional pain syndromes: new pathophysiological concepts and therapies. Eur J Neurol. 2010;17(5):649–60.

14. Huygen FJ, Ramdhani N, van Toorenenbergen A, Klein J, Zijlstra FJ. Mast cells are involved in inflammatory reactions during complex regional pain syndrome type 1. Immunol Lett. 2004;91(2–3):147–54.
15. Russo MA, Fiore NT, van Vreden C, Bailey D, Santarelli DM, McGuire HM, Fazekas de St Groth B, Austin PJ. Expansion and activation of distinct central memory T lymphocyte subsets in complex regional pain syndrome. J Neuroinflammation. 2019;16(1):63.
16. Kohr D, Singh P, Tschernatsch M, Kaps M, Pouokam E, Diener M, Kummer W, Birklein F, Vincent A, Goebel A, Wallukat G, Blaes F. Autoimmunity against the β2 adrenergic receptor and muscarinic-2 receptor in complex regional pain syndrome. Pain. 2011;152(12):2690–700.
17. Dubuis E, Thompson V, Leite MI, Blaes F, Maihöfner C, Greensmith D, Vincent A, Shenker N, Kuttikat A, Leuwer M, Goebel A. Longstanding complex regional pain syndrome is associated with activating autoantibodies against alpha-1a adrenoceptors. Pain. 2014;155(11):2408–17.
18. David Clark J, Tawfik VL, Tajerian M, Kingery WS. Autoinflammatory and autoimmune contributions to complex regional pain syndrome. Mol Pain. 2018;14:1–13.
19. Goebel A, Baranowski A, Maurer K, Ghiai A, McCabe C, Ambler G. Intravenous immunoglobulin treatment of the complex regional pain syndrome: a randomized trial. Ann Intern Med. 2010;152(3):152–8.
20. Elsharydah A, Loo NH, Minhajuddin A, Kandil ES. Complex regional pain syndrome type 1 predictors - epidemiological perspective from a national database analysis. J Clin Anesth. 2017;39:34–7.
21. Sharma A, Agarwal S, Broatch J, Raja SN. A web-based cross-sectional epidemiological survey of complex regional pain syndrome. Reg Anesth Pain Med. 2009;34(2):110–5.
22. Jo YH, Kim K, Lee BG, Kim JH, Lee CH, Lee KH. Incidence of and risk factors for complex regional pain syndrome type 1 after surgery for distal radius fractures: a population-based study. Sci Rep. 2019;9(1):4871.
23. Beerthuizen A, Stronks DL, Van't Spijker A, Yaksh A, Hanraets BM, Klein J, Huygen FJPM. Demographic and medical parameters in the development of complex regional pain syndrome type 1 (CRPS1): prospective study on 596 patients with a fracture. Pain. 2012;153(6):1187–92.
24. Lloyd ECO, Dempsey B, Romero L. Complex regional pain syndrome. Am Fam Physician. 2021;104(1):49–55.
25. Shirani P, Jawaid A, Moretti P, Lahijani E, Salamone AR, Schulz PE, Edmondson EA. Familial occurrence of complex regional pain syndrome. Can J Neurol Sci. 2010;37(3):389–94.
26. de Rooij AM, de Mos M, van Hilten JJ, Sturkenboom MC, Gosso MF, van den Maagdenberg AM, Marinus J. Increased risk of complex regional pain syndrome in siblings of patients? J Pain. 2009;10(12):1250–5.
27. Gallagher JJ, Tajerian M, Guo T, Shi X, Li W, Zheng M, Peltz G, Kingery WS, Clark JD. Acute and chronic phases of complex regional pain syndrome in mice are accompanied by distinct transcriptional changes in the spinal cord. Mol Pain. 2013;9:40.
28. Bruehl S. An update on the pathophysiology of complex regional pain syndrome. Anesthesiology. 2010;113(3):713–25.
29. van Rijn MA, Marinus J, Putter H, Bosselaar SR, Moseley GL, van Hilten JJ. Spreading of complex regional pain syndrome: not a random process. J Neural Transm (Vienna). 2011;118(9):1301–9.
30. Drummond PD. Sensory disturbances in complex regional pain syndrome: clinical observations, autonomic interactions, and possible mechanisms. Pain Med. 2010;11:1257–66.
31. Schwartzman R. Complex regional pain syndrome: systemic complications. Pract Pain Manag. 2013;13(3):2.
32. Serpell MG, Neuropathic Pain Study Group. Gabapentin in neuropathic pain syndromes: a randomised, double-blind, placebo-controlled trial. Pain. 2002;99(3):557–66.
33. van de Vusse AC, Stomp-van den Berg SG, Kessels AH, Weber WE. Randomised controlled trial of gabapentin in complex regional pain syndrome type 1 [ISRCTN84121379]. BMC Neurol. 2004;4:13.

34. Brown S, Johnston B, Amaria K, Watkins J, Campbell F, Pehora C, McGrath P. A randomized controlled trial of amitriptyline versus gabapentin for complex regional pain syndrome type I and neuropathic pain in children. Scand J Pain. 2016;13:156–63.
35. Saltık S, Sözen HG, Basgul S, Karatoprak EY, Içağasıoğlu A. Pregabalin treatment of a patient with complex regional pain syndrome. Pediatr Neurol. 2016;54:88–90.
36. Millecamps M, Coderre TJ. Rats with chronic post-ischemia pain exhibit an analgesic sensitivity profile similar to human patients with complex regional pain syndrome—type I. Eur J Pharmacol. 2008;583(1):97–102.
37. Zhao Z, Chen SR, Eisenach JC, Busija DW, Pan HL. Spinal cyclooxygenase-2 is involved in development of allodynia after nerve injury in rats. Neuroscience. 2000;97(4):743–8.
38. Resmini G, Ratti C, Canton G, Murena L, Moretti A, Iolascon G. Treatment of complex regional pain syndrome. Clin Cases Miner Bone Metab. 2015;12(Suppl 1):26–30.
39. Christensen K, Jensen EM, Noer I. The reflex dystrophy syndrome response to treatment with systemic corticosteroids. Acta Chir Scand. 1982;148(8):653–5.
40. Kalita J, Vajpayee A, Misra UK. Comparison of prednisolone with piroxicam in complex regional pain syndrome following stroke: a randomized controlled trial. QJM. 2006;99(2):89–95.
41. Cipriani A, Koesters M, Furukawa TA, Nosè M, Purgato M, Omori IM, Trespidi C, Barbui C. Duloxetine versus other anti-depressive agents for depression. Cochrane Database Syst Rev. 2012;10:CD006533.
42. Gilron I, Bailey JM, Tu D, Holden RR, Jackson AC, Houlden RL. Nortriptyline and gabapentin, alone and in combination for neuropathic pain: a double-blind, randomised controlled crossover trial. Lancet. 2009;374(9697):1252–61.
43. Baldini A, Von Korff M, Lin EH. A review of potential adverse effects of long-term opioid therapy: a practitioner's guide. Prim Care Companion CNS Disord. 2012;14(3):PCC.11m01326.
44. Harke H, Gretenkort P, Ladleif HU, Rahman S, Harke O. The response of neuropathic pain and pain in complex regional pain syndrome I to carbamazepine and sustained-release morphine in patients pretreated with spinal cord stimulation: a doubleblinded randomized study. Anesth Analg. 2001;92(2):488–95.
45. Tompkins DA, Campbell CM. Opioid-induced hyperalgesia: clinically relevant or extraneous research phenomenon? Curr Pain Headache Rep. 2011;15(2):129–36.
46. Schwartzman RJ, Alexander GM, Grothusen JR, Paylor T, Reichenberger E, Perreault M. Outpatient intravenous ketamine for the treatment of complex regional pain syndrome: a double-blind placebo controlled study. Pain. 2009;147(1–3):107–15.
47. Niesters M, Martini C, Dahan A. Ketamine for chronic pain: risks and benefits. Br J Clin Pharmacol. 2014;77(2):357–67.
48. Sinis N, Birbaumer N, Schwarz A, Gustin S, Unertl K, Schaller HE, Haerle M. Memantine and complex regional pain syndrome (CRPS): effects of treatment and cortical reorganisation. Handchir Mikrochir Plast Chir. 2006;38(3):164–71.
49. Ahmad-Sabry MH, Shareghi G. Effects of memantine on pain in patients with complex regional pain syndrome-a retrospective study. Middle East J Anaesthesiol. 2015;23(1):51–4.
50. Ferrara JM. CRPS-related neurogenic edema responsive to dextromethorphan/quinidine. Pain Med. 2014;15(11):1981–3.
51. Calderón E, Calderón-Seoane ME, García-Hernández R, Torres LM. 5% lidocaine-medicated plaster for the treatment of chronic peripheral neuropathic pain: complex regional pain syndrome and other neuropathic conditions. J Pain Res. 2016;9:763–70.
52. Rowbotham MC, Davies PS, Verkempinck C, Galer BS. Lidocaine patch: double-blind controlled study of a new treatment method for post-herpetic neuralgia. Pain. 1996;65(1):39–44.
53. Robbins WR, Staats PS, Levine J, Fields HL, Allen RW, Campbell JN, Pappagallo M. Treatment of intractable pain with topical large-dose capsaicin: preliminary report. Anesth Analg. 1998;86(3):579–83.
54. Girtler R, Kloimstein H, Gustorff B. Pronounced symptom deterioration in complex regional pain syndrome type II after isolated application of a highly concentrated capsaicin patch. A case report. Schmerz. 2013;27(1):67–71.

55. Price DD, Long S, Wilsey B, Rafii A. Analysis of peak magnitude and duration of analgesia produced by local anesthetics injected into sympathetic ganglia of complex regional pain syndrome patients. Clin J Pain. 1998;14(3):216–26.
56. Raja SN, Treede RD, Davis KD, Campbell JN. Systemic alpha-adrenergic blockade with phentolamine: a diagnostic test for sympathetically maintained pain. Anesthesiology. 1991;74(4):691–8.
57. Carroll I, Clark JD, Mackey S. Sympathetic block with botulinum toxin to treat complex regional pain syndrome. Ann Neurol. 2009;65(3):348–51.
58. Stanton-Hicks M, Burton A, Bruehl S, et al. An updated interdisciplinary clinical pathway for CRPS: report of an expert panel. Pain Pract. 2002;2(1):1–16.
59. Kemler MA, Barendse GAM, van Kleef M, et al. Spinal cord stimulation in patients with chronic reflex sympathetic dystrophy. N Engl J Med. 2000;343(9):618–24.
60. Kemler M, De Vet H, Barendse G, Van Den Wildenberg F, van Cleef M. The effect of spinal cord stimulation in patients with chronic reflex sympathetic dystrophy: two years follow-up of the randomized controlled trial. Ann Neurol. 2004;55(1):13–8.
61. Kemler MA, de Vet HC, Barendse GA, van den Wildenberg FA, van Kleef M. Spinal cord stimulation for chronic reflex sympathetic dystrophy—five-year follow-up. N Engl J Med. 2006;354(22):2394–6.
62. Visnjevac O, Costandi S, Patel BA, Azer G, Agarwal P, Bolash R, Mekhail NA. A comprehensive outcome-specific review of the use of spinal cord stimulation for complex regional pain syndrome. Pain Pract. 2017;17(4):533–45.
63. Deer TR, Levy RM, Kramer J, et al. Dorsal root ganglion stimulation yielded higher treatment success rate for complex regional pain syndrome and causalgia at 3 and 12 months: a randomized comparative trial. Pain. 2017;158(4):669–81.
64. Herring EZ, Frizon LA, Hogue O, Mejia JU, Rosenquist R, Bolash RB, Machado AG, Nagel SJ. Long-term outcomes using intrathecal drug delivery systems in complex regional pain syndrome. Pain Med. 2019;20(3):515–20.
65. van Rijn MA, Munts AG, Marinus J, Voormolen JH, de Boer KS, Teepe-Twiss IM, van Dasselaar NT, Delhaas EM, van Hilten JJ. Intrathecal baclofen for dystonia of complex regional pain syndrome. Pain. 2009;143(1-2):41–7.
66. Pleger B, Janssen F, Schwenkreis P, Völker B, Maier C, Tegenthoff M. Repetitive transcranial magnetic stimulation of the motor cortex attenuates pain perception in complex regional pain syndrome type I. Neurosci Lett. 2004;356(2):87–90.
67. Picarelli H, Teixeira MJ, de Andrade DC, Myczkowski ML, Luvisotto TB, Yeng LT, Fonoff ET, Pridmore S, Marcolin MA. Repetitive transcranial magnetic stimulation is efficacious as an add-on to pharmacological therapy in complex regional pain syndrome (CRPS) type I. J Pain. 2010;11(11):1203–10.
68. Schmid AC, Hummel FC, Birbaumer N. Pain reduction in a CRPS patient due to tDCS and sensorimotor training. A single case study. Clin Neurophysiol. 2011;122:S144.
69. Houde F, Harvey MP, Tremblay Labrecque PF, Lamarche F, Lefebvre A, Leonard G. Combining transcranial direct current stimulation and transcutaneous electrical nerve stimulation to relieve persistent pain in a patient suffering from complex regional pain syndrome: a case report. J Pain Res. 2020;13:467–73.
70. Bilgili A, Çakır T, Doğan ŞK, Erçalık T, Filiz MB, Toraman F. The effectiveness of transcutaneous electrical nerve stimulation in the management of patients with complex regional pain syndrome: a randomized, double-blinded, placebo-controlled prospective study. J Back Musculoskelet Rehabil. 2016;29(4):661–71.
71. Johnson JP, Ahn SS, Choi WC, Masciopinto JE, Kim KD, Filler AG, Desalles AA. Thoracoscopic sympathectomy: techniques and outcomes. Neurosurg Focus. 1998;4(2):e4.
72. Wilkinson HA. Percutaneous radiofrequency upper thoracic sympathectomy. Neurosurgery. 1996;38(4):715–25.
73. Mockus MB, Rutherford RB, Rosales C, Pearce WH. Sympathectomy for causalgia. Patient selection and long-term results. Arch Surg. 1987;122(6):668–72.

Non-operative Back Pain

9

Mazin Al Tamimi, Yves Jordan Kenfack, Emerson Lout, Umaru Barrie, and Salah G. Aoun

Introduction

Musculoskeletal conditions affect a staggering number of individuals across the globe, with approximately 1.71 billion people grappling with these ailments [1]. These conditions have emerged as the primary cause of disability worldwide, with back pain alone identified as the leading cause of disability in 160 countries. Particularly in the United States, patients with back pain expend a disproportionate percentage of healthcare resources, further underscoring the significance of musculoskeletal conditions [2]. Their profound impact on mobility often leads to early retirement, decreased well-being, and limited participation and productivity in society. Compounded by an increase in growth and relative aging of the population, the prevalence of musculoskeletal conditions and associated functional decline is rapidly increasing [3]. Understanding the characteristics and presentation of patients with back pain is crucial for healthcare professionals to provide accurate diagnoses and effective treatment. While surgical interventions may be necessary in certain cases, nonoperative management approaches play an even more significant role in the initial treatment and continual care of patients with back pain. This chapter aims to explore the various aspects of patient presentations of back pain, encompassing clinical features, physical examination findings, current guidelines, and relevant diagnostic tests. By delving into the comprehensive assessment of patients with back pain, healthcare providers can enhance their diagnostic skills and optimize patient care. In addition, our chapter provides a thorough review of treatment modalities and escalation of care in the management of back pain.

M. Al Tamimi (✉) · Y. J. Kenfack · E. Lout · U. Barrie · S. G. Aoun
UT Southwestern Medical Center, Dallas, TX, USA
e-mail: mazin.altamimi@utsouthwestern.edu

C. E. Noe (ed.), *Musculoskeletal Pain*,
https://doi.org/10.1007/978-3-031-86057-7_9

Clinical Features

Risk Factors

Age is a significant factor, as the first onset of low back pain often occurs between the ages of 30 and 50, and its prevalence tends to increase with advancing age [4]. Poor fitness level is another risk factor, as individuals who are not physically fit may have weaker muscles that fail to adequately support the spine. Weight gain and obesity also contribute to back pain, as the additional weight places stress on the back and can lead to pain [5]. Some forms of back pain, such as ankylosing spondylitis, have a genetic component, highlighting the influence of genetics on back pain susceptibility [6]. Job-related factors, such as heavy lifting, prolonged sitting, and poor posture, can contribute to back pain by placing strain on the spine [7]. Mental health factors, including anxiety, mood disorders, and depression, can impact the perception of back pain and contribute to muscle tension. Smoking is another risk factor, as it restricts blood flow and oxygen supply to the spinal discs, thus accelerating degeneration [8]. Understanding these risk factors is crucial in preventing and managing back pain effectively. Guidelines adapted from the NASS low back pain treatment guidelines pertaining to the evidence-based assessment of low back pain are detailed in Table 9.1 [9].

Pain Characteristics and Associated Symptoms

Patients with back pain commonly experience different types of pain, including dull, achy, or sharp sensations. The pain may be localized to a specific area or radiate to other regions such as the buttocks, legs, or even the arms. Additionally, the pain intensity can vary from mild discomfort to severe debilitating episodes. Duration of back pain can range from acute (less than 6 weeks), subacute (6–12 weeks), to chronic (more than 12 weeks) [10]. Some patients may report intermittent episodes of pain, while others may describe continuous discomfort

Table 9.1 Evidence based assessment of low back pain

Conversion from acute to chronic pain:
Psychosocial and workplace factors may be risk factors for conversion to chronic
Pain severity should be used to stratify patients according to risk of conversion
Prognostic factors:
Diffuse low back pain and tenderness may be associated with a nonstructural etiology of low back pain
Kinesiophobia is a negative prognostic factor
Discography:
Discography with manometric measurements correlate with pain reproduction in patients with degenerative disk disease and end plate abnormalities in patients with MRI findings of end plate abnormalities on MRI
Bony vibration provocation may correlate with discography

MRI magnetic resonance imaging

[11]. Understanding the duration and patterns of back pain aids in determining appropriate treatment strategies. Patients with back pain may present with a varying array of associated symptoms, including muscle stiffness, limited range of motion, numbness or tingling sensations, weakness, or bowel and bladder dysfunction. These symptoms can provide valuable clues regarding potential underlying causes of the back pain and will be discussed below in association with specific etiologies, concerns for cervical myelopathy, and red flag symptoms.

Physical Examination

Gait and Posture

Observing a patient's posture and gait can provide valuable insights into their back pain as there is strong evidence indicating differences in gait when comparing patients with back pain and those with healthy backs [12]. Antalgic or guarded postures may indicate pain-related compensatory mechanisms as it is an anomalous walking pattern resulting from pain, leading to a noticeable limp or favoring of one side [13]. This abnormality may suggest underlying musculoskeletal or neurological involvement.

Range of Motion

Assessing the patient's range of motion helps identify limitations and provokes pain. Active and passive movements of the spine, including flexion, extension, lateral bending, and rotation, should be evaluated in every patient presenting with back pain. Pain induced with specific movements can clue to different diagnosis [14]. Limited range of motion may indicate musculoskeletal or spinal joint pathology. During the physical examination, certain findings can suggest the presence of radicular pain. These include positive straight leg raising, crossed straight leg raising, blunted reflexes, weakness, or sensory loss. These signs may indicate nerve root involvement and warrant further investigation.

Muscle Strength and Reflexes

Evaluating muscle strength and reflexes is crucial in detecting any neurological involvement associated with back pain. Manual muscle testing of the lower extremities, assessment of deep tendon reflexes, and sensory examination aid in identifying potential nerve root compression or spinal cord abnormalities. The Medical Research Council Manual Muscle Testing scale is widely recognized as the primary approach for assessing muscle strength. This technique entails examining specific muscles in the upper and lower extremities and assessing their strength by applying resistance. The patient's strength is then graded on a scale of 0–5 based on the

Table 9.2 Medical Research Council Manual Muscle Testing Scale

Score	Physical exam finding
0	No muscle activation
1	Trace muscle activation, such as a twitch, without achieving full range of motion
2	Muscle activation with gravity eliminated, achieving full range of motion
3	Muscle activation against gravity, full range of motion
4	Muscle activation against some resistance, full range of motion
5	Muscle activation against examiner's full resistance, full range of motion

observed response [15]. Table 9.2 describes the six gradations of the Medical Research Council Manual Muscle Testing scale and their associated physical exam findings.

Red Flags

These are several indicators that may suggest underlying serious conditions requiring further investigation or immediate medical attention. Recognizing these red flags allows for timely intervention and appropriate management. During the physical examination for nonoperative back pain, several red flags should be considered. A comprehensive overview of major red flags and likely diagnoses is provided in Table 9.3. Assessing neurological deficits is crucial, looking for signs of nerve root compression, weakness, sensory loss, or abnormal reflexes, which may indicate conditions like spinal cord compression, cauda equina syndrome, or nerve root impingement. Severe or progressively worsening neurological symptoms, such as rapid muscle weakness, bladder or bowel dysfunction, sexual dysfunction, bilateral radiculopathy, or saddle anesthesia, require immediate attention for risk of cauda equine syndrome [16]. Fever or systemic illness accompanying back pain may suggest an inflammatory process or infection, such as a spinal epidural abscess, warranting prompt work-up and treatment [17]. Further, history findings of significant immunosuppression, IV drug use, or concurrent infection should prompt further examination for infectious etiology. Back pain in the setting of trauma or a history of cancer should be carefully evaluated for concerns of spinal fractures or spinal metastases. Unexplained weight loss with back pain raises concerns about malignancy or systemic illness, necessitating cancer screening and evaluation [18]. Breast, lung, prostate, and renal malignancies are the most common to yield spinal metastases, and back pain in patients with diagnosed primary tumors should raise high clinical suspicion [19]. Regarding spinal fractures, elderly patients with a history of osteoporosis or known risk factors are at high risk for potential vertebral compression fractures or osteoporotic fractures [20]. These risk factors presenting with acute onset back pain and a history of an inciting event or prior fractures pose a very high clinical likelihood for spinal fracture [21]. Additionally, cervical

Table 9.3 Red flags for specific etiologies of back pain

Etiologies	Red flags
Malignancy	Unexplained weight loss
	Current or prior malignancy
	Breast, lung, prostate, or renal (top 4 most common metastases)
Cauda equina syndrome	Urinary retention/overflow incontinence
	Saddle anesthesia
	Loss of anal sphincter tone/fecal incontinence
	Progressive lower extremity weakness
	Sexual dysfunction
	Loss of perineal sensation
	Bilateral radiculopathy
Fracture	Acute onset
	History of trauma or inciting factor
	High risk for osteoporosis
	Female (post-menopausal), chronic steroid use, elderly
	Prior vertebral fractures
Spinal abscess/infection	Fever
	Immunosuppression
	IV Drug use
	Active infection
	UTI, bacteremia, cellulitis
	Recent spinal intervention

IV Intravenous, *UTI* Urinary tract infection

spondylotic myelopathy should be considered early, as its symptoms can mimic other common conditions. When any of these red flags are present, additional diagnostic tests, imaging, or consultation with specialists, such as spine surgeons or neurologists, should be pursued to determine the cause of the back pain and provide appropriate management.

In cases where symptoms or examination findings are progressively worse or when there is suspicion of malignancy, serious disease processes, or the need for surgical intervention, urgent imaging should be performed. Additionally, imaging should be considered if patients do not respond to conventional treatments or when surgical intervention or spinal injections are being contemplated. By recognizing these signs of radicular pain and appropriately utilizing imaging, healthcare professionals can obtain crucial diagnostic information. This aids in guiding treatment decisions, identifying potential underlying causes, and ensuring timely interventions for improved patient outcomes [22].

History and Physical Examination Review

To identify the common causes of back pain, it is essential to consider the history and physical exam findings. Degenerative disk disease can often be observed on plain radiographs, although it does not have a specific history of present illness or examination findings associated with it. However, patients with a disk herniation

Table 9.4 Findings concerning for myelopathy on review of back pain

	Gross motor	Fine motor/ functional	Sensory	Reflexes
History	Weakness Gait/balance issues Falls Lower extremity involvement	Loss of dexterity Bladder symptoms (50%)	Neck or arm pain Numbness or sensory disturbance (39%) Paresthesia Stereoanesthesia	–
Physical exam	Weakness (50%) Atrophy Altered tone Spastic gait Unsteady tandem gait Abnormal Grip and release test[a]	Finger escape sign present	Lhermitte's sign	Babinski (50%) Hoffmann sign, dynamic Hoffmann Hyperreflexia below the lesion (87%) Clonus Inverted radial reflex Hyperactive pectoralis reflex

[a]Normal grip and release test = 20 repetitions in 10 seconds
(%) = Prevalence of finding in patients with back pain.

commonly experience sciatica and may display blunted patellar or ankle reflexes, positive straight leg raising or cross straight leg raising, as well as weakness or sensory loss during the examination. Conversely, individuals with spinal stenosis typically complain of leg pain that worsens with ambulation but improves when sitting or flexing the lumbar spine. It is worth noting that lumbar extension may produce thigh pain [22]. Table 9.4 further provides an in-depth adaptation from Lavelle et al.'s 2007 publication on the pertinent history and physical exam findings indicative of cervical myelopathy [23]. By analyzing the history and physical examination findings, healthcare professionals can effectively determine the underlying causes of back pain, such as disk herniation and spinal stenosis. This knowledge aids in accurate diagnosis and appropriate management of back pain, leading to improved patient outcomes.

Diagnostic Tests

Imaging Studies

Acute low back pain is generally a self-limiting condition that does not necessitate imaging for uncomplicated cases. Uncomplicated cases are typically characterized by the absence of red flag signs, symptoms, and concerns, with symptoms typically resolving within 6 weeks through conservative medical treatment. For low back pain, imaging can usually be deferred safely until a reassessment after initial treatment. Early imaging is associated with overutilization and work absence [22]. Radiographic imaging, such as X-rays, can provide an overview of the spinal structures, including vertebral alignment and potential degenerative changes. Magnetic resonance imaging (MRI) offers more detailed visualization of soft tissues, intervertebral discs, and nerves, aiding in the identification of malignancies, herniated discs, spinal stenosis, or other structural abnormalities. Computed tomography (CT) scans should be prioritized for patients who have contraindications to magnetic resonance imaging (MRI) [24]. MR Imaging should be completed if any red flag symptoms (Table 9.3) are present. If no high-risk factors or red flags, imaging can likely be deferred.

Conservative Management

Patient Education, Self-Care, and Behavioral Interventions

Patients should also be encouraged to maintain an active lifestyle, engage in regular physical activity, and adopt strategies to manage stress, as these factors can significantly impact their back pain outcomes [25]. Richard and Shea 2011 provide specific delineations for patient self-care, which was further extrapolated by Kongsted et al. 2021 to focus on three important patient factors in the management of low back pain—self-care, self-management, and symptom monitoring [25, 26]. Symptom monitoring is primarily patient actions to avoid symptoms, whilst self-management takes it one step further to manage the actual or potential impact of their disease. Finally, overall self-care is identified as the most encompassing mindset patients can take by pursuing overall healthy lifestyle modifications. These play a crucial role in the management of nonoperative back pain. Educating patients about their condition, its natural course, and the importance of self-care can empower them to actively participate in their recovery process. Providing information on proper body mechanics and lifestyle modifications can help prevent exacerbations and promote a healthy spine. Psychological and behavioral interventions can significantly impact the management of nonoperative back pain. Techniques such as cognitive behavioral therapy (CBT), mindfulness-based stress reduction (MBSR), and relaxation training can help individuals develop coping strategies, modify pain-related thoughts and behaviors, and enhance overall well-being [27].

Physical Therapy and Exercise Programs

Physical therapy and exercise serve as core components of the conservative management of nonoperative back pain. These interventions aim to improve strength, flexibility, posture, and overall functional capacity. Physical therapists can tailor exercises based on the individual's specific needs and capabilities, incorporating stretching, strengthening, and stabilization exercises [28]. Complementary and alternative medicine (CAM) approaches, such as acupuncture, spinal manipulation, tai chi, or yoga, are sometimes considered in the management of nonoperative back pain [29]. These interventions may offer additional options for pain relief and functional improvement, particularly for individuals who prefer nonpharmacological or

Table 9.5 Nonpharmacologic conservative management of low back pain

Topical/manipulation	Exercise/therapy	Psychological/behavioral
Topical capsicum is recommended for use <3 months duration Heat is effective for acute low back pain Spinal manipulative therapy produced short-term benefit for acute low back pain	Aerobic exercise is beneficial for patients with non-specific low back pain Specific stabilization exercises may be as effective as a generalized exercise program Yoga may be beneficial for patients with chronic back pain Patients with acute low back pain who exercise more at baseline and use exercise to recover have better functional outcomes compared to patients who do not Patients who remain active with acute low back pain have similar outcomes to patients who are treated with bed rest McKenzie method of exercise may help chronic back pain	CBT with PT is recommended for chronic back pain for analgesia, functional improvement and return to work Targeting fear avoidance along with PT may improve pain during the first 6 months of a back pain episode Work hardening may help patients return to work

Chronic = > 12 months
CBT Cognitive behavioral therapy, *PT* physical therapy

noninvasive treatments. However, the evidence supporting the effectiveness of CAM approaches for nonoperative back pain is variable, and individual responses may vary. An overview of nonpharmacologic conservative therapies for low back pain, adapted from the NASS clinical guidelines for the treatment of low back pain, is provided in Table 9.5 [9].

Manual Therapy Techniques

Spinal manipulation or mobilization can be valuable adjuncts to conservative management. These hands-on interventions aim to improve joint mobility, reduce pain, and restore function [30]. Manual therapy is typically performed by skilled physical therapists, chiropractors, or osteopathic physicians. However, careful consideration should be given to the individual patient's characteristics, preferences, and potential contraindications.

Alternative Stimulation Modalities

Heat, cold, and electrical stimulation modalities such as heat therapy, cold therapy, and electrical stimulation can provide symptomatic relief and promote healing in nonoperative back pain. Heat therapy, including hot packs or warm showers, helps relax muscles, improve blood flow, and alleviate pain. Cold therapy, such as ice packs or cold compresses, can reduce inflammation and numb the area [31].

Electrical stimulation techniques, such as transcutaneous electrical nerve stimulation (TENS) or interferential current therapy, may modulate pain signals and promote pain reduction by activating descending inhibitory systems in the central nervous system to reduce hyperalgesia [32].

Pharmacological Interventions

Pharmacological management may be considered in the management of nonoperative back pain, particularly when pain is moderate to severe or significantly affects the individual's ability to function. An overview of first and second-line pharmacological therapies is provided in Table 9.6. Nonsteroidal anti-inflammatory drugs (NSAIDs) (ibuprofen, naproxen) are commonly used as first-line pharmacotherapy to reduce pain and inflammation. Analgesics such as acetaminophen can also provide symptomatic relief. Acetaminophen alone is not very effective, but it is an excellent co-analgesic with NSAID [33]. The mechanism of action for acetaminophen remained unknown for decades but is now thought to work in endogenous cannabinoid systems to produce analgesia [22, 34]. In certain cases, myorelaxants or low-dose antidepressants may be prescribed to address specific symptoms or comorbidities. However, while benzodiazepines are sometimes indicated in the management of acute low back pain, they are not indicated in the management of chronic pain [35]. Duloxetine is approved by the FDA for the treatment of chronic musculoskeletal pain [36]. In the management of chronic back pain, a combination of duloxetine and acetaminophen can be utilized as a baseline analgesic, while nonsteroidal anti-inflammatory drugs (NSAIDs) can be used for breakthrough pain. For patients with renal insufficiency, venlafaxine and desipramine are viable alternatives to duloxetine. Additionally, while gabapentin is commonly prescribed for chronic pain, it is not effective for axial back pain. These should be used with caution in patients with renal diseases. It is important to note that opioids are not recommended as the initial choice of medication for either acute or chronic back pain. The use of opioids in the management of back pain is associated with various risks and potential adverse effects, including dependence, addiction, respiratory depression, and overdose [37]. Moreover, opioids have not been found to provide significant long-term benefits for chronic back pain and may even lead to the development of opioid dependence and abuse.

Table 9.6 Pharmacologic management of low back pain

Acute	Chronic
First-line: NSAIDs (naproxen, ibuprofen), Acetaminophen	*First-line:* NSAIDs (naproxen, ibuprofen), Acetaminophen
Second-line: Myorelaxants (including benzodiazepines), opioids only recommended for short-term use	*Second-line:* Duloxetine, venlafaxine/desipramine (renal insufficiency), myorelaxants (not including benzodiazepines)

Multidisciplinary Teams

Collaborative Care Team

A collaborative care team and a multidisciplinary strategy are crucial in the management of nonoperative back pain. The members of this team are often a variety of medical specialists that collaborate to offer comprehensive care and address the various facets of the patient's condition. Primary care doctors, rehabilitation specialists, pain management specialists, psychologists, and other mental health specialists could all be part of the collaborative care team.

Role of Primary Care Physicians

The treatment of nonoperative back pain requires the involvement of primary care physicians. They oversee the first assessment, diagnosis, and therapy and are frequently the first point of contact for patients. Primary care physicians are in a good position to launch conservative treatment options, offer self-care advice, and educate patients. They are essential in coordinating care with other specialists and keeping track of the patient's development during therapy.

Rehabilitation Specialists

The collaborative care team must include rehabilitation specialists like physical therapists and occupational therapists. They specialize in helping people with back pain regain function, lessen discomfort, and generally improve their quality of life. Specialists in rehabilitation evaluate the patient's physical capabilities and create individualized exercise regimens and therapies to address certain deficits [28]. These programs could include posture correction methods, stretching regimens, strengthening exercises, and ergonomic adjustments.

Pain Management Specialists

Specialists with experience in treating complex pain disorders, such as nonoperative back pain. To reduce pain and pain management and increase the patient's functional capacity, they use a number of therapies and modalities. Pharmacological treatments, such as non-opioid analgesics or adjuvant drugs, as well as interventional techniques, like epidural steroid injections or nerve blocks, may be among them [38]. Specialists in pain management work collaboratively with other members of the care team to create customized treatment regimens and enhance pain management.

Psychologists and Mental Health Professionals

The psychological and emotional aspects of nonoperative back pain should not be overlooked, as they can significantly impact a patient's experience and outcomes. Psychologists and mental health professionals play a vital role in addressing the psychosocial factors associated with back pain. They provide support, counseling, and behavioral interventions to help patients cope with pain, manage stress, improve sleep, and enhance overall well-being. Their expertise in CBT and other evidence-based approaches can be valuable in improving pain-related outcomes.

Ensuring optimal patient care requires effective communication and coordination within the collaborative care team. To achieve this, it is crucial to conduct regular interdisciplinary meetings and implement shared decision-making processes. These practices promote the exchange of vital information, foster continuity of care, and ultimately improve treatment outcomes. By maintaining open lines of communication, the team can develop a comprehensive understanding of the patient's needs, make timely adjustments to the treatment plan, and address all aspects of the patient's condition in a coordinated manner. Patients with nonoperative back pain might gain from a thorough and all-encompassing management strategy by using a multidisciplinary approach and encouraging teamwork among healthcare experts. This method considers the variety of back pain and treats its functional, psychological, and physical elements, improving patient results overall.

Evidence-Based Guidelines and Recommendations

Review of Clinical Practice Guidelines

For the treatment of nonoperative back pain management, numerous clinical practice guidelines have been developed based on the best available evidence. These guidelines provide healthcare professionals with valuable recommendations and evidence-based strategies to guide their clinical decision-making. It is essential for clinicians to review and familiarize themselves with these guidelines to ensure that their management approach aligns with the most current and effective practices.

Best Practices in Conservative Management

Conservative management plays a central role in the treatment of nonoperative back pain, and adhering to best practices is crucial for optimal patient outcomes. These best practices are derived from a synthesis of the available evidence, clinical expertise, and patient preferences. They represent the most effective evidence-based strategies for managing back pain without resorting to surgical interventions.

Best practices in conservative management encompass a range of approaches, including patient education and self-care, physical therapy, exercise programs, pharmacological interventions, manual therapy techniques, modalities (such as heat, cold, and electrical stimulation), psychological and behavioral interventions, and complementary/alternative medicine approaches. The American College of Physicians' guidelines for noninvasive treatments for acute low back pain recommend heat, massage, acupuncture, and spinal manipulation for nonpharmacological therapies and NSAIDs and muscle relaxers [39].

Prevention of low back pain is also achievable through the practice of regular exercise. Additionally, there are various factors that have been associated with low back pain and disability. These factors include heavy lifting, twisting, vibration, physical inactivity, obesity, arthritis, osteoporosis, pregnancy, being over the age of 30, poor posture, stress, depression, and smoking. By addressing these risk factors through patients' own self-care, individuals can significantly reduce their chances of experiencing low back pain and related disabilities [22].

Adhering to best practices involves tailoring treatment plans to individual patients based on their specific needs and characteristics. It is important to consider factors such as the duration and severity of symptoms, functional limitations, psychosocial factors, and treatment preferences. By following evidence-based best practices, healthcare professionals can optimize the effectiveness of conservative management strategies and improve patient outcomes. By incorporating evidence-based guidelines and best practices into clinical decision-making, healthcare professionals can provide high-quality care for patients with nonoperative back pain. This approach ensures that management strategies are based on the best available evidence, align with current recommendations, and ultimately lead to improved patient outcomes and satisfaction.

Take Home Messages

1. Axial neck and back pain are often best managed without prescription drugs and invasive procedures.
2. Magnetic resonance imaging is usually not required to evaluate axial spine pain.
3. Myelopathy should be included in the differential diagnosis.
4. Nonpharmacological analgesic techniques are safe and effective.
5. Over-the-counter analgesics (ibuprofen, naproxen) are first-line medications.
6. Many recommended medications (NSAIDS, gabapentin, duloxetine) must be used with caution in patients with renal disease.
7. Opioids are not first-line drugs for acute or chronic back pain.
8. Medical treatment with psychological and physiotherapy (multidisciplinary treatment) is safe and effective for patients with chronic axial neck and back pain.
9. Patients with radicular pain or other red flags are outside the scope of the guidelines for axial neck and back pain.

References

1. Cieza A, Causey K, Kamenov K, Hanson SW, Chatterji S, Vos T. Global estimates of the need for rehabilitation based on the global burden of disease study 2019: a systematic analysis for the global burden of disease study 2019. Lancet. 2021;396(10267):2006–17. https://doi.org/10.1016/s0140-6736(20)32340-0.
2. Dieleman JL, Cao J, Chapin A, et al. US health care spending by payer and health condition, 1996–2016. JAMA. 2020;323(9):863–84. https://doi.org/10.1001/jama.2020.0734.
3. Hartvigsen J, Hancock MJ, Kongsted A, et al. What low back pain is and why we need to pay attention. Lancet. 2018;391(10137):2356–67. https://doi.org/10.1016/s0140-6736(18)30480-x.
4. Wong AYL, Karppinen J, Samartzis D. Low back pain in older adults: risk factors, management options and future directions. Scoliosis Spinal Disord. 2017;12:14. https://doi.org/10.1186/s13013-017-0121-3.
5. Lee CA, Jang HD, Moon JE, Han S. The relationship between change of weight and chronic low back pain in population over 50 years of age: a nationwide cross-sectional study. Int J Environ Res Public Health. 2021;18(8) https://doi.org/10.3390/ijerph18083969.
6. Kenyon M, Maguire S, Rueda Pujol A, O'Shea F, McManus R. The genetic backbone of ankylosing spondylitis: how knowledge of genetic susceptibility informs our understanding and management of disease. Rheumatol Int. 2022;42(12):2085–95. https://doi.org/10.1007/s00296-022-05174-5.
7. Heneweer H, Staes F, Aufdemkampe G, van Rijn M, Vanhees L. Physical activity and low back pain: a systematic review of recent literature. Eur Spine J. 2011;20(6):826–45. https://doi.org/10.1007/s00586-010-1680-7.
8. Rajesh N, Moudgil-Joshi J, Kaliaperumal C. Smoking and degenerative spinal disease: a systematic review. Brain Spine. 2022;2:100916. https://doi.org/10.1016/j.bas.2022.100916.
9. Kreiner DS, Matz P, Bono CM, et al. Guideline summary review: an evidence-based clinical guideline for the diagnosis and treatment of low back pain. Spine J. 2020;20(7):998–1024. https://doi.org/10.1016/j.spinee.2020.04.006.
10. Fatoye F, Gebrye T, Odeyemi I. Real-world incidence and prevalence of low back pain using routinely collected data. Rheumatol Int. 2019;39(4):619–26. https://doi.org/10.1007/s00296-019-04273-0.
11. Chiodo AE, Bhat SN, Van Harrison R, et al. Michigan medicine clinical care guidelines. Low Back Pain. Michigan Medicine University of Michigan. © Regents of the University of Michigan; 2020.
12. Smith JA, Stabbert H, Bagwell JJ, Teng HL, Wade V, Lee SP. Do people with low back pain walk differently? A systematic review and meta-analysis. J Sport Health Sci. 2022;11(4):450–65. https://doi.org/10.1016/j.jshs.2022.02.001.
13. Auerbach N, Tadi P. Antalgic gait in adults. StatPearls. StatPearls Publishing. Copyright © 2023, StatPearls Publishing LLC; 2023.
14. Bratton RL. Assessment and management of acute low back pain. Am Fam Physician. 1999;60(8):2299–308.
15. Naqvi U, Sherman AL. Muscle strength grading. StatPearls. StatPearls Publishing. Copyright © 2023, StatPearls Publishing LLC; 2023.
16. Todd NV. Guidelines for cauda equina syndrome. Red flags and white flags. Systematic review and implications for triage. Br J Neurosurg. 2017;31(3):336–9. https://doi.org/10.1080/02688697.2017.1297364.
17. Ameer MA, Knorr TL, Munakomi S, Mesfin FB. Spinal epidural abscess. StatPearls. StatPearls Publishing. Copyright © 2023, StatPearls Publishing LLC; 2023.
18. Ziu E, Viswanathan VK, Mesfin FB. Spinal Metastasis. StatPearls. StatPearls Publishing. Copyright © 2023, StatPearls Publishing LLC; 2023.

19. Mundy GR. Metastasis to bone: causes, consequences and therapeutic opportunities. Nat Rev Cancer. 2002;2(8):584–93. https://doi.org/10.1038/nrc867.
20. Whitney E, Alastra AJ. Vertebral fracture. StatPearls. StatPearls Publishing. Copyright © 2023, StatPearls Publishing LLC; 2023.
21. Roux C, Fechtenbaum J, Kolta S, Briot K, Girard M. Mild prevalent and incident vertebral fractures are risk factors for new fractures. Osteoporos Int. 2007;18(12):1617–24. https://doi.org/10.1007/s00198-007-0413-1.
22. Chou R. Low back pain. Ann Intern Med. 2021;174(8):ITC113–28. https://doi.org/10.7326/AITC202108170.
23. Lavelle WF, Bell GR. Cervical myelopathy: history and physical examination. Semin Spine Surg. 2007;19(1):6–11. https://doi.org/10.1053/j.semss.2007.01.004.
24. Lancaster B, Goldman J, Kobayashi Y, Gottschalk AW. When is imaging appropriate for a patient with low back pain? Ochsner J Fall. 2020;20(3):248–9. https://doi.org/10.31486/toj.20.0077.
25. Kongsted A, Ris I, Kjaer P, Hartvigsen J. Self-management at the core of back pain care: 10 key points for clinicians. Braz J Phys Ther. 2021;25(4):396–406. https://doi.org/10.1016/j.bjpt.2021.05.002.
26. Richard AA, Shea K. Delineation of self-care and associated concepts. J Nurs Scholarsh. 2011;43(3):255–64. https://doi.org/10.1111/j.1547-5069.2011.01404.x.
27. Cherkin DC, Sherman KJ, Balderson BH, et al. Effect of mindfulness-based stress reduction vs cognitive behavioral therapy or usual care on Back pain and functional limitations in adults with chronic low back pain: a randomized clinical trial. JAMA. 2016;315(12):1240–9. https://doi.org/10.1001/jama.2016.2323.
28. Shipton EA. Physical therapy approaches in the treatment of low back pain. Pain Ther. 2018;7(2):127–37. https://doi.org/10.1007/s40122-018-0105-x.
29. Kanga I, Severn M. CADTH rapid response reports. Manual therapy for recent-onset or persistent non-specific lower back pain: a review of clinical effectiveness and guidelines. Canadian Agency for Drugs and Technologies in Health. Copyright © 2017 Canadian Agency for Drugs and Technologies in Health; 2017.
30. Bronfort G, Haas M, Evans RL, Bouter LM. Efficacy of spinal manipulation and mobilization for low back pain and neck pain: a systematic review and best evidence synthesis. Spine J. 2004;4(3):335–56. https://doi.org/10.1016/j.spinee.2003.06.002.
31. Cheville AL, Basford JR. Role of rehabilitation medicine and physical agents in the treatment of cancer-associated pain. J Clin Oncol. 2014;32(16):1691–702. https://doi.org/10.1200/jco.2013.53.6680.
32. Vance CG, Dailey DL, Rakel BA, Sluka KA. Using TENS for pain control: the state of the evidence. Pain Manag. 2014;4(3):197–209. https://doi.org/10.2217/pmt.14.13.
33. Ong CK, Seymour RA, Lirk P, Merry AF. Combining paracetamol (acetaminophen) with nonsteroidal antiinflammatory drugs: a qualitative systematic review of analgesic efficacy for acute postoperative pain. Anesth Analg. 2010;110(4):1170–9. https://doi.org/10.1213/ANE.0b013e3181cf9281.
34. Klinger-Gratz PP, Ralvenius WT, Neumann E, et al. Acetaminophen relieves inflammatory pain through CB(1) cannabinoid receptors in the rostral ventromedial medulla. J Neurosci. 2018;38(2):322–34. https://doi.org/10.1523/jneurosci.1945-17.2017.
35. Ketenci A, Zure M. Pharmacological and non-pharmacological treatment approaches to chronic lumbar back pain. Turk J Phys Med Rehabil. 2021;67(1):1–10. https://doi.org/10.5606/tftrd.2021.8216.
36. Smith HS, Smith EJ, Smith BR. Duloxetine in the management of chronic musculoskeletal pain. Ther Clin Risk Manag. 2012;8:267–77. https://doi.org/10.2147/tcrm.S17428.

37. Deyo RA, Von Korff M, Duhrkoop D. Opioids for low back pain. BMJ. 2015;350:g6380. https://doi.org/10.1136/bmj.g6380.
38. El-Tallawy SN, Nalamasu R, Salem GI, LeQuang JAK, Pergolizzi JV, Christo PJ. Management of musculoskeletal pain: an update with emphasis on chronic musculoskeletal pain. Pain Ther. 2021;10(1):181–209. https://doi.org/10.1007/s40122-021-00235-2.
39. Qaseem A, Wilt TJ, McLean RM, et al. Noninvasive treatments for acute, subacute, and chronic low back pain: a clinical practice guideline from the American College of Physicians. Ann Intern Med. 2017;166(7):514–30. https://doi.org/10.7326/m16-2367.

The Diagnosis and Management of Common Shoulder Pathology

10

Hayden Schuette, B. Gage Griswold, John B. Schrock, Armodios M. Hatzidakis, and Michael Khazzam

Shoulder Impingement and Stiffness

Subacromial Impingement

Introduction

Shoulder pain associated with subacromial impingement is a prevalent issue [1]. The potential sources of shoulder pain linked to subacromial impingement encompass a spectrum, including inflammation of the subacromial bursa, tendinopathy of the rotator cuff, and partial- or full-thickness rotator cuff tears. Many researchers posit that external compression from the anterior acromion, coracoacromial ligament (CAL), and acromioclavicular joint significantly contributes to rotator cuff disease through extrinsic compression [2–4]. However, there is intrinsic tendon degeneration, which may be the underlying reason for this pathological pain [5, 6].

Extrinsic Compression

Neer's dissection of 100 cadaver scapulae revealed osteophytes and excrescences on the undersurface of the anterior acromion [7]. These changes, resulting from the impingement of the rotator cuff and humeral head against the anterior acromion and

H. Schuette · B. Gage Griswold
Western Orthopaedics, Denver, CO, USA

J. B. Schrock
OhioHealth/Doctors Hospital, Columbus, OH, USA

A. M. Hatzidakis
Western Orthopaedics & Rose Medical Center, Denver, CO, USA

M. Khazzam (✉)
Baylor Scott & White Orthopaedic Associates of Dallas Complex Shoulder Institute, Grapevine, TX, USA
e-mail: michael.khazzam@bswhealth.org

C. E. Noe (ed.), *Musculoskeletal Pain*,
https://doi.org/10.1007/978-3-031-86057-7_10

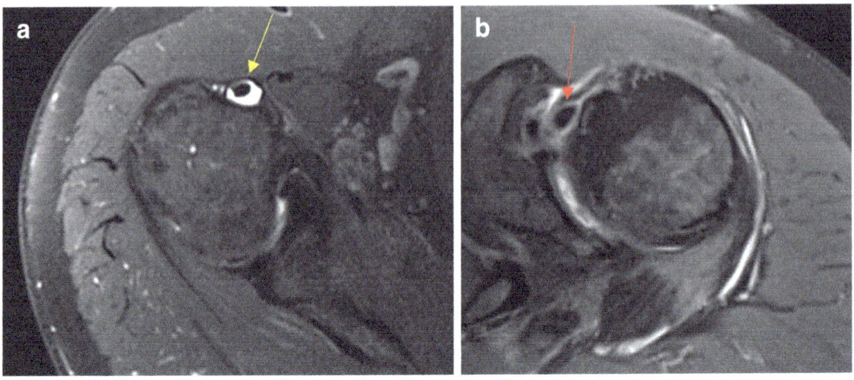

Fig. 10.1 (**a**) Axial MRI without contrast of the right shoulder demonstrating intraarticular fluid within the biceps sheath (yellow arrow). (**b**) Axial MRI without contrast of a left shoulder demonstrating a medially subluxed LHBT (red arrow) with associated subscapularis tendon tear

CAL, were primarily anterior and not lateral. Some propose that the osteophytes and excrescences result from ossification of the CAL insertion [7]. Chambler et al. suggested that this ossification is secondary to tensile forces on the ligament, demonstrating that shoulder abduction places a tensile force on the ligament, which could create a traction enthesophyte [8]. A cadaver study suggests that repetitive contact and bending of the CAL may lead to degenerative changes, including acromial osteophytes [9]. Variations in acromial morphology, initially described by Bigliani et al., were classified into three types based on shape: type I, flat; type II, curved; and type III, hooked Fig. 10.1. The authors also associate a hook-shaped acromion with cuff degeneration [10].

Intrinsic Degeneration

Some authors argue that extrinsic compression is not the primary cause of rotator cuff disease, emphasizing intrinsic factors such as diminished vascular supply, aging, and tensile forces. In this model, degenerative changes or trauma weaken the supraspinatus, preventing it from centering the humeral head on the glenoid. This migration of the humeral head upward narrows the subacromial space, causing osteophytic changes of the acromion and tuberosity erosion [11]. There is a hypovascular critical zone of the supraspinatus tendon that might also contribute as an intrinsic factor leading to tendon degeneration, as identified in a cadaver study by Lohr and Uhthoff [6].

Clinical Presentation

Accurate identification of impingement necessitates a comprehensive examination, including a detailed medical history, physical assessment, and relevant imaging. Patients experiencing impingement often describe symptoms associated with rotator cuff pathologies, such as anterolateral arm pain. This pain pattern was highlighted in Gerber et al.'s study on pain patterns stemming from subacromial space irritation [12]. Symptoms are frequently aggravated during shoulder elevation at or exceeding 90° or when lifting objects away from the body. Utilizing various imaging modalities can be instrumental in pinpointing potential sources of mechanical impingement. The diagnosis of subacromial impingement typically involves a combined approach employing physical examination and radiographic assessments.

Physical Examination

Commonly employed, the Neer and Hawkins tests serve as essential tools for assessing evidence of impingement, demonstrating high sensitivity but limited specificity [13]. In a study by Roberts et al. involving 10 subjects with normal shoulders (average age of 32 years), it was found that the rotator cuff insertion was closest to the anteroinferior acromion at 90° of flexion (Hawkins sign position) but not at full elevation (Neer sign position) [14]. A cross-sectional analysis of nine cadaver specimens in Neer and Hawkins positions showed similar outcomes, with soft tissue contact observed between the shoulders in the Neer position and the medial acromion, and soft tissue contact between shoulders in the Hawkins position and the CAL [15].

Diagnostic Studies

Radiographic evaluations, including AP and Grashey views, are crucial for identifying bony abnormalities in the coracoacromial arch. Additional views such as outlet and axillary views play a significant role, with the outlet view offering insights into acromial morphology and the axillary view providing evidence of os acromiale, potentially contributing to secondary impingement. Radiographic findings associated with impingement include acromioclavicular osteoarthritis with inferior osteophyte formation, acromial enthesophytes or sclerosis, and cystic changes in the humeral head. However, controversy arises as these findings may also be present in asymptomatic individuals. Magnetic resonance imaging is effective in revealing ossification of the CAL or the presence of a subacromial prominence, best visualized in the sagittal oblique plane. Yet, distinguishing between pathological osseous changes and a normal CAL can present challenges.

Management

Management options encompass various injections, physical therapy, and surgical interventions such as bursectomy or subacromial decompression. Nonsurgical approaches have shown success, with studies reporting positive outcomes in a significant percentage of patients [16]. Exercise has been effective in reducing pain and improving function [17]. Surgical interventions become relevant for persistent pain after failed nonsurgical attempts. Arthroscopic subacromial decompression has evolved as a successful surgical technique, providing good long-term results [18].

Nonoperative Management of Subacromial Impingement

The conservative management of subacromial impingement demonstrates widespread success among patients [2, 16]. In a prospective study by Cummins et al., 100 consecutive subacromial impingement patients underwent a nonsurgical treatment regimen, including subacromial cortisone injections and physical therapy.

After a 2-year follow-up, an encouraging 79% of patients did not necessitate surgical intervention [16]. Kuhn's systematic review of 11 randomized controlled trials (RCTs) explored the effectiveness of exercise in addressing rotator cuff impingement, revealing statistically and clinically significant reductions in pain and improvements in function, although no substantial impact on range of motion or strength was observed [17]. Kang et al. investigated the accuracy and effectiveness of subacromial injections in a study involving 60 shoulders with impingement syndrome. Despite a 70% accuracy rate for each injection portal in radiographic assessments, clinical improvement did not consistently correlate with injection accuracy [19]. A double-blind RCT comparing the efficacy of subacromial injections of tenoxicam, a nonsteroidal anti-inflammatory drug, versus corticosteroid injections demonstrated significant superiority of corticosteroids in terms of Constant and Disabilities of the Arm, Shoulder, and Hand scores at the 6-week evaluation point [20].

Operative Management of Subacromial Impingement

Surgery becomes a consideration for patients experiencing persistent pain despite unsuccessful nonsurgical interventions. The advent of arthroscopic shoulder surgery has shifted from open anterior acromioplasty to arthroscopic subacromial decompression and acromioplasty. Arthroscopic decompression allows for direct visualization of arch abrasion and targeted management of potential impingement sources. In a retrospective study evaluating 162 patients who underwent arthroscopic subacromial decompression without rotator cuff repair over a 10- to 13-year follow-up, the authors concluded that isolated supraspinatus tears did not exhibit clinical progression, affirming the favorable long-term outcomes of subacromial decompression for subacromial impingement [21]. In a prospective study by Henkus et al., 57 patients with primary subacromial impingement failing nonsurgical management were randomized to either bursectomy alone or bursectomy with acromioplasty. Both interventions exhibited good clinical results at a mean follow-up of 2.5 years, with a trend favoring acromioplasty, though statistical significance was not reached due to the study's underpowered nature. The type of acromion and symptom severity emerged as more predictive of clinical outcomes than the specific treatment chosen [22].

Summary

Subacromial impingement stands out as a prevalent cause of shoulder pain, sparking ongoing debates within the orthopedic surgery community. The multifactorial nature of subacromial impingement, involving both extrinsic compression and intrinsic degenerative factors, is acknowledged. Surgical intervention proves successful for patients unresponsive to nonsurgical treatments, emphasizing the need for a comprehensive approach to address this common shoulder ailment.

Adhesive Capsulitis

Introduction

Adhesive capsulitis is characterized by pain and a gradual restriction of both active and passive shoulder movements. Patients experiencing a painful and stiff shoulder are commonly diagnosed with "frozen shoulder," a term initially coined by Codman [23]. Adhesive capsulitis, however, represents a distinct pathological condition marked by persistent inflammation in the capsule's synovial layer, leading to thickening, fibrosis, and adherence of the capsule to itself and the anatomic neck of the humerus [24]. This contracted and adherent capsule not only induces pain, particularly during sudden stretches, but also imposes a mechanical limitation on shoulder mobility.

Pathology

In 1945, Neviaser provided a comprehensive description of both the gross and histologic pathology observed in a series of cases, introducing the term "adhesive capsulitis" to characterize the findings precisely. Adhesive capsulitis manifests as a thickened and taut glenohumeral joint capsule, featuring adhesions that obliterate the typically open axillary fold. The fibrotic capsule adheres to both itself and the anatomic neck of the humerus, resulting in minimal synovial fluid within the joint and an overall reduction in joint volume. Microscopic analysis of the capsule revealed a chronic inflammatory infiltrate, the absence of synovial lining, and moderate to extensive synovial fibrosis. Additionally, perivascular lymphocytic reactions are evident [24]. The disease progression is delineated into four stages based on arthroscopic observations of the joint capsule, advancing from capsular inflammation to fibrosis.

Stage 1, the preadhesive stage, is characterized by a fibrinous inflammatory synovitic reaction without adhesion formation. Patients in this stage typically maintain full motion but report pain, particularly at night, presenting with nonspecific symptoms that may lead to misdiagnosis.

Stage 2 involves acute adhesive synovitis marked by synovial proliferation and early adhesion formation, notably in the dependent inferior capsular fold. Prominent pain is accompanied by mild motion loss.

Stage 3, the maturation stage, exhibits reduced synovitis and increased fibrosis, resulting in the obliteration of the axillary fold. Pain intensity may decrease compared to stages 1 and 2, but there is a significant restriction in motion.

Stage 4, the chronic stage, is when fully mature adhesions lead to severe motion restriction, making it challenging to identify intra-articular structures during arthroscopy. Patients may experience a painless but limited range of motion, with pain occurring when the arm is abruptly moved beyond the scarred capsule's limits [25].

Clinical Presentation

Adhesive capsulitis predominantly affects women between the ages of 40 and 60 years, with a higher likelihood of the nondominant arm being more severely impacted [26–29]. Several systemic conditions, including cardiovascular disease, thyroid dysfunction, and a history of breast cancer treatment, are associated with this shoulder ailment. Individuals with a history of cerebrovascular accidents, myocardial infarctions, and diabetes face an elevated risk of developing adhesive capsulitis [30–33]. Diabetes, in particular, is linked to a less favorable prognosis, an increased need for surgery, and suboptimal treatment outcomes [34]. Patients typically present with gradually developing pain persisting for several months, distinguishing it from the more abrupt onset seen in other shoulder conditions. The pain, often radiating to the origin of the deltoid, is especially pronounced at night. Concurrent with, or, in rare instances, preceding the onset of pain, there is a noticeable loss of shoulder motion that tends to worsen with disease progression. Individuals may encounter challenges in daily activities such as dressing, combing hair, reaching into a back pocket, or fastening a brassiere. In stages 3 and 4, the loss of motion becomes severe, impacting movement in all directions. While pain diminishes, it may only become apparent when the shoulder is moved beyond the limits allowed by the contracted capsule [24].

Physical Examination

There is no specific point of tenderness identified. On occasion, tenderness may be observed in the long head of the biceps tendon due to its synovial connection with the glenohumeral joint. Rotator cuff strength typically remains within the normal range. The hallmark of adhesive capsulitis lies in the mechanical restriction of passive motion, with the most noticeable impact seen during passive external rotation when the arm is at the side [24].

Diagnostic Studies

Although radiographs commonly appear normal, they play a crucial role in ruling out alternative causes such as arthritis, calcific tendinitis, and potential shoulder dislocation. While advanced imaging does not serve as the primary diagnostic tool, its utility lies in recognizing features indicative of adhesive capsulitis. Magnetic resonance arthrography proves beneficial in identifying the thickening of the joint capsule and reduced filling of the axillary pouch as diagnostic criteria. Emig et al. highlighted that a capsule and synovium thickness exceeding 4 mm adjacent to the axillary recess is highly specific for adhesive capsulitis; however, changes in the coracohumeral ligament were not consistently observed [35]. Other studies have indicated scarring within the rotator interval as a more prevalent finding [36, 37]. These imaging modalities are particularly valuable for excluding alternative causes of symptoms, such as full and partial-thickness rotator cuff tears, calcific tendinitis, glenohumeral or acromioclavicular arthritis, and cervical radiculopathy.

Management

The natural course of adhesive capsulitis sparks ongoing debates, with potential spontaneous improvement, but the reported outcomes of minimal interventions exhibit significant variability, heavily contingent on the measurement criteria employed. Subjective outcome measures tend to yield more favorable results than objective measures. For instance, in one study, 90% of patients under minimal therapy expressed satisfaction with their shoulder function [38]. However, another study utilizing objective outcomes indicated that 50% of patients still experienced residual pain, and 60% exhibited impaired motion [39].

Nonoperative Management of Adhesive Capsulitis

Irrespective of the disease stage, physical therapy, coupled with a home exercise program, stands as the cornerstone of treatment. Physical therapy does not need to be aggressive or painful, and strenuous strengthening exercises are required [40]. Gentle, progressive stretching proves to be optimal and effective in most cases. It is crucial to counsel patients on the expectation of a prolonged recovery period. While nonsteroidal anti-inflammatory drugs may enhance sleep and therapy tolerability, their impact on recovery remains limited. Both oral and intra-articular steroid injections have been extensively studied. Despite theoretical promise due to the inflammatory nature of early disease stages, most studies reveal only a transient pain reduction (e.g., 3 to 6 weeks) with no concurrent improvement in motion [41–46]. Longer-term follow-ups indicate no notable difference between patients treated with steroids and control subjects. Some reports suggest success with suprascapular nerve blocks and hydrodilatation as alternative approaches [47, 48]. Quraishi et al. conducted a randomized trial involving 17 patients undergoing manipulation under anesthesia and 19 patients undergoing hydrodilatation. The procedure involved injecting a mixture of steroid (30 mg triamcinolone) and local anesthetic (2% lidocaine), with varying volumes of saline required to rupture the capsule. Patient satisfaction rates were notably higher with hydrodilatation compared to manipulation under anesthesia, standing at 94% versus 81%, as observed during the 6-month final follow-up [47]. There is no direct comparison between hydrodilatation and arthroscopic arthrolysis. Nevertheless, existing evidence indicates that some patients may necessitate arthroscopic arthrolysis following suboptimal outcomes from hydrodilatation procedures [49].

Operative Management of Adhesive Capsulitis

Surgical intervention becomes necessary for patients who do not exhibit improvement with physical therapy. According to Levine et al., individuals with severe initial symptoms, younger age at onset, and a reduction in motion despite 4 months of compliant therapy are more likely to undergo surgery [29]. Arthroscopic capsular release has emerged as the primary surgical approach, surpassing manipulation under anesthesia due to its advantages, including complete joint inspection, confirmation of diagnosis, and a more precise capsulotomy without associated manipulation risks. Comparative to manipulation under anesthesia, arthroscopic capsular division has demonstrated enhanced pain relief and functional restoration over a 2- to 5-year period, with sustained results even in longer-term follow-ups [50]. Arthroscopic capsular release can be performed in either the beach chair position or lateral decubitus position. The posterolateral portal is established, and electrocautery inserted through an anterior portal is utilized for releasing the anterior capsule and rotator interval, excluding the subscapularis. Electrocautery use is ceased upon identification of the plane between the capsule and subscapularis tendon and always stopped before reaching the lower border of the subscapularis to safeguard the axillary nerve. After the anterior and anterior-inferior releases, the shoulder undergoes external rotation and abduction, followed by internal rotation to verify the adequacy of the release. The diseased coracohumeral ligament can also be released in the subacromial space if there is still a deficiency in external rotation.

The decision to release the posterior capsule remains controversial. Some advocate for circumferential release or selective posterior release if persistent loss of internal rotation occurs after the anterior release. Comparison studies between anterior release and circumferential release yield mixed results, with early benefits demonstrated in routine posterior capsule release studies; however, long-term outcomes are similar to those with isolated anterior release [51, 52]. Postoperative physical therapy is crucial, emphasizing early, diligent efforts aimed at preventing recurrent stiffness.

Summary
The patient presenting with a painful and stiff shoulder requires a comprehensive evaluation for an accurate differential diagnosis, guiding appropriate treatment based on the underlying pathology. The initial approach involves gentle physical therapy, prioritizing a pain-free range of motion. Despite the success of nonsurgical treatment, patients may endure months of persistent symptoms. While pharmacologic interventions like intra-articular steroid injections do not significantly reduce symptom duration, they might offer some early pain relief. Candidates not showing improvement after 6 months of dedicated therapy are suitable for further intervention. Arthroscopic capsular release emerges as a precise intervention, avoiding potential complications associated with manipulation. Postoperative therapy remains essential to achieve complete active motion and prevent recurrence.

Rotator Cuff Disorders

Rotator Cuff Tears

Incidence and Prevalence
Around 4.5 million patient consultations are recorded annually in the United States due to shoulder pain [53]. A significant majority of individuals undergoing rotator cuff repair are in the workforce. The incidence of rotator cuff tears increases with

age, with approximately 54% of individuals aged 60 or older exhibiting either partial or complete tears on magnetic resonance imaging, even if they are asymptomatic [54]. Studies utilizing ultrasonography indicate that 13% of individuals in their 50 s, 20% in their 60 s, and 31% in their 70 s have rotator cuff tears [55].

Factors Contributing to Rotator Cuff Tears

Individuals engaging in repetitive lifting or overhead tasks face an increased risk of experiencing rotator cuff tears. Athletes, in particular, are prone to overuse injuries, commonly observed among tennis players and baseball pitchers due to repetitive microtrauma. Professions involving overhead work, such as painting and carpentry, also elevate the likelihood of developing tears. While overuse injuries stemming from sports or overhead activities are prevalent among younger individuals, traumatic incidents such as falls or shoulder dislocations are the primary causes of tears in young adults [56].

Physical Examination

The examination of the shoulder commences with a thorough inspection of the affected shoulder girdle in comparison to the opposite side. It is essential for the patient to remove their shirt (ensuring the chest is covered for female patients) to facilitate examination of the shoulder and periscapular region at rest, allowing for the detection of asymmetry, scapular malposition, atrophy of the deltoid or rotator cuff, as well as signs of ecchymosis, erythema, wounds, or surgical incisions, all of which offer valuable diagnostic cues.

Subsequently, osseous landmarks are methodically palpated for tenderness, deformity, or signs of fracture. These landmarks include the sternoclavicular joint, clavicle, acromioclavicular joint, acromion, coracoid process, and scapular spine. Additionally, soft-tissue landmarks such as the lateral shoulder, periscapular region, and the long head of the biceps tendon are assessed through palpation. Evaluation of distal pulses, capillary refill, and finger temperature is also warranted. Dermatomal sensation and resisted isometric strength in the C5-T1 distribution are then tested and compared bilaterally.

Further assessment involves evaluating both active and passive glenohumeral range of motion. Key movements assessed include forward elevation, isolated glenohumeral abduction with scapular stabilization, external rotation with the arm at the side, and internal rotation (measured by reaching up the spine), with normal values typically considered as 180°, 90°, 80° to 90°, and T5-T8, respectively. However, individual variations exist, necessitating comparison with the contralateral side for accurate interpretation [57, 58].

Subacromial Impingement Assessment

Neer Test

The Neer sign is conducted by stabilizing scapular rotation with one hand while the other hand of the examiner passively elevates the arm forward, eliciting pain in the anterior or lateral shoulder, indicating a positive result [13, 59, 60]. In addition, the

Neer test can involve the administration of a local anesthetic under the anterior acromion, with a positive outcome noted if there is a reduction or elimination of pain [13].

Hawkins Test

The Hawkins test entails raising the shoulder to 90° while internally rotating the arm. A positive result is indicated by pain localized at the anterior edge of the acromion [13, 59–61].

Supraspinatus Assessment

Jobe Test

During the Jobe test, the patient positions their arm at 90° of abduction, 30° of horizontal adduction, and complete internal rotation while resisting downward pressure from the examiner's hand. A positive outcome is characterized by the presence of pain and/or weakness [59, 60, 62, 63].

Drop Arm Test

In the Drop Arm test, the patient actively abducts their shoulder to 90° and then slowly lowers the arm. A positive result is observed when the patient is unable to lower the arm gradually and instead drops it immediately due to pain [64].

Infraspinatus/Teres Minor Assessment

External Rotation Test

For the External Rotation test, the patient's elbow is flexed at 90°, with the arm by their side initially internally rotated by 45°, followed by external rotation against resistance provided by the examiner.

Hornblower Test

During the Hornblower test, the examiner stabilizes the patient's elbow at 90° of flexion with the arm abducted in the scapular plane while the patient attempts to externally rotate the arm against resistance. A positive outcome is indicated by the inability to externally rotate against resistance [60, 65].

External Rotation Lag Sign

To conduct the External Rotation Lag sign, position the patient's elbow at 90° of flexion with the arm beside the body, then externally rotate the arm by 45°. A positive outcome is observed when the patient cannot maintain the externally rotated position after the examiner releases the forearm, causing the arm to lag back to a neutral external rotation [65].

Liftoff Test

In the Liftoff test, instruct the patient to place the hand of the affected arm on the back at the midlumbar spine level and internally rotate the arm to lift the hand off the back posteriorly. A positive indication is noted if the patient struggles to lift the arm off the back posteriorly or resorts to extending the elbow or shoulder to achieve this movement [66].

Belly Press Test

For the Belly Press test, position the affected arm at the side with the elbow flexed to 90° and ask the patient to press the palm into their abdomen while maintaining maximal internal rotation, positioning the elbow in front of the trunk [66]. This test yields a negative result if the patient can press the hand against the stomach with the wrist fully extended. Conversely, it is considered positive if the elbow or shoulder extends or if the wrist flexes, indicating subscapularis deficiency compensated by the posterior deltoid. An advantage of the Belly Press test over the Liftoff test is its ability to assess the subscapularis even in stiff and painful shoulders, as the Liftoff test's position of internal rotation behind the back can be uncomfortable and compromise testing [66, 67].

Guidelines for Nonoperative Treatment of Rotator Cuff Tears

Partial-Thickness Rotator Cuff Tears

Conservative approaches are typically employed for impingement and partial-thickness tears of the rotator cuff. Rehabilitation aims to restore the full range of motion, synchronize the firing of the rotator cuff and periscapular muscles, and normalize glenohumeral and scapulothoracic kinematics. Addressing posterior capsular contractures reduces anterosuperior shoulder translation, thereby minimizing contact between the rotator cuff and the acromion [68]. Strengthening the infraspinatus, teres minor, and subscapularis muscles facilitates coordinated action against superior humeral head translation, potentially alleviating subacromial impingement. Manual physical therapy techniques, such as joint mobilization, combined with supervised exercises, have demonstrated superior efficacy over exercises alone in enhancing strength, reducing pain, and improving function [69, 70].

Full-Thickness Rotator Cuff Tear

While conservative management can yield success with rotator cuff tears, predicting outcomes reliably remains challenging. Some patients regain function with minimal or no pain post-injury, while others experience significant disability. The primary objective of management is to establish a balanced axial plane force between the anterior subscapularis muscle and the posterior infraspinatus and teres minor muscles. Nonsurgical management aims to alleviate pain and restore function, initially focusing on inflammation reduction and motion restoration. Addressing contractures lowers the risk of subacromial impingement. Subsequent rotator cuff strengthening enables intact musculature to compensate for the torn tendon(s). In cases where conservative treatment proves ineffective, many professionals advocate for surgical intervention, believing that postoperative recovery is smoother in shoulders with preoperative suppleness compared to those with stiffness [71].

Operative Management of Rotator Cuff Tears

If nonsurgical interventions prove ineffective, the patient may then be considered for a rotator cuff repair procedure. Fixation techniques employed in arthroscopic rotator cuff repair aim to restore anatomy, recreate biomechanics with robust fixation, promote healing, and enhance function [72]. To achieve these objectives, various fixation methods have been developed, differing in anchor quantity, suture material, fixation region, and biomechanical qualities [73]. Following diagnostic arthroscopy, identification of the tear pattern and tendon mobilization anchors are strategically placed. Medial anchors, when utilized, are positioned just lateral to the articular margin, while lateral row anchors are situated at the lateral aspect of the greater tuberosity, taking advantage of optimal bone quality in the humeral head [74–76].

Common techniques include single-row and double-row repairs, with double-row repairs generally considered biomechanically superior [72, 75]. Studies have raised concerns regarding single-row repairs, with recurrent defects observed in approximately 94% of cases in some studies. Additionally, there is a significant deterioration in functional outcomes between 12- and 24-month follow-ups [77]. It has been noted that single-row repairs may not adequately reproduce the surface area of the tendon on the greater tuberosity, potentially hindering healing. Some suggest that the lack of healing with arthroscopic repair could be attributed to the reduced restoration of the anatomical surface area ("footprint") [78]. However, some comparative studies have shown improved surface area restoration with similar strength in load-to-failure tests between single-row and double-row techniques. However, biomechanical testing alone does not fully determine outcomes, as the biological quality of repair through a larger tendon-to-footprint surface is also crucial [79]. Several meta-analyses have demonstrated comparable clinical results and significantly lower retear rates with the double-row technique compared to single-row repairs. However, it is important to note that some studies have not found significant differences in clinical scores between the two techniques. While MRI has been used to confirm retear rates, it has limitations in distinguishing between a retear and a lack of healing from the initial repair [80, 81].

Millett et al. were pioneers in describing the linking of medial and lateral rows, introducing a crisscross method that has since become the standard approach in arthroscopic repair. This technique optimizes anatomy, biomechanics, and biology by maximizing tendon-bone contact area, placing anchors in high-quality bone, compressing the tendon onto the bone with sutures on the bursal surface, minimizing foreign material at the cuff bone interface, allowing resistance to multivector loads due to the crisscrossing suture configuration, and enhancing bone resistance to tendon failure by dissipating forces over the entire construct [82].

Calcific Tendinitis

Epidemiology

Calcific tendinitis is a common shoulder pathology causing pain. In a study involving 6061 office workers (equivalent to 12,122 shoulders), Bosworth discovered that the prevalence of calcific deposits in a predominantly younger population under 40 years old was 2.7%, with 35% of shoulders exhibiting symptoms [83]. Calcific tendinitis typically manifests in individuals aged 30 to 60 years, with a higher incidence in women compared to men. While the right shoulder is more commonly affected than the left, bilateral presentation is also possible. Radiographic and ultrasound investigations have consistently shown the supraspinatus tendon to be the most frequently involved [83–88]. Harvie et al. explored the natural progression of calcific tendinitis and its association with endocrine disorders. Their findings indicated a notably high prevalence of concurrent endocrine abnormalities, particularly hypothyroidism, in individuals with calcific tendinitis. Moreover, a substantial percentage of female participants (69%) had a history of menstrual disorders, suggesting a potential role of estrogen in the condition's pathogenesis. Patients with endocrine abnormalities tend to develop symptoms at a younger age, experience prolonged symptom duration, and ultimately undergo surgery at a higher rate compared to those without such conditions [89].

Pathogenesis

The underlying causes of calcific tendinitis remain elusive, with various theories proposed. It is important to distinguish calcific tendinitis from insertional calcific tendinitis [90]. While degenerative theories were previously favored, Uhthoff and Loehr introduced the concept of an active, cell-mediated process, which is now widely accepted. Unlike earlier theories suggesting a degenerating tendon that later calcified, Uhthoff and Loehr described a reactive process involving cartilage metaplasia within an active biological environment. They delineated three main stages of calcification: precalcific, calcific, and postcalcific. Within the calcific stage, three distinct phases were identified: formative, resting, and resorptive [84].

During the precalcific stage, fibrocartilaginous metaplasia predominantly occurs, likely within less vascularized regions of the tendon. In the formative phase of the calcific stage, matrix vesicles aggregate to form calcific deposits, interspersed with fibrocartilage or fibrocollagenous tissue. The resting phase is characterized by dormancy, with minimal inflammation or vascular activity. Eventually, resorption occurs, coinciding with the emergence of thin-walled vascular channels, as well as macrophages and multinucleated giant cells. Following resorption, fibroblasts and granulation tissue appear at the site of the previous deposit [84, 90].

Clinical Presentation and Physical Examination

Calcific tendinitis typically manifests as shoulder pain, resembling the clinical presentation of subacromial impingement. Many individuals with calcific tendinitis experience reduced active range of motion and adapt their shoulder mechanics to alleviate discomfort.

During the formative phase of calcific tendinitis, patients commonly report chronic pain. Deposits in this phase are often described as having a chalk-like appearance [91]. Pain intensity may fluctuate during the resting phase but tends to be particularly severe during the resorptive phase. In the latter phase, patients may present with a sudden onset of shoulder pain without any traumatic incident, which can resemble symptoms of infection. Additionally, the expression of deposits during the resorptive phase often resembles a toothpaste-like material [84].

Diagnostic Studies

The standard radiographic assessment typically includes plain radiographs, comprising anteroposterior (AP), supraspinatus outlet, and axillary views. Internal and external rotation views may also be obtained to better delineate the deposit's location. Typically, the calcific deposit is situated approximately 1.5 to 2 cm from the insertion point near the tendon's critical zone, an area characterized by reduced vascularity near the superior rotator cuff's insertion [92].

In cases of persistent or resistant pain, MRI may be utilized to identify any accompanying pathologies, such as rotator cuff tears, that could be exacerbating symptoms. Calcific deposits typically exhibit low signal intensity across all MRI sequences, with possible surrounding edema evident on fluid-sensitive sequences. On ultrasonography, calcific deposits present as hyperechoic areas. In patients with symptomatic calcific tendinitis, ultrasonography often reveals large fragmented deposits, a positive power Doppler signal, and widening of the subacromial bursal space [85].

Nonoperative Management of Calcific Tendinitis

Nonsurgical approaches are typically the initial choice for managing calcific tendinitis, with anti-inflammatories, physical therapy, and corticosteroid injections constituting primary interventions. Ogon et al. conducted a study involving 488 shoulders to assess prognostic factors for nonsurgical management of calcific tendinitis following initial treatment failure. Failure was defined as persistent symptoms lasting at least 6 months, with 3 months of standardized treatment at the institution. The study found an overall failure rate of 27%, with the likelihood of failure increasing in cases of bilateral or large calcifications, deposits located beneath the anterior third of the acromion, and extension of calcific deposits medial to the acromion. However, a Gärtner type III calcific deposit was identified as a positive prognostic factor [93]. In a study by Cho et al. involving 87 patients (92 shoulders) treated nonsurgically for calcific tendinopathy with a mean follow-up of 16 months, significant improvements were noted in shoulder outcome scores. Following treatment consisting solely of NSAIDs and passive range of motion exercises, 66 shoulders (72%) achieved good to excellent results. Additionally, deposits in 57 shoulders (62%) either disappeared or decreased in size during the follow-up period [93].

Extracorporeal Shock Wave Therapy (ESWT)

Research on ESWT for managing calcific tendinitis of the rotator cuff has demonstrated considerable variability in parameters such as energy flux density, number of impulses, and treatment sessions. However, studies have consistently shown that high-energy ESWT effectively improves overall shoulder function and reduces pain scores. Refractory calcific tendinitis, particularly outside the acute resorptive phase, has shown promising responses to ESWT compared to conventional treatments in short- and medium-term studies [94–96].

Short-term randomized trials comparing ESWT to placebo treatment have revealed dose-dependent improvements with ESWT. Despite its efficacy, ESWT may not always provide complete resolution, necessitating further long-term investigation [95, 97]. In a study by Daecke et al., 20% of patients with calcific tendinitis treated with ESWT underwent shoulder surgery within 4 years post-treatment [98]. Several randomized controlled trials have compared high- and low-energy ESWT to placebo [99, 100]. Gerdesmeyer et al. conducted a study with 144 patients randomized into three groups: high-energy ESWT, low-energy ESWT, and placebo. Both ESWT groups demonstrated significant and clinically relevant improvements in Constant and visual analog scale (VAS) scores at 6 months compared to the placebo group. The high-energy group exhibited superior outcomes compared to the low-energy group, with larger reductions in VAS scores and greater decreases in calcific deposit size and resorption rates. These superior outcomes persisted at the 12-month follow-up, highlighting the efficacy of high-energy ESWT for calcific tendinitis of the rotator cuff [99].

Peters et al. conducted a randomized controlled trial involving 90 patients treated with either high- or low-energy ESWT or a placebo, yielding similar findings. The high-energy group required significantly fewer treatments on average compared to the low-energy group (mean 1.2 versus 4.1) to alleviate pain and improve mobility—a clinically significant discrepancy. However, the high-energy group experienced a higher level of procedural discomfort compared to the low-energy group, with no requirement for procedural anesthesia. Conversely, the placebo group reported no discomfort and derived no benefit from the procedure [100].

Numerous studies have indicated a relationship between treatment effectiveness and reduction in the size of calcific deposits. However, Albert et al. found no significant change in resorption rates among patients treated with high- or low-energy ESWT at a mean follow-up of 4 months. Despite persistent calcifications, the high-energy group still demonstrated statistically significant improvement in Constant scores (alongside increased pain during treatment) compared to the low-energy group [94]. A meta-analysis by Ioppolo et al. reported a higher incidence of total and partial resorption of calcific deposits 6 months after ESWT compared to placebo treatment [97]. Complications associated with ESWT have been documented, including procedural discomfort, particularly at higher energy flux densities. Common adverse reactions include local responses such as petechiae, ecchymosis, hematoma, and erythema.

Ultrasound-Guided Needle Lavage (UGNL)

Ultrasound is used to pinpoint the location of the calcific deposit, after which local anesthesia is administered, typically into the subacromial bursa and surrounding soft tissue. Guided by ultrasound, a needle is then inserted either adjacent to or directly into the calcification. Some studies suggest using a single needle for aspiration and lavage, while others employ two needles to establish an outflow system for lavage [101–103].

A solution of saline or a mixture of anesthetic and saline is injected near the calcification, and the calcific material is aspirated. Lavage continues until the irrigation runs clear. While some authors advocate puncturing multiple sites (needling) to manually break up the deposit, [104, 105] others recommend keeping the needle in the same position to minimize potential damage to the rotator cuff [101]. Following the procedure, the needle is typically retracted into the subacromial bursa under ultrasound guidance, and a steroid is injected.

In a randomized controlled trial, de Witte et al. compared needle lavage and subacromial injection with subacromial injection alone. They found that both groups showed improvement, but the needle lavage group had higher Constant scores and smaller mean calcification size. After 6 months, more patients in the initial injection group opted for needle lavage or surgery compared to those in the initial needle lavage group [104]. Similarly, Krasny et al. compared UGNL and ESWT with ESWT alone in two groups. At the 4-month follow-up, both groups showed statistically and clinically significant improvement in Constant scores, with the UGNL and ESWT group reporting a higher rate of deposit elimination, less pain during ESWT, and a lower final rate of arthroscopic surgery compared to the ESWT alone group [105]. UGNL is considered an effective, well-tolerated, and cost-effective procedure, making it a reasonable treatment option when less invasive approaches fail. However, as with many studies of ESWT, interpreting outcomes of UGNL can be challenging due to the characteristic spontaneous improvement seen in the natural progression of the disease [103].

Operative Management of Calcific Tendinitis

Multiple investigations have examined the outcomes of arthroscopic removal of calcific deposits. In one study involving 54 patients who underwent this procedure, the overall results were positive, with 92% of patients achieving excellent outcomes at a 2-year follow-up. However, various controversies persist regarding the surgical management of calcific tendinitis, such as the optimal extent of calcification removal, the long-term effects on the tendon, and the potential benefits of subacromial decompression. Further well-designed studies assessing different treatments for calcific tendinitis are necessary to determine their comparative effectiveness accurately [106, 107].

Subacromial decompression remains a subject of debate in the management of calcific tendinitis It is typically considered when there is evidence of fraying of the coracoacromial ligament or erosions on the undersurface of the acromion [108]. Research by Porcellini et al. suggests that acromioplasty may not always be necessary, as simply removing the deposit can often alleviate mechanical impingement symptoms [109]. For instance, a study by Maier et al. followed 93 patients (99 shoulders) over an average of 3 years after arthroscopic removal of calcific deposits without acromioplasty or rotator cuff repair. They found that 91% of patients achieved good to excellent results. Similarly, Marder et al. conducted a retrospective case-control study involving 50 patients with calcific tendinitis treated surgically by two different surgeons. One group underwent acromioplasty and subacromial decompression, while the other underwent deposit removal alone. The study revealed that the group undergoing subacromial decompression had a longer average time to return to work (18 weeks vs. 11 weeks), but overall long-term outcomes were comparable between the two groups [110].

Comparative investigations have assessed the efficacy of surgery in comparison to alternative treatments. In a study conducted by Wittenberg et al., a matched-pair analysis was conducted involving 100 patients who received either surgical or non-surgical interventions. Open surgery entailed the resection of the coracoacromial (CA) ligament in all cases, with acromioplasty performed in only 20% of instances. Results revealed that patients undergoing surgical intervention exhibited higher satisfaction rates and functional scores during 3- to 5-year follow-ups. The authors concluded that the removal of the calcific deposit constituted a significant aspect of the surgical procedure [111]. Rompe et al. conducted a comparative study between surgery and ESWT for the treatment of calcific tendinitis. The surgical group comprised 29 patients who underwent open procedures, while the ESWT group consisted of 50 patients, selected based on the insurance company's coverage for ESWT. The study exclusively included patients with Gärtner type I or II calcific tendinitis. ESWT entailed a single treatment session comprising 3000 impulses at 0.60 mJ/mm^2. Although the ESWT group demonstrated a swifter recovery and return to work, both cohorts exhibited significant improvement at the 1-year follow-up. By the 2-year follow-up, patients who underwent surgery showed higher University of California Los Angeles (UCLA) scores compared to those treated with ESWT. Moreover, the rate of calcific deposit resorption was higher in patients with Gärtner type II deposits compared to type I deposits. In patients with type II deposits, comparable outcomes were observed between surgery and ESWT. However, for patients with type I deposits, surgery yielded statistically and clinically superior results, with 75% and 92% reporting good to excellent outcomes at 1- and 2-year follow-ups, respectively, in contrast to 48% and 53% in the ESWT group [112]. Several studies have examined the results of arthroscopic removal of calcific deposits. Rebuzzi et al. compared arthroscopic surgery with ESWT for managing chronic calcific tendinitis of the shoulder. Arthroscopic removal of calcifications was conducted in 22 cases, while ESWT was administered in 24 cases, with the choice of treatment based on insurance coverage. ESWT involved an average of three sessions comprising 1500 pulses at an energy flux density ranging from 0.10 to 0.13 mJ/mm^2. At the 2-year follow-up, significant enhancement in the UCLA scores was observed in both groups, with the degree of resorption correlating with overall patient improvement. The authors concluded that the two treatments yielded comparable outcomes. However, the study was constrained by its small sample size, the nearly significant difference in the baseline groups ($P = 0.09$ for initial UCLA scores, suggesting incomplete similarity between the two groups), and the absence of a power analysis [106].

Summary
Musculoskeletal specialists often come across cases of calcific tendinitis. The primary approach involves nonsurgical methods, accompanied by patient education about the condition. However, understanding the natural progression of improvement over time is crucial as it can confound the interpretation of clinical studies, as outcomes may vary depending on the disease stage and duration of follow-up. There is a need for a deeper understanding of the mechanisms underlying the disease to develop more effective treatment strategies. Large-scale, meticulously designed, controlled studies comparing treatment options at comparable disease stages are essential to determine the most optimal treatments.

Proximal Biceps Tendon Pathology

Epidemiology

The long head of the biceps tendon (LHBT) can be a significant source of shoulder pain in both younger and elderly patients. LHBT pathology can include tendinitis, partial tears, complete ruptures, subluxation, and biceps-labral complex pathology such as a superior labrum anterior to posterior (SLAP) tear. LHBT pathology is highly associated with rotator cuff pathology [113] and has been reported to have an incidence ranging from 36% to 82% in the setting of rotator cuff tears [114–117]. While primary LHBT tendonitis, or better termed inflammatory tenosynovitis, can occur, it is much less common than LHBT tendonitis in the setting of concomitant shoulder pathology [118]. Similarly, isolated LHBT ruptures infrequently occur, with the true incidence being unknown. The prevalence of SLAP tears on MRI has been found to be as high as 81% in the elderly population [119, 120]; however, the incidence of SLAP lesions during shoulder arthroscopy has been reported at much lower rates, typically less than 25% [121, 122].

Relevant Anatomy

The LHBT originates within the glenohumeral joint at the supraglenoid tubercle and superior labrum. After traversing the glenohumeral joint, the LHBT exits the joint through the bicipital groove in the proximal humerus. The LHBT is stabilized in the bicipital groove by the biceps sling or pulley, which is a tendoligamentous structure composed of the subscapularis tendon, supraspinatus tendon, coracohumeral ligament, and the superior glenohumeral ligament. Additionally, the transverse humeral ligament and pectoralis major tendon help to stabilize the LHBT. While the contribution of the LHBT to shoulder function has been debated, it is thought to act as a humeral head depressor as well as assist in glenohumeral joint stabilization and forward flexion [123–127].

Clinical Presentation

Patients with LHBT pathology typically present with anterior shoulder pain that may radiate down the anterior arm [113, 118]. Typically, symptoms are worse with repetitive overhead activities as well as activities that require elbow flexion and forearm supination. In the case of LHBT instability, patients may experience mechanical symptoms such as popping or catching. In older patients, concomitant rotator cuff symptoms may be present, such as lateral deltoid pain, shoulder weakness, or pain at night. In the younger overhead athletes, isolated LHBT symptoms are more likely. In the setting of LHBT rupture, patients may experience biceps cramping, ecchymosis of the arm which may track distally, as well as a Popeye deformity of the biceps [113]. Patients with SLAP tears may report an acute traumatic event or repetitive overhead motion [128]. Most commonly, SLAP tears will present with shoulder pain during overhead motions as well as subjective shoulder instability, catching, and popping [122, 128].

Physical Examination

Physical examination should consist of direct palpation over the bicipital groove and LHBT, as well as several specific provocative tests. Additionally, a gross deformity or ecchymosis may be observed in the setting of an LHBT rupture. Provocative tests for LHBT and SLAP pathology include Speed's test, Yergason's test, and the O'Brien active compression test. Speed's test is considered positive when the patient experiences pain localized to the anterior shoulder with resisted shoulder forward elevation with the forearm supinated. Yergason's test is considered positive when the patient experiences pain localized to the anterior shoulder with resisted forearm supination while the elbow is flexed to 90°. While Speed's and Yergason's tests have been found to be specific for LHBT and SLAP pathology, they are limited by their low sensitivity [129]. The O'Brien active compression test is performed by having the patient resist downward pressure on their arm when the patient's shoulder is positioned at 90° of forward flexion and 10° of adduction. A positive O'Brien active compression test will result in deep shoulder pain. According to meta-analysis data, the O'Brien active compression test has been noted to have a sensitivity ranging from 47% to 78% and a specificity from 11% to 73% for the diagnosis of SLAP lesions [130]. It is important to localize the pain with the O'Brien active compression test, as the test can also be positive with acromioclavicular joint pathology. Due to the varying sensitivity and specificity of provocative tests, a combination of the abovementioned tests and findings should be used to diagnose LHBT and SLAP pathology.

Diagnostic Studies

Diagnostic imaging for LHBT and SLAP pathology should begin with a complete radiographic series of the shoulder to evaluate for concomitant pathology, although patients with isolated LHBT and SLAP pathology will often have normal radiographs [113]. A shoulder MRI is the diagnostic study of choice when evaluating the LHBT and the biceps-labral complex. Specific pathologic findings on MRI may include fluid within the biceps sheath (Fig. 10.1a), medial LHBT subluxation (Fig. 10.1b), tearing of the LHBT, absence of the LHBT, or a SLAP tear. Contrast-enhanced MRIs will show fluid in the biceps sheath, which may not be pathologic; however, contrast-enhanced MRIs may better identify SLAP lesions [118] (Fig. 10.1a, b).

Table 10.1 Nonoperative outcomes for proximal biceps pathology

Study	Diagnosis	Methods	Results
Deutch et al. [134]	LHBT rupture	11 patients treated nonoperatively	Mean follow-up of 1.7 years 23% decrease in supination strength, 29% decrease in pronation strength, 29% decrease in elbow flexion strength All patients experienced continued pain or disability at final follow-up
Mariani et al. [133]	LHBT rupture	31 patients treated nonoperatively compared to 27 patients treated operatively with biceps tenodesis	Mean follow-up of 4.6 years for nonoperative group No difference in pain and shoulder or elbow range or motion Nonoperaative group had an 8% decrease in elbow flexion strength and 21% decrease in forearm supination strength 11 nonsurgical patients were unable to return to full work capacity, compared to only 2 in the surgical group
McDevitt et al. [135]	Chronic tendinopathy	Case series of 10 patients treated by physical therapist with stretching, exercises, and dry needling	Patients had significant improvement in numeric pain rating scale, Quick Disabilities of the Arm, Shoulder, and Hand score, and Global Rating of Change score

(continued)

Table 10.1 (continued)

Study	Diagnosis	Methods	Results
Edward et al [136].	SLAP tear	39 patients were reviewed	Mean follow-up of 3.1 years 19 patients (49%) with successful nonoperative treatment had significantly improvement in ASES, SST, VAS scores All 19 returned to sport 20 patients (51%) underwent surgical intervention
Jang et al. [137]	SLAP tear	63 patients treated with physical therapy and activity modifications	Mean follow-up of 21 months
		Minimum 6-month follow-up	ASES, VAS score significantly improved in 71.4% of patients 28.5% of patients failed nonoperative treatment due to being dissatisfied or going on to have surgery
Yiannakopoulos et al. [139]	LHBT tendinopathy	44 patients randomized to undergoing bicipital sheath injection under ultrasound guidance (22 patients) versus free-hand technique (22 patients)	Significant improvement in VAS, SANE and QuickDASH scores improved in both groups and 4 weeks and 6 months
		Clinical follow-up at 4 weeks and 6 months following injections	Significantly better improvement in the ultrasound-guided group
Zhang et al. [140]	LHBT tendinopathy	Compared outcomes of biceps sheath corticosteroid injection in 45 patients using a free-hand technique and 53 patients using ultrasound-guided technique	Mean follow-up of 33 weeks
		Minimum follow-up of 24 months	Both groups reported significantly improved VAS and Constant-Murley scores 91% of the ultrasound-guided group had improvement in pain and function 80% in the free-hand technique group had improvement in pain and function

In addition to MRI imaging, ultrasound has also been advocated as a useful diagnostic modality for the evaluation of the LHBT. Ultrasound has been shown to be accurate in diagnosing full thickness LHBT tears, LHBT subluxation or dislocation, and a normal LHBT; however, it is much less accurate in identifying partial thickness LHBT tears [126, 131, 132].

Nonoperative Management of Proximal Biceps Pathology

Management of symptomatic LHBT and SLAP pathology should begin with nonoperative management including rest, activity modifications, physical therapy, and nonsteroidal anti-inflammatory medications [113, 118, 126]. Studies evaluating nonoperative management of LHBT pathology are limited and have demonstrated mixed results [133–135]; however, these results seem to be dependent on the LHBT pathology. There has been some evidence that nonoperative management of SLAP tears results in acceptable rates of return to sport and work [137, 138]. Corticosteroid injections, either into the subacromial space, glenohumeral joint, or biceps sheath have also been advocated as an acceptable nonoperative treatment for LHBT tendinopathy [113, 118, 126]. While limited in number, studies have shown good short term symptomatic relief following corticosteroid injections for LHBT tendinopathy, and have also shown ultrasound-guided injections to be superior to a free-hand technique [139, 140]. The outcomes of nonoperative treatment are outlined in Table 10.1.

Operative Management of Proximal Biceps Pathology

Operative management for LHBT pathology is reserved for patients who have failed to improve with nonoperative treatment and typically entails biceps tenotomy or tenodesis, in addition to addressing concomitant shoulder pathology [113, 118, 126]. Biceps tenotomy entails cutting the LHBT at its origin on the superior labrum while biceps tenodesis involves cutting the LHBT at its origin on the superior labrum and then reattaching it to the proximal humerus either in an arthroscopic or open technique. There has been much debate regarding biceps tenotomy versus biceps tenodesis. Multiple meta-analyses and systematic reviews have found biceps tenodesis to have less cosmetic deformity, or Popeye deformity; however, differences in clinical outcome scores appear to be similar [141–144]. In addition to a Popeye deformity, muscle cramping and fatigue may also be a concern in the younger patient population following a biceps tenotomy, with one study reporting fatigue and cramping in 38% of patients [145]. Proponents of biceps tenotomy note the lower cost and operative time as potential advantages [146]. The outcomes of several randomized controlled trials [147–149] have are outlines in Table 10.2.

Table 10.2 Operative management of proximal biceps pathology

Study	Diagnosis	Methods	Results
Belay et al. [147]	LHBT tendinopathy	Randomized controlled trial of 14 patients undergoing tenodesis and 20 patients undergoing tenotomy	Clinical outcome scores demonstrated no significant difference between the groups at final follow-up; however, pain score at 3 months was significantly better in the tenotomy group
		Minimum follow-up of 24 months	Cosmetic deformity occurred in 7% of the tenodesis group and 25% of the tenotomy group
MacDonald et al. [148]	LHBT pathology	Randomized controlled trial of 57 patients undergoing tenodesis (open or arthroscopic) and 57 patients undergoing tenotomy	Clinical outcome scores significantly improved in both groups with no significant difference between the groups
		Minimum follow-up of 24 months	Cosmetic deformity occurred in 10% of the tenodesis group and 33% of the tenotomy group No significant difference in cramping or strength
Lee et al. [149]	LHBT pathology (partial tear, subluxation, dislocation)	Randomized controlled trial of 72 patients undergoing tenodesis and 56 patients undergoing tenotomy	Clinical outcome scores significantly improved in both groups with no significant difference between the groups
		Minimum follow-up of 12 months	Cosmetic deformity occurred in 5.6% of the tenodesis group and 19.6% of the tenotomy group Tenodesis group had greater forearm supination power at final follow-up, but no difference in elbow flexion or forearm pronation power
Ide et al. [155]	SLAP tears	40 overhead-throwing athletes retrospectively reviewed following SLAP repair	Clinical outcome scores significantly improved
		Minimum follow-up of 24 months	75% of patients reported an excellent outcome 63% return to play in baseball players 86% return to play in other overhead athletes

(continued)

Table 10.2 (continued)

Study	Diagnosis	Methods	Results
Park et al. [157]	SLAP tears	24 elite overhead athletes retrospectively reviewed following SLAP repair Minimum follow-up of 24 months	Clinical outcome scores significantly improved 38% return to play in baseball players 75% return to play in other overhead athletes
Provencher et al. [158]	SLAP tears	179 patients prospectively followed following arthroscopic SLAP repair Minimum 26 months follow-up	Mean clinical scores significantly improved 36.8% of patients met failure criteria 28% of patients underwent revision surgery Age greater than 36 years was associated with a higher rate of failure
Boileau et al. [153]	SLAP tears	25 patients with average age of 52 years old were retrospectively reviewed following either SLAP repair (10 patients) or biceps tenodesis (15) Minimum 24 months follow-up	60% of patients in the repair group were disappointed and only 20% returned to their previous level of sports participation 93% of patients in the tenodesis group were satisfied or very satisfied and 87% returned to their previous level of sports participation
Lacheta et al. [156]	SLAP tears	38 patients under the age of 35 years old were retrospectively reviewed following either SLAP repair (24 patients) or subpectoral biceps tenodesis (24) Minimum 24 months follow-up	Clinical outcome scores significantly improved with no significant differences between both groups 79% in the SLAP repair group returned to previous level of sport 85% in the tenodesis group returned to previous level of sport

Surgical management options for SLAP tears include arthroscopic debridement, arthroscopic repair, and biceps tenodesis or tenotomy [113, 128]. Several recent studies looking at the trend of surgical management of SLAP tears have shown a decrease in SLAP repairs and an increase in biceps tenodesis or tenotomy over the last two decades [150–152]. This trend has been largely driven by recent literature showing superior outcomes and patient satisfaction following biceps tenodesis for the management of SLAP tears in older patients [153, 154]. Despite this, SLAP repair remains a popular treatment choice for the younger patient and throwing athlete; however, return to play rates have varied widely in the literature [113, 128, 155–157]. Table 10.2 also outlines the literature investigating the surgical management of SLAP tears.

Acromioclavicular Joint Pathology

Acromioclavicular Joint Separations

Epidemiology and Etiology

Acromioclavicular (AC) joint separations are infrequent injuries that tend to occur during trauma from contact activities. In the general population, the annual incidence of AC joint separations is estimated to range from 0.8 to 4.6 per 10,000 [159–162], with an incidence as high as 9.2 to 26.1 per 10,000 in at risk populations such as football players and military personnel [163, 164]. Additionally, AC joint separations most frequently occur in males [159, 161, 164].

Injury to the AC joint most often occurs from a superior to inferior directed force onto the shoulder. Clinically, this is most often seen from a direct fall onto the shoulder or an impact injury during contact with another person or object. Injury typically occurs with the shoulder in an adducted position [165].

Relevant Anatomy

The AC joint is a diarthrodial joint composed of the lateral clavicle and the medial acromion, with a fibrocartilaginous intra-articular disc. Both static and dynamic structures stabilize the AC joint. The AC ligaments, which have superior, inferior, anterior, and posterior components, are responsible for horizontal or anterior to posterior stability [166]. The coracoclavicular (CC) ligaments, including the conoid ligament and the trapezoid ligament, help to control vertical or superior to inferior stability [166]. When considering surgical reconstruction, it is important to note the conoid ligaments attach, on average, 4.6 cm medial to the lateral edge of the clavicle, while the trapezoid ligament attaches 2.5 cm medial to the lateral edge of the clavicle [167]. In addition to its ligamentous support, the AC joint is also stabilized by muscular attachments, including the deltoid laterally and the trapezius posteriorly and superiorly.

Injury Classification

When classifying AC joint injuries according to the Rockwood Classification (Table 10.3), both the injured anatomic structures as well as the amount and direction of displacement are considered.

Clinical Presentation

Patients typically present following an acute trauma to the shoulder, although iatrogenic AC instability following distal clavicle resection has also been reported [168–170]. Patients will typically complain of pain isolated to the anterior and superior shoulder, which is worse with cross-body abduction and overhead activities.

Table 10.3 Rockwood classification of AC joint injury

Type	AC ligament injury	CC ligament injury	Displacement
I	Partial tear	Intact	None
II	Complete tear	Intact	Less than 25% increased CC distance
III	Complete tear	Complete tear	25–100% increased CC distance
IV	Complete tear	Complete tear	Posterior displacement
V	Complete tear	Complete tear	Greater than 100% increased CC distance
VI	Complete tear	Complete tear	Inferior displacement below the coracoid process

Physical Examination

Physical examination should begin with an inspection of the injured and contralateral shoulder. In some injury patterns, a visible prominence of the lateral clavicle and abnormal shoulder contour will be noted. Additionally, any skin tenting should be noted. Direct palpation will show tenderness over the lateral clavicle and AC joint. The ability to reduce the lateral clavicle to its anatomic position should be noted. This can be done by directly attempting to reduce the lateral clavicle with direct pressure or by having the patient shrug their shoulders. In a Type III injury, the lateral clavicle will reduce, but in a Type V injury, the lateral clavicle will remain superiorly displaced [171].

Special tests for AC separations include the cross-body abduction test and O'Brien's active compression test. The cross-body abduction test involves forward flexing the shoulder to 90 degrees and then maximally adducting the shoulder. A positive test will produce pain at the AC joint and has been shown to have a sensitivity of 77% [172] for AC injuries. O'Brien's active compression test is performed by having the patient resist the downward pressure of their arm when the patient's shoulder is positioned at 90° of forward flexion and 10° of adduction. While less sensitive, this test has been found to be highly specific for AC joint injuries [172, 173].

Diagnostic Studies

Initial diagnostic studies should include standard radiographs of the shoulder and AC joint. Bilateral anterior-posterior views of the AC joints are important to evaluate the contralateral AC joint in comparison to the injured side, and bilateral weighted radiographs have been recommended to classify AC joint separations more accurately [174]. Additionally, a Zanca view, or 10-degree cephalic tilt view, can aid in better visualizing the AC joint by decreasing the effect of superimposed structures. Lastly, an axillary view is needed to diagnose a type IV AC separation with posterior displacement. While infrequently needed for the diagnosis and management of AC joint separations, an MRI may be obtained if there is concern for concomitant injuries about the shoulder.

Nonoperative Treatment of Type I and II AC Separations

It has been widely accepted that the mainstay of treatment for type I and II AC separation is nonoperative [165, 171, 175]. Nonoperative management for type I and II AC separations typically involves a brief period of immobilization followed by physical therapy to improve range of motion and ultimately strength. Park et al. [176] found that patients with type I and II injuries were disabled for only a period of 6 weeks and had excellent outcomes. Despite a strong consensus on nonoperative management for type I and II AC separations, literature has also shown a high incidence of residual symptoms at long-term follow-up, although these symptoms are typically minimal. In a study evaluating long-term outcomes following nonoperative management of type I and II injuries, Mikek [177] found that 52% of patients will have occasional, mild AC joint symptoms at an average 10-year follow-up. Similarly, Mouhsine et al. [178] found that at a mean follow-up of 6.3 years, 48% of patients remained symptomatic. Additionally, 27% of patients required subsequent surgery for chronic AC joint pathology [178]. Shaw et al. [179] found that 6 months after nonoperative management of type I and II AC separations, up to 40% of patients will suffer from significant pain, although this rate improved to 14% at final follow-up [179]. Table 10.4 summarized the clinical results of type 1 and II AC separations managed nonoperatively.

Table 10.4 Nonoperative management of type I and II AC joint separations

Authors	Rockwood classification	Methods	Results
Park et al. [176]	Type I, II	24 patients with type I separations immobilized for a mean of 19.5 days 25 patients with type II separations immobilized for a mean of 27 days Recovery graded on a scale of 0–100%	Average follow-up of 6.3 years (range 1–19 years) Type I separations resulted in 6 weeks of disability and 94% recovery at final follow-up Type II separations resulted in 6 weeks of disability and 90% recovery at final follow-up
Mikek et al. [177]	Type I, II	23 patients (12 with type 1 separations, 11 with type II separations) Treated with sling, rest, ice, oral anti-inflammatory's and standard physical therapy	Average follow-up of 10.2 years 52% with mild occasional subjective symptoms No patients sought further treatment due to these symptoms
Mouhsine et al. [178]	Type I, II	33 patients with type I and II separations Treated with sling and oral anti-inflammatory's	Average follow-up of 63 years 48% of patients reported symptoms at final follow-up Mean Constant score of 82 points 54% of patients showed radiographic degenerative changes 27% of patients required eventual surgical treatment and were excluded from analysis

(continued)

Table 10.4 (continued)

Authors	Rockwood classification	Methods	Results
Shaw et al. [179]	Type I, II	47 patients	40% with significant pain at 6 months which decreased to 14% at final follow-up
		Treated with sling and oral anti-inflammatory's	20% with restricted range of motion at 6-month follow-up 9% found symptoms affected daily activities 6% had to change sporting activities

Treatment of Type III AC Joint Separations

There is less consensus on the optimal treatment of type III AC joint separations. In general, good-to-excellent outcomes have been found with nonoperative management of type III AC joint injuries [175, 180–183] and is typically recommended as the first-line treatment for type III AC joint injuries. However, due to concern for overhead strength and endurance, some authors have recommended surgical management of acute type III AC separation in more high-demand patients [184]. Despite this, conclusive evidence supporting operative intervention for acute type III AC joint injuries is lacking [171, 185]. Table 10.5 summarized the clinical outcomes of the management of type II AC separations.

Treatment of Type IV, V, and VI AC Separations

There is a much stronger consensus on the recommendation for surgical intervention of Type IV, V, and VI AC separations, although some will still advocate for nonoperative management of some Type IV AC separations [171, 185]. Although beyond the scope of this chapter, more than 60 surgical techniques have been described to address AC joint injuries [171, 185], which must be considered when evaluating the operative literature for AC joint injuries. Table 10.6 outlines the surgical outcomes of various techniques for Type IV, V, and VI AC separations.

Acromioclavicular Joint Degenerative Conditions

Epidemiology and Etiology

Degenerative conditions of the acromioclavicular joint are most frequently due to osteoarthritis, post-traumatic arthritis, or distal clavicle osteolysis [192]. While symptomatic primary osteoarthritis of the AC joint is relatively rare, radiographic and MR imaging has shown rates to be as high as 75% in asymptomatic patients [193, 194]. Post-traumatic arthritis of the AC joint is common following AC joint separations and distal clavicle fractures. Following low-grade AC joint separations, post-traumatic arthritis has been reported at rates as high as 42% [195]. Distal clavicle osteolysis (DCO) is another cause of AC joint degeneration. DCO is most commonly seen in younger males who participate in frequent weightlifting and results from repetitive microtrauma [192, 196].

Table 10.5 Operative and nonoperative management of type III AC joint separations

Authors	Rockwood classification	Methods	Results
Dias et al. [181]	Type III	53 patients managed nonoperatively	Average follow-up of 5.3 years 55% of patients with mild discomfort 4.7% of patients with moderate discomfort
Finsterwald et al. [182]	Type III	18 patients randomized to nonoperative treatment with a brace and 17 patients managed with nonoperative treatment to a sling	Both groups experienced similarly good subjective outcomes scores at 12 weeks 1 patient underwent operative stabilization at 4 months due to persistent pain
Schlegel et al. [183]	Type III	25 patients managed nonoperatively with sling and early progression range motion	80% of patients were subjectively satisfied with their result
		1-year minimum follow-up	No patients had limited shoulder motion compared to their contralateral shoulder Patients who required repetitive overhead use noted decreased strength and endurance
Gstettner et al. [184]	Type III	17 patients treated nonoperatively	34-month follow-up
		24 patients treated surgically	Nonoperative patients with 59% good to excellent results Surgical patients with 87.5% of patients with good to excellent results
Bannister et al. [186]	Type III	33 patients randomized to nonoperative treatment	At 1 year, 88% of nonsurgical patients with good to excellent result and 77% of surgical patients with good to excellent results
		27 patients randomized to operative treatment	At 4 years, 100% of nonsurgical patients with good to excellent result and 74% of surgical patients with good to excellent results
Larsen et al. [187]	Type III	40 patients randomized to nonoperative treatment	13-month follow-up
		39 patients randomized to operative treatment	Both groups have 98% good to excellent results Surgical group took more time off from work
Boström Windhamre et al. [188]	Type III	33 patients randomized to nonoperative treatment	24-month minimum follow-up
		30 patients randomized to operative treatment with a hook plate	At 24 months no significant difference in Constant score between nonoperative (88) and operative (91) patients 6 patients assigned to nonoperative treatment underwent surgery within 19 months

Table 10.6 Operative outcomes of type IV, V, and VI AC joint separations

Authors	Rockwood classification	Methods	Results
Liu et al. [189]	Type V	57 patients treated with hook plate	46-month average follow-up Outcomes scores all showed significant improvement compared to preoperative scores Patient reported excellent result of 35.1% Patient reported good result of 54.1% Complication rate of 15.8% (impingement, acromial osteolysis, reduction loss, AC osteoarthritis, calcification)
Feichtinger et al. [190]	Type IV	27 patients with 18 receiving operative management and 9 receiving nonoperative management	4.8 years average follow-up Significantly better AC Joint Instability score in operative group No differences between arthroscopic and open procedures
Huang et al. [191]	Type V	25 patients treated with tape fixation 24 patients treated with clavicle hook plate	26-month average follow-up 36% reduction loss with tape fixation Significantly better coracoclavicular distance in hook plate group both before and after hook plate removal No significant difference in complications or clinical outcomes
Boström Windhamre et al. [188]	Type V	30 patients randomized to nonoperative treatment 31 patients randomized to operative treatment with a hook plate	24-month minimum follow-up At 24 months no significant difference in Constant score between nonoperative (90) and operative (91) patients 5 patients assigned to nonoperative treatment underwent surgery within 19 months

Relevant Anatomy

As previously discussed, the AC joint is a diarthrodial joint composed of the lateral clavicle and the medial acromion, with a fibrocartilaginous intraarticular disc. It has been shown that this degeneration of this fibrocartilaginous disc may occur as early as the second decade of life [192]. The small articular surface area of the AC joint and the relatively high axial and rotational loads across the joint lead to high-contact forces and, therefore, degeneration.

Clinical Presentation

Patients with symptomatic AC joint degeneration typically complain of pain over the superior and anterior aspect of the shoulder with both active and passive shoulder motion. Typically, symptoms are worse with cross-body adduction as well as overhead motion. In addition to pain, patients may also complain of mechanical symptoms such as popping, catching, and grinding [192]. In younger athletes with DCO, pain will be common with pushing exercises such as bench press, push-up, and dips [197].

It is important to note that patients will frequently present with concomitant shoulder pathology such as rotator cuff pathology, labral tears, glenohumeral degeneration, biceps tendinitis, or subacromial impingement [198]; therefore, a thorough history and physical examination are imperative to identify and address all contributing pathologies.

Physical Examination

In addition to a general shoulder and cervical spine examination to identify any concomitant pathology, a focused examination of the AC joint should be performed. Due to the rather subcutaneous location of the AC joint, often a prominence over the AC joint can be seen. Additionally, there may be tenderness to palpation of the AC joint. AC joint tenderness has been found to be sensitive but rather nonspecific [59]. The range of motion will typically be unrestricted; however, crepitus and popping can be felt with active and passive motion of the shoulder.

Pain with the crossbody adduction test has been found to be the most sensitive test for AC joint pathology [172]. As discussed in the previous section on AC joint separations, this test is performed by forward flexing the shoulder to 90° and then maximally adducting the shoulder across the body. The O'Brien's active compression test has been shown to be less sensitive than the crossbody adduction test but more specific [172, 173]. It is performed by having the patient resist the downward pressure of their arm when the patient's shoulder is positioned at 90° of forward flexion and 10° of adduction.

Diagnostic Studies

While AC joint degeneration can be noted on standard AP and grashey views of the shoulder, a Zanca view, or 10-degree cephalic tilt view, can aid in better visualizing the AC joint by decreasing the effect of superimposed structures. Typical findings of degeneration will be noted, including sclerosis, joint space narrowing, subchondral cysts, and osteophyte formation. In DCO, radiographs may show widening of the joint space, relative osteopenia, and loss of subchondral bone detail [192]. MRI is a common diagnostic imaging technique for shoulder pathology. MRI will provide valuable information such as the presence of subchondral edema, effusion, and synovial hypertrophy [196]. MRI findings should be judiciously correlated with physical examination findings, as MRI evidence of degenerative changes is frequently found in asymptomatic patients [194].

Diagnostic AC joint injections with a local anesthetic can be a valuable diagnostic tool. Improvement or resolution of pain within minutes or hours of injection can help differentiate symptomatic AC joint degeneration versus non-AC joint shoulder pain [199]. AC joint injections can be easily performed under sterile conditions in the office with 1 or 2 mL of local anesthetic. The bony landmarks are easily palpated, and the needle can be introduced into the AC joint via an anterior or superior approach. The use of ultrasound guidance has been shown to increase the accuracy of reaching the intra-articular space [200, 201]. It is important to have the patient note any improvement in symptoms in the days following a diagnostic AC joint injection.

Nonoperative Treatment of AC Joint Degenerative Conditions

In the setting of isolated AC joint degeneration, nonoperative management should be thoroughly exhausted prior to surgical intervention. Nonoperative management most commonly consists of activity modifications, physical therapy, nonsteroidal anti-inflammatory medications, and intra-articular steroid injections [192, 196, 199]. Activity modification typically involves avoidance of aggravating movements such as cross-body and overhead lifting, pushing, and pulling. Physical therapy, while less successful in the setting of isolated AC joint degeneration, can be particularly useful if concomitant impingement or rotator cuff pathology is present. While studies assessing the effectiveness of physical therapy for AC joint degeneration are limited, several studies [202–204] have looked at the effectiveness of AC joint injections and have found mixed results (Table 10.7). While one study [202] found sustained long-term relief after AC joint steroid injections, others have failed to demonstrate a high rate of long-term efficacy [203, 204].

Table 10.7 Outcomes of intra-articular injections for AC joint degenerative conditions

Authors	Methods	Results
Hossain et al. [202]	Prospective study of 25 shoulders receiving AC joint steroid injections for primary AC arthritis	Significant improvements in Constant score were noted at 6 and 12 months
	Minimum follow-up of 5 years	Deterioration in Constant score at 5 years but still significant improvement compared to reinjection scores Younger patients and women had a greater improvement in scores
Jacob et al. [203]	Retrospective study of 27 patients with AC joint arthropathy receiving AC joint steroid injection	93% of patients reported improvement in pain and function which lasted on overage 20 days
	Average 19-month follow-up	81% of patients failed to obtain long-term relief from the injection 18 patients (67%) underwent distal clavicle excision on average of 4 months after infection
van Riet et al. [204]	Prospective study of 58 patients receiving AC joint steroid injections for isolated AC joint symptoms	16/58 patients (27.5%) had satisfactory resolution of symptoms at 1 month
	All patients evaluated at 1 month and average final follow-up of 42 months	Of these 16 patients, at final follow-up, 1 had recurrence which required surgery, and 4 reported occasional mild pain

Operative Treatment of AC Joint Degenerative Conditions

Operative intervention for degenerative conditions of the AC joint is typically reserved for patients who have failed 6 months of conservative treatment [192, 199]. Additionally, patients undergoing shoulder surgery for concomitant shoulder pathology may benefit from operative management of their AC joint degeneration if it is a clear contributor to their shoulder symptoms. Operative management consists of either open or arthroscopic distal clavicle excision (DCE). While both open and arthroscopic DCE provide successful outcomes (Table 10.8), some authors [205, 206] have noted superior pain relief with arthroscopic DCE compared to open DCE; however, others have not demonstrated such a difference [207].

Table 10.8 Outcomes of distal clavicle excision for AC joint degenerative conditions

Authors	Methods	Results
Freedman et al. [205]	17 patients randomized to open or arthroscopic DCE Minimum 1-year follow-up	VAS improved in both groups at 6 months and 1 year VAS improvement at 1 year was statistically significant for the arthroscopic group, but not the open group At 1 year, 50% of the open group and 100% of the arthroscopic group returned to their normal level of sports and physical activity
Robertson et al. [206]	17 patients undergoing open DCE compared to 32 patients undergoing arthroscopic DCE were retrospectively compared Minimum 5-year follow-up	Arthroscopic DCE resulted in significantly lower VAS pain score (0.61 vs. 1.59) at final follow-up No significant difference between open and arthroscopic DCE ASES scores (87.5 vs. 94.6) at final follow-up No significant difference between open and arthroscopic DCE percentage of normal shoulder function (89.7% vs. 92.9%) at final follow-up
Elhassan et al. [207]	Retrospective review of 81 patients undergoing arthroscopic DCE compared to 24 patients undergoing open DCE Minimum 1-year follow-up	Constant scores significantly improved both arthroscopic and open DCE groups with no difference between the 2 groups Pain with cross-body adduction and palpation improved in 94% of arthroscopic patients and 92% of open patients Revision DCE occurred 1 patient (4.2%) in the open group and 5 patients (6.2%) in the arthroscopic group

(continued)

Table 10.8 (continued)

Authors	Methods	Results
Eskola et al. [208]	73 patients treated with open DCE for AC osteoarthritis 4-year minimum follow-up	Median follow-up of 9 years 20 patients (27.4%) reported a good result 29 patients (39.7%) reported a satisfactory result 23 patients (31.5%) reported a poor result Patients who had a smaller amount of distal clavicle resected (10 mm or less) had less pain than those who had a large amount resected
Leon et al. [209]	Prospective study of 59 patients undergoing isolated arthroscopic DCE for AC osteoarthritis or DCO Minimum 24-month follow-up	Median follow-up of 5.7 years Significant improvement in ROM and patient reported outcome scores All patients returned to work (average of 1.72 months) All but 1 patient returned to sport (average of 3.02 months) 4 patients (6.8%) had ongoing high pain (VAS > 5) at final follow-up

Glenohumeral Joint Degenerative Conditions

Epidemiology and Etiology

Common causes of glenohumeral joint degenerative disease include primary osteoarthritis (OA), rotator cuff arthropathy, humeral head avascular necrosis (AVN), post-traumatic arthritis, and inflammatory arthritis, as well as less common causes such as neuropathic arthropathy. The true prevalence of glenohumeral OA is difficult to estimate; however, several studies have found close to 20% of patients 60 years of age or older to have glenohumeral OA [210–212]. In patients older than 80 years of age, rates have been reported as high as 94% in women and 85% in men [213]. Well-known risk factors for the development of primary glenohumeral OA include female sex, Caucasian race, obesity, and advancing age [214, 215]. Post-traumatic arthritis can be seen in the setting of previous shoulder instability as well as proximal humerus fractures. Several studies have found radiographic arthritic changes at long-term follow-up in as high as 68% of patients with a history of anterior shoulder instability [216, 217], while others have found rates closer to 20% [218, 219]. Proximal humerus fractures can result in rates of post-traumatic arthritis ranging from 9 to 38% and AVN rates ranging from 30 to 40% of patients with three- and four-part fractures [220]. In addition to previous trauma, other common risk factors for humeral head AVN include systematic steroid use, alcohol abuse, chemotherapy, systemic lupus erythematosus, and sick cell disease [221].

Rotator cuff arthropathy (RCA), which is defined by rotator cuff insufficiency, degenerative changes of the glenohumeral joint, and superior migration of the humeral head, is another common cause of glenohumeral degeneration [222]. Several theories have been proposed to explain the etiology of RCA; however, most believe its cause to be a combination of mechanical and nutritional factors [222, 223]. With massive rotator cuff tears, the humeral head escapes anterosuperiorly, causing abnormal mechanical forces and cartilage wear. Additionally, with a massive rotator cuff tear, nutrient factors can escape from the glenohumeral joint, which is proposed to cause cartilage atrophy [222, 223]. Typically, RCA affects females in their seventh decade and is most commonly seen in the dominant extremity [223, 224]. Rheumatoid arthritis is the most common type of inflammatory arthritis seen in the shoulder and may present as bilateral glenohumeral osteoarthritis [215]. In patients with rheumatoid arthritis for greater than 5 years, 90% will have affected shoulders [214].

Relevant Anatomy

The glenohumeral joint is a complex joint with significant mobility due to the relatively small contact area of the humeral head on the glenoid. Because of this, the glenohumeral joint relies on both dynamic and static stabilizers. The rotator cuff muscles, including the subscapularis, supraspinatus, infraspinatus, and teres minor, as well as the long head of the biceps, are important dynamic stabilizers, while the glenohumeral ligaments, glenoid labrum, and glenohumeral capsule play an important role in static stabilization. The rotator cuff muscles act to compress the humeral head into the glenoid cavity- a concept referred to as concavity-compression [222]. With this concavity-compression mechanism imposed by the rotator cuff musculature, the deltoid muscle has a stable fulcrum to enact its superior force without resulting in superior migration of the humeral head. The loss of this concavity-compression mechanism results in an unstable fulcrum and superior humeral head migration with altered glenohumeral joint biomechanics [222].

Clinical Presentation

Patients with glenohumeral joint degeneration will present with shoulder pain that is typically deep and posterior, stiffness, crepitus or catching with movement, loss of function, and often report difficulty sleeping. Additionally, patients with RCA may complain of profound weakness with active forward flexion of less than 45° but maintained passive ROM; this has been termed pseudoparalysis [225]. Additionally, RCA patients may present with less pain than patients with other glenohumeral degeneration conditions. A thorough history should be obtained with a focus on previous trauma, surgery, comorbidities, and other joint pain. Additionally, a history of chemotherapy, alcohol abuse, or chronic steroid use should be noted.

Physical Examination

Physical examination begins with a thorough inspection. While glenohumeral OA may not present with signs upon inspection, in the presence of RCA, muscle atrophy may be noted as well as a bony prominence form anterosuperior humeral escape or swelling at the AC joint (Geyser sign) from synovial fluid escaping superiorly through the rotator cuff tear and AC joint [215, 222, 223]. Active and passive shoulder range of motion should be assessed and compared to the contralateral shoulder; any crepitus should be noted. Rotator cuff strength testing should be thoroughly assessed. Additionally, a thorough cervical spine examination should be performed to rule out cervical pathology, which may present as shoulder pain.

Diagnostic Studies

The diagnostic workup for glenohumeral joint degeneration begins with a complete shoulder radiographic series, including anterior-posterior, Grashey (Fig. 10.2), scapular y, and axillary views. Radiographic findings of glenohumeral osteoarthritis may include joint space narrowing, osteophyte formation, subchondral sclerosis and cysts, and posterior glenoid wear [214, 215]. With glenohumeral OA, patients classically develop an inferomedial humeral neck osteophyte termed a "Goats-Beard" osteophyte [214, 215]. In more advanced glenohumeral OA or humeral head AVN, humeral head collapse may be noted. In RCA, radiographic findings may include superior humeral head migration, erosion of the greater tuberosity, erosion of the undersurface of the acromion, and superior erosion of the glenoid [222, 223]. Advanced imaging such as an MRI or CT scan is rarely needed for diagnostic

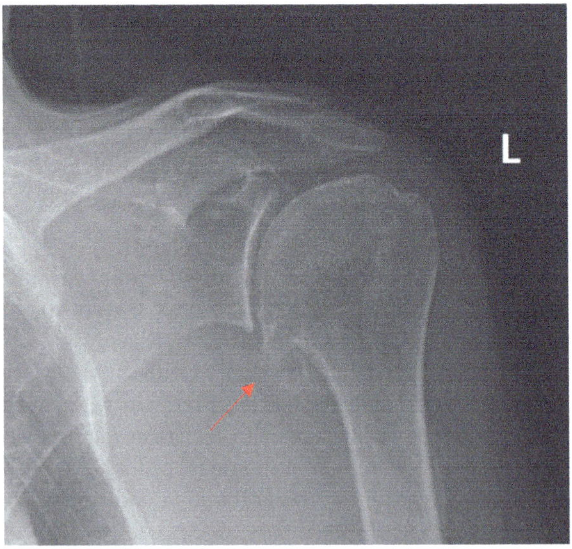

Fig. 10.2 Grashey radiograph of a left shoulder demonstrating moderate glenohumeral osteoarthritic change with a "Goats-Bear" (red arrow) osteophyte

purposes but can be very useful in staging and preoperative planning. Surgical treatment decisions are often based on the integrity of the rotator cuff as well as the deformity of the glenoid, so advanced imaging is often used to assess these factors.

Nonoperative Management of Glenohumeral Joint Degenerative Conditions

The management of glenohumeral degenerative joint disease typically begins with a multimodal nonoperative approach, including NSAIDs, activity modifications, physical therapy, and intra-articular corticosteroid injections (Table 10.9). Physical therapy for glenohumeral OA typically aims to improve shoulder motion and stiffness; however, aggressive strengthening should be avoided as this may exacerbate

Table 10.9 Nonoperative outcomes for glenohumeral joint degenerative conditions

Study	Diagnosis	Methods	Results
Kwon et al. [227]	Glenohumeral OA	150 patients randomized to hyaluronic acid (HA) injections and 150 randomized to saline injection 26-week minimum follow-up	Both groups showed improvement in pain and function outcomes scores but there was no statistical difference between the groups
Kim et al. [228]	Glenohumeral OA	311 shoulders were reviewed after receiving an intraarticular corticosteroid injection of the shoulder Minimum 3-year follow-up	37.3% of patients eventually underwent arthroplasty 21.9% had further injections 33.4% had no further treatment
Metzger et al. [229]	Glenohumeral OA	30 shoulders were reviewed after receiving an intraarticular corticosteroid injection of the shoulder Minimum 12-month follow-up	Significant improvement in Oxford Shoulder Score between baseline and months 1–4 Significant improvement in pain score between baseline and months 1–4, 6, 9, and 12
Guo et al. [232]	Glenohumeral OA	129 patients over the age of 65 years were prospectively evaluated following multimodal treatment with therapy, NSAIDs, and corticosteroid/hyaluronic acid injections Minimum 3-year follow-up	Most patients reported significant improvement in pain scores, self-assessed shoulder function, and mental health Scores declined at 6 months and 12 months but then improved between 12 months and 36 months
Agarwala et al. [231]	Humeral head AVN	5 patients with humeral head AVN treated with oral alendronate 70 mg weekly and intravenous zoledronic acid for 1 year	80% (4 patients) progressed within 4 years

symptoms [226]. In contrast, physical therapy for RCA focuses on strengthening the deltoid and scapular musculature. Intra-articular injections including corticosteroid and hyaluronic acid have been advocated, and while there is some evidence that hyaluronic acid injections may have some benefit for glenohumeral OA [227], currently it is not approved for use in shoulders by the US Food and Drug nor is it recommended according to the clinical practice guidelines set forth by the American Academy of Orthopedic Surgeons [213]. While several studies have shown beneficial effects of intra-articular corticosteroid injections for glenohumeral degenerative conditions [228, 229] it is typically recommended to limit the total amount of injections to three in order to decrease the risk of infection following future surgical procedures [226].

Similar to glenohumeral OA and RCA, a trial of nonoperative management is appropriate for early stages of humeral head AVN; however, conservative management for later-stage humeral head AVN typically has poor results [230]. While bisphosphonate therapy has shown promising outcomes in the early stages of femoral AVN, the same has not been shown with humeral head AVN [231].

Operative Management of Glenohumeral Joint Degenerative Conditions

For patients who have failed nonoperative management, operative intervention is indicated, and select studies outlining different operative outcomes are shown in Table 10.10. For most degenerative conditions of the glenohumeral joint, anatomic total shoulder arthroplasty (TSA) or reverse total shoulder arthroplasty (RSA) provide excellent clinical outcomes and survivorship. In patients with a preserved rotator cuff and good glenoid bone stock, TSA is typically preferred. While in patients with RCA or significant bone loss, RSA is favored due to its inherent stability as well as improved glenoid fixation when compared to TSA.

Long-term survivorship of TSA for the treatment of glenohumeral degenerative conditions is excellent, with many studies demonstrating 10-year survivorship of 90% and 20-year survivorship of 80% [233, 235]. Additionally, short-term results of RSA for glenohumeral OA have also shown excellent outcomes, which appear similar to TSA [236, 237]. In the management of RCA, TSA results are typically poor due to the increased forces on the glenoid component, which lead to early glenoid failure [223]. Due to this, RSA is the arthroplasty of choice for RCA, and long-term results have shown significant improvement in outcome scores and motion for patients with RCA [238–240].

In younger patients with glenohumeral degenerative conditions, alternative treatment options, including hemiarthroplasty and arthroscopic techniques, may be appropriate. Hemiarthroplasty has been advocated in younger or high-demand patients due to the concern for glenoid component failure in this patient population following TSA; however, with traditional metallic hemiarthroplasty, native glenoid wear is also of concern [241]. Pyrocarbon hemiarthroplasty is an alternative bearing surface that has recently been approved for use in the United States and shows

Table 10.10 Operative outcomes for glenohumeral joint degenerative conditions

Study	Diagnosis	Procedure	Methods	Results
Fox et al. [234]	Glenohumeral OA	TSA	Review of 1542 primary TSAs	5-, 10-, and 15-year survivorship for 497 all poly glenoid components was 99%, 94%, and 89%, respectively
	Rheumatoid arthritis Post-traumatic arthritis AVN		Evaluated based on glenoid component type	Similar findings for all other glenoid components except for a specific metal backed glenoid which had 5, 10, and 15-year survivorship of 86%, 79%, and 67%, respectively
Singh et al. [235]	Glenohumeral OA	TSA	Review of prospectively collected data on 2588 patients undergoing TSA	Overall 5-, 10-, and 20-year implant survivorship of 94.2%, 90.2%, and 81.4%, respectively
	Rheumatoid arthritis Trauma Other			For diagnosis of OA, 5-, 10-, and 20-year implant survivorship of 93.9%, 89.2%, and 76.6%, respectively
Kirsch et al. [236]	Glenohumeral OA	TSA and RSA	Retrospective matched-cohort study of 67 TSAs and 67 RSAs	Average follow-up of 30 months
			Minimum 2-year follow-up	No difference in pain or functional outcomes scores between TSA and RSA at final follow-up TSA had significantly better postoperative forward elevation, external rotation, and internal rotation Overall complication rate of 4.5% with no difference between TSA and RSA groups
Wright et al. [237]	Glenohumeral OA	TSA and RSA	Retrospective cohort study of 102 TSAs and 33 RSAs Minimum 2-year follow-up	No difference in pain or functional outcome scores between TSA and RSA at final follow-up No significant difference in complication or revision rates between TSA and RSA at final follow-up No difference in satisfaction rates for TSA (86.1%) or RSA (91.8%) at final follow-up

(continued)

Table 10.10 (continued)

Study	Diagnosis	Procedure	Methods	Results
Bacle et al. [238]	RCA Massive irreparable rotator cuff tear Glenohumeral OA with rotator cuff compromise Failed previous arthroplasty	RSA	Retrospective review of 87 RSAs Minimum 10-year follow-up	10-year survivorship of 93% Significant decrease in clinical outcome scores from 2 years to 10 years
Cuff et al. [239]	RCA Massive irreparable rotator cuff tear	RSA	Retrospective review of 42 patients undergoing RSA Minimum 10-year follow-up	10-year survivorship of 90.7% Significant improvement in functional outcome scores compared to baseline which were maintained between 5 and 10 years Small decrease in shoulder motion between 5-year follow-up and 10-year follow-up
Garret et al. [242]	Glenohuemral OA AVN Rheumatoid arthritis Post-traumatic OA	Pyrocarbon hemiarthroplasty	Retrospective review of 37 patients undergoing pyrocarbon hemiarthroplasty Minimum 2–4-year follow-up and 5–9-year follow-up available	Significant improvement in outcome scores at 2–4 years which were maintained at 5–9 years At final follow-up, glenoid erosion was severe in 8.1% of patients and moderate in 24% of shoulders
Kleim et al. [243]	Glenohumeral OA Post-traumatic arthritis	Pyrocarbon hemiarthroplasty	Retrospective review of 31 patients undergoing pyrocarbon hemiarthroplasty Minimum 3-year follow-up	Average follow-up of 5.5 years Survivorship of 100% Significant improvement in pain and functional outcome scores Mean medial glenoid erosion of 1.4 millimeters at final follow-up
Millett et al. [244]	Glenohumeral OA	Arthroscopic CAM procedure	30 shoulders with a mean age of 52 years underwent arthroscopic CAM procedure	20% of patients progressed to an arthroplasty at a mean of 1.9 years For those who did not progress to arthroplasty, there was a significant improvement in outcome scores and pain levels

promising mid-term outcomes with less native glenoid wear compared to traditional metallic hemiarthroplasty [242, 243]. An arthroscopic technique, known as comprehensive arthroscopic management (CAM Procedure), has been described by Millet et al. [244] for the treatment of glenohumeral OA in younger patients. This technique involves extensive capsular release, osteophyte resection from the humeral head, treatment of concomitant SLAP or biceps pathology, and axillary nerve neurolysis.

Shoulder Instability

Epidemiology and Etiology

Traumatic anterior shoulder instability is a common injury and accounts for 45% of all dislocations presenting to emergency rooms [245]. Anterior instability accounts for 96% of all glenohumeral dislocations [246]. The incidence in the general population is approximately 1.7% [247]. It occurs most frequently in young males, athletes, and military personnel, where incidence approaches 3% per year [248, 249]. It is especially common in those participating in contact sports. The incidence of these injuries has been reported to be 14.8% in high school rugby athletes [250]. Anterior shoulder dislocations are three times more common in men than women, and approximately 90% of patients are between the ages of 21 and 30 [245]. Recurrent instability is common in nonsurgically treated shoulders and has been reported to be as high as 75%, with 19% requiring repeated closed reduction [251].

Anterior shoulder dislocations generally occur from trauma with anteriorly directed forces on an abducted, extended, and externally rotated shoulder [252]. This can be seen clinically with falls onto an outstretched hand and can result in injury to a number of structures in the shoulder; including: the capsule, labrum, glenohumeral ligaments, rotator cuff, bony glenoid, and humeral head [253]. Instability can also be caused by repetitive microtrauma and subluxations without frank dislocation [254].

Posterior shoulder instability is an increasingly recognized cause of pain and dysfunction and can be caused by acute traumatic instability, atraumatic instability, or repetitive microtrauma [255]. Posterior instability makes up approximately 2–10% of all cases of shoulder instability [256]. It can be seen frequently in certain athletes such as football players, rugby players, weight lifters, paddling sport athletes, and climbers [256].

A less common entity, but important to recognize and differentiate from unidirectional instability, is multidirectional instability of the shoulder (MDI). MDI has been defined as instability in two to three directions and can be seen in those with generalized ligamentous laxity, connective tissue disorders, or repetitive microtrauma [257].

Relevant Anatomy

The glenohumeral joint is a synovial ball-and-socket joint and has the most range of motion of any joint in the body [258, 259]. The downside to increased motion is inherent instability [247]. There are a number of structures whose interplay helps create stability. Primary static support is provided by glenohumeral congruency between the articular surfaces of the humeral head and glenoid fossa, as well as the glenoid labrum, glenohumeral ligaments (GHLs), and the negative intra-articular pressure of the joint capsule [247].

The labrum is a fibrocartilaginous structure that serves as an attachment site for the glenohumeral ligaments and increases the depth of the glenoid socket by one-third, thereby increasing contact surface area with the humeral head [247, 259].

There are three glenohumeral ligaments: the superior, middle, and inferior. These are important passive stabilizers, and each functions at different ranges of motion. The superior GHL resists inferior and posterior subluxation when the shoulder is adducted or neutral [260]. The middle GHL becomes responsible for static stability as the arm is abducted to approximately 45 degrees [260]. The inferior GHL is responsible for stability as the arm is abducted to 90 degrees [260] and is most often injured during anterior shoulder dislocation [259]. The GHLs are lax in the mid-ranges of motion, where dynamic stabilizers become more important for glenohumeral stability [259]. The posterior capsule, which includes the posterior inferior glenohumeral ligament and the glenoid version, becomes important in the setting of posterior instability [256].

Several structures are responsible for dynamic stability and include the rotator cuff muscles, pectoralis major, latissimus dorsi, periscapular muscles, and the long head of the biceps tendon [260]. The rotator cuff muscles help center and compress the humeral head on the glenoid through muscle contraction and are of high importance for stability in the midrange of shoulder abduction motion [259]. The function of the subscapularis is especially important in posterior instability as it is the primary dynamic stabilizer in preventing posterior shoulder translation [256].

Clinical Presentation

There are important details of the patient history when suspecting anterior shoulder instability, including whether or not the patient has generalized ligamentous laxity, previous instability events and how many, mechanism of injury, previous treatment, activity level, and expectations for treatment [261]. Patients with anterior shoulder instability commonly complain of joint instability and pain associated with activity.

Those with posterior instability vary in their presentation. Some will have an acute traumatic injury that precedes the symptoms, as can be seen in football linemen who sustain a blocking injury or as the result of electrocution or seizures [256]. Others will present with atraumatic instability and are usually seen in patients with generalized ligamentous laxity [256].

MDI patients can have a wide range of symptoms, including non-focal shoulder pain to recurrent subluxation or dislocations [257]. There are aspects of the history that can aid in determining the direction of instability; for example, inferior instability can be exacerbated with carrying heavy objects [257].

Physical Examination

Physical examination should include an assessment of both shoulders in order to identify any asymmetries in appearance, motion, or strength. Differentiating between anterior, posterior, and multidirectional instability is important as treatment algorithms differ, given the underlying pathology [261]. There are special clinical exams that aid in making the correct diagnosis [261]. The Beighton score can be used to assess joint hypermobility [262]. A thorough neurovascular exam is also warranted as an anterior shoulder dislocation can place the axillary nerve at risk. Assessment of axillary nerve motor function can be difficult in the acute dislocation setting due to limited range of motion and pain. The sensation function can be assessed over the lateral aspect of the deltoid [261]. Vascular injury should also be assessed and include signs such as expanding or pulsatile hematoma, distal ischemia, and absent or weak pulses [263].

Diagnostic Studies

Radiographs of the shoulder with anteroposterior (AP), Grashey (true AP), and scapular-Y lateral views are recommended imaging in the initial presentation of suspected shoulder instability. In addition, either an axillary or Velpeau view is recommended to confirm the presence and direction of dislocation, as well as the confirmation of adequate reduction [261]. The axillary can also be used to assess glenoid version changes, as posterior version can be seen with posterior instability [256].

A computerized tomography (CT) scan helps determine the size and orientation of bone loss to the humeral head and/or anterior or posterior glenoid, which is important in determining treatment decision-making and preoperative planning [261]. The anterior glenoid fracture, or bony Bankart lesion, is a common sequela of anterior shoulder dislocation. The size and morphology of the bone fragment have treatment implications, as large defects are more likely to result in recurrent instability if not addressed [264]. It has been shown that recurrent instability leads to larger glenoid bone defects [265]. CT can also be used to assess glenoid hypoplasia and/or glenoid retroversion [256].

The Hill-Sachs lesion is a compression fracture of the posterosuperolateral humeral head and is another sequelae of traumatic anterior shoulder dislocation [266]. It occurs as the humeral head comes into forceful contact with the anterior glenoid after dislocation. The incidence of Hill-Sachs lesions has been reported to be 40–90% of primary instability and approaches 100% with recurrent instability

[266]. The reverse Hill-Sachs lesion occurs with posterior shoulder dislocation and has been shown to be evident in up to 86% of posterior instability cases [266].

A bipolar lesion refers to both the bony Bankart lesion and the Hill-Sachs lesion. Recognizing bipolar lesions and understanding the shape, size, and morphology of these lesions have treatment implications as larger bone defects to the anterior glenoid and/or humeral head can increase the risk of recurrent instability, and combined defects have an additive and negative effect on glenohumeral stability [267]. The concept of engaging vs. non-engaging lesions is helpful to understand how these lesions influence instability recurrence. An engaging lesion is one in which the humeral head defect engages the anterior rim of the glenoid while the shoulder is abducted and externally rotated, which leads to instability [268, 269]. A non-engaging lesion is one in which the humeral head lesion is not parallel with the rim of the glenoid as the shoulder is abducted and externally rotated and has a lower likelihood of causing recurrent instability [264]. The glenoid track is the contact area between the humeral head and the glenoid. An off-track Hill-Sachs lesion is one in which the lesion engages the anterior glenoid; it is on-track if it does not engage the glenoid [266]. The CT scan with 3D reconstruction is a valuable tool for assessing these bony defects [267].

In addition to bony pathology, there are a number of soft tissue structures that are damaged during anterior or posterior shoulder instability and are best evaluated with magnetic resonance imaging (MRI). As the humeral head is forced anteriorly, the capsulolabral structures are stretched and often torn, resulting in the Bankart lesion. These structures become further attenuated with each recurrent dislocation or subluxation event [266]. In addition, the posterior components should be evaluated in the setting of posterior instability. The labrum is important in conferring stability to the glenohumeral joint by creating a negative-pressure seal, which is lost when the labrum is disrupted [270].

In addition to the Bankart lesion, there are a number of other structures that can be injured during anterior shoulder dislocation and are best assessed with MRI. The humeral avulsion of the glenohumeral ligament (HAGL) is a specific injury commonly observed following anterior shoulder dislocation [271]. In this injury, the inferior glenohumeral ligament (IGHL) tears away from its attachment point on the humerus, leading to instability in the shoulder joint and incompetence of the IGHL. HAGL injuries can result in significant pain, weakness, and limited range of motion in the affected shoulder. Patients tend to complain of pain more so than recurrent instability with these injuries [271].

Superior labrum anterior to posterior (SLAP) injuries can occur concurrently with anterior shoulder dislocations [272]. A SLAP injury involves a tear or detachment of the superior aspect of the labrum where the long head of the biceps tendon attaches. In cases of anterior shoulder dislocation, forceful movement can cause shearing or tearing of this area. SLAP injuries after traumatic anterior shoulder dislocation have been observed in up to 22% of patients [273].

The anterior labroligamentous periosteal sleeve avulsion (ALPSA) lesion is a specific type of injury that can occur after anterior shoulder dislocation. In this injury, the anterior-inferior labrum becomes detached from the glenoid rim and flips inward, forming a "sleeve" that remains attached to the periosteum of the glenoid rim [274]. The ALPSA lesion differs from a Bankart lesion in that the labrum remains attached to the periosteum rather than the glenoid rim [274]. This injury can lead to recurrent shoulder instability and pain [261].

The glenolabral articular disruption (GLAD) lesion is a specific injury in which the anterior-inferior labrum becomes detached from the glenoid rim and avulses with a portion of the adjacent articular cartilage, which remains attached to the humerus [275]. The GLAD lesion is associated with anterior shoulder instability and can contribute to recurrent dislocations or subluxations [275].

The Kim lesion is an incomplete avulsion of the posterior labrum and can be seen on MRI or MRA [256]. This is important to evaluate in the setting of posterior instability as those with labral injuries tend to have successful outcomes after surgical intervention [256].

Rotator cuff injuries associated with shoulder instability occur more frequently in older patients (>40 years old) and are associated with symptoms such as persistent pain, dysfunction, and weakness [276]. The MRI is a useful tool in evaluating the integrity of the rotator cuff in these patients [276].

Treatment and Management

In addition to the patient's history, clinical examination, and imaging results, there are a couple of factors that are important to consider when deciding the management of shoulder instability. These factors include the patient's age, gender, expectations, and physical requirements, such as sports participation and labor [261]. Whether the patient has had previous dislocations or instability events is also important to consider. Most treatment algorithms involve a period of immobilization followed by rehabilitation and a delayed return to activity.

First-time dislocation management presents a challenge. Surgery is recommended for younger patients with apprehension and bone loss and those at high risk of re-dislocation. Recurrent instability becomes more common with younger patients [277]. There are reports of a 100% re-dislocation rate in patients younger than 10 years of age, over 90% in 10–20-year olds, and up to 80% between the ages of 20 and 30 [277]. In addition, what activities/sports the patient participates in and when during the season the initial injury occurred plays a factor in treatment. Athletes in the middle of their season can be expected to return to play in 2–3 weeks [278] and complete their season. However, 37–90% will experience at least one additional episode of instability during that season [278]. In general, athletes should be pain-free with symmetric shoulder strength and functional range of motion before returning to sport or activity [278].

Patients with posterior instability should initially be treated with nonoperative management, which includes physical therapy and rehabilitation [256]. These programs should emphasize strength training as well as proprioception training, as these have been shown to diminish pain and/or improve stability in up to 66% of patients with posterior instability [279]. Strengthening of the subscapularis muscle is important as this confers stability to posterior translation [256].

The standard of care for MDI is nonoperative treatment with a comprehensive rehabilitation program, with a focus on strengthening the rotator cuff and addressing scapular dyskinesis [257]. The success of nonoperative treatment for nontraumatic MDI ranges greatly from 47% to 80% with satisfactory results [279, 280].

Operative Management

Surgical stabilization of anterior shoulder dislocation reduces the risk of recurrent instability and improves the likelihood of return to sport [281]. High-level contact athletes who undergo surgical repair are more likely to return to sport without subsequent instability events the following season than those treated nonoperatively [282]. However, there is conflicting evidence for optimal surgical treatment [283]. Surgical techniques can be categorized as soft tissue or bony procedures, and further as performed through an open incision or arthroscopically. A Bankart procedure repairs the injured labrum and is the most widely used technique for anterior shoulder instability [283]. The Bankart repair is best utilized for shoulders with little to no glenoid bone loss, as increased bone loss is a risk factor for failure after an all-soft tissue repair [283]. Additional soft tissue procedures include capsular plication and the remplissage procedure, which involves tenodesis of the infraspinatus into the Hill-Sachs lesion, which adds stability to bipolar lesions [283].

The most popular bony procedure is the Latarjet, which involves moving the coracoid to the anterior glenoid. It is most commonly performed for recurrent instability associated with glenoid bone loss [283]. Appreciating glenoid bone loss and bipolar lesions appears to be most important when choosing between soft tissue and bony procedures for anterior shoulder instability [283]. Bone loss between 0 and 10% results in similar outcomes across all procedures, whereas the open Latarjet procedure shows the lowest incidence of recurrent instability when glenoid bone loss is greater than 10% [283].

Surgical intervention should be reserved for posterior instability patients with persistent symptoms after a trial of nonoperative treatment [256]. Open surgical treatment of posterior instability does not have the same success rate as is seen in anterior instability, with failure rate up between 30 and 70% [256]. Therefore, arthroscopic treatment alone for posterior instability without significant glenoid bone loss is the treatment of choice [256]. In the setting of substantial glenoid bone loss, open procedures such as glenoid osteotomy, bone blocks, or rotational osteotomy of the proximal humerus are advocated [256].

Surgical treatment should be considered for MDI patients who fail a comprehensive rehabilitation program and have persistent symptoms [257]. The surgical treatment options include open inferior capsular shift and arthroscopic plication. Open inferior capsular shift has demonstrated good to excellent results in 94–97% of patients with recurrent instability less than 11% [257, 284]. Arthroscopic capsular plication also demonstrates good to excellent results and involves addressing the redundancy of the anteroinferior and posteroinferior capsule [257]. Comparison studies of open and arthroscopic techniques for MDI have demonstrated similar rates of recurrent instability, complications, revision surgeries, return to sport, and postoperative range of motion [285, 286].

References

1. Michener LA, McClure PW, Karduna AR. Anatomical and biomechanical mechanisms of subacromial impingement syndrome. Clin Biomech (Bristol, Avon). 2003;18(5):369–79. https://doi.org/10.1016/s0268-0033(03)00047-0.
2. Bigliani LU, Levine WN. Subacromial impingement syndrome. J Bone Joint Surg Am. 1997;79(12):1854–68.
3. Neer CS 2nd. Impingement lesions. Clin Orthop Relat Res. 1983;173:70–7.
4. Vaz S, Soyer J, Pries P, Clarac JP. Subacromial impingement: influence of coracoacromial arch geometry on shoulder function. Joint Bone Spine. 2000;67(4):305–9.
5. Chansky HA, Iannotti JP. The vascularity of the rotator cuff. Clin Sports Med. 1991;10(4):807–22.
6. Lohr JF, Uhthoff HK. The microvascular pattern of the supraspinatus tendon. Clin Orthop Relat Res. 1990;254:35–8.
7. Neer CS 2nd. Anterior acromioplasty for the chronic impingement syndrome in the shoulder: a preliminary report. J Bone Joint Surg Am. 1972;54(1):41–50.
8. Chambler AF, Bull AM, Reilly P, Amis AA, Emery RJ. Coracoacromial ligament tension in vivo. J Shoulder Elb Surg. 2003;12(4):365–7. https://doi.org/10.1016/s1058-2746(03)00031-4.
9. Yamamoto N, Muraki T, Sperling JW, et al. Contact between the coracoacromial arch and the rotator cuff tendons in nonpathologic situations: a cadaveric study. J Shoulder Elb Surg. 2010;19(5):681–7. https://doi.org/10.1016/j.jse.2009.12.006.
10. Balke M, Schmidt C, Dedy N, Banerjee M, Bouillon B, Liem D. Correlation of acromial morphology with impingement syndrome and rotator cuff tears. Acta Orthop. 2013;84(2):178–83. https://doi.org/10.3109/17453674.2013.773413.
11. Budoff JE, Nirschl RP, Guidi EJ. Debridement of partial-thickness tears of the rotator cuff without acromioplasty. Long-term follow-up and review of the literature. J Bone Joint Surg Am. 1998;80(5):733–48. https://doi.org/10.2106/00004623-199805000-00016.
12. Gerber C, Galantay RV, Hersche O. The pattern of pain produced by irritation of the acromioclavicular joint and the subacromial space. J Shoulder Elb Surg. 1998;7(4):352–5. https://doi.org/10.1016/s1058-2746(98)90022-2.
13. Park HB, Yokota A, Gill HS, El Rassi G, McFarland EG. Diagnostic accuracy of clinical tests for the different degrees of subacromial impingement syndrome. J Bone Joint Surg Am. 2005;87(7):1446–55. https://doi.org/10.2106/JBJS.D.02335.
14. Roberts CS, Davila JN, Hushek SG, Tillett ED, Corrigan TM. Magnetic resonance imaging analysis of the subacromial space in the impingement sign positions. J Shoulder Elb Surg. 2002;11(6):595–9. https://doi.org/10.1067/mse.2002.127095.
15. Valadie AL 3rd, Jobe CM, Pink MM, Ekman EF, Jobe FW. Anatomy of provocative tests for impingement syndrome of the shoulder. J Shoulder Elb Surg. 2000;9(1):36–46. https://doi.org/10.1016/s1058-2746(00)90008-9.
16. Cummins CA, Sasso LM, Nicholson D. Impingement syndrome: temporal outcomes of nonoperative treatment. J Shoulder Elb Surg. 2009;18(2):172–7. https://doi.org/10.1016/j.jse.2008.09.005.
17. Kuhn JE. Exercise in the treatment of rotator cuff impingement: a systematic review and a synthesized evidence-based rehabilitation protocol. J Shoulder Elb Surg. 2009;18(1):138–60. https://doi.org/10.1016/j.jse.2008.06.004.

18. Odenbring S, Wagner P, Atroshi I. Long-term outcomes of arthroscopic acromioplasty for chronic shoulder impingement syndrome: a prospective cohort study with a minimum of 12 years' follow-up. Arthroscopy. 2008;24(10):1092–8. https://doi.org/10.1016/j.arthro.2008.04.073.
19. Kang MN, Rizio L, Prybicien M, Middlemas DA, Blacksin MF. The accuracy of subacromial corticosteroid injections: a comparison of multiple methods. J Shoulder Elb Surg. 2008;17(1 Suppl):61S–6S. https://doi.org/10.1016/j.jse.2007.07.010.
20. Karthikeyan S, Kwong HT, Upadhyay PK, Parsons N, Drew SJ, Griffin D. A double-blind randomised controlled study comparing subacromial injection of tenoxicam or methylprednisolone in patients with subacromial impingement. J Bone Joint Surg Br. 2010;92(1):77–82. https://doi.org/10.1302/0301-620X.92B1.22137.
21. Norlin R, Adolfsson L. Small full-thickness tears do well ten to thirteen years after arthroscopic subacromial decompression. J Shoulder Elb Surg. 2008;17(1 Suppl):12S–6S. https://doi.org/10.1016/j.jse.2007.06.020.
22. Henkus HE, de Witte PB, Nelissen RG, Brand R, van Arkel ER. Bursectomy compared with acromioplasty in the management of subacromial impingement syndrome: a prospective randomised study. J Bone Joint Surg Br. 2009;91(4):504–10. https://doi.org/10.1302/0301-620X.91B4.21442.
23. Codman E. The shoulder: rupture of the supraspinatus tendon and other lesions in or about the subacromial bursa; 1934. p. 514.
24. Neviaser AS, Neviaser RJ. Adhesive capsulitis of the shoulder. J Am Acad Orthop Surg. 2011;19(9):536–42. https://doi.org/10.5435/00124635-201109000-00004.
25. Neviaser RJ, Neviaser TJ. The frozen shoulder. Diagnosis and management. Clin Orthop Relat Res. 1987;223:59–64.
26. Lloyd-Roberts GC, French PR. Periarthritis of the shoulder: a study of the disease and its treatment. Br Med J. 1959;1(5137):1569–71. https://doi.org/10.1136/bmj.1.5137.1569.
27. Binder A, Hazleman BL, Parr G, Roberts S. A controlled study of oral prednisolone in frozen shoulder. Br J Rheumatol. 1986;25(3):288–92. https://doi.org/10.1093/rheumatology/25.3.288.
28. Hand C, Clipsham K, Rees JL, Carr AJ. Long-term outcome of frozen shoulder. J Shoulder Elb Surg. 2008;17(2):231–6. https://doi.org/10.1016/j.jse.2007.05.009.
29. Levine WN, Kashyap CP, Bak SF, Ahmad CS, Blaine TA, Bigliani LU. Nonoperative management of idiopathic adhesive capsulitis. J Shoulder Elb Surg. 2007;16(5):569–73. https://doi.org/10.1016/j.jse.2006.12.007.
30. Minter WT 3rd. The shoulder-hand syndrome in coronary disease. J Med Assoc Ga. 1967;56(2):45–9.
31. Wohlgethan JR. Frozen shoulder in hyperthyroidism. Arthritis Rheum. 1987;30(8):936–9. https://doi.org/10.1002/art.1780300815.
32. Cheville AL, Tchou J. Barriers to rehabilitation following surgery for primary breast cancer. J Surg Oncol. 2007;95(5):409–18. https://doi.org/10.1002/jso.20782.
33. Bowman CA, Jeffcoate WJ, Pattrick M, Doherty M. Bilateral adhesive capsulitis, oligoarthritis and proximal myopathy as presentation of hypothyroidism. Br J Rheumatol. 1988;27(1):62–4. https://doi.org/10.1093/rheumatology/27.1.62.
34. Arkkila PE, Kantola IM, Viikari JS, Ronnemaa T. Shoulder capsulitis in type I and II diabetic patients: association with diabetic complications and related diseases. Ann Rheum Dis. 1996;55(12):907–14. https://doi.org/10.1136/ard.55.12.907.
35. Emig EW, Schweitzer ME, Karasick D, Lubowitz J. Adhesive capsulitis of the shoulder: MR diagnosis. AJR Am J Roentgenol. 1995;164(6):1457–9. https://doi.org/10.2214/ajr.164.6.7754892.
36. Sofka CM, Ciavarra GA, Hannafin JA, Cordasco FA, Potter HG. Magnetic resonance imaging of adhesive capsulitis: correlation with clinical staging. HSS J. 2008;4(2):164–9. https://doi.org/10.1007/s11420-008-9088-1.

37. Lefevre-Colau MM, Drape JL, Fayad F, et al. Magnetic resonance imaging of shoulders with idiopathic adhesive capsulitis: reliability of measures. Eur Radiol. 2005;15(12):2415–22. https://doi.org/10.1007/s00330-005-2830-x.
38. Griggs SM, Ahn A, Green A. Idiopathic adhesive capsulitis. A prospective functional outcome study of nonoperative treatment. J Bone Joint Surg Am. 2000;82(10):1398–407.
39. Shaffer B, Tibone JE, Kerlan RK. Frozen shoulder. A long-term follow-up. J Bone Joint Surg Am. 1992;74(5):738–46.
40. van den Hout WB, Vermeulen HM, Rozing PM, Vliet Vlieland TP. Impact of adhesive capsulitis and economic evaluation of high-grade and low-grade mobilisation techniques. Aust J Physiother. 2005;51(3):141–9. https://doi.org/10.1016/s0004-9514(05)70020-9.
41. Bulgen DY, Binder AI, Hazleman BL, Dutton J, Roberts S. Frozen shoulder: prospective clinical study with an evaluation of three treatment regimens. Ann Rheum Dis. 1984;43(3):353–60. https://doi.org/10.1136/ard.43.3.353.
42. Rizk TE, Pinals RS, Talaiver AS. Corticosteroid injections in adhesive capsulitis: investigation of their value and site. Arch Phys Med Rehabil. 1991;72(1):20–2.
43. Lee M, Haq AM, Wright V, Longton EB. Periarthritis of the shoulder: a controlled trial of physiotherapy. Physiotherapy. 1973;59(10):312–5.
44. van der Windt DA, Koes BW, Deville W, Boeke AJ, de Jong BA, Bouter LM. Effectiveness of corticosteroid injections versus physiotherapy for treatment of painful stiff shoulder in primary care: randomised trial. BMJ. 1998;317(7168):1292–6. https://doi.org/10.1136/bmj.317.7168.1292.
45. Carette S, Moffet H, Tardif J, et al. Intraarticular corticosteroids, supervised physiotherapy, or a combination of the two in the treatment of adhesive capsulitis of the shoulder: a placebo-controlled trial. Arthritis Rheum. 2003;48(3):829–38. https://doi.org/10.1002/art.10954.
46. Buchbinder R, Green S, Youd JM. Corticosteroid injections for shoulder pain. Cochrane Database Syst Rev. 2003;2003(1):CD004016. https://doi.org/10.1002/14651858.CD004016.
47. Quraishi NA, Johnston P, Bayer J, Crowe M, Chakrabarti AJ. Thawing the frozen shoulder. A randomised trial comparing manipulation under anaesthesia with hydrodilatation. J Bone Joint Surg Br. 2007;89(9):1197–200. https://doi.org/10.1302/0301-620X.89B9.18863.
48. Dahan TH, Fortin L, Pelletier M, Petit M, Vadeboncoeur R, Suissa S. Double blind randomized clinical trial examining the efficacy of bupivacaine suprascapular nerve blocks in frozen shoulder. J Rheumatol. 2000;27(6):1464–9.
49. Brinker MR, Cuomo JS, Popham GJ, O'Connor DP, Barrack RL. An examination of bias in shoulder scoring instruments among healthy collegiate and recreational athletes. J Shoulder Elb Surg. 2002;11(5):463–9. https://doi.org/10.1067/mse.2002.126209.
50. Ide J, Takagi K. Early and long-term results of arthroscopic treatment for shoulder stiffness. J Shoulder Elb Surg. 2004;13(2):174–9. https://doi.org/10.1016/j.jse.2003.11.001.
51. Snow M, Boutros I, Funk L. Posterior arthroscopic capsular release in frozen shoulder. Arthroscopy. 2009;25(1):19–23. https://doi.org/10.1016/j.arthro.2008.08.006.
52. Chen J, Chen S, Li Y, Hua Y, Li H. Is the extended release of the inferior glenohumeral ligament necessary for frozen shoulder? Arthroscopy. 2010;26(4):529–35. https://doi.org/10.1016/j.arthro.2010.02.020.
53. Mather RC 3rd, Koenig L, Acevedo D, et al. The societal and economic value of rotator cuff repair. J Bone Joint Surg Am. 2013;95(22):1993–2000. https://doi.org/10.2106/JBJS.L.01495.
54. Sher JS, Uribe JW, Posada A, Murphy BJ, Zlatkin MB. Abnormal findings on magnetic resonance images of asymptomatic shoulders. J Bone Joint Surg Am. 1995;77(1):10–5. https://doi.org/10.2106/00004623-199501000-00002.
55. Tempelhof S, Rupp S, Seil R. Age-related prevalence of rotator cuff tears in asymptomatic shoulders. J Shoulder Elb Surg. 1999;8(4):296–9. https://doi.org/10.1016/s1058-2746(99)90148-9.
56. RC: O. American Academy of Orthopaedic Surgeons.
57. DeLee JDD, Miller MD, Thompson SR. DeLee & Drez's orthopaedic sports medicine: principles and practice. 4th ed; 2015.

58. Hippensteel KJ, Brophy R, Smith MV, Wright RW. A comprehensive review of physical examination tests of the cervical spine, scapula, and rotator cuff. J Am Acad Orthop Surg. 2019;27(11):385–94. https://doi.org/10.5435/JAAOS-D-17-00090.
59. Hegedus EJ, Goode A, Campbell S, et al. Physical examination tests of the shoulder: a systematic review with meta-analysis of individual tests. Br J Sports Med. 2008;42(2):80–92.; discussion 92. https://doi.org/10.1136/bjsm.2007.038406.
60. Hughes PC, Taylor NF, Green RA. Most clinical tests cannot accurately diagnose rotator cuff pathology: a systematic review. Aust J Physiother. 2008;54(3):159–70. https://doi.org/10.1016/s0004-9514(08)70022-9.
61. MacDonald PB, Clark P, Sutherland K. An analysis of the diagnostic accuracy of the Hawkins and Neer subacromial impingement signs. J Shoulder Elb Surg. 2000;9(4):299–301. https://doi.org/10.1067/mse.2000.106918.
62. Holtby R, Razmjou H. Validity of the supraspinatus test as a single clinical test in diagnosing patients with rotator cuff pathology. J Orthop Sports Phys Ther. 2004;34(4):194–200. https://doi.org/10.2519/jospt.2004.34.4.194.
63. Jobe FW, Moynes DR. Delineation of diagnostic criteria and a rehabilitation program for rotator cuff injuries. Am J Sports Med. 1982;10(6):336–9. https://doi.org/10.1177/036354658201000602.
64. Calis M, Akgun K, Birtane M, Karacan I, Calis H, Tuzun F. Diagnostic values of clinical diagnostic tests in subacromial impingement syndrome. Ann Rheum Dis. 2000;59(1):44–7. https://doi.org/10.1136/ard.59.1.44.
65. Walch G, Boulahia A, Calderone S, Robinson AH. The 'dropping' and 'hornblower's' signs in evaluation of rotator-cuff tears. J Bone Joint Surg Br. 1998;80(4):624–8. https://doi.org/10.1302/0301-620x.80b4.8651.
66. Gerber C, Hersche O, Farron A. Isolated rupture of the subscapularis tendon. J Bone Joint Surg Am. 1996;78(7):1015–23. https://doi.org/10.2106/00004623-199607000-00005.
67. Barth JR, Burkhart SS, De Beer JF. The bear-hug test: a new and sensitive test for diagnosing a subscapularis tear. Arthroscopy. 2006;22(10):1076–84. https://doi.org/10.1016/j.arthro.2006.05.005.
68. Goldberg BA, Scarlat MM, Harryman DT 2nd. Management of the stiff shoulder. J Orthop Sci. 1999;4(6):462–71. https://doi.org/10.1007/s007760050131.
69. Bang MD, Deyle GD. Comparison of supervised exercise with and without manual physical therapy for patients with shoulder impingement syndrome. J Orthop Sports Phys Ther. 2000;30(3):126–37. https://doi.org/10.2519/jospt.2000.30.3.126.
70. Conroy DE, Hayes KW. The effect of joint mobilization as a component of comprehensive treatment for primary shoulder impingement syndrome. J Orthop Sports Phys Ther. 1998;28(1):3–14. https://doi.org/10.2519/jospt.1998.28.1.3.
71. Millett PJ, Wilcox RB 3rd, O'Holleran JD, Warner JJ. Rehabilitation of the rotator cuff: an evaluation-based approach. J Am Acad Orthop Surg. 2006;14(11):599–609. https://doi.org/10.5435/00124635-200610000-00002.
72. Vaishnav S, Millett PJ. Arthroscopic rotator cuff repair: scientific rationale, surgical technique, and early clinical and functional results of a knotless self-reinforcing double-row rotator cuff repair system. J Shoulder Elb Surg. 2010;19(2 Suppl):83–90. https://doi.org/10.1016/j.jse.2009.12.012.
73. Nho SJ, Slabaugh MA, Seroyer ST, et al. Does the literature support double-row suture anchor fixation for arthroscopic rotator cuff repair? A systematic review comparing double-row and single-row suture anchor configuration. Arthroscopy. 2009;25(11):1319–28. https://doi.org/10.1016/j.arthro.2009.02.005.
74. Randelli P, Cucchi D, Ragone V, de Girolamo L, Cabitza P, Randelli M. History of rotator cuff surgery. Knee Surg Sports Traumatol Arthrosc. 2015;23(2):344–62. https://doi.org/10.1007/s00167-014-3445-z.
75. Lo IK, Burkhart SS. Double-row arthroscopic rotator cuff repair: re-establishing the footprint of the rotator cuff. Arthroscopy. 2003;19(9):1035–42. https://doi.org/10.1016/j.arthro.2003.09.036.

76. Tingart MJ, Apreleva M, Lehtinen J, Zurakowski D, Warner JJ. Anchor design and bone mineral density affect the pull-out strength of suture anchors in rotator cuff repair: which anchors are best to use in patients with low bone quality? Am J Sports Med. 2004;32(6):1466–73. https://doi.org/10.1177/0363546503262644.
77. Galatz LM, Ball CM, Teefey SA, Middleton WD, Yamaguchi K. The outcome and repair integrity of completely arthroscopically repaired large and massive rotator cuff tears. J Bone Joint Surg Am. 2004;86(2):219–24. https://doi.org/10.2106/00004623-200402000-00002.
78. Dugas JR, Campbell DA, Warren RF, Robie BH, Millett PJ. Anatomy and dimensions of rotator cuff insertions. J Shoulder Elb Surg. 2002;11(5):498–503. https://doi.org/10.1067/mse.2002.126208.
79. Mazzocca AD, Millett PJ, Guanche CA, Santangelo SA, Arciero RA. Arthroscopic single-row versus double-row suture anchor rotator cuff repair. Am J Sports Med. 2005;33(12):1861–8. https://doi.org/10.1177/0363546505279575.
80. Duquin TR, Buyea C, Bisson LJ. Which method of rotator cuff repair leads to the highest rate of structural healing? A systematic review. Am J Sports Med. 2010;38(4):835–41. https://doi.org/10.1177/0363546509359679.
81. Millett PJ, Warth RJ, Dornan GJ, Lee JT, Spiegl UJ. Clinical and structural outcomes after arthroscopic single-row versus double-row rotator cuff repair: a systematic review and meta-analysis of level I randomized clinical trials. J Shoulder Elb Surg. 2014;23(4):586–97. https://doi.org/10.1016/j.jse.2013.10.006.
82. Millett PJ, Mazzocca A, Guanche CA. Mattress double anchor footprint repair: a novel, arthroscopic rotator cuff repair technique. Arthroscopy. 2004;20(8):875–9. https://doi.org/10.1016/j.arthro.2004.07.015.
83. Bosworth BM. Calcium deposits in the shoulder and subacromial bursitis: a survey of 12,122 shoulders. JAMA J Am Med Assoc. 1941;116(22):2477–82. https://doi.org/10.1001/jama.1941.02820220019004.
84. Uhthoff HK, Loehr JW. Calcific tendinopathy of the rotator cuff: pathogenesis, diagnosis, and management. J Am Acad Orthop Surg. 1997;5(4):183–91. https://doi.org/10.5435/00124635-199707000-00001.
85. Le Goff B, Berthelot JM, Guillot P, Glemarec J, Maugars Y. Assessment of calcific tendonitis of rotator cuff by ultrasonography: comparison between symptomatic and asymptomatic shoulders. Joint Bone Spine. 2010;77(3):258–63. https://doi.org/10.1016/j.jbspin.2010.01.012.
86. Lin CH, Chao HL, Chiou HJ. Calcified plaque resorptive status as determined by high-resolution ultrasound is predictive of successful conservative management of calcific tendinosis. Eur J Radiol. 2012;81(8):1776–81. https://doi.org/10.1016/j.ejrad.2011.05.018.
87. Cho NS, Lee BG, Rhee YG. Radiologic course of the calcific deposits in calcific tendinitis of the shoulder: does the initial radiologic aspect affect the final results? J Shoulder Elb Surg. 2010;19(2):267–72. https://doi.org/10.1016/j.jse.2009.07.008.
88. Yoo JC, Park WH, Koh KH, Kim SM. Arthroscopic treatment of chronic calcific tendinitis with complete removal and rotator cuff tendon repair. Knee Surg Sports Traumatol Arthrosc. 2010;18(12):1694–9. https://doi.org/10.1007/s00167-010-1067-7.
89. Harvie P, Pollard TC, Carr AJ. Calcific tendinitis: natural history and association with endocrine disorders. J Shoulder Elb Surg. 2007;16(2):169–73. https://doi.org/10.1016/j.jse.2006.06.007.
90. Oliva F, Via AG, Maffulli N. Physiopathology of intratendinous calcific deposition. BMC Med. 2012;10:95. https://doi.org/10.1186/1741-7015-10-95.
91. Uhthoff HK, Sarkar K, Maynard JA. Calcifying tendinitis: a new concept of its pathogenesis. Clin Orthop Relat Res. 1976;118:164–8.
92. Moseley HF, Goldie I. The arterial pattern of the rotator cuff of the shoulder. J Bone Joint Surg Br. 1963;45(4):780–9.
93. Ogon P, Suedkamp NP, Jaeger M, Izadpanah K, Koestler W, Maier D. Prognostic factors in nonoperative therapy for chronic symptomatic calcific tendinitis of the shoulder. Arthritis Rheum. 2009;60(10):2978–84. https://doi.org/10.1002/art.24845.

94. Albert JD, Meadeb J, Guggenbuhl P, et al. High-energy extracorporeal shock-wave therapy for calcifying tendinitis of the rotator cuff: a randomised trial. J Bone Joint Surg Br. 2007;89(3):335–41. https://doi.org/10.1302/0301-620X.89B3.18249.
95. Wang CJ, Yang KD, Wang FS, Chen HH, Wang JW. Shock wave therapy for calcific tendinitis of the shoulder: a prospective clinical study with two-year follow-up. Am J Sports Med. 2003;31(3):425–30. https://doi.org/10.1177/03635465030310031701.
96. Hsu CJ, Wang DY, Tseng KF, Fong YC, Hsu HC, Jim YF. Extracorporeal shock wave therapy for calcifying tendinitis of the shoulder. J Shoulder Elb Surg. 2008;17(1):55–9. https://doi.org/10.1016/j.jse.2007.03.023.
97. Ioppolo F, Tattoli M, Di Sante L, et al. Clinical improvement and resorption of calcifications in calcific tendinitis of the shoulder after shock wave therapy at 6 months' follow-up: a systematic review and meta-analysis. Arch Phys Med Rehabil. 2013;94(9):1699–706. https://doi.org/10.1016/j.apmr.2013.01.030.
98. Daecke W, Kusnierczak D, Loew M. Long-term effects of extracorporeal shockwave therapy in chronic calcific tendinitis of the shoulder. J Shoulder Elb Surg. 2002;11(5):476–80. https://doi.org/10.1067/mse.2002.126614.
99. Gerdesmeyer L, Wagenpfeil S, Haake M, et al. Extracorporeal shock wave therapy for the treatment of chronic calcifying tendonitis of the rotator cuff: a randomized controlled trial. JAMA. 2003;290(19):2573–80. https://doi.org/10.1001/jama.290.19.2573.
100. Peters J, Luboldt W, Schwarz W, Jacobi V, Herzog C, Vogl TJ. Extracorporeal shock wave therapy in calcific tendinitis of the shoulder. Skeletal Radiol. 2004;33(12):712–8. https://doi.org/10.1007/s00256-004-0849-8.
101. del Cura JL, Torre I, Zabala R, Legorburu A. Sonographically guided percutaneous needle lavage in calcific tendinitis of the shoulder: short- and long-term results. AJR Am J Roentgenol. 2007;189(3):W128–34. https://doi.org/10.2214/AJR.07.2254.
102. Yoo JC, Koh KH, Park WH, Park JC, Kim SM, Yoon YC. The outcome of ultrasound-guided needle decompression and steroid injection in calcific tendinitis. J Shoulder Elb Surg. 2010;19(4):596–600. https://doi.org/10.1016/j.jse.2009.09.002.
103. Serafini G, Sconfienza LM, Lacelli F, Silvestri E, Aliprandi A, Sardanelli F. Rotator cuff calcific tendonitis: short-term and 10-year outcomes after two-needle us-guided percutaneous treatment – nonrandomized controlled trial. Radiology. 2009;252(1):157–64. https://doi.org/10.1148/radiol.2521081816.
104. de Witte PB, Selten JW, Navas A, et al. Calcific tendinitis of the rotator cuff: a randomized controlled trial of ultrasound-guided needling and lavage versus subacromial corticosteroids. Am J Sports Med. 2013;41(7):1665–73. https://doi.org/10.1177/0363546513487066.
105. Krasny C, Enenkel M, Aigner N, Wlk M, Landsiedl F. Ultrasound-guided needling combined with shock-wave therapy for the treatment of calcifying tendonitis of the shoulder. J Bone Joint Surg Br. 2005;87(4):501–7. https://doi.org/10.1302/0301-620X.87B4.15769.
106. Rebuzzi E, Coletti N, Schiavetti S, Giusto F. Arthroscopy surgery versus shock wave therapy for chronic calcifying tendinitis of the shoulder. J Orthop Traumatol. 2008;9(4):179–85. https://doi.org/10.1007/s10195-008-0024-4.
107. Seil R, Litzenburger H, Kohn D, Rupp S. Arthroscopic treatment of chronically painful calcifying tendinitis of the supraspinatus tendon. Arthroscopy. 2006;22(5):521–7. https://doi.org/10.1016/j.arthro.2006.01.012.
108. Balke M, Bielefeld R, Schmidt C, Dedy N, Liem D. Calcifying tendinitis of the shoulder: midterm results after arthroscopic treatment. Am J Sports Med. 2012;40(3):657–61. https://doi.org/10.1177/0363546511430202.
109. Porcellini G, Paladini P, Campi F, Paganelli M. Arthroscopic treatment of calcifying tendinitis of the shoulder: clinical and ultrasonographic follow-up findings at two to five years. J Shoulder Elb Surg. 2004;13(5):503–8. https://doi.org/10.1016/j.jse.2004.04.001.
110. Maier D, Jaeger M, Izadpanah K, Bornebusch L, Suedkamp NP, Ogon P. Rotator cuff preservation in arthroscopic treatment of calcific tendinitis. Arthroscopy. 2013;29(5):824–31. https://doi.org/10.1016/j.arthro.2013.01.031.

111. Wittenberg RH, Rubenthaler F, Wolk T, Ludwig J, Willburger RE, Steffen R. Surgical or conservative treatment for chronic rotator cuff calcifying tendinitis – a matched-pair analysis of 100 patients. Arch Orthop Trauma Surg. 2001;121(1–2):56–9. https://doi.org/10.1007/s004020000195.
112. Rompe JD, Zoellner J, Nafe B. Shock wave therapy versus conventional surgery in the treatment of calcifying tendinitis of the shoulder. Clin Orthop Relat Res. 2001;387:72–82. https://doi.org/10.1097/00003086-200106000-00010.
113. Frank RM, Cotter EJ, Strauss EJ, et al. Management of biceps tendon pathology: from the glenoid to the radial tuberosity. J Am Acad Orthop Surg. 2018;26(4):e77–89.
114. Candela V, Standoli JP, Carbone S, et al. Shoulder long head biceps tendon pathology is associated with increasing rotator cuff tear size. Arthrosc Sports Med Rehabil. 2021;3(5):e1517–23.
115. Desai SS, Mata HK. Long head of biceps tendon pathology and results of tenotomy in full-thickness reparable rotator cuff tear. Arthroscopy. 2017;33(11):1971–6.
116. Lafosse L, Reiland Y, Baier GP, et al. Anterior and posterior instability of the long head of the biceps tendon in rotator cuff tears: a new classification based on arthroscopic observations. Arthroscopy. 2007;23(1):73–80.
117. Murthi AM, Vosburgh CL, Neviaser TJ. The incidence of pathologic changes of the long head of the biceps tendon. J Shoulder Elbow Surg. 2000;9(5):382–5.
118. Nho SJ, Strauss EJ, Lenart BA, et al. Long head of the biceps tendinopathy: diagnosis and management. J Am Acad Orthop Surg. 2010;18(11):645–56.
119. Lansdown DA, Bendich I, Motamedi D, Feeley BT. Imaging-based prevalence of superior labral anterior-posterior tears significantly increases in the aging shoulder. Orthop J Sports Med. 2018;6(9):2325967118797065.
120. Schwartzberg R, Reuss BL, Burkhart BG, Butterfield M, et al. High prevalence of superior labral tears diagnosed by MRI in middle-aged patients with asymptomatic shoulders. Orthop J Sports Med. 2016;4(1):2325967115623212.
121. Kim TK, Queale WS, Cosgarea AJ, McFarland EG. Clinical features of the different type of SLAP lesions: an analysis of one hundred and thirty-nine cases. J Bone Joint Surg Am. 2003;85(1):66–71.
122. Maffet MW, Garsman GM, Moseley B. Superior labrum-biceps tendon complex lesions of the shoulder. Am J Sports Med. 1995;23(1):93–8.
123. Snyder SJ, Banas MP, Karzel RP. An analysis of 140 injuries to the superior glenoid labrum. J Shoulder Elb Surg. 1995;4(4):243–8.
124. Andrews JR, Carson WG Jr, McLeod WD. Glenoid labrum tears related to the long head of the biceps. Am J Sports Med. 1985;13(5):337–41.
125. Chalmers PN, Cip J, Trombley R, et al. Glenohumeral function of the long head of the biceps muscle: an electromyographic analysis. Orthop J Sports Med. 2014;2(2):2325967114523902.
126. Khazzam M, George MS, Churchill RS, Kuhn JE. Disorders of the long head of biceps tendon. J Shoulder Elb Surg. 2011;21(1):136–45.
127. Pagnani MJ, Deng XH, Warren RF, et al. Role of the long head of the biceps brachii in glenohumeral stability: a biomechanical study in cadavera. J Shoulder Elb Surg. 1996;5(4):255–62.
128. LeVasseur MR, Mancini MR, Hawthorne BC, et al. SLAP tears and return to sport and work: current concepts. J ISAKOS. 2021;6(4):204–11.
129. Holtby R, Razmjou H. Accuracy of the speed's and Yergason's test in detecting biceps pathology and SLAP lesion: comparison with arthroscopic findings. Arthroscopy. 2004;20(3):231–16.
130. Meserve BB, Cleland JA, Boucher TR, et al. A meta-analysis examining clinical test utility for assessing superior labral anterior posterior lesions. Am J Sports Med. 2009;37(11):2252–8.
131. Armstrong A, Teefey SA, Wu T, et al. The efficacy of ultrasound in the diagnosis of long head of the biceps tendon pathology. J Shoulder Elb Surg. 2006;15(1):7–11.
132. Skendzel JG, Jacobson JA, Carpenter JE, Miller BS. Long head of biceps brachii tendon evaluation: accuracy of preoperative ultrasound. AJR Am J Roentgenol. 2011;197(4):942–8.
133. Mariani EM, Cofield RH, Askew LJ, et al. Rupture of the tendon of the long head of the biceps brachii. Surgical versus nonsurgical treatment. Clin Orthop Relat Res. 1988;228:233–9.

134. Deutch S, Gelineck J, Johannsen H, Sneppen O. Permanent disabilities in the displaced muscle from rupture of the long head tendon of the biceps. Scand J Sci Sports. 2005;15(3):159–62.
135. McDevitt AW, Snodgrass SJ, Cleland JA, et al. Treatment of individuals with chronic bicipital tendinopathy using dry needling, eccentric-concentric exercise and stretching; a case series. Physiother Theory Prac. 2020;36(3):397–407.
136. Edwards SL, Lee JA, Bell JE, Packer JD, Ahmad CS, Levine WN, Bigliani LU, Blaine TA. Nonoperative treatment of superior labrum anterior posterior tears: improvements in pain, function, and quality of life. Am J Sports Med. 2010;38(7):1456–61. https://doi.org/10.1177/0363546510370937. Epub 2010 Jun 3. PMID: 20522835.
137. Jang SH, Seo JG, Jang HS, et al. Predictive factors associated with failure of nonoperative treatment of superior labrum anterior-posterior tears. J Shoulder Elb Surg. 2016;25(3):428–34.
138. Steinmetz RG, Guth JJ, Matava MJ, et al. Return to play following nonsurgical management of superior labrum anterior-posterior tears: a systematic review. J Shoulder Elb Surg. 2022;31(6):1323–33.
139. Yiannakopoulos CK, Megaloikonomos PD, Foufa K, Gliatis J. Ultrasound-guided versus palpation-guided corticosteroid injections for tendinosis of the long head of the biceps: a randomized comparative study. Skeletal Radiol. 2020;49(4):585–91.
140. Zhang J, Ebraheim N, Lause GE. Ultrasound-guided injection for the biceps brachii tendinitis: results and experience. Ultrasound Med Biol. 2011;37(5):729–33.
141. Belk JW, Kraeutler MJ, Houck DA, et al. Biceps tenodesis versus tenotomy: a systematic review and meta-analysis of level I randomized controlled trials. J Shoulder Elb Surg. 2021;30(5):951–60.
142. Daou JP, Nagaya DY, Matsunaga FT, Tamaoki MJS. Does biceps tenotomy or tenodesis have better results after surgery? A systematic review and meta-analysis. Clin Orthop Relat Res. 2021;479(7):1561–73.
143. Na Y, Zhu Y, Shi Y, et al. A meta-analysis comparing tenotomy or tenodesis for lesions of the long head of the biceps tendon with concomitant reparable rotator cuff tears. J Orthop Surg Res. 2019;14(1):370.
144. Zhou P, Liu J, Deng X, Li Z. Biceps tenotomy versus tenodesis for lesions of the long head of the biceps tendon: a systematic review and meta-analysis of randomized controlled trials. Medicine (Baltimore). 2021;100(3):e23993.
145. Kelly AM, Drakos MC, Fealy S, et al. Arthroscopic release of the long head of the biceps tendon: function outcome and clinical results. Am J Sports Med. 2005;33(2):208–13.
146. O'Brien MJ. Editorial commentary: shoulder biceps tenotomy versus tenodesis surgical decision making must be individualized for each patient. Arthroscopy. 2021;37(6):1777–8.
147. Belay ES, Wittstein JR, Garrigues GE, et al. Biceps tenotomy has earlier pain relief compared to biceps tenodesis: a randomized prospective study. Knee Surg Sports Traumatol Arthrosc. 2019;27(12):4032–7.
148. MacDonald P, Verhulst F, McRae S, et al. Biceps tenodesis versus tenotomy in the treatment of lesions of the long head of the biceps tendon in patients undergoing arthroscopic shoulder surgery: a prospective double-blinded randomized controlled trial. Am J Sports Med. 2020;48(6):1439–49.
149. Lee HJ, Jeong JY, Kim CK, Kim YS. Surgical treatment of lesions of the long head of the biceps brachii tendon with rotator cuff tear: a prospective randomized clinical trial comparing the clinical results of tenotomy and tenodesis. J Shoulder Elb Surg. 2016;25(7):1107–14.
150. Cvetanovich GL, Gowd AK, Frantz TL. Superior labral anterior posterior repair and biceps tenodesis surgery: trends of the American Board of Orthopedic Surgery database. Am J Sports Med. 2020;48(7):1583–9.
151. Erickson BJ, Jain A, Abrams GD, et al. SLAP lesions: trends in treatment. Arthroscopy. 2016;32(6):976–81.
152. Patterson BM, Creighton RA, Spang JT, et al. Surgical trends in the treatment of superior labrum anterior and posterior lesions of the shoulder: analysis of data from the American Board of Orthopedic Surgery certification examination database. Am J Sports Med. 2014;42(8):1904–10.

153. Boileau P, Parratte S, Chuinard C, et al. Arthroscopic treatment of isolated type II SLAP lesions: biceps tenodesis as an alternative to reinsertion. Am J Sports Med. 2009;37(5):929–36.
154. Denard PJ, Lädermann A, Parsley BK, Burkhard SS. Arthroscopic biceps tenodesis compared with repair of isolated type II slap lesions in patients older than 35 years. Orthopedics. 2014;37(3):e292–7.
155. Ide J, Maeda S, Takagi K. Sports activity after arthroscopic superior labral repair using suture anchors in overhead-throwing athletes. Am J Sports Med. 2005;33(4):507–14.
156. Lacheta L, Horan MP, Nolte PC, et al. SLAP repair versus subpectoral biceps tenodesis for isolated SLAP type 2 lesions in overhead athletes younger than 35 years: comparison of minimum 2-year outcomes. Orthop J Sports Med. 2022;10(6):23259671221105239.
157. Park JY, Chung SW, Jeon SH, et al. Clinical and radiological outcomes of type 2 superior labral anterior posterior repairs in elite overhead athletes. Am J Sports Med. 2013;41(6):1372–9.
158. Provencher MT, McCormick F, Dewing C, et al. A prospective analysis of 179 type 2 superior labrum anterior and posterior repairs: outcomes and factors associated with success and failure. Am J Sports Med. 2013;41(4):880–6.
159. Chillemi C, Franceschini V, Dei Guidici L, et al. Epidemiology of isolated acromioclavicular joint dislocation. Emerg Med Int. 2013;2013:171608. https://doi.org/10.1155/2013/171609.
160. Enger M, Skjaker SA, Melhuus K, et al. Shoulder injuries from birth to old age: a 1-year prospective study of 3031 shoulder injuries in an urban population. Injury. 2018;49(7):1324–9. https://doi.org/10.1016/j.injury.2018.05.013.
161. Hibberd EE, Kerr ZY, Roos KG, et al. Epidemiology of acromioclavicular joint sprains in 25 National Collegiate Athletic Associations Sports: 2009–2010 to 2014–2015 academic years. Am J Sports Med. 2016;44(10):2667–74. https://doi.org/10.1177/0363546516643721.
162. Lunsjö K, Olsson O, Nordin JS. Acromioclavicular joint dislocations: incidence, injury profile, and patient characteristics from a prospective case series. JSES Int. 2020;4(2):246–50. https://doi.org/10.1016/j.jseint.2020.01.009.
163. Lynch TS, Saltzman MD, Ghodasra JH, Bilimoria KY, Bowen MK, Nuber GW. Acromioclavicular joint injuries in the National Football League: epidemiology and management. Am J Sports Med. 2013;41:2904–8.
164. Pallis M, Cameron KL, Svoboda SJ, Owens BD. Epidemiology of acromioclavicular joint injury in young athletes. Am J Sports Med. 2012;40(9):2072–7. https://doi.org/10.1177/0363546512450162.
165. Mazzocca AD, Arciero RA, Bicos J. Evaluation and treatment of acromioclavicular joint injuries. Am J Sports Med. 2007;35:316–29.
166. Fakuda K, Craug EV, An KN, et al. Biomechanical study of the ligamentous system of the acromioclavicular joint. J Bone Joint Surg Am. 1986;68(3):434–40.
167. Rios CG, Arciero RA, Mazzocca AD. Anatomy of the clavicle and coracoid process for reconstruction of the coracoclavicular ligaments. Am J Sports Med. 2007;35:811–7.
168. Blazar PE, Iannotti JP, Williams GR. Anteroposteiror instability of the distal clavicle after distal clavicle resection. Clin Orthop Relat Res. 1998;348:114–20.
169. Geyer S, Achtnich AE, Voss A, et al. Iatrogenic instability of the acromioclavicular joint leads to ongoing impairment of shoulder function even following secondary surgical stabilization. Arch Orthop Trauma Surg. 2023;143(4):1877–86.
170. Labson JD, Anderson KA, Marder RA. Acromioclavicular dislocation after arthroscopic distal clavicle resection: a case report. J Shoulder Elb Surg. 2011;20(2):e10–2.
171. Frank RM, Cotter EJ, Leroux TS, Romeao AA. Acromioclavicular joint injuries: evidence-based treatment. J Am Acad Orthop Surg. 2019;17:e-775–e788.
172. Chronopoulos E, Kim TK, Park HB, Ashenbrenner D, McFarland EG. Diagnostic value of physical tests for isolated chronic acromioclavicular lesion. Am J Sports Med. 2004;32(3):655–61.
173. Krill MK, Rosas S, Kwon K, Dakkak A, Nwachukwu BU, McCormick R. A concise evidence-based physical examination for diagnosis of acromioclavicular joint pathology: a systematic review. Phys Sportsmed. 2018;46(1):98–104.

174. Ibrahim EF, Forrest NP, Forester A. Bilateral weighted radiographs are required for accurate classification of acromioclavicular separation: an observational study of 59 cases. Injury. 2015;46(10):1900–19005.
175. Beitzel K, Cote MP, Apostolakos J, et al. Current concepts in the treatment of acromioclavicular joint dislocations. Arthroscopy. 2013;29(2):387–97.
176. Park JP, Arnold JA, Coker TP, Harris WD, Becker DA. Treatment of acromioclavicular separations: a retrospective study. Am J Sports Med. 1980;8(4):251–6.
177. Mikek M. Long-term shoulder function after type I and II acromioclavicular joint disruption. Am J Sports Med. 2008;36(11):2147–50.
178. Mouhsine E, Garofalo R, Crevoisier X, Farron A. Grade I and II acromioclavicular dislocations: results of conservative treatment. J Shoulder Elb Surg. 2003;12:599–602.
179. Shaw MB, McInerney JJ, Dias JJ, Evans PA. Acromioclavicular joint sprains: the post-injury recovery intervals. Injury. 2003;34:438–42.
180. Calvo E, López-Franco M, Arribas IM. Clinical and radiographic outcomes of surgical and conservative treatment of type III acromioclavicular joint injury. J Shoulder Elb Surg. 2006;15(3):300–5.
181. Dias JJ, Steingold RF, Richardson RA, et al. The conservative treatment of acromioclavicular dislocation: review after five years. J Bone Joint Surg Br. 1987;69:719–22.
182. Finsterwald M, Dao Trong ML, Hollo D, Müller AM, Riede U, Bouaicha S. Conservative treatment of Rockwood type III acromioclavicular joint separation: a randomized controlled trial sling vs. brace. JSES Int. 2023;7(4):527–31.
183. Schlegel TF, Burks RT, Marcus RL, Dunn HK. A prospective evaluation of untreated acute grade III acromioclavicular separations. Am J Sports Med. 2001;29:699–703.
184. Gstettner C, Tauber M, Hitzl W, Resch H. Rockwood type III acromioclavicular dislocation: surgical versus conservative treatment. J Shoulder Elb Surg. 2008;17(2):220–5.
185. Li X, Ma R, Bedi A, et al. Management of acromioclavicular joint injuries. J Bone Joint Surg Am. 2014;96(1):73–84.
186. Bannister GC, Wallace WA, Stableforth PG, Hutson MA. The management of acute acromioclavicular dislocation. A randomized prospective controlled trial. J Bone Joint Surg Br. 1989;71(5):848–50.
187. Larsen E, Bjerg-Nielsen A, Christensen P. Conservative or surgical treatment of acromioclavicular dislocation. A prospective, controlled, randomized study. J Bone Joint Surg Am. 1986;68(4):552–5.
188. Boström Windhamre H, von Heideken J, Une-Larsson V, et al. No difference in clinical outcomes at 2-year follow-up in patients with type III and V acromioclavicular joint dislocation treated with hook plate or physiotherapy: a randomized controlled trial. J Shoulder Elb Surg. 2022;31(6):1122–36.
189. Liu G, Hu Y, Ye F, et al. Clavicular hook plate for acute high-grade acromioclavicular dislocation involving Rockwood type V: clinical and radiological outcomes and complications evaluation. Int Orhtop. 2022;46(10):2405–11.
190. Feichtinger X, Dahm F, Schallmayer D, et al. Surgery improves the clinical and radiological outcome in Rockwood type IV dislocations, whereas Rockwood type III dislocations benefit from conservative treatment. Knee Surg Sports Traumatol Arthrosc. 2021;29(7):2143–51.
191. Huan YC, Yang SW, Cy C, et al. Single coracoclavicular suture fixation with Mersilene tape versus hook plate in the treatment of acute type V acromioclavicular dislocation: a retrospective analysis. J Orthop Surg Res. 2018;13(1):110.
192. Shaffer BS. Painful conditions of the acromioclavicular joint. J Am Acad Orthop Surg. 1999;7(3):176–88.
193. Horvath F, Kery L. Degenerative deformations of the acromioclavicular joint in the elderly. Arch Gerontol Geriatr. 1984;3:259–65.
194. Needell SD, Zlatkin MB, Sher JK, et al. MR imaging of the rotator cuff: peritendinous and bone abnormalities in an asymptomatic population. AJR Am J Roentgenol. 1996;166:863–7.
195. Taft T, Wilson FC, Oglesby JW. Dislocation of the acromioclavicular joint. An end-result study. Bone Joint Surg Am. 1987;69(7):1045–51.

196. Mall NA, Foley E, Chalmers PN, et al. Degenerative joint disease of the acromioclavicular joint: a review. Am J Sports Med. 2013;14(11):2684–92.
197. Cahill BR. Osteolysis of the distal part of the clavicle in male athletes. J Bone Joint Surg Am. 1982;64:1053–8.
198. Brown JN, Roberts SN, Hayes MG, Sales AD. Shoulder pathology associated with symptomatic acromioclavicular joint degeneration. J Shoulder Elb Surg. 2000;9(3):173–6.
199. Docimo S Jr, Kornitsky D, Futterman B, Elkowitz DE. Surgical treatment for acromioclavicular joint osteoarthritis: patient selection, surgical options, complications, and outcomes. Curr Rev Musculoskelet Med. 2008;1(2):154–60.
200. Borbas P, Kraus T, Clement H, et al. The influence of ultrasound guidance in the rate of success of acromioclavicular joint injection: an experimental study on human cadavers. J Shoulder Elb Surg. 2012;21(12):1694–7.
201. Daley EL, Bajaj S, Bisson LJ, Cole BJ. Improving injection accuracy of the elbow, knee, and shoulder: dose injection site and imaging make a difference? A systematic review. Am J Sports Med. 2011;39(3):656–62.
202. Hossain S, Jacobs LG, Hashmi R. The long-term effectiveness of steroid injection sin primary acromioclavicular joint arthritis: a five-year prospective study. J Shoulder Elb Surg. 2008;17(4):535–8.
203. Jacob AK, Sallay PI. Therapeutic efficacy of corticosteroid injections in the acromioclavicular joint. Biomed Sci Instrum. 1997;34:380–5.
204. van Riet RP, Goehre T, Bell SN. The long term effect of an intra-articular injection of corticosteroids in the acromioclavicular joint. J Shoulder Elb Surg. 2012;21(3):376–9.
205. Freedman BA, Javernick MA, O'Brien FP, et al. Arthroscopic versus open distal clavicle excision: comparative results at six months and one year from a randomized, prospective clinical trial. J Shoulder Elb Surg. 2007;16(4):413–8.
206. Robertson WJ, Griffith MH, Carrol K, et al. Arthroscopic versus open distal clavicle excision: a comparative assessment at intermediate-term follow-up. Am J Sports Med. 2011;39(11):2415–20.
207. Elhassan B, Ozbaydar M, Diller D, et al. Open versus arthroscopic acromioclavicular joint resection: a retrospective comparison study. Arthroscopy. 2009;25(11):1224–12232.
208. Eskola A, Santavirta S, Viljakka HT, et al. The results of operative resection of the lateral end of the clavicle. J Bone Joint Surg Am. 1996;78(4):584–7.
209. Leon JKV, Hermans D, Venkatesha V, Duckworth DG. Patient outcomes following arthroscopic distal clavicle excision: a prospective case series. JSES Int. 2023;7(6):2400–5.
210. Kerr R, Resnick D, Pineda C, Haghighi P. Osteoarthritis of the glenohumeral joint: a radiographic-pathologic study. Am J Roentgenol. 1985;144:967–72.
211. Kobayashi T, Takagishi K, Shitara H. Prevalence of and risk factors for shoulder osteoarthritis in Japanese middle-aged and elderly populations. J Shoulder Elb Surg. 2014;23(5):613–9.
212. Oh JH, Chung SW, Oh CH, et al. The prevalence of shoulder osteoarthritis in the elderly Korean population: association with risk factors and function. J Shoulder Elb Surg. 2011;20(5):756–63.
213. Khazzam M, Gee AO, Pearl M. Management of glenohumeral joint osteoarthritis. J Am Acad Orthop Surg. 2020;28(19):781–9.
214. Ansok CB, Muh SJ. Optimal management of glenohumeral osteoarthritis. Orthop Res Rev. 2018;10:9–18.
215. Ibounig T, Simons T, Launonen A, Paavola M. Glenohumeral osteoarthritis: an overview of etiology and diagnostics. Scand J Surg. 2021;110(3):441–51.
216. Hovelius L, Saeboe M. Neer Awar 2008: arthropathy after primary anterior should dislocation – 223 shoulders prospectively followed up for twenty-five years. J Shoulder Elb Surg. 2009;18(3):339–47.
217. Kavaja L, Pajarinen J, Sinisaari I, et al. Arthrosis of glenohumeral joint after arthroscopic Bankart repair: a long-term follow-up of 13 years. J Shoulder Elb Surg. 2012;21(3):350–5.

218. Buscayret F, Edward TB, Szabo I, et al. Glenohumeral arthrosis in anterior instability before and after surgical treatment: incidence and contributing factors. Am J Sports Med. 2004;32(5):1165–72.
219. Kruckeberg BM, Leland DP, Bernard CD, et al. Incidence of and risk factors for glenohumeral osteoarthritis after anterior shoulder instability: a US population-based study with average 15-year follow-up. Orthop J Sports Med. 2020;8(11):2325967120962515.
220. Cancio-Bello AM, Barlow JD. Avascular necrosis and posttraumatic arthritis after proximal humerus fracture internal fixation: evaluation and management. Curr Rev Musculoskeletl Med. 2023;16(2):66–74.
221. Harreld KL, Marker DR, Wiesler ER, et al. Osteonecrosis of the humeral head. J Am Acad Orthop Surg. 2009;17(6):345–55.
222. Nam D, Maak TG, Raphael BS, et al. Rotator cuff tear arthropathy: evaluation, diagnosis, and treatment. J Bone Joint Surg Am. 2012;94(6):e34.
223. Feeley BT, Gallo RA, Craig EV. Cuff tear arthropathy: current trends in diagnosis and surgical management. J Shoulder Elb Surg. 2009;18(3):484–94.
224. Zeman CA, Arcand MA, Cantrell, et al. The rotator cuff-deficient arthritic shoulder: diagnosis and surgical management. J Am Acad Orthop Surg. 1998;6(6):337–48.
225. Reddy RP, Sabzevari S, Karimi A, et al. Pseudoparesis and pseudoparalysis in the setting of massive irreparable rotator cuff tear: demographic, anatomic, and radiographic risk factors. J Shoulder Elb Surg. 2024;33(2):e88–96.
226. Yamamoto N, Szymski D, Voss A, et al. Non-operative management of shoulder osteoarthritis: current concepts. J ISAKOS. 2023;8(5):289–95.
227. Kwon YW, Eisenberg G, Zuckerman JD. Sodium hyaluronate for the treatment of chronic shoulder pain associated with glenohumeral osteoarthritis: a multicenter, randomized, double blind, placebo-controlled trial. J Shoulder Elb Surg. 2013;22(5):584–94.
228. Kim HM, Muhammad M, Heil SD, Smith MJ. Clinical fate of glenohumeral osteoarthritis following intraarticular corticosteroid injection: an analysis of 311 shoulders. J Shoulder Elbow Arthroplast. 2022;6:24715492221075446.
229. Metzger CM, Farooq H, Merrell GA, et al. Efficacy of a single, image-guided corticosteroid injection for glenohumeral arthritis. J Shoulder Elb Surg. 2021;30(5):1128–34.
230. Lee WQ, Lie HM, Lie DTT. Diagnosis and treatment of avascular necrosis of the humeral head: current concepts. J ISAKOS. 2023;8(2):108–13.
231. Agarwala S, Vijayvargiya M. Bisphosphonate combination therapy for non-femoral avascular necrosis. J Orthop Surg Res. 2019;14(1):112.
232. Guo JJ, Wu K, Guan H, et al. Three-year follow-up of conservative treatments of shoulder osteoarthritis in older patients. Orthopedics. 2016;39(4):e634–41.
233. Piper C, Neviaser A. Survivorship of anatomic total shoulder arthroplasty. J Am Acad Orthop Surg. 2022;30(10):457–65.
234. Fox TJ, Cil A, Sperling JW, Sanchez-Sotelo J, Schleck CD, Cofield RH. Survival of the glenoid component in shoulder arthroplasty. J Shoulder Elbow Surg. 2009;18:859–63.
235. Singh JA, Sperling JW, Cofield RH. Revision surgery following total shoulder arthroplasty: analysis of 2588 shoulders over three decades (1976 to 2008). J Bone Joint Surg Br. 2011;93(11):1513–7.
236. Kirsch JM, Puzzitiello RN, Swanson D, et al. Outcomes after anatomic and reverse shoulder arthroplasty for the treatment of glenohumeral osteoarthritis: a propensity score-matched analysis. J Bone Joint Surg. 2022;104(15):1362–9.
237. Wright MA, Keener JD, Chamberlain AM. Comparison of clinical outcomes after anatomic total shoulder arthroplasty and reverse shoulder arthroplasty in patients 70 years and older with glenohumeral osteoarthritis and an intact rotator cuff. J Am Acad Orthop Surg. 2020;28(5):e222–9.
238. Bacle G, Nové-Josserand L, Garaud P, Walch G. Long-term outcomes of reverse total shoulder arthroplasty: a follow-up of a previous study. J Bone Joint Surg Am. 2017;99(6):454–61.

239. Cuff DJ, Pupello DR, Santoni BG, et al. Reverse shoulder arthroplasty for the treatment of rotator cuff deficiency: a concise follow-up, at a minimum of 10 years, of previous reports. J Bone Joint Surg Am. 2017;99(22):1895–9.
240. Ernstbrunner L, Andronic O, Grubhofer F, et al. Long-term results of reverse total shoulder arthroplasty for rotator cuff dysfunction: a systematic review of longitudinal outcomes. J Shoulder Elb Surg. 2019;28(4):774–81.
241. Park CN, Zhang GX, Chang J, et al. Pyrocarbon hemiarthroplasty of the shoulder: a systematic review and meta-analysis of clinical results. J Shoulder Elb Surg. 2023;32(6):1323–32.
242. Garret J, Cuinet T, Ducharne L, et al. Pyrocarbon humeral heads for hemishoulder arthroplasty grant satisfactory clinical scores with minimal glenoid erosion at 5–9 years of follow-up. J Shoulder Elb Surg. 2024;33(2):328–34.
243. Kleim BD, Zolotar A, Hinz M, et al. Pyrocarbon hemiprostheses show little glenoid erosion and good clinical function at 5.5 years of follow-up. J Shoulder Elb Surg. 2024;33(1):55–64.
244. Millett PJ, Horan MP, Pennock AT, Rios D. Comprehensive arthroscopic management (CAM) procedure: clinical results of a joint-preserving arthroscopic treatment for young, active patients with advanced shoulder osteoarthritis. Arthroscopy. 2013;29(3):440–8.
245. Khiami F, Gérometta A, Loriaut P. Management of recent first-time anterior shoulder dislocations. Orthop Traumatol Surg Res. 2015;101(1 Suppl):S51–7. https://doi.org/10.1016/j.otsr.2014.06.027.
246. Goss TP. Anterior glenohumeral instability. Orthopedics. 1988;11(1):87–95. https://doi.org/10.3928/0147-7447-19880101-10.
247. Dumont GD, Russell RD, Robertson WJ. Anterior shoulder instability: a review of pathoanatomy, diagnosis and treatment. Curr Rev Musculoskelet Med. 2011;4(4):200–7. https://doi.org/10.1007/s12178-011-9092-9.
248. Nazzal EM, Herman ZJ, Engler ID, Dalton JF, Freehill MT, Lin A. First-time traumatic anterior shoulder dislocation: current concepts. J ISAKOS. 2023;8(2):101–7. https://doi.org/10.1016/j.jisako.2023.01.002.
249. Waterman B, Owens BD, Tokish JM. Anterior shoulder instability in the military athlete. Sports Health. 2016;8(6):514–9. https://doi.org/10.1177/1941738116672161.
250. Kawasaki T, Ota C, Urayama S, Maki N, Nagayama M, Kaketa T, Takazawa Y, Kaneko K. Incidence of and risk factors for traumatic anterior shoulder dislocation: an epidemiologic study in high-school rugby players. J Shoulder Elb Surg. 2014;23(11):1624–30. https://doi.org/10.1016/j.jse.2014.05.007.
251. Leroux T, Wasserstein D, Veillette C, Khoshbin A, Henry P, Chahal J, Austin P, Mahomed N, Ogilvie-Harris D. Epidemiology of primary anterior shoulder dislocation requiring closed reduction in Ontario, Canada. Am J Sports Med. 2014;42(2):442–50. https://doi.org/10.1177/0363546513510391.
252. Tanaka M, Koizumi K, Kakiuchi M, Hayashida K. Evaluation of dislocation position in patients with recurrent anterior shoulder dislocation. J Shoulder Elb Surg. 2012;21(11):1588–92. https://doi.org/10.1016/j.jse.2011.11.020.
253. Wang SI. Management of the first-time traumatic anterior shoulder dislocation. Clin Shoulder Elb. 2018;21(3):169–75. https://doi.org/10.5397/cise.2018.21.3.169.
254. Burns TC, Owens BD. Management of shoulder instability in in-season athletes. Phys Sportsmed. 2010;38(3):55–60. https://doi.org/10.3810/psm.2010.10.1808.
255. Frank RM, Romeo AA, Provencher MT. Posterior glenohumeral instability: evidence based treatment. J Am Acad Orthop Surg. 2017;25(9):610–23. https://doi.org/10.5435/JAAOS-D-15-00631.
256. Provencher MT, LeClere LE, King S, McDonald LS, Frank RM, Mologne TS, Ghodadra NS, Romeo AA. Posterior instability of the shoulder: diagnosis and management. Am J Sports Med. 2011;39(4):874–86. https://doi.org/10.1177/0363546510384232.
257. Hippensteel KJ, Uppstrom TJ, Rodeo SA, Warren RF. Comprehensive review of multidirectional instability of the shoulder. J Am Acad Orthop Surg. 2023;31(16):871–80. https://doi.org/10.5435/JAAOS-D-22-00983.

258. Abrams JS, Jeffrey S, Abrams MD. "Pathoanatomy of first-time, traumatic, anterior glenohumeral subluxation events" by Lieutenant Colonel Brett D. Owens, MD, et al. J Bone Joint Surg Am. 2010;92(7):e5. https://doi.org/10.2106/JBJS.J.00736.
259. Ladd LM, Crews M, Maertz NA. Glenohumeral joint instability: a review of anatomy, clinical presentation, and imaging. Clin Sports Med. 2021;40(4):585–99. https://doi.org/10.1016/j.csm.2021.05.001.
260. Burkart AC, Debski RE. Anatomy and function of the glenohumeral ligaments in anterior shoulder instability. Clin Orthop Relat Res. 2002;400:32–9. https://doi.org/10.1097/00003086-200207000-00005.
261. Provencher MT, Midtgaard KS, Owens BD, Tokish JM. Diagnosis and management of traumatic anterior shoulder instability. J Am Acad Orthop Surg. 2021;29(2):e51–61. https://doi.org/10.5435/JAAOS-D-20-00202.
262. Beighton PH, Solomon L, Soskolne CL. Articular mobility in an African population. Ann Rheum Dis. 1973;32(5):413.
263. Kane P, Bifano SM, Dodson CC, Freedman KB. Approach to the treatment of primary anterior shoulder dislocation: a review. Phys Sportsmed. 2015;43(1):54–64. https://doi.org/10.1080/00913847.2015.1001713.
264. Burkhart SS, De Beer JF. Traumatic glenohumeral bone defects and their relationship to failure of arthroscopic Bankart repair: significance of the inverted-pear glenoid and the humeral engaging Hill-Sachs lesion. Arthroscopy. 2000;16:677–94.
265. Nakagawa S, Ozaki R, Take Y, et al. Enlargement of glenoid defects in traumatic anterior shoulder instability: influence of the number of recurrences and type of sports. Orthop J Sports Med. 2014;2(4):2325967114529920.
266. Provencher MT, Frank RM, Leclere LE, Metzger PD, Ryu JJ, Bernhardson A, Romeo AA. The Hill-Sachs lesion: diagnosis, classification, and management. J Am Acad Orthop Surg. 2012;20(4):242–52. https://doi.org/10.5435/JAAOS-20-04-242.
267. Arciero RA, Parrino A, Bernhardson AS, et al. The effect of a combined glenoid and Hill-Sachs defect on glenohumeral stability: a biomechanical cadaveric study using 3-dimensional modeling of 142 patients. Am J Sports Med. 2015;43:1422–9.
268. Burkhart SS, De Beer JF. Traumatic glenohumeral bone defects and their relationship to failure of arthroscopic Bankart repairs: significance of the inverted-pear glenoid and the humeral engaging Hill-Sachs lesion. Arthroscopy. 2000;16(7):677–94. https://doi.org/10.1053/jars.2000.17715.
269. Palmer I, Widen A. The bone block method for recurrent dislocation of the shoulder joint. J Bone Joint Surg Br. 1948;30B(1):53–8.
270. Habermeyer P, Schuller U, Wiedemann E. The intra-articular pressure of the shoulder: an experimental study on the role of the glenoid labrum in stabilizing the joint. Arthroscopy. 1992;8(2):166–72. https://doi.org/10.1016/0749-8063(92)90031-6.
271. Provencher MT, McCormick F, Leclere L, Sanchez G, Golijanin P, Anthony S, Dewing CB. Prospective evaluation of surgical treatment of humeral avulsions of the glenohumeral ligament. Am J Sports Med. 2017;45(5):1134–40.
272. Feng S, Song Y, Li H, Chen J, Chen J, Chen S. Outcomes for arthroscopic repair of combined Bankart/SLAP lesions in the treatment of anterior shoulder instability: a systematic review and meta-analysis. Orthop J Sports Med. 2019;7(10):2325967119877804.
273. Taylor DC, Arciero RA. Pathologic changes associated with shoulder dislocations: arthroscopic and physical examination findings in first-time, traumatic anterior dislocations. Am J Sports Med. 1997;25(3):306–11.
274. Neviaser TJ. The anterior labroligamentous periosteal sleeve avulsion lesion: a cause of anterior instability of the shoulder. Arthroscopy. 1993;9(1):17–21.
275. Pogorzelski J, et al. Failure following arthroscopic Bankart repair for traumatic anteroinferior instability of the shoulder: is a glenoid labral articular disruption (GLAD) lesion a risk factor for recurrent instability? J Shoulder Elb Surg. 2018;27(8):e235–42.
276. Gombera MM, Sekiya JK. Rotator cuff tear and glenohumeral instability: a systematic review. Clin Orthop Relat Res. 2014;472(8):2448–56. https://doi.org/10.1007/s11999-013-3290-2.

Erratum in: Clin Orthop Relat Res 2015;473(2):751. Gomberawalla, M Mustafa [corrected to Gombera, Mufaddal Mustafa]

277. Rowe CR. Acute and recurrent anterior dislocations of the shoulder. Orthop Clin North Am. 1980;11(2):253–70.
278. Watson S, Allen B, Grant JA. A clinical review of return-to-play considerations after anterior shoulder dislocation. Sports Health. 2016;8(4):336–41. https://doi.org/10.1177/1941738116651956.
279. Burkhead WZ Jr, Rockwood CA Jr. Treatment of instability of the shoulder with an exercise program. J Bone Joint Surg Am. 1992;74(6):890–6.
280. Misamore GW, Sallay PI, Didelot W. A longitudinal study of patients with multidirectional instability of the shoulder with seven- to ten-year follow-up. J Shoulder Elb Surg. 2005;14(5):466–70. https://doi.org/10.1016/j.jse.2004.11.006.
281. Bottoni CR, Wilckens JH, DeBerardino TM, D'Alleyrand JC, Rooney RC, Harpstrite JK, Arciero RA. A prospective, randomized evaluation of arthroscopic stabilization versus nonoperative treatment in patients with acute, traumatic, first-time shoulder dislocations. Am J Sports Med. 2002;30(4):576–80. https://doi.org/10.1177/03635465020300041801.
282. Dickens JF, Rue JP, Cameron KL, Tokish JM, Peck KY, Allred CD, Svoboda SJ, Sullivan R, Kilcoyne KG, Owens BD. Successful return to sport after arthroscopic shoulder stabilization versus nonoperative management in contact athletes with anterior shoulder instability: a prospective multicenter study. Am J Sports Med. 2017;45(11):2540–6. https://doi.org/10.1177/0363546517712505.
283. Masud S, Momtaz D, Betsch M, Migliorini F, Ghali A, Popa A, Gouveia K, Leroux T, Degen R, Khan M. A comprehensive comparison and evaluation of surgical techniques for anterior shoulder instability: a Bayesian network meta-analysis. J Shoulder Elb Surg. 2023;32(11):e531–47. https://doi.org/10.1016/j.jse.2023.07.004.
284. Altchek DW, Warren RF, Skyhar MJ, Ortiz G. T-plasty modification of the Bankart procedure for multidirectional instability of the anterior and inferior types. J Bone Joint Surg Am. 1991;73(1):105–12.
285. Chen D, Goldberg J, Herald J, Critchley I, Barmare A. Effects of surgical management on multidirectional instability of the shoulder: a meta-analysis. Knee Surg Sports Traumatol Arthrosc. 2016;24(2):630–9. https://doi.org/10.1007/s00167-015-3901-4.
286. Longo UG, et al. Multidirectional instability of the shoulder: a systematic review. Arthroscopy. 2015;31(12):2431–43.

The Wrist and Hand

11

Edward Lawson and Jennifer Kargel

Traumatic Injury

Hand and upper extremity injuries account for 26% of all injuries [1] presenting to the emergency room. These include fractures, sprains, dislocations, and lacerations that result from falls, crushing injuries, or twisting injuries. Pain is localized to the site of injury and is often associated with edema and ecchymosis. In fractures, sensory nerve fibers containing mechanosensitive C and A-delta nociceptors found within the periosteum surrounding the bony cortex are stimulated with mechanical distortion and increased intraosseous pressure [2]. This noxious stimulus is then transmitted to the central nervous system, eliciting a pain response. Subsequent mobilization of the injured site results in repeated distortion of these nerve fibers, which, in combination with released cell mediators, such as prostaglandins, bradykinin, endothelins, and nerve growth factors, which sensitize and upregulate nociceptors, leads to persistent pain even after the initial event.

Assessment involves the identification of sensory deficits, areas of point tenderness that often correspond with the site of bony injury, and abnormalities in position, including angulation or rotation and instability with motion. Treatment is tailored to the injury, with nondisplaced fractures often responding favorably to a limited period of splint or cast immobilization to allow edema to resolve and sites to heal. Unstable or displaced fractures are treated with surgical reduction and fixation. Sprains and dislocations are usually treated with a combination of short-term immobilization for pain relief and subsequent gentle guided motion. Skin and soft

E. Lawson
Loma Linda University, Loma Linda, CA, USA
e-mail: edlawson@students.llu.edu

J. Kargel (✉)
Department of Plastic Surgery, UT Southwestern Medical Center, Dallas, TX, USA
e-mail: Jennifer.Kargel@utsouthwestern.edu

C. E. Noe (ed.), *Musculoskeletal Pain*,
https://doi.org/10.1007/978-3-031-86057-7_11

tissue lacerations may be treated with closure under local anesthetic at the time of the injury, and tendon lacerations require repair within 1–2 weeks of injury to avoid the need for further reconstruction.

Overuse and Inflammatory Conditions

Tendonitis and tendinopathy are frequently encountered in the hand and wrist, with tendon disorders representing over 30% of all musculoskeletal consultations [3]. Microscopically, tendons are composed of tenoblasts and mature tenocytes, as well as an extracellular matrix composed of collagen, fibronectin, and proteoglycans [4]. Tendonitis and tendinopathy are related to overuse and associated with pain, swelling, and subsequent functional limitation. During the initial period of this condition, inflammatory markers can be found that trigger a pain response, and over time, as seen in tendinopathies, the affected collagen fibers lose their organized parallel fiber arrangement, and there is an increased proportion of extracellular matrix.

Common overuse injuries seen in the hand and wrist include De Quervain stenosing tenosynovitis and intersection syndrome, extensor digitorum communis tendonitis, extensor carpi ulnaris tendonitis and tendinopathy, and trigger fingers. De Quervain involves thickening of the tendon sheaths of the first dorsal compartment by up to five times that of control subjects [5] with painful limitation of movement of the abductor pollicis longus and extensor pollicis brevis tendons within the approximately 2 cm length retinaculum of the first dorsal compartment. Patients present with radial-sided wrist pain, which worsens with thumb abduction, wrist extension, and radial deviation. Diagnostic maneuvers include pain on direct palpation of the radial styloid and a positive Finkelstein test in which the thumb is flexed into the palm and the wrist ulnar deviated, eliciting pain. Nonoperative treatment includes splinting and corticosteroid injection [6], with surgical release of the first dorsal compartment reserved for patients who have failed conservative treatment.

Intersection syndrome is a rare overuse injury localized over the dorsal wrist at the point where the first dorsal compartment tendons intersect at a 60-degree angle with the second dorsal compartment contents. Often seen in sports such as rowing, canoeing, skiing, weightlifting, and racket sports, symptoms of pain and palpable crepitus are noted 4–8 centimeters proximal to the radial styloid [7, 8]. Diagnostic maneuvers also include pain on resisted wrist extension. Treatment involves wrist immobilization, oral anti-inflammatories, activity modification, and corticosteroid injection. Up to 60% of cases will be resolved with conservative management within 2–3 weeks. Surgical treatment is reserved for refractory cases and involves the release of the second dorsal extensor compartment.

Extensor digitorum communis (EDC) tenosynovitis is localized to the fourth dorsal extensor compartment. This can occur in a variety of inflammatory conditions, including overuse, autoimmune synovitis such as rheumatoid arthritis, and following trauma or arthritis of the wrist. Patients present with dorsal wrist swelling and tenderness over the fourth compartment. As with the previously described dorsal extensor compartment overuse diagnoses, successful treatment involves immobilization, anti-inflammatories, and steroid injection. When there is underlying associated pathology, such as arthritis, treatment of the underlying condition is often required to prevent recurrence.

Extensor carpi ulnaris (ECU) tenosynovitis is a common cause of ulnar-sided wrist pain with a differential diagnosis that includes ECU subluxation and triangulofibrocartilage complex (TFCC) ligament injury. Patients present with point tenderness directly over the tendon. Provocative maneuvers such as pain with resisted ulnar deviation while in pronation and with resisted wrist extension while in supination can be used to assist in diagnosis. Conservative treatments are often successful and include rest, activity modification, and corticosteroid injection.

Trigger finger, also known as stenosis tenosynovitis of the A-1 pulley, affects women six times more often than men, with the prevalence of trigger digit noted to be 2–3% in the general population, increasing to 10–20% in the diabetic patient population [8]. Patients with this condition present with painful "locking" of the digit with attempted extension following full flexion. This is due to the thickening of the A1 pulley and the flexor tendons, which results in the limitation of the normally smooth gliding mechanism that occurs with active tendon motion. In more advanced diseases, this can be associated with pain radiating distally to the proximal interphalangeal (PIP) joint or proximally to the forearm. Diagnostic maneuvers include pain on palpation of the A1 pulley localized over the volar metacarpal head of the affected digit, as well as a palpable nodule and active locking on attempted active ranging of the finger. Nonoperative treatment is often very successful, with a resolution rate of 60–90% following corticosteroid injection. This is often combined with nighttime extension splinting of the digit. Surgical treatment, which involves direct or percutaneous release of the A-1 pulley, can be performed under local anesthetic in a sterile environment to treat refractory cases.

Infection

Infections in the hand and wrist can cause significant pain, particularly in the setting of abscess formation. While inflammatory mediators trigger pain through the action of proteins such as cytokines and growth factors, prostaglandins, and other mediators, it has also been shown that bacteria can directly activate nociceptors through bacterial metabolic byproducts called N-formyl peptides [9]. Additionally, the protein flagellin, which is found in bacterial flagella, activates A-fiber sensory neurons. Separate from tissue swelling, as bacterial load increases, hyperalgesia can also increase. The Gram-positive pathogen *Staphylococcus aureus* is a common cause of skin infections. It produces pain by releasing the toxin α-hemolysin, which in turn creates membrane pore-formation, leading to the generation of action potentials that cause mechanical and thermal allodynia [10].

Hand infections require prompt diagnosis and treatment to prevent compromised function. Patients that are particularly susceptible include diabetics, immunocompromised patients, IV drug users, and patients on long-term steroids. The most common organisms identified are *Staphylococcus aureus* and *beta-hemolytic Streptococci species* [11]. While hand infections can present in many forms, the most easily recognized is cellulitis, which is an infection involving the skin and subcutaneous tissue without the presence of purulence. It presents as erythema, swelling, and pain over the infected site. The additional presence of red streaking extending up the extremity is called lymphangitis and can signify a more severe infection. Lymphatic channels within the deep dermal and subdermal tissue planes become inflamed, leading to its classic appearance. Cellulitis is treated with oral and/or intravenous antibiotics.

Localized abscesses involving the finger include paronychia, which is confined to the nail fold, and felon, which involves the distal pulp of the fingertip. Both present with swelling, pain, erythema, and fluctuance. The bacteria itself, as well as the increased pressure associated with purulent fluid accumulation, leads to significant pain at the site. They are treated with incision and drainage under local anesthetic, as well as antibiotics. In the case of paronychia, this may require at least partial elevation of the nail plate to allow adequate drainage. As with most hand infections, the most common causative agent is *Staphylococcus aureus*.

Herpetic whitlow can present similarly in the finger. It is caused by Herpes simplex virus type 1 or 2 (HSV-1 and HSV-2) as a direct exogenous or autogenous inoculation through viral invasion and replication in epidermal and dermal cells. The virus then travels to the sensory dorsal root ganglion for a latency period. A prodromal phase of pain and paresthesia occurs 24–72 h prior to the development of vesicles on the pulp or lateral aspect of the digit, after which they coalesce into honeycomb-like bullae. Surrounding erythema and edema are noted. Diagnosis is clinical and can be confirmed with a positive Tzanck smear test. Treatment is limited, as the condition spontaneously resolves within 2–4 weeks, and incision and drainage can lead to viremia and bacterial superinfection [12].

Bite wounds of the hand may be human-related, such as clenched fist injuries or "fight bite," which occurs when someone strikes another individual in the mouth with a closed fist, resulting in tooth penetration over the dorsal metacarpophalangeal (MCP) joint. As the fingers are later extended, the inoculated tendon and soft tissue are then retracted proximally into the hand. These injuries can cause damage to the extensor tendon and penetration of the joint capsule, resulting in significant infection. This is due to the overlying skin and soft tissue barrier being thin, the relative avascular nature of the tendon and joint, and the high bacterial load in the human mouth [13]. These patients often present in a delayed fashion with pain, swelling, and erythema over the injury site and require antibiotics, irrigation, and debridement of the site. Animal-related bite wounds are most commonly associated with dogs and cats. While dog bite wounds are more frequent and associated with more trauma to the surrounding tissue, cat bites have a much higher risk of infection, with a rate of 50% versus 4% in dog bites [14]. This is due to their more needle-like teeth being able to penetrate joint capsules and bone more easily, which can result in septic arthritis and osteomyelitis. As with human bites, these infections present with swelling, erythema, and pain, particularly with axial loading and ranging of the joint. They are treated with antibiotics that cover *Staphylococcus, Pasteurella,* and *Streptococcus* species and, if not responsive or if there is evidence of joint involvement, operative debridement.

More severe infections require operative interventions in addition to antibiotic therapy. Pyogenic flexor tenosynovitis (FTS) is a closed space infection within the flexor sheath that is most commonly caused by penetrating trauma and inoculation by skin flora. The sheath is composed of a superficial parietal paratenon and a deeper visceral paratenon, which is adherent to the tendon surface. In infection, the space between these two layers fills with purulent fluid. As fluid and pressure increase, this leads to ischemia and eventual tendon necrosis if not treated in a timely manner. FTS is diagnosed clinically by the presence of Kanavel signs [15], including fusiform swelling, localized tenderness to palpation of the volar surface of the digit, flexed posture of the digit, and pain with attempted passive extension of the digit. This pain is due to increased pressure within the sheath as the finger extends and the potential space decreases. Treatment requires surgical irrigation and debridement in combination with IV antibiotics. The thumb and small finger flexor sheaths are continuous with radial and ulnar bursae, which extend proximally into the carpal tunnel sheath and into the space of Parona. There are potential deep spaces within the thenar eminence, the hypothenar eminence, and the midpalmar space. When infected, they present with significant swelling and pain. Infections that extend into these deeper areas require urgent operative intervention for washout and debridement.

Septic arthritis of the hand and wrist joints presents as closed-space infections caused by direct inoculation, contiguous spread, or hematogenous spread. It presents as a hot, swollen, erythematous joint with pain on active and passive movement and with joint loading. Definitive diagnosis requires joint aspiration and analysis of the fluid for a white blood cell count greater than 50,000, greater than 75% polymorphonuclear leukocytes, and glucose level less than 40 mg/dL. Mimickers include non-infectious arthritis and crystalline arthropathies. Without timely intervention, including open versus arthroscopic irrigation and debridement [16], articular destruction from proteolytic enzymes and bacterial toxins occurs rapidly, and this condition can result in significant morbidity and mortality. This can include osteomyelitis or infection of the bone. Osteomyelitis presents with painful swelling and localized erythema, as well as possible draining of the sinus tract. This most often involves the distal interphalangeal joint [12]. Treatment requires the use of prolonged antibiotics over 6–8 weeks in most cases, with possible debridement if failed oral therapy or if there is an associated draining sinus or wound.

Neuropathy

Neuropathic pain occurs with injury or inflammation of peripheral nerves, resulting in stimulation of nociceptors that send signals to the central nervous system. This information can become dysregulated, leading to central sensitization and amplification of the pain response and sensation of pain beyond the expected area of injury. Complex regional pain syndrome is a well-known neuropathic pain condition that can occur following a traumatic event to an extremity, in which an exaggerated inflammatory response following trauma leads to persistent swelling, temperature changes, and vasodilation. Inflammatory mediators, growth factors, catecholamines, and autoantibodies stimulate trophic changes and sensitize nociceptors. This leads to increased pain with any motion, hypersensitivity to heat, hyperalgesia, and allodynia in the skin and deeper tissue due to sensitization of second-order neurons in the spinal cord [17]. Two forms of the syndrome have been described. Type I, previously called reflex sympathetic dystrophy, occurs after an injury or illness that does not directly injure the nerves in the affected extremity. The majority of complex regional pain syndrome falls in this category. Type 2, also referred to as causalgia, occurs following direct known injury to a nerve.

Patients experience sensory symptoms, vasomotor differences in the affected extremities such as temperature and skin color changes, the presence of limb edema and sweating changes, and trauma-related motor changes or trophic changes of skin, hair, and nail growth. Diagnosis requires a history of symptoms in at least three of the four categories and signs in at least two of the four categories. Treatment focuses on occupational and physical therapy to improve edema control and range of motion, as well as desensitization, combined with medications such as non-opioid analgesics, vasodilators, steroids, and sympathetic nerve blocks [19].

Nerve compressions can occur anywhere along the length of the major nerves of the upper extremity. Compression at one point can then cause intraneural changes and edema, leading to an increased risk of developing compression at additional points, a process called the double-crush phenomenon [18]. With mild compression, venous outflow is obstructed, leading to congestion and edema. Inflammatory cytokines such as interleukin-1, interleukin-6, substance P, tumor necrosis factor-alpha, bradykinin, and prostaglandins are released. Fibrosis can occur, which worsens the effects of mechanical compression, and eventual demyelination leads to axonal signaling abnormalities. Median nerve compression at the level of the wrist is referred to as carpal tunnel syndrome. It is the most common form of nerve compression and presents with pain and paresthesia in the thumb, index finger, long finger, and radial aspect of the ring finger. With severe disease, thenar atrophy occurs, and thumb opposition and palmar abduction are weakened. Patients with carpal tunnel syndrome often note worsening of symptoms with repetitive activities and can exhibit the flick sign in which they are awakened with symptoms and must shake their hands to resolve them. Provocative maneuvers support the diagnosis and include the Tinel sign, which is a reproduction of symptoms when gently striking the volar wrist, Phalen's test, which reproduces symptoms with wrist flexion for at least 60 s, and Durkin's test, which reproduces symptoms with external compression of the median nerve at the wrist for 30 s [20]. In some cases, electrodiagnostic tests such as electromyography and nerve conduction studies are also obtained. Not only can this confirm a suspected diagnosis, but it can exclude other causes, such as more proximal compressions, polyneuropathy, and radiculopathy. Treatment of mild carpal tunnel syndrome focuses on activity and wrist position modification with nighttime wrist extension splints, oral anti-inflammatories, and steroid injections. More severe diseases are treated with surgical decompression, either endoscopic or open. While the ulnar nerve can be compressed within Guyon's canal at the level of the wrist and hand, symptoms are paresthesia or numbness and possibly intrinsic muscle weakness rather than pain. The radial nerve can also be compressed at the level of the wrist, a diagnosis called Wartenberg syndrome and cheiralgia paresthetica. In this condition, the superficial sensory branch of the radial nerve is compressed within proximity of the radial styloid due to trauma such as distal radius fracture, external compression such as a tight watch or a bracelet, and internal compression by lipomas or ganglion cysts. Patients present with abnormal sensation to light touch and pain over the dorsum of the radial hand proximal to the thumb and the index finger. Conservative treatment is highly successful with desensitization and therapy exercises, as well as the removal of potential external sources of compression.

Osteoarthritis

Osteoarthritis is the most common joint disease worldwide. It is a degenerative disease in which the articular cartilage is worn away, exposing the underlying cortical bone to unbuffered friction and force. The joint surface is normally innervated by sensory and sympathetic fibers that participate in nociception, proprioception, and vasoregulation. Mechanoreceptors on these sensory nerve terminals have reduced activation threshold in arthritic joints, resulting in otherwise innocuous stimulation causing magnified responses. Additionally, with exposure to inflammatory mediators released into the joint, native nociceptors become sensitized and amplify painful signaling [21]. In osteoarthritis, nociceptive and sympathetic nerve endings have also been shown to sprout into the degenerated cartilage and periosteum, causing neuropathic pain with compression of the cartilage with mobilization and axial loading. Patients present with stiff, swollen, and painful joints worsened with changes in weather and limited motion. Imaging is utilized to confirm arthritic changes in the joints, and treatment initially focuses on inflammation control with the use of nonsteroidal anti-inflammatories and glucocorticoids. Surgical intervention is utilized when conservative measures fail, with the goal of treatment focused on pain control by stabilization of the joint via osteophyte excision, resurfacing, or fusion.

Autoimmune Conditions

Autoimmune and inflammatory diseases of the hand and wrist can cause debilitating pain and limitation of function. These can involve the joint surface, synovial tissue, skin and soft tissue, and vasculature. The most common autoimmune arthropathy is rheumatoid arthritis (RA), a chronic progressive heritable disease that involves the synovial membrane. This inflammation is initiated by a genetic predisposition that results in the generation of autoreactive T and B cells combined with a triggering event that causes activated antigen-presenting cells (APC) to activate the previously generated autoreactive lymphocytes. Autoantibodies such as rheumatoid factor (RF) and anti-citrullinated protein antibodies (ACPA) are identified in the earliest stages of the disease [22], and since these ubiquitous antigens are always present, there is continuous immune cell activation. Over time, synovial tissue becomes chronically inflamed by infiltrating T cells, B cells, and monocytes and develops a pannus which then erodes adjacent cartilage and bone [23].

Inflamed synovium generates mediators such as prostaglandins and bradykinin that directly activate fine, unmyelinated sensory nerves within the synovium and cause pain. Additional cytokines like TNF-alpha, interleukin-1, and interleukin-6 are upregulated in the tissue, and they sensitize peripheral nerves. As the osteochondral junction is eroded, additional subchondral nerves are exposed to circulating activating and sensitizing synovial fluid biological factors [24].

Initial evaluation focuses on a combination of clinical history, physical examination, family history, and assessment of laboratory markers such as RF, ACPA, CRP, and ESR. Formal diagnosis is based on grading using the American College of Rheumatology-European League against Rheumatism (ACR-EULAR) scale, which looks at the number and size of joints involved, presence of RA-specific autoantibodies, abnormal levels of inflammatory markers, and duration of disease symptoms. Treatment is primarily pharmacologic, targeting multiple sources of inflammation. Medications include non-steroidal anti-inflammatories, glucocorticoids, and disease-modifying anti-rheumatic drug (DMARD) therapy. NSAIDs inhibit prostanoid biosynthesis and improve joint function but do not prevent additional joint damage. Glucocorticoids suppress gene expression and slow progression in early disease stages. Synthetic DMARDs, which include methotrexate, hydrochloroquine, and sulfadiazine, and biologic DMARDs, which include TNF-receptor inhibitors, IL-6, B-cell depleting antibodies, and co-stimulatory molecule inhibitors, diminish symptoms and prevent disease progression through targeted pathways.

Systemic sclerosis is an autoimmune condition that affects the connective tissue and vasculature. It is divided into three types, which include limited cutaneous systemic sclerosis or calcinosis cutis, Raynaud syndrome, esophageal dysmotility, sclerodactyly, and telangiectasias (CREST) syndrome, generalized systemic sclerosis form, and systemic sclerosis sine scleroderma which spares the skin. An initial vascular insult leads to endothelial cell activation, which in turn contributes to the activation of platelets and thrombotic and fibrinolytic cascades, as well as the activation of fibroblasts. Patients develop chronic tissue hypoxia, oxidative stress, and dysregulation of immune responses, which ultimately leads to interstitial and vascular fibrosis. Raynaud's phenomenon is often seen, in which cold-induced vasospasm leads to ischemic changes followed by reactive hyperemia. Vessels are fibrosed and lack flexibility and ischemic ulcers develop on the fingers. With skin involvement, the associated inflammation and edema lead to compression of underlying structures and neuropathic pain. As tissue becomes more fibrosed, there is decreased mobility of joints, and symptoms of arthralgia and myalgia are present. Diagnosis is based on a combination of clinical exam findings and confirmatory laboratory markers such as antinuclear antibodies (ANA), anticentromere, anti-Scl-70, and anti-RNA polymerase III, using another of the American College of

Rheumatology-European League against Rheumatism (ACR-EULAR) scale for classification of systemic sclerosis. Treatment is system-specific and includes immunosuppressants for lung disease, a combination of medication and surgical debridement for calcinosis, calcium channel blockers, IV prostaglandin E1 infusions, and sympathetic blocks for the treatment of Raynaud syndrome.

Various forms of vascular disorders involve the fingers and hands. Raynaud phenomenon is an exaggerated response to cold exposure or stress with significant pain and color changes to the digits, associated with underlying autoimmune conditions such as collagen vascular disease, connective tissue disease, rheumatoid arthritis, and systemic lupus erythematosus. Due to the vasoconstriction response, patients present with color changes corresponding to the degree of blood flow (white with ischemia, purple or blue with low oxygen level, and red with return of blood flow) and significant pain corresponding to tissue ischemia. Diagnosis is based on clinical exam, and initial treatment involves pharmacologic therapy, including oral calcium channel blockers, stellate ganglion blocks, and botulinum toxin A injection. When the condition progresses to digital ulceration that does not resolve with conservative treatment, surgical treatment is considered. Periarterial sympathectomy and arterial bypass vein grafts have shown resolution of symptoms to varying degrees [25]. Another vascular disease that warrants mention is Buerger disease, also known as thromboangiitis obliterans. This progressive inflammatory condition affects small and medium-sized arteries of the extremities with thrombosis and eventual vessel fibrosis, impacting all three layers of the arterial wall. It is associated with nicotine use in patients with immunologic dysfunction and tobacco hypersensitivity. Patients initially present with claudication of the distal extremity, including feet and hands, and eventually progress to ischemic rest pain and ulcerations on the digits. The cornerstone of management is nicotine cessation and symptomatic management with calcium channel blockers, vasodilators, and prostanoid therapy [26].

Crystalline Arthropathies

There are two primary forms of crystalline arthropathies that affect the hand and wrist: gout and pseudogout. Gout occurs with the deposition of uric acid crystals in joints and connective tissue following saturation of serum with urate, the final breakdown product of purine metabolism. This can occur as a result of either overproduction or under-excretion of uric acid [27]. The supersaturation of urate in joint fluid attracts polymorphonuclear neutrophils (PMNs). The PMNs attempt to phagocytize the crystals, rupturing cells and releasing cytokines and enzymes. The uric acid crystals stimulate an inflammatory response and attract more PMNs. During this process, the pH of the fluid is lowered, leading to increased crystal precipitation. Symptoms of gout include swelling, erythema, increased warmth, and excruciating pain around the involved joint. In chronic disease, uric acid crystals deposit in the soft tissue and can cause erosion of the skin. The differential diagnosis of an acute gouty flare-up is septic arthritis, and examination of laboratory values and joint aspiration to assess for the presence of bacteria versus positively birefringent uric acid crystals may be required. Treatment begins with lifestyle and dietary modifications, medications to reduce uric acid levels such as allopurinol, nonsteroidal anti-inflammatories including colchicine, and glucocorticoids. Surgical treatment is reserved for refractory disease despite maximal medical therapy, poorly controlled pain, nerve compression or entrapment, recurrent infection, skin ulceration, and joint instability or impaired motion [28].

Pseudogout is also known as calcium pyrophosphate dihydrate arthropathy. It is caused by the deposition of calcium pyrophosphate dihydrate (CPPD) in and around joints. While the exact mechanism is not entirely understood, this condition occurs with the overproduction of pyrophosphate (PPi) by chondrocytes, which form the substrate for CPPD crystals that are deposited in the cartilaginous matrix. Acute attacks of joint pain, edema, and erythema are similar to gout, although with slower onset and longer duration, and are believed to result from auto-inflammatory responses to the crystals with the generation of several pro-inflammatory cytokines, including interleukin 1 beta by macrophages and monocytes, with the influx of neutrophils, fibroblast-like synoviocytes and recruitment of other inflammatory pathways via tumor necrosis factor-alpha (TNF alpha). Definitive diagnosis requires the presence of CPPD crystals in synovial fluid. Treatment is primarily pharmacologic symptomatic relief with nonsteroidal anti-inflammatories and glucocorticoids and preventative medications that target the inflammasomes, such as methotrexate and anti-TNF alpha medication [29].

Tumors

While bone has been reported as one of the most common sites of cancer metastasis, the hand is a rare location with frequent misdiagnosis and is associated with poor prognosis. The majority of primary malignancies in these cases are found in the lung, gastrointestinal tract, and kidney. The most frequently presenting symptom is pain [30]. Diagnosis is assisted by magnetic resonance imaging and definitively confirmed with incisional versus excisional biopsy. There is no standardized treatment, as it is tailored to each case and may include analgesia, radiotherapy, excision, or amputation.

Glomus tumors are benign vascular neoplasms involving the glomus body, often presenting in the subungual region of a finger where they are highly concentrated [31]. Patients present with pain, tenderness to palpation, and cold sensitivity. The source of pain is hypothesized to occur either due to the tumor capsules being sensitive to pressure, the high concentration of mast cells that release heparin, 5-hydroxytryptamin, and histamine which sensitize pressure and cold stimulation receptors, and/or the excess of non-myelinated nerve fibers that penetrate into the tumors [32]. Diagnosis is based on clinical exam and confirmatory diagnostic tests that include Hildreth's test, in which exsanguination and ischemia of the digit decrease pain, cold sensitivity test, in which cold water or ice applied to the site elicits pain, and Love's pin test, in which direct pressure over the mass itself causes isolated pain [33]. Treatment is direct surgical excision.

Hand and Wrist Pain Emergencies

Many hand and wrist conditions are associated with pain. However, there are two conditions that are considered hand and wrist pain emergencies. Failure to recognize and effectively treat these conditions can result in extreme morbidity and death.

Compartment syndrome occurs when the pressure inside a muscle compartment increases to the point that it inhibits blood flow and oxygenation. Causes can be trauma-related, in association with fractures, dislocations, and crush injuries, reperfusion-related following revascularization of an extremity with prolonged ischemia, increased pressure from IV infiltration, or in patients with abnormal bleeding diatheses. As interstitial pressure increases, the venous outflow is limited, and the arterial inflow collapses. The metabolic needs of muscles and nerves are not met, resulting in myocyte lysis, capillary leakage, and further increased intracompartmental pressure [34]. Diagnosis is usually based on clinical presentation and exam with noted pain out of proportion, worsened with passive stretch, pallor, paresthesia, paralysis, and pulselessness. In patients who are unconscious or unable to participate in the exam, intramuscular pressure measurement provides an objective assessment with a value of delta pressure (i.e., diastolic pressure minus compartment pressure) less than 30, being highly suggestive of compartment syndrome. Treatment is acute surgical decompression, as damage is irreversible after 6 to 8 h.

Necrotizing fasciitis is a medical emergency that can result in loss of limb or life if left untreated. It is characterized by angiothrombotic microbial invasion and liquefactive necrosis. The source of infection may be polymicrobial but most often is associated with *Streptococcus pyogenes*. Patients at most risk are immunocompromised, IV drug users, alcoholics, diabetics, and patients with peripheral vascular disease. On initial examination, patients will present with low-grade cellulitis and pain out of proportion. This will rapidly progress to severe pain, bullae, crepitus, and skin necrosis. Treatment requires a combination of supportive therapy, including fluid resuscitation and empiric IV antibiotics, and rapid and repeated surgical debridement and amputation when indicated [35].

Bullet points

- Hand and wrist fractures are associated with pain due to stimulation of nociceptors within the periosteum. Management entails stabilization to decrease pain and edema while allowing osteosynthesis.
- Tendonitis and tendinopathy are related to overuse and associated with pain and swelling. Initially, inflammatory markers trigger a pain response. Over time, the affected collagen fibers lose their organized parallel fiber arrangement.
- The most common hand infections are felons and paronychia, and the most frequently isolated bacteria are *S. aureus* and *beta-hemolytic streptococci.*
- Patients with complex regional pain syndrome must have 3 of 4 criteria: sensory symptoms, vasomotor differences in the affected extremity such as temperature

and skin color changes, presence of limb edema and sweating changes, and trauma-related motor changes or trophic changes of skin, hair, and nail growth.
- Osteoarthritis of the hand and wrist is one of the most common causes of pain and symptomatic treatment focuses on the reduction of inflammation.
- The most common autoimmune arthropathy is rheumatoid arthritis (RA), which specifically targets the synovial membrane of joints. Treatment is primarily pharmacologic, including NSAIDs, glucocorticoids, and DMARDs.
- Gout occurs with the deposit of uric acid crystals within the joint. Management focuses on decreasing serum urate levels and symptom management with NSAIDs and glucocorticoids.
- The most common sources of primary malignancy in bony hand metastases are lung, gastrointestinal tract, and kidney.
- Hand and wrist pain emergencies include compartment syndrome and necrotizing fasciitis. These conditions require urgent recognition and surgical treatment to decrease morbidity and mortality.

References

1. Gordon AM, Malik AT, Goyal KS. Trends of hand injuries presenting to US emergency departments: a 10-year national analysis. *Am J Emerg Med*. 2021;50:466–71.
2. Mitchell SAT, Majuta LA, Mantyh PW. New insights in understanding and treating bone gracture pain. Curr Osteoporos Rep. 2018;16(4):325–32.
3. Loiacono C, Palermi S, Massa B, Belviso I, Romano V, Gregorio AD, Sirico F, Sacco AM. Tendinopathy: pathophysiology, therapeutic options, and role of nutraceutics. A narrative literature review. *Medicina (Kaunas)*. 2019;55(8):447–59.
4. Sharma P, Maffulli N. Biology of tendon injury: healing, modeling and remodeling. *J Musculoskelet Neuronal Interact*. 2006;6(2):181–90.
5. Pensak MJ, Bayron J, Wolf JM. Current treatment of De Quervain tendinopathy. *J Hand Surg Am*. 2013;38(11):2247–9.
6. Hassan K, Sohn A, Shi L, Lee M, Wolf JM. De Quervain tenosynovitis: an evaluation of the epidemiology and utility of multiple injections using a national database. *J Hand Surg Am*. 2022;47(3):284.e1–6.
7. Balakatounis K, Angoules AG, Angoules NA, Panagiotopoulou K. Synthesis of evidence or the treatment of intersection syndrome. *World J Orthop*. 2017;8(8):619–23.
8. Adams JE, Habbu R. Tendinopathies of the hand and wrist. *J Am Acad Orthop Surg*. 2015;23(12):741–50.
9. Chiu IM, Heesters BA, Ghasemlou N, Von Hehn CA, Zhao F, Tran J, Wainger B, Strominger A, Muralidharan S, Horswill AR, Wardenburg JB, Hwang SW, Carroll MC, Woolf CJ. Bacteria activate sensory neurons that modulate pain and inflammation. *Nature*. 2013;501(7465):52–7.
10. Chiu IM, Pino-Ribeiro F, Woolf CJ. Pain and infection: pathogen detection by nociceptors. *Pain*. 2016;157(6):1192–3.
11. Osterman M, Draeger R, Stern P. Acute hand infections. *J Hand Surg Am*. 2014;39(8):1628–35.
12. Flevas DA, Syngouna S, Fandridis E, Tsiodras SM, Mavrogenis AF. Infections of the hand: an overview. *EFORT Open Rev*. 2019;4(5):183–93.
13. Perron AD, Miller MD, Brady WJ. Orthopedic pitalls in the ED: fight bite. *Am J Emerg Med*. 2002;20(2):114–7.
14. Ong YS, Levin LS. Hand infections. *Plast Reconstr Surg*. 2009;124(4):225e–33e.
15. Chapman T, Ilyas AM. Pyogenic flexor tenosynovitis: evaluation and treatment strategies. *J Hand Surg Am*. 2019;44(11):981–5.

16. Sammer DM, Shin AY. Comparison of arthroscopic and open treatment of septic arthritis of the wrist. *J Bone Joint Surg Am*. 2009;91(6):1387–93.
17. Birklein F, Ajit SK, Goebel A, Perez RSGM, Sommer C. Complex regional pain syndrome—phenotypic characteristics and potential biomarkers. *Nat Rev Neurol*. 2018;14(5):272–84.
18. Poppler L, Mackinnon S. The role of the peripheral nerve surgeon in treatment of pain. Neurotherapeutics. 2019;16(1):9–25.
19. Rand SE, Basu S, Khalid S. Complexion regional pain syndrome: current diagnostic and treatment considerations. *Curr Sports Med Rep*. 2019;18(9):325–9.
20. Wipperman J, Goerl K. Carpal tunnel syndrome: diagnosis and management. *Am Fam Physician*. 2016;94(12):993–9.
21. Bharde S, Caxaria S, Dell'Accio F, Sikandar S. Update on pain in arthritis. *Curr Opin Support Palliat Care*. 2021;15(2):99–107.
22. Zhao J, Guo S, Schrodi SJ, He D. Molecular and cellular heterogeneity in rheumatoid arthritis: mechanisms and clinical implications. *Front Immunol*. 2021;12(790122):1–21.
23. Lin Y, Anzaghe M, Schulke S. Update on the pathomechanism, diagnosis, and treatment options for rheumatoid arthritis. *Cells*. 2020;9(4):880.
24. Walsh DA, McWilliams DF. Pain in rheumatoid arthritis. *Curr Pain Headache Rep*. 2012;16(6):509–17.
25. Porter SB, Murray PM. Raynaud phenomonen. *J Hand Surg Am*. 2013;38(2):375–8.
26. Klein-Weigel P, Volz TS, Zange L, Richter J. Buerger's disease: providing integrated care. *J Multidiscip Healthc*. 2016;12(9):511–8.
27. Underwood M. Diagnosis and management of gout. *BMJ*. 2006;332(7553):1315–9.
28. Kasper IR, Juriga MD, Giurini JM, Shmerling RH. Treatment of tophaceous gout: when medication is not enough. *Semin Arthritis Rheum*. 2016;45(6):669–74.
29. MacMullan P, McCarthy G. Treatment and management of pseudogout: insights for the clinician. *Ther Adv Musculoskelet Dis*. 2012;4(2):121–31.
30. Morris G, Evans S, Stevenson J, Kotecha A, Parry M, Jeys L, Grimer R. Bone metastases of the hand. *Ann R Coll Surg Engl*. 2017;99(7):563–7.
31. Santoshi JA, Kori VK, Khurana U. Glomus tumor of the fingertips: a frequently missed diagnosis. *J Family Med Prim Care*. 2019;8(3):904–8.
32. Senhaji G, Gallouj S, El Jouari O, Lamouaffaq A, Rimani M, Mernissi FZ. Rare tumor in unusual location—glomus tumor of the finger pulp (clinical and dermoscopic features): a case report. *J Med Case Rep*. 2018;12(1):196–200.
33. Tang CYK, Tipoe T, Fung B. Where is the lesion? Glomus tumours of the hand. *Arch Plast Surg*. 2013;40(5):492–5.
34. Leversedge FJ, Moore TJ, Peterson BC, Seiler JG III. Compartment syndrome of the upper extremity. *J Hand Surg Am*. 2011;36(3):544–59.
35. Chauhan A, Wigton MD, Palmer BA. Necrotizing fasciitis. *J Hand Surg Am*. 2014;39(8):1598–601.

Myofascial Pelvic Pain

12

Evidence-Based Musculoskeletal Medicine

Rupali Kumar

Background/Epidemiology

Myofascial pelvic pain refers to nonarticular musculoskeletal pain originating from the pelvic floor muscles and their surrounding connective tissue and fascia [1, 2]. This includes the superficial pelvic floor muscles or urogenital diaphragm (bulbospongiosus, ischiocavernosus, and transverse perineal muscles) and the deep pelvic floor muscles or pelvic diaphragm, consisting of the levator ani muscles (puborectalis, pubococcygeus, iliococcygeus) and the tendinous arch to which they are anchored, the coccygeus muscles, and the obturator internus muscles. Myofascial pelvic pain is characterized by myofascial trigger points located within taut bands of over-contracted muscle within the pelvic floor [1]. This pelvic floor muscle overactivity can occur in response to biomechanical factors (e.g. repetitive motion, hypermobility, joint pain), trauma (e.g. surgery, pregnancy/childbirth), nearby visceral pathology (e.g. endometriosis, inflammatory bowel disease), nerve entrapment or injury, or psychological stress (e.g. anxiety, history of abuse) [3]. In addition to causing local or referred pain in the lower abdomen, groin, penis, scrotum, vulva, vagina, perineum, anus, rectum, buttocks, or coccyx, hypertonicity in the pelvic floor muscles can result in urinary, defecatory, and sexual dysfunction.

Pelvic floor myofascial pain is an often overlooked etiology for pain in the pelvis. This is despite the fact that musculoskeletal etiologies of pelvic pain are highly prevalent among patients with chronic pelvic pain (CPP), often coexisting with other sources of CPP, such as gynecological, urological, or colorectal pathologies [4, 5]. It is difficult to accurately estimate the number of patients with pelvic pain for whom the etiology is myofascial pain, in part because pelvic floor muscles are

R. Kumar (✉)
Department of Physical Medicine and Rehabilitation, UT Southwestern Medical Center, Dallas, TX, USA
e-mail: rupali.kumar@utsouthwestern.edu

C. E. Noe (ed.), *Musculoskeletal Pain*,
https://doi.org/10.1007/978-3-031-86057-7_12

not routinely evaluated by the providers to whom pelvic pain patients most often present, such as gynecologists and urologists. Initial studies estimated that 14–22% of women with chronic pelvic pain have an underlying musculoskeletal etiology, but in clinical settings where musculoskeletal pelvic floor evaluations are routinely performed for patients with pelvic pain, 50–90% are noted to have pain of a musculoskeletal origin [3]. In a study of women with CPP, 89% had levator ani tenderness, 50.8% had piriformis tenderness, and 31.7% had obturator internus tenderness [6]. Myofascial pelvic pain is not specific to females– in a study of 72 men with chronic prostatitis/chronic pelvic pain syndrome, palpation of the pelvic floor and abdominal muscle trigger points reproduced their pelvic pain greater than 75% of the time [7].

Diagnosis

Part of the difficulty in ascertaining the prevalence of myofascial pelvic pain is that there are no standardized diagnostic criteria for this condition [8]. The mainstay for evaluation is physical examination with direct palpation of the superficial and deep pelvic floor muscles, including internal vaginal and rectal examination, assessing for muscle tone, tenderness or trigger points, strength, range of motion, and coordination of these muscles. Complete evaluation of this condition should also include neurological and musculoskeletal examination of the lumbar spine, pelvis, and hips, including assessment of alignment, range of motion, sensation, strength, and reflexes [2, 9]. While ultrasound or dry needling have been explored as methods of evaluating for myofascial trigger points, and electromyography (EMG) has been used to assess for pelvic floor myofascial dysfunction, these methods are not routinely used or required to diagnose myofascial pelvic pain [2]. Depending on the presenting symptoms, the usual diagnostic testing for urological, gynecological, colorectal, or spine and hip pathology, such as urinalysis, vaginal discharge evaluation, spinal or abdominopelvic imaging, or colonoscopy, are often useful in identifying associated pathologies that may be driving or influencing the myofascial pelvic pain [3].

Treatment

As in other musculoskeletal pain conditions, a multimodal approach is fundamental in treating myofascial pelvic pain. This should begin with patient education on the condition, use of modalities such as heat or ice, targeted therapeutic exercise (including physical therapy and home exercise program), and recognition and management of contributing psychological factors, and can progress to include pharmacologic and interventional treatment options if indicated [10]. As myofascial pelvic pain frequently coexists with other musculoskeletal, neurological, visceral, and psychological pathologies of the pelvis, treatment of these associated pelvic conditions is essential to treating the myofascial pelvic pain, and should be undertaken concurrently to maximize improvement in the patient's overall pain. As such, the treatment of myofascial pelvic pain should ideally involve a multidisciplinary team approach including the relevant medical specialists as well as physical therapists [2].

Pelvic Floor Physical Therapy

The mainstay of treatment for myofascial pelvic pain is pelvic floor physical therapy with a highly trained pelvic floor physical therapist, involving thorough assessment and individualized treatment of the patient's specific condition. Given the diversity in patient presentations, there is no standardized treatment protocol that applies to all patients with myofascial pelvic pain. The evidence base in this area is limited, as it is challenging to take the holistic evaluation and tailored treatment approach of pelvic floor physical therapy and break it down into individual components that are easily studied and generalizable. However, there are some general principles that apply to most patients with myofascial pelvic pain. As this is a condition of muscle overactivity, therapeutic interventions should primarily focus on lengthening and relaxation of pelvic floor muscles, an approach referred to as pelvic floor "downtraining." It is essential for patients and providers to recognize that pelvic floor physical therapy is not a passive modality– it is not simply "pelvic floor massage." The goal of therapy should be not only to improve in baseline pelvic floor muscle hypertonicity, but also for the patient to learn about the function of their pelvic floor muscles and the role they play in pain, gain kinesthetic and proprioceptive awareness of the pelvic floor, and become empowered to use a combination of exercises, strategies, and tools to self-manage their myofascial pelvic pain going forward. A few of these methods are detailed below.

Downtraining

Pelvic floor muscle downtraining techniques, including diaphragmatic breathing, stretches, and active pelvic floor lengthening exercises known as perineal bulges or reverse Kegels, are the mainstay of reducing pelvic floor overactivity. However, there are limited studies evaluating these techniques individually. Pelvic floor downtraining techniques have been shown to improve pelvic pain related to overactive pelvic floor muscles in men with prostate cancer post-prostatectomy [11]. These techniques can be utilized alone or in conjunction with biofeedback modalities described below.

Biofeedback

Biofeedback therapy refers to the recording of bodily activities for the patient to observe via visual or auditory feedback in real-time to improve their awareness of their own bodily functions, and is useful in reducing pelvic floor overactivity-associated pain [12]. It is often undertaken in the form of surface EMG electrodes placed over the superficial pelvic floor muscles or on an internal vaginal or rectal probe, with a monitor displaying to the patient their own baseline and dynamic pelvic floor muscle activity. With this setup, patients can be coached to work on pelvic floor downtraining techniques. In a randomized controlled trial of 157 patients with levator ani syndrome (i.e., painful pelvic floor spasm), 57.7% of those who received biofeedback therapy reported adequate pain relief after 12 months—this was superior to the rate of adequate pain relief in a group who received electrogalvanic stimulation alone (26.5%) and massage alone (20.8%) [13]. Tailoring the use of biofeedback to the type and extent of pelvic floor muscle dysfunction noted is essential to the effectiveness of this treatment modality [14].

Myofascial Release

A key technique in reducing pelvic floor muscle tension is myofascial release, which is done by applying direct pressure to overactive muscles of the pelvic floor and surrounding musculature. This is performed manually by pelvic physical therapists and patients, and tools such as a pelvic wand can also be utilized by a patient individually. In a study of 374 patients with chronic pelvic pain who were taught to use a pelvic wand for pelvic floor trigger point myofascial release, the majority of subjects experienced a reduction in pelvic pain symptoms after 6 months, and the percentage of patients using pain medications to manage their pelvic pain dropped from 63.6 to 40.1% [15].

Dilators

Vaginal and rectal dilators are tube-like medical devices that come in sets of increasing diameter and are inserted internally to provide passive stretch. Dilators play an essential role in myofascial pelvic pain, not only in providing gentle and graduated lengthening of pelvic floor muscles, but also in desensitizing the surrounding soft tissue to stretch, as well as decreasing anxiety and pain relating to penetration [16].

Dry Needling

Dry needling is a treatment commonly used by physical therapists to treat myofascial trigger points all over the body. In this technique, a thin microfilament needle is inserted directly into muscle trigger points in order to deactivate them, increase blood flow, and reduce pain. In a case series of two female patients with chronic myofascial pelvic pain, dry needling of pelvic floor muscles led to the resolution of pain and improvement of associated disability [17].

Electrical Stimulation

Transcutaneous electrical nerve stimulation (TENS) is a common and effective pain relief modality for musculoskeletal pain generally and has been shown to be beneficial in idiopathic chronic pelvic pain, which, as noted earlier, is very frequently musculoskeletal in origin [18]. As described earlier, most of these interventions work best in concert with each other and not individually, as evidenced by a recent study showing that the addition of self-myofascial release to biofeedback and electrical stimulation resulted in superior pain relief [19].

Medications

Topical Analgesics

Though not well studied, the use of topical analgesics in myofascial pelvic pain is common and can help patients tolerate other treatment modalities, such as myofascial release and dilators. Topical lidocaine may show some benefit in patients with provoked vestibulodynia and dyspareunia, conditions that commonly coexist with myofascial pelvic pain, but is not recommended to be used long-term. Other topical treatments, such as topical tricyclics and NSAIDs, have a plausible mechanism for efficacy but are not well-studied [20].

Muscle Relaxants

There is limited high-quality data supporting the use of oral skeletal muscle relaxants, including antispastic medications (e.g., baclofen, dantrolene), antispasmodic medications (e.g., cyclobenzaprine, methocarbamol), or antispastic-antispasmodic medications (e.g., diazepam, tizanidine), in myofascial pelvic pain [21].

Intravaginal or intrarectal suppositories containing either diazepam, baclofen, or various other compounds of muscle relaxant and analgesic medications have been utilized in the treatment of pelvic floor myofascial pain. However, evidence as to their efficacy is mixed. A recent systematic review of two observational studies and three small randomized controlled trials (RCTs) on vaginal diazepam showed no consistent effect on pain, sexual function, or quality of life indices nor resting tone on EMG compared to placebo suppositories [22–24].

Neuropathic Pain Medications

Neuropathic pain medications such as gabapentinoids, tricyclic antidepressants, and serotonin-norepinephrine reuptake inhibitors are utilized in the management of neuropathic pain and chronic pain generally, and can be beneficial in patients with myofascial pelvic pain [2, 20].

Psychological Interventions

Myofascial pelvic pain is closely correlated with psychosocial stressors and comorbid psychiatric conditions, such as anxiety, depression, and history of physical or sexual trauma. These conditions must be screened for in patients with myofascial pelvic pain. Treatment of psychiatric comorbidities via pharmacologic management, CBT, and relaxation techniques can help reduce the experience of myofascial pelvic pain [2]. Interestingly, further illustrating the strong connection between myofascial pelvic pain and psychological comorbidities, the converse has also been demonstrated– myofascial therapy for pelvic floor pain can help improve psychological outcomes [25].

Trigger Point Injections

Trigger point injections are widely utilized for myofascial pain throughout the body and can be performed on muscles either transvaginally, paravaginally, or transperineally to address pelvic floor myofascial pain. The mechanism of action of trigger point injections is not fully known, but it is theorized that the local anesthetic infiltration may disrupt tight muscle fibers, halt the pain feedback loop, and/or dilute out nociceptive substances in the local area, resulting in short-term reduction of pain, with further potential anti-inflammatory effect brought on if steroid is also injected [2].

There are several retrospective reviews assessing the effectiveness of trigger point injections to the pelvic floor muscles, which generally show favorable results. In one retrospective review of 101 patients with chronic pelvic pain who underwent transvaginal trigger point injections with local anesthetic, often with the addition of triamcinolone, there was significant improvement in pain scores in subsequent visits, with only minor adverse events noted [26].

Magnesium-based pelvic floor trigger point injections have also been explored, based on the proposed mechanism of magnesium inhibiting calcium release in order to stop myocyte contraction in hypertonic muscles. In a small RCT comparing magnesium-based pelvic floor trigger point injections to local anesthetic, improvement in pain with function and quality of life was seen in the magnesium group when compared to the waitlist group, but there was no significant difference when compared with the lidocaine-only group [27].

Botulinum Toxin Injections

Botulinum toxin injections to the pelvic floor are performed utilizing a similar technique to trigger point injections. These work by inducing temporary muscle weakness or paralysis lasting about 3–6 months while also inhibiting the release of pain-sensitizing neuropeptides in afferent C fibers [28]. These mechanisms of action would theoretically give the patient a reprieve from painful pelvic floor muscle hypertonicity, allowing them to make easier progress with pelvic physical therapy. A 2022 systematic review and meta-analysis looked at eight studies and 289 participants who received pelvic floor botulinum toxin A injections and noted a statistically significant improvement in visual analog scale pain scores in those who received the injections [28].

Other Interventions

Other less studied interventions for myofascial pelvic pain include radiofrequency modulation [29], biomimetic physiotherapy [30], and pelvic floor magnetic stimulation, all with limited data on their efficacy.

References

1. Aredo JV, Heyrana KJ, Karp BI, Shah JP, Stratton P. Relating chronic pelvic pain and endometriosis to signs of sensitization and myofascial pain and dysfunction. Semin Reprod Med. 2017;35(1):88–97. https://doi.org/10.1055/s-0036-1597123.
2. Bonder JH, Chi M, Rispoli L. Myofascial pelvic pain and related disorders. Phys Med Rehabil Clin N Am. 2017;28(3):501–15. https://doi.org/10.1016/j.pmr.2017.03.005.
3. Lamvu G, Carrillo J, Witzeman K, Alappattu M. Musculoskeletal considerations in female patients with chronic pelvic pain. Semin Reprod Med. 2018;36(2):107–15. https://doi.org/10.1055/s-0038-1676085.
4. Ross V, Detterman C, Hallisey A. Myofascial pelvic pain: an overlooked and treatable cause of chronic pelvic pain. J Midwifery Womens Health. 2021;66(2):148–60. https://doi.org/10.1111/jmwh.13224.
5. Neville CE, Fitzgerald CM, Mallinson T, Badillo S, Hynes C, Tu F. A preliminary report of musculoskeletal dysfunction in female chronic pelvic pain: a blinded study of examination findings. J Bodyw Mov Ther. 2012;16(1):50–6. https://doi.org/10.1016/j.jbmt.2011.06.002.
6. de Souza Montenegro MLL, Mateus-Vasconcelos ECL, Silva JCR e, Nogueira AA, Reis FJCD, Poli Neto OB. Importance of pelvic muscle tenderness evaluation in women with chronic pelvic pain. Pain Med Malden Mass. 2010;11(2):224–8. https://doi.org/10.1111/j.1526-4637.2009.00758.x.
7. Anderson RU, Sawyer T, Wise D, Morey A, Nathanson BH. Painful myofascial trigger points and pain sites in men with chronic prostatitis/chronic pelvic pain syndrome. J Urol. 2009;182(6):2753–8. https://doi.org/10.1016/j.juro.2009.08.033.
8. Meister MR, Sutcliffe S, Ghetti C, et al. Development of a standardized, reproducible screening examination for assessment of pelvic floor myofascial pain. Am J Obstet Gynecol. 2019;220(3):255.e1–9. https://doi.org/10.1016/j.ajog.2018.11.1106.
9. Dune TJ, Griffin A, Hoffman EG, et al. Importance of internal vaginal pelvic floor muscle exams for women with external lumbar/hip/pelvic girdle pain: International urogynecology journal. Int Urogynecol J. 2023;34(7):1471–6. https://doi.org/10.1007/s00192-022-05390-4.
10. El-Tallawy SN, Nalamasu R, Salem GI, LeQuang JAK, Pergolizzi JV, Christo PJ. Management of musculoskeletal pain: an update with emphasis on chronic musculoskeletal pain. Pain Ther. 2021;10(1):181–209. https://doi.org/10.1007/s40122-021-00235-2.
11. Scott KM, Gosai E, Bradley MH, et al. Individualized pelvic physical therapy for the treatment of post-prostatectomy stress urinary incontinence and pelvic pain. Int Urol Nephrol. 2020;52(4):655–9. https://doi.org/10.1007/s11255-019-02343-7.
12. Hite M, Curran T. Pelvic floor disorders: biofeedback for pelvic floor disorders. Clin Colon Rectal Surg. 2021;34(1):56. https://doi.org/10.1055/s-0040-1714287.
13. Chiarioni G, Nardo A, Vantini I, Romito A, Whitehead WE. Biofeedback is superior to electrogalvanic stimulation and massage for treatment of levator ani syndrome. Gastroenterology. 2010;138(4):1321. https://doi.org/10.1053/j.gastro.2009.12.040.
14. Pedraza R, Nieto J, Ibarra S, Haas EM. Pelvic muscle rehabilitation: a standardized protocol for pelvic floor dysfunction. Adv Urol. Published online January 1, 2014. https://doi.org/10.1155/2014/487436
15. Anderson RU, Harvey RH, Wise D, Nevin Smith J, Nathanson BH, Sawyer T. Chronic pelvic pain syndrome: reduction of medication use after pelvic floor physical therapy with an internal myofascial trigger point wand. Appl Psychophysiol Biofeedback. 2015;40(1):45–52. https://doi.org/10.1007/s10484-015-9273-1.
16. Liu M, Juravic M, Mazza G, Krychman ML. Vaginal dilators: issues and answers. Sex Med Rev. 2021;9(2):212–20. https://doi.org/10.1016/j.sxmr.2019.11.005.
17. George A, VanEtten L, Briggs M. Dry needling for female chronic pelvic pain: a case series. J Womens Pelvic Health Phys Ther. 2018;42(1):8. https://doi.org/10.1097/JWH.0000000000000093.

18. Sharma N, Rekha K, Srinivasan JK. Efficacy of transcutaneous electrical nerve stimulation in the treatment of chronic pelvic pain. J -Life Health. 2017;8(1):36. https://doi.org/10.4103/jmh.JMH_60_16.
19. Xu J, Chen K, Ding B, et al. Effectiveness of self-myofascial release combined with biofeedback and electrical stimulation for the management of myofascial pelvic pain: a randomized controlled trial. Eur J Pain. 2022;26(2):405–16. https://doi.org/10.1002/ejp.1867.
20. Atashroo DT, Cockrum R. Pharmacological with management pelvic pain of patients. *Manag Chronic Pelvic Pain Pract Man*. Published online 2021:50.
21. Flatow V, Uy-Kroh J, Carey ET, Ascher-Walsh C, Khalil S. Skeletal muscle relaxants for the treatment of myofascial pelvic pain and high tone pelvic floor disorders. Curr Opin Obstet Gynecol. 2023;35(4):311. https://doi.org/10.1097/GCO.0000000000000894.
22. Crisp CC, Vaccaro CM, Estanol MV, et al. Intra-vaginal diazepam for high-tone pelvic floor dysfunction: a randomized placebo-controlled trial. Int Urogynecol J. 2013;24(11):1915–23. https://doi.org/10.1007/s00192-013-2108-9.
23. Stone RH, Abousaud M, Abousaud A, Kobak W. A systematic review of intravaginal diazepam for the treatment of pelvic floor hypertonic disorder. J Clin Pharmacol. 2020;60(S2):S110–20. https://doi.org/10.1002/jcph.1775.
24. Holland MA, Joyce JS, Brennaman LM, Drobnis EZ, Starr JA, Foster RTS. Intravaginal diazepam for the treatment of pelvic floor hypertonic disorder: a double-blind, randomized, placebo-controlled trial. Urogynecology. 2019;25(1):76. https://doi.org/10.1097/SPV.0000000000000514.
25. Diaz-Mohedo E, Hita-Contreras F, Castro-Martin E, Pilat A, Perez-Dominguez B, Valenza-Peña G. Using myofascial therapy to improve psychological outcomes, quality of life, and sexual function in women with chronic pelvic pain—a case series. Healthcare. 2024;12(3):304. https://doi.org/10.3390/healthcare12030304.
26. Bartley J, Han E, Gupta P, et al. Transvaginal trigger point injections improve pain scores in women with pelvic floor hypertonicity and pelvic pain conditions. Urogynecology. 2019;25(5):392. https://doi.org/10.1097/SPV.0000000000000581.
27. Leitch J, Webb A, Pudwell J, Chamberlain S, Henry R, Nitsch R. Magnesium-based trigger point infiltrations versus local anaesthetic infiltrations in chronic pelvic myofascial pain: a randomized, double-blind, Controlled Study. J Obstet Gynaecol Can. 2022;44(8):877–85. https://doi.org/10.1016/j.jogc.2022.02.129.
28. Spruijt MA, Klerkx WM, Kelder JC, Kluivers KB, Kerkhof MH. The efficacy of botulinum toxin a injections in pelvic floor muscles in chronic pelvic pain patients: a systematic review and meta-analysis. Int Urogynecol J. 2022;33(11):2951–61. https://doi.org/10.1007/s00192-022-05115-7.
29. Ashtiani EM, Shokouhi N, Mohseni M, Saedi N, Haeri-Mehrizi AA, Bakhtiyari M. A novel radiofrequency modulation therapy versus routine physiotherapy modalities in treatment of myofascial pelvic pain syndrome: a pilot randomized trial. Obstet Gynecol Sci. 2023;66(3):230–40. https://doi.org/10.5468/ogs.22171.
30. Su X, Liu J, Yang H, et al. Observations on the therapeutic efficacy of biomimetic physiotherapy combined with manipulation therapy in managing myofascial pelvic pain syndrome in women. Altern Ther Health Med. Published online April 18, 2024. Accessed May 10, 2024. https://pubmed.ncbi.nlm.nih.gov/38639618/

The Hip

13

Georges Bounajem

History

Multiple characteristics of the hip pain should be elicited from the patient, including location, onset, quality, aggravating and alleviating factors, and change over time. Pain radiating into the thigh and/or knee may indicate lumbar radiculopathy, but may also be caused by referred pain from intra-articular hip pathology. Mechanical symptoms such as locking or catching in the hip can be due to a labral tear, osteoarthritis, or a loose body in the hip joint. A fall or other trauma preceding the pain may be suggestive of a fracture, or of acute aggravation of chronic underlying disease such as osteoarthritis. The co-occurrence of cutaneous, gastrointestinal, or ocular symptoms may indicate a rheumatologic cause for hip pain. The location of pain is frequently helpful in narrowing the differential diagnosis, and can often be categorized as anterior, lateral, or posterior.

Physical Exam

A thorough physical exam of the hip entails observing the patient's gait, as well as performance of specific tests with the patient supine on the exam table. Common gait conditions and exam maneuvers are listed in Table 13.1.

G. Bounajem (✉)
UT Southwestern Medical Center, Dallas, TX, USA
e-mail: georges.bounajem@utsouthwestern.edu

C. E. Noe (ed.), *Musculoskeletal Pain*,
https://doi.org/10.1007/978-3-031-86057-7_13

Table 13.1 Physical exam of the hip

Test	Position	Findings	Differential Diagnosis
Gait testing	Standing	Antalgic (shortened stance phase on affected side), Trendelenburg (contralateral side of pelvis droops during stance on ipsilateral side), stiff-legged (avoidance of simultaneous hip flexion and knee extension), non-weight-bearing	Antalgic: Osteoarthritis, osteonecrosis, inflammatory arthropathy, FAI/labral tear, GTPS, transient osteoporosis, hip pointer, tumor Trendelenburg: Greater trochanteric pain syndrome/abductor tendon injury Stiff-legged: Hamstring injuries Non-weight-bearing: Septic arthritis, fracture/dislocation
Range of motion	Sitting, supine, or prone	Pain, reduced range of motion (normal internal rotation: 30–40°, normal external rotation: 40–60°, crepitus	Pain: Osteoarthritis, osteonecrosis, inflammatory arthropathy, septic arthritis, FAI/labral tear, GTPS, transient osteoporosis, hip pointer, fracture/dislocation, tumor Crepitus: Osteoarthritis, osteonecrosis, fracture
FADIR (hip flexion, adduction, internal rotation)	Supine	Pain	Osteoarthritis, osteonecrosis, inflammatory arthropathy, septic arthritis, FAI/labral tear, hip pointer, fracture, tumor
FABER (hip flexion, abduction, external rotation), also known as Patrick's test	Supine	Pain	Osteoarthritis, osteonecrosis, inflammatory arthropathy, septic arthritis, FAI/labral tear, GTPS, iliopsoas syndrome, hip pointer, fracture, tumor
Scour test (hip axially loaded while passively internally and externally rotated in varying degrees of flexion and adduction/abduction	Supine	Pain	Osteoarthritis, osteonecrosis, inflammatory arthropathy, septic arthritis, FAI/labral tear, hip pointer, fracture, tumor

Stinchfield test (Resisted active hip flexion between 30–45 degrees while knee is extended)	Supine	Pain	Osteoarthritis, osteonecrosis, inflammatory arthropathy, septic arthritis, FAI/labral tear, hip pointer, fracture, tumor
Ober's test (examiner stabilizes pelvis and extends/abducts hip, then allows slow adduction with gravity until motion is restricted)	Lateral with affected side up, unaffected hip and knee flexed	Leg remains in adducted position, lateral pain	GTPS, ITB tightness
Resisted sit-up, resisted hip adduction	Supine	Pain	Sports hernia
Resisted external derotation test (active internal rotation from an externally rotated position against examiner's resistance)	Supine	Pain	GTPS
Modified bent knee stretch (rapid passive extension of knee)	Supine with hip and knee maximally flexed	Buttock/posterior thigh pain	Hamstring injury
Modified Thomas test (passive hip extension off table)	Supine with unaffected leg supported at 90 degrees of hip flexion	Affected thigh does not fall parallel to table	Hip flexor tightness/iliopsoas syndrome

FAI femoroacetabular impingement, *GTPS* greater trochanteric pain syndrome, *ITB* iliotibial band

Imaging

Radiography Radiographs are a helpful component of the initial evaluation of the painful hip. Adequate assessment requires orthogonal views in the form of an anteroposterior (AP) view and a lateral view. Radiographs can be helpful in identifying conditions such as osteoarthritis, osteonecrosis, fracture, and malignancy, although additional imaging studies may be necessary depending on the specific diagnosis.

Ultrasonography Ultrasonography is useful in the evaluation of suspected muscle and/or tendon disorders around the hip. It allows for real-time evaluation of mechanical symptoms such as snapping. Ultrasonography can be more limited in utility when evaluating deeper intra-articular structures of the hip joint, particularly in patients with larger body habitus. It has the advantage of not exposing patients to ionizing radiation, but does require adequate training to perform and assess.

Computed Tomography Computed tomography (CT) provides detailed imaging of osseous anatomy. It is also quick to technically perform, making it favorable for assessment of patients in the emergency trauma setting. However, it exposes patients to significant ionizing radiation, and because it has lower sensitivity compared to magnetic resonance imaging for many pathologic conditions of the hip, its utility in the initial management of hip pain is limited.

Magnetic Resonance Imaging Magnetic resonance imaging (MRI) provides superior assessment of soft tissue anatomy. It is also the imaging modality of choice for evaluation of suspected stress fractures, with a sensitivity of nearly 100%, and is helpful in further evaluation of suspected malignancy lesions that may be first identified on radiographs. MRI can be combined with arthrography, in which contrast media is injected into the hip joint, to increase the sensitivity for intra-articular pathology such as labral tears. It does not expose patients to ionizing radiation, but is greater in cost compared to other imaging modalities.

Common Hip Diagnoses

Osteoarthritis

Description Osteoarthritis is a degenerative disease that results in loss of articular cartilage. Hip osteoarthritis more commonly occurs in patients of older age, and may be associated with history of prior trauma to the hip, heavy labor, and high-impact sports. Osteoarthritis is associated with loss of proteoglycan content in articular cartilage, destruction of cartilage matrix by proteolytic enzymes, and inflammation of synovial tissue. In severe cases, hip osteoarthritis can lead to functionally debilitating pain.

Clinical Presentation Pain is the most common symptom of hip osteoarthritis, and occurs most commonly in the groin. Patients may use the "c-sign," in which the hand is wrapped around the greater trochanter with the fingers anterior and the thumb posterior, to describe the location of pain. Buttock pain, thigh pain, and knee pain can also occur. Pain is commonly aggravated by weight-bearing activities such as standing, walking, and climbing stairs and may be alleviated by rest. Rotation of the hip typically aggravates pain. Patients may describe walking with a limp and may notice the affected leg feeling shorter than the unaffected leg. Stiffness is another common symptom and may result in difficulty with donning socks and shoes.

Physical Examination Patients with hip osteoarthritis may present with an antalgic gait. Leg lengths should be examined with the patient supine, as loss of joint space with advanced osteoarthritis can lead to superior migration of the entire extremity. Passive internal rotation of the hip frequently aggravates pain and may be limited due to stiffness. In severe disease, audible and palpable crepitus can sometimes be observed with active and/or passive movement of the hip. Flexion contracture of the hip may also be present and is observed when the patient's thigh is unable to lay flat on the exam table with the patient supine.

Diagnostic Workup Radiographs should be obtained, including a standing anteroposterior (AP) pelvis and lateral view of the hip. Hip joint space narrowing, subchondral sclerosis and cysts, and osteophyte formation may be present. MRI may be used in equivocal cases to better characterize the articular cartilage but is frequently unnecessary. A diagnostic corticosteroid injection may also be valuable in equivocal cases, as an improvement in pain after injection supports the assertion that an intra-articular cause of pain is present, even if relief is temporary.

Treatment The American Academy of Orthopaedic Surgeons has published evidence-based clinical practice guidelines to help guide treatment of hip osteoarthritis. Nonoperative treatment is recommended for initial management. Non-narcotic medications, such as nonsteroidal anti-inflammatory medications, are strongly recommended, while long-term prescription opioid medications are not recommended. Strong evidence supports physical therapy as a treatment that can reduce pain and improve function. Intra-articular corticosteroid injections may also be helpful in providing short-term relief. Weight loss is also recommended for patients who are overweight, as reduced chronic stress on the hip joint can help improve pain and function. Surgery may be necessary if nonoperative treatment fails to provide sufficient improvement. Total hip arthroplasty has been shown to provide significant improvements in pain and quality of life for many patients with hip osteoarthritis.

References [1–7]

Osteonecrosis

Description Osteonecrosis, also referred to as avascular necrosis, is a condition in which impaired blood flow to bone leads to the death of osteocytes. In the case of hip osteonecrosis, lack of adequate blood supply to the femoral heads can lead to eventual femoral head collapse and secondary hip osteoarthritis. Multiple risk factors for this diagnosis exist, including a history of trauma to the hip, hematologic disease, irradiation, chemotherapy, corticosteroid use, and alcoholism. The choice of treatment is driven by the stage of disease, and like osteoarthritis, advanced stages of osteonecrosis can lead to severe and functionally debilitating pain.

Clinical Presentation Because risk factors for osteonecrosis can occur at any age, patients with osteonecrosis can often be much younger than patients who typically present with osteoarthritis. However, the clinical presentation is often similar. Groin pain is the most common sign of hip osteonecrosis, and as with osteoarthritis patients, the "c-sign" may be used to describe the pain's location. Buttock pain, thigh pain, and knee pain can also occur. Pain often worsens with weight-bearing physical activity and hip rotation and may improve with rest.

Physical Examination Patients may present with an antalgic gait. Passive internal rotation of the hip frequently aggravates pain and may be limited due to stiffness. In advanced disease with femoral head collapse, audible and palpable crepitus may be observed with active and/or passive movement of the hip.

Diagnostic Workup Standing AP pelvis and lateral view x-rays of the hip should be used for initial assessment. The early stages of osteonecrosis may be accompanied by normal X-rays, but cystic and sclerotic changes are often observed prior to the disease stage reaching femoral head collapse. After collapse has occurred, the weight-bearing region of the femoral head flattens, and sphericity is progressively lost. In advanced stages, cartilage loss results in evident joint space narrowing. MRI has high sensitivity and specificity as a diagnostic tool for osteonecrosis and is the imaging modality of choice if osteonecrosis is suspected in the setting of unremarkable X-rays. It is also helpful in evaluating the extent of the disease. MRI typically shows low-intensity signal demarcating the affected region in T1-weighted images and alternating high-and low-intensity signal on T2-weighted images.

Treatment Optimal treatment of pre-collapse osteonecrosis of the hip has not been well-established. Studies have investigated the use of multiple pharmacologic agents such as bisphosphonates and anticoagulants, as well as modalities such as extracorporeal shock wave therapy. While these treatments have shown promise in some studies, there is a lack of consensus on efficacy and treatment approach. Surgical options include femoral head-preserving procedures and hip arthroplasty procedures. Core decompression is a head-preserving procedure that involves drilling one or multiple tracts into the necrotic region of the femoral head with the intention of stimulating angiogenesis and relieving intraosseous hypertension in the area. This can be augmented with bone graft, bone substitute, or other adjunctive therapies and may help slow the progression of the disease. Rotational osteotomy is another head-preserving procedure that can be used to rotate the necrotic region of bone away from the weight-bearing surface of the hip. For patients with collapsed osteonecrosis of the hip, arthroplasty is often preferred.

References [8–13]

Inflammatory Arthropathy

Description Rheumatoid arthritis, seronegative spondyloarthropathies, and crystal arthropathies are examples of inflammatory arthropathies that can affect the hip joint. Rheumatoid arthritis is a systemic autoimmune disease that is characterized by an immune response, most commonly mediated by IgM antibodies, that leads to progressive synovial inflammation and cartilage destruction. Seronegative spondyloarthropathies are associated with the HLA-B27 allele and include conditions such as ankylosing spondylitis, psoriatic arthritis, and reactive arthritis. Gout and pseudogout are crystal arthropathies caused by monosodium urate crystals and calcium pyrophosphate dihydrate crystals, respectively.

Clinical Presentation The American College of Rheumatology has published diagnostic criteria for rheumatoid arthritis. Patients may describe morning stiffness, joint swelling, subcutaneous nodules, and hand/wrist symptoms. Those with seronegative spondyloarthropathies may exhibit similar symptoms, with some variability depending on the specific disease. Ankylosing spondylitis may present with complaints of back and/or neck pain, psoriatic arthritis with the presence of silvery cutaneous plaques, and reactive arthritis with urethral and ocular inflammation. While reactive arthritis itself is a noninfectious process, it can be triggered by infection elsewhere in the body. Gout flares may be provoked by trauma, surgery, fatty foods, and alcohol consumption. Trauma, surgery, and medical illness may also provoke pseudogout, but many patients with radiographically evident pseudogout are asymptomatic.

Physical Examination As with other intra-articular causes of hip pain, passive rotation of the hip joint can recreate groin or buttock pain. Stiffness can cause difficulty with putting on socks and shoes. Examination of the hands and wrists is an important component of establishing the diagnosis of rheumatoid arthritis and may reveal joint swelling. Patients with ankylosing spondylitis may exhibit kyphotic deformity of the spine, as well as a reduced ability to perform lumbar flexion. Examination of the extensor surfaces of the extremities for cutaneous plaques should be performed in patients suspected of having psoriatic arthritis. The presence of conjunctivitis or uveitis in patients with hip pain may be suggestive of reactive arthritis. Severe pain can occur in patients with flares of gout and pseudogout, but the typical warmth and erythema that occur in other joints affected by these conditions are often absent in the hip due to the deeper nature of this joint.

Diagnostic Workup Standing AP pelvis and lateral view x-rays are helpful in ruling out more common causes of hip pain, such as osteoarthritis, and may also demonstrate joint space narrowing in more severe cases of inflammatory arthropathy. Periarticular erosions, which appear as focal loss of cortical bone and adjacent trabecular bone, can be seen in inflammatory arthropathy. Calcification of articular cartilage, also referred to as chondrocalcinosis, can occur in patients with pseudogout. Serum labs to identify the presence of anti-cyclic citrullinated peptide (CCP) antibodies and rheumatoid factor (RF) can be helpful. Serum HLA-B27 may be positive in patients with seronegative spondyloarthropathy, while RF and anti-CCP are often negative. Erythrocyte sedimentation rate (ESR) and c-reactive protein (CRP) may be elevated in various forms of inflammatory arthropathy, although these labs are nonspecific. Gout is definitively diagnosed by joint aspiration and crystal analysis, which shows negatively birefringent needle-shaped monosodium urate crystals. Because gout flares can occur in patients with low serum urate levels, serum urate is not required to make the diagnosis of gout. Pseudogout is similarly diagnosed with joint aspiration, with positively birefringent rhomboid-shaped crystals on crystal analysis. Importantly, the presence of crystals in synovial fluid does not rule out the possibility of concomitant infection, and septic arthritis should be ruled out in patients presenting with a suspected crystal arthropathy flare.

Treatment Pharmacologic treatment is commonly used for the initial management of inflammatory arthropathy. Multiple drugs, including corticosteroids and disease-modifying antirheumatic drugs (DMARDs), may be used in the treatment of rheumatoid arthritis and psoriatic arthritis. Ankylosing spondylitis is commonly treated first with nonsteroidal anti-inflammatory medications and physical therapy to maintain flexibility, but antitumor necrosis factor (TNF) medications may also be utilized. Antibiotics are recommended for the treatment of the underlying infectious cause of reactive arthritis. Anti-inflammatory medications, including corticosteroids, may be used for gout and pseudogout flares after the diagnosis of infection has been excluded. Urate-lowering agents such as allopurinol are helpful for the prevention of recurrent gout flares.

References [14–21]

Septic Arthritis

Description Septic arthritis of the hip entails inflammation of the hip joint due to infection by a pathogen. It is considered an orthopedic emergency due to the potential for rapid cartilage degradation within hours of onset, and rapid diagnosis and treatment are important to maximize the chance of a favorable outcome. Staphylococcus aureus is the most common organism responsible for septic arthritis of the hip overall, but other organisms such as *Streptococcus* and Gram-negative bacteria can also be responsible. Depending on the individual clinical scenario, infection is thought to occur by direct inoculation from trauma or surgery, as an extension of osteomyelitis, or by hematogenous seeding.

Clinical Presentation Patients with acute septic arthritis of the hip typically present with sudden severe pain aggravated by hip range of motion, avoidance of weight-bearing on the affected extremity, and inability to ambulate. The pain is often located in the groin region but can be located in the buttock or thigh. Chronic septic arthritis may present with less severe pain. Risk factors for septic arthritis of the hip include immune-compromising conditions such as diabetes mellitus, liver disease, infection with human immunodeficiency virus (HIV), and history of intravenous drug use. Even in the absence of known risk factors, septic arthritis can occur in healthy individuals. Fever may be present but is commonly absent.

Physical Examination Active and passive motion of the affected hip commonly causes severe pain in patients with septic arthritis. The patient may prefer to position the hip in a flexed, abducted, and externally rotated position, which is the position of least pressure within the hip capsule. Swelling, warmth, and tenderness around the hip are often not appreciated because of the deep location of the hip joint.

Diagnostic Workup Radiographs should be obtained to rule out other causes of hip pain, such as fracture, but are often normal in early cases of septic arthritis apart from a possible effusion. With persistence of the disease, periarticular osteopenia and erosions, and ultimately joint space narrowing due to cartilage loss, will occur. Advanced imaging is typically not necessary and often delays treatment. Pertinent lab work includes c-reactive protein (normal <1 mg/dL), erythrocyte sedimentation rate (normal <30 mm/hr), and white blood cell count (normal <11,000 cells /μL), with CRP the most sensitive of the three. Joint aspiration frequently allows for definitive diagnosis, and synovial fluid white blood cell count, gram stain, crystal analysis, and cultures should be obtained. White blood cell count >50,000 cells /μL is frequently used as the diagnostic threshold for septic arthritis, although infection can occur in patients with lower white blood cell counts as well. If septic arthritis of the hip is suspected in the outpatient clinical setting, immediate presentation to the emergency department is recommended for orthopedic and infectious diseases evaluation.

Treatment Urgent surgical treatment is essential for maximizing the likelihood of saving the native hip joint and reducing the risk of rapid chondrocyte death. (1) Arthroscopic irrigation and debridement, (2) open irrigation and debridement, and (3) hip resection and antibiotic spacer placement followed by eventual total hip arthroplasty are the primary surgical options. Which surgery is chosen depends on factors such as surgeon skill set, patient age, presence of arthritis, disease chronicity, and extent of disease involvement. Culture-driven intravenous antibiotics help increase the likelihood of infection eradication.

References [22–26]

Labral Tear, Hip Dysplasia, and Femoroacetabular Impingement

Description The labrum of the hip joint is a fibrocartilaginous structure that is located at the periphery of the acetabulum. It increases the contact surface area between the femoral head and acetabulum, helping to distribute forces across the hip joint. It also effectively deepens the hip joint and improves hip stability. Tears of the labrum can occur by acute injury or by degenerative change over time and are more likely to occur in patients with anatomic variations such as hip dysplasia or femoroacetabular impingement. Hip dysplasia is the lack of adequate acetabular coverage of the femoral head and is accompanied by a large, hypertrophic labrum that is more prone to tearing; femoroacetabular impingement describes abnormal contact between the acetabulum and femur due to the presence of excessive bone, resulting in damage to the intervening labrum. Femoroacetabular impingement occurs in various forms and may be described as cam-type (excessive femoral bone), pincer-type (excessive acetabular bone), and mixed-type (excessive femoral and acetabular bone). Hip dysplasia and impingement describe conceptually opposite entities, but both can result in labral tears. Osteoarthritis of the hip commonly results in labral tears due to the loss of joint space and impingement of the labrum by osteophytes. While labral tears can be asymptomatic, they can also cause significant hip pain.

Clinical Presentation Symptoms can occur due to an acute injury, often when the hip is subjected to an extreme position during flexion or rotation. Conversely, chronic degenerative tears may be associated with no pain or vague, insidious pain. Pain may be aggravated by movement of the hip and weight-bearing activities. The "c-sign" may be used to describe the pain. The pain can also be located at the lateral or posterior hip. Activities involving extremes of hip motion, commonly hip flexion and internal rotation, tend to aggravate the pain. Mechanical symptoms such as locking, catching, and snapping may be present.

Physical Examination Impingement tests are used to help detect the presence of a labral tear and are performed with the patient supine on the exam table. Passive hip flexion, adduction, and internal rotation (FADIR) of the affected hip may cause groin pain in patients with anterior labral tears, while passive hip flexion, abduction, and external rotation (FABER, also known as Patrick's test) may cause posterior hip pain in patients with posterior labral tears. The scour test, in which the hip is axially loaded while passively and internally and externally rotating the hip in varying degrees of hip flexion and adduction/abduction, may also recreate pain. The Stinchfield test involves resisted hip flexion between 30–45 degrees while the knee is extended, which may recreate hip pain.

Diagnostic Workup Radiographs comprise the initial imaging workup and help rule out other possible causes of hip pain. AP pelvis, cross-table lateral, frog-leg lateral, Dunn, and false profile views are helpful in the radiographic assessment. Various radiographic measurements, including the lateral center-edge angle, anterior center-edge angle, Tönnis angle, and alpha angle, are used to assess the osseous anatomy of the hip. In hip dysplasia, inadequate acetabular coverage of the femoral head is recognized by low lateral center-edge angle and anterior center-edge angle (< 20°) and high Tönnis angle (> 10°). Patients with femoroacetabular impingement may have a high lateral center-edge angle (> 40°) or high anterior center-edge angle (> 45°), which indicates excessive acetabular coverage, or high alpha angle (> 50–60°), which indicates femoral bone prominence. MRI is the imaging modality of choice for the detection of labral tears, and MRI combined with arthrography has been shown to have superior sensitivity. If degenerative change in the form of arthritis is visible on X-ray, MRI generally does not change management and is not recommended for the sole purpose of diagnosing a labral tear.

Treatment Current literature suggests that non-operative management in the form of physical therapy, anti-inflammatory medications, and activity modification can improve pain and function in patients with labral tears, although there is no widely accepted protocol for nonoperative treatment. For patients with persistent pain, surgery is considered. Patients with labral tears are more frequently being treated with arthroscopic surgery, namely, for labral repair or reconstruction. Some studies have shown improved outcomes for patients with combined arthroscopic surgery and physical therapy compared to physical therapy alone. For patients with femoroacetabular impingement, acetabuloplasty and/or femoroplasty is performed to remove the bone causing impingement. Young patients with concomitant labral tear and hip dysplasia are most likely to benefit from combined labral repair and periacetabular osteotomy, which reorients the acetabulum and provides additional coverage of the femoral head. When degenerative osteoarthritis is present, hip preservation surgery is less likely to result in satisfactory outcomes, and hip arthroplasty may be considered.

References [27–33]

Sports Hernia

Description Sports hernias are overuse injuries caused by repetitive, chronic stress to the musculotendinous structures of the groin region. The term is a misnomer, as the condition is not caused by a defect in a wall of the body but is characterized by pain in the inguinal region. Pain in other nearby structures, including the iliopsoas, adductor longus, and pubic symphysis, can be variably present. Alternative names that have been used to describe a sports hernia include "athletic pubalgia" and "hockey groin," owing to the fact that the condition is more commonly found in athletes. They typically occur in sports in which the athletic stance is utilized, which describes a position of hip flexion, hip abduction, and knee flexion. Multiple etiologies have been proposed for sports hernias, but most agree upon the presence of abnormal strain in the inguinal canal. The imbalance between the opposing abdominal muscles and adductor muscles may contribute to chronic stress, overuse, and pain in this region. Irritation of the nearby ilioinguinal, iliohypogastric, and genital branch of the genitofemoral nerve can also contribute to pain. Femoroacetabular impingement may coincide and predispose to the development of a sports hernia.

Clinical Presentation Patients are often athletes who present with inguinal pain that may involve the pubic symphysis, rectus abdominis, and/or adductor longus. The pain can be aggravated by high-intensity activities such as kicking and sprinting, as well as by increases in intra-abdominal pressure caused by coughing and sneezing.

Physical Examination Tenderness at the inguinal region is present. Superficial inguinal ring palpation during a hernia exam may aggravate pain as well, although a true hernia is typically not identified. Having the patient perform a resisted sit-up often reproduces pain. Tenderness may also be present at the adductor longus origin, iliopsoas, and pubic symphysis. Resisted hip adduction can aggravate adductor longus pain, and passive extension of the hip can aggravate iliopsoas pain.

Diagnostic Workup Radiographs are obtained to rule out other causes of hip pain but are typically normal. MRI is the imaging modality of choice for most providers and may show strains or tears of the rectus abdominis, adductor longus, or pectineus. Evidence of edema within the pubic symphysis may be present. A large field of view is helpful in imaging the various structures that may be affected. A skilled ultrasonographer may be able to identify similar findings via ultrasound, and an injection with a local anesthetic can also help elucidate the diagnosis.

Treatment Initial treatment with aggravation avoidance, anti-inflammatory medications, and physical therapy is recommended. Physical therapy should focus on core and hip strengthening to help improve stability during functional movement. The recommended duration of attempted nonoperative treatment is variable, but if 2–6 months of physical therapy do not improve symptoms, surgery may be considered. The described surgical treatments are variable but may consist of hernia-type repair with or without mesh, adductor tenotomy, and/or nerve decompression, often dependent on the structures believed to be pathologically involved. Most studies show high rates of return to sport at a similar level of performance following recovery after surgery.

References [34–39]

Greater Trochanteric Pain Syndrome

Description Greater trochanteric pain syndrome encompasses a spectrum of conditions, including gluteus medius and minimus tendinopathy, trochanteric bursitis, and external coxa saltans. Historically, many patients with lateral hip pain had received the diagnosis of trochanteric bursitis, but an improved understanding of peritrochanteric pathology has shown that many of these patients may, in fact, be experiencing symptoms of gluteus medius and minimus pathology. These gluteal muscles are frequently referred to as the hip abductors, as one of their primary functions is to initiate hip abduction. They also function to help stabilize the femoral head within the acetabulum. Multiple fluid-filled bursae are present in the vicinity of the greater trochanter, which help to provide smooth gliding of soft tissue structures of the hip during movement. The subgluteus maximus bursa is located medial to the gluteus maximus and lateral to the greater trochanter and is the primary bursa involved in what is typically referred to as trochanteric bursitis. External coxa saltans entails snapping of the iliotibial band (ITB) over the greater trochanter when the hip transitions between flexion and extension.

Clinical Presentation Patients typically describe lateral hip pain in the region of the greater trochanter. Weight-bearing activities, bending and twisting, prolonged time in one position, and lying down on the affected side can aggravate the pain. The pain can also extend along the lateral thigh, along the ITB. Patients may describe their hip popping, snapping, or demonstrating other mechanical symptoms around the affected hip. ITB snapping is often described as the hip "dislocating."

Physical Examination A gait exam should be performed, which may reveal an antalgic or Trendelenburg gait. An antalgic gait describes a shortened stance phase of gait on the ipsilateral side. A Trendelenburg gait involves the leaning of the torso toward the ipsilateral side and the downward tilt of the pelvis on the contralateral side when the ipsilateral foot is in the stance phase of gait; it is the result of abductor weakness and the body's compensatory mechanisms to shift the center of gravity toward the affected hip. The greater trochanter on the affected side is typically tender to palpation, and tenderness at the lateral thigh along the ITB can also be present. Pain with resisted external derotation, in which the patient internally rotates the hip from an externally rotated position against the examiner's resistance, suggests gluteal tendinopathy. Lateral hip pain may occur with flexion, abduction, and external rotation (FABER) of the hip. Ober's test may be positive, which entails lateral pain or decreased hip adduction with gravity when the patient is positioned laterally with the affected side up. Palpable and visible snapping of the ITB may occur over the greater trochanter when the hip is actively moved between a flexed and extended position. Passive range of motion of the hip is often normal in isolated greater trochanteric pain syndrome, although patients may describe peritrochanteric pain during range of motion testing.

Diagnostic Workup Radiographs are used to help rule out other causes of pain that may radiate to the lateral hip, including osteoarthritis. Calcifications within the abductor tendons and/or peritrochanteric bursae may be visualized but are not specific nor necessary for the diagnosis of greater trochanteric pain syndrome. Ultrasonography may be helpful and allows for dynamic evaluation. Tenderness of the abductor tendons and snapping of the ITB may be observed during the exam. The most common finding in ultrasonography is gluteus medius and/or minimus tendinosis; ITB thickening and subgluteus maximus bursitis may also be observed. MRI is the gold standard imaging modality, with thickening and increased signal on T2-weighted images indicative of tendinosis. Varying degrees of tendon tears may be observed. An increased signal in the subgluteus maximus bursa is a sign of bursitis.

Treatment Initial treatment consists of anti-inflammatory medications, physical therapy, and corticosteroid injections, and this treatment regimen is successful in most patients. Injections may be administered with or without ultrasound guidance, but patients with large body habitus may be better served with ultrasound guidance for increased accuracy. Extracorporeal shockwave therapy has also been shown to improve pain and function in patients with greater trochanteric pain syndrome. Platelet-rich plasma (PRP) injections are derived from the patient's own blood and contain growth factors that may augment healing. While some studies show promising results from PRP injections, varying PRP formulations and preparation methods make comparing the results of multiple studies challenging. For patients with persistent symptoms despite 6–12 months of nonoperative treatment, surgery may be considered. Surgery is dependent on the pathological structures involved but typically involves abductor tendon repair or reconstruction, ITB release, and/or bursectomy. Both open and endoscopic techniques have been described with success.

References [40–46]

Hamstring Injuries

Description Hamstring injuries occur commonly in athletes and other active individuals but can also occur in patients who do not participate in sporting activities. Three muscles comprise the hamstrings: the semitendinosus, semimembranosus, and biceps femoris. Together, they act to extend the hip and flex the knee. A spectrum of injuries to the hamstrings exists, including hamstring tendinopathy, strains, and tendon tears. Most injuries occur at the myotendinous junction but may occur anywhere along the muscle-tendon unit. Proximal hamstring tendinopathy represents a chronic overuse injury to the hamstring origin at the ischial tuberosity. Hamstring muscle strains are common in athletes and are caused by eccentric load during hip flexion and knee extension. Tears of the hamstring origin can occur as partial tears or complete tears.

Clinical Presentation Hamstring injuries may present as acute or chronic problems. Proximal tendinopathy and tendon tears may be associated with complaints of pain in the buttock region, and prolonged sitting may aggravate the pain. The pain may also be present in the posterior thigh. Patients with acute development of symptoms may describe having experienced a pop in the hip or buttock at symptom onset; this may have occurred during running or jumping in athletes. The pain can also present with insidious onset and no clear injury mechanism.

Physical Examination A stiff-legged gait with avoidance of simultaneous hip flexion and knee extension on the affected side may be observed, as this combination of movements increases tension within the hamstrings. Tenderness at the ischial tuberosity is often present. Ecchymosis at the posterior thigh may be observed in patients with tendon tears, and a localized mass of retracted muscle may be palpable in patients with complete tendon tears. Hamstring strength can be tested by having the patient flex the knee from 90 degrees against resistance while in a prone position, and it may be decreased compared to the unaffected side. The modified bent knee stretch involves positioning the patient supine with the hip and knee maximally flexed, followed by the examiner rapidly extending the knee; if pain is experienced in the buttock or proximal posterior thigh, the test is considered positive and suggestive of a hamstring injury. Due to its proximity to the hamstrings, the sciatic nerve may be affected in acute or chronic hamstring injuries. As a result, tibial and peroneal nerve motor and sensory exams should be performed, and may reveal abnormalities such as a foot drop in rare cases.

Diagnostic Workup Radiographs may show avulsion of bone from the ischial tuberosity in some instances of hamstring tendon tears. Enthesophytes, which are proliferations of bone along soft tissue attachments, may be observed at the hamstring tendon origin in cases of chronic tendinopathy. However, in most cases of hamstring injury, radiographs are unremarkable. Ultrasonography may be used to help establish the diagnosis and allows for dynamic assessment during hamstring contraction. MRI is the imaging modality of choice for the definitive diagnosis of a hamstring injury. It allows for determining the grade of injury, which hamstring muscles are involved, and degree of retraction if a complete tear is present. Of note, hamstring pathology on imaging is highly prevalent in the general population and is often asymptomatic, and MRI is therefore typically reserved for when nonoperative treatment has been unsuccessful or if a complete tear is suspected.

Treatment An initial period of rest, ice, and anti-inflammatory medications, followed by physical therapy, is the recommended treatment for most low-grade hamstring injuries, particularly those occurring at the musculotendinous junction. An elastic wrap may be used to provide gentle compression. Isometric and eccentric strengthening, dynamic stretching, and neuromuscular training are among the common approaches used in rehabilitating the hamstrings. PRP injections have shown promise in some studies that have demonstrated lower pain scores and earlier return-to-play times, but other studies have shown no significant benefit. There is currently no consensus on the utility of PRP injections in the context of hamstring injuries. Ultrasound-guided corticosteroid injections may help improve pain and facilitate a return to play. While corticosteroid injections have largely been reported to be safe, there is theoretical concern for tendon rupture with repeated use, and these injections are generally used as an adjunct to other treatment if needed. Other treatment modalities, such as dry needling and extracorporeal shockwave therapy, have shown promise, but additional studies are necessary to establish their role in the treatment of hamstring injuries. For patients who have proximal avulsion injuries, 2+ tendon involvement and significant tendon retraction, or persistent symptoms despite several months of nonoperative treatment, surgical repair may be undertaken.

References [47–52]

Iliopsoas Syndrome

Description The iliopsoas is a powerful hip flexor and is composed of the iliacus and psoas major. Conditions that affect the iliopsoas can cause acute or chronic groin pain and can also cause painful snapping during movement of the hip. These conditions include iliopsoas tendinopathy, iliopsoas bursitis, and internal coxa saltans, and due to their frequent coexistence, the term "iliopsoas syndrome" has been used to describe them. Iliopsoas tendinopathy and bursitis are commonly believed to occur due to abnormal snapping of the iliopsoas tendon over the iliopectineal eminence or femoral head, which causes chronic microtrauma to the iliopsoas tendon and inflammation of the intervening iliopsoas bursa. Prior hip surgery can also predispose to iliopsoas pathology. Coxa saltans describes the snapping hip, with iliopsoas-related snapping considered the internal variety. External coxa saltans refers to the snapping of the ITB over the greater trochanter of the femur and is discussed in the greater trochanteric pain syndrome section.

Clinical Presentation Patients experiencing iliopsoas pathology are frequently athletes who may participate in soccer, hockey, or dance. Symptoms may or may not be preceded by trauma or hip surgery. Patients often describe groin pain, which may be aggravated by lifting the leg or by kicking motions in athletes. Painful snapping in the hip during movement may also be described. This may occur during athletic activities, but can also occur during positional changes and ambulation. Patients sometimes complain of concomitant low back pain, which can be aggravated by stiffness of the iliopsoas.

Physical Examination Active movement of the affected hip from a flexed, abducted, externally rotated (FABER) position to an extended, adducted, internally rotated position may recreate hip snapping. In some cases, the snapping may be audible. With the patient seated, active flexion of the hip against the examiner's resistance may cause groin pain. The modified Thomas test may be used to assess hip flexor tightness; with the patient lying supine with the gluteal folds at the edge of the bed and legs off the bed, the unaffected leg is supported with the patient's hands at 90 degrees of hip flexion. The affected hip is allowed to extend, and if the thigh does not fall parallel to the table, then iliopsoas tightness may be present. When assessing for iliopsoas snapping, external coxa saltans should be ruled out, which may be detected by palpable snapping of the ITB over the greater trochanter during hip flexion and extension.

Diagnostic Workup Radiographs are frequently normal but may be obtained to rule out other hip pathologies. For patients with ipsilateral total hip arthroplasty, a cross-table lateral X-ray helps assess for possible anterior prominence of the acetabular component, which may result in iliopsoas irritation. Ultrasound may be used to confirm the diagnosis and may demonstrate snapping of the iliopsoas tendon during movement from the FABER position to extension, adduction, and internal rotation. MRI is typically unnecessary, but may show increased signal in T2-weighted images consistent with iliopsoas bursitis, and may also be used to rule out intra-articular pathology as the cause for hip pain. Iliopsoas bursography, which entails injection of contrast into the iliopsoas bursa, may reveal snapping back and forth under fluoroscopy during provocative testing.

Treatment Patients with iliopsoas syndrome are often successfully treated nonoperatively. Painless audible popping requires no specific treatment and may be observed. For painful iliopsoas syndrome, activity modification and physical therapy are the mainstays of treatment. Rehabilitation may entail progression from isometric to eccentric and concentric strengthening, neuromuscular training, and a stretching regimen. Manual therapy and posture correction may also be employed. Corticosteroid injections may be used adjunctly to help reduce pain and inflammation. While most patients improve with a nonoperative regimen, those with persistent symptoms despite several months of treatment may benefit from an orthopedic referral for possible iliopsoas lengthening or release.

References [53–58]

Meralgia Paresthetica

Description Meralgia paresthetica is a compressive neuropathy of the lateral femoral cutaneous nerve (LFCN). The term is derived from the Greek words *meros*, meaning "thigh," and *algos*, meaning "pain." The LFCN is a sensory nerve that typically originates from the L1 to L3 nerve roots and follows a retroperitoneal path along the ilium toward the anterior superior iliac spine (ASIS). The nerve has been found to have variable courses as it passes the inguinal ligament to the anterior thigh, and this region is where compression most commonly occurs in symptomatic patients. Distally, it branches into anterior and posterior divisions that innervate the anterior and lateral thigh, respectively. Meralgia paresthetica can affect patients of all ages and may occur spontaneously or iatrogenically after surgery. Anatomic variations, where the nerve traverses lateral to the ASIS or is enveloped by the inguinal ligament or sartorius tendon, may predispose to meralgia paresthetica. Compression from tight clothing, pregnancy, large body habitus, and tumors can also lead to symptoms.

Clinical Presentation A thorough history should be obtained to identify risk factors for nerve compression, including recent weight gain, pregnancy, use of tight clothing or belts, repetitive heavy lifting, recent trauma, and previous surgery. Patients often describe pain, tingling, and/or numbness at the anterolateral thigh. Some patients may describe increased sensitivity to light touch in this area. Activity involving repetitive hip extension, including prolonged walking, may aggravate the pain. Patients may describe trying to massage the area to improve symptoms, typically without success. The diagnosis of meralgia paresthetica is supported only by symptoms that occur in the anterolateral thigh; posterior thigh or distal leg symptoms should prompt consideration of alternative diagnoses such as lumbosacral spine or plexus pathology.

Physical Examination Diminished sensation to light touch and/or pinprick in the anterolateral thigh may be present. Tapping the lateral aspect of the inguinal ligament (just inferomedial to the ASIS) may reproduce symptoms, indicating a positive Tinel's sign. However, due to anatomic variability of the LFCN as it crosses the inguinal ligament, Tinel's sign may be negative. The Valsalva maneuver may also reproduce symptoms. Strength and reflex testing of the lower extremity is normal.

Diagnostic Workup The diagnosis of meralgia paresthetica is primarily clinical. However, in uncertain cases, electrodiagnostic studies may be obtained. Nerve conduction studies may be abnormal, and when performed, testing of the unaffected side is also recommended to improve test sensitivity. Needle electromyography (EMG) is normal, and an abnormal EMG suggests an alternate diagnosis. An ultrasound-guided injection of local anesthetic and/or corticosteroid can also be both diagnostic and therapeutic. Imaging is typically unnecessary for diagnosis, but lumbar spine or plexus MRI may be helpful in ruling out radiculopathy as the cause of symptoms.

Treatment Meralgia paresthetica is often successfully treated without surgery. Treatment is aimed at the cause of compression. Weight loss, avoidance of tight belts and clothing, and padding the area for occupation-related compression can be helpful. Pregnancy-induced symptoms often improve after delivery. Anti-inflammatory medications, anticonvulsants, and antidepressants may be used as adjunctive treatment. An ultrasound-guided injection may provide temporary relief. Occasionally, persistent symptoms may prompt surgical treatment, which entails neurolysis or neurectomy. Neurolysis involves the release of structures compressing the nerve, while neurectomy entails transecting and excising a portion of the nerve. Neurolysis poses the advantage of maintaining the sensory function of the nerve, but some studies show lower rates of symptom resolution compared to neurectomy.

Neurectomy may be more reliable, but it results in permanent loss of sensation in the region innervated by the LFCN. To date, there is no clear consensus on which surgical approach is recommended.

References [59–63]

Transient Osteoporosis of the Hip

Description Transient osteoporosis of the hip is typically a self-limiting disease that, as the name implies, is characterized by a temporary reduction in bone density of the femoral head. It has sometimes also been referred to as regional migratory osteoporosis, bone marrow edema syndrome, and reflex sympathetic dystrophy. Patients across a wide spectrum of ages may be affected, but men with the disease are commonly middle-aged, while women are often in the third trimester of pregnancy. While many etiologies have been proposed, no consensus on pathogenesis exists to date.

Clinical Presentation Patients may otherwise be healthy, without clear predisposition for acute or degenerative hip conditions. The onset of pain may be acute or insidious and is typically not associated with a history of recent trauma to the hip. Unilateral occurrence is most common, but pain may occur bilaterally in some patients. The location of pain is often the groin and/or thigh. Weight-bearing activity tends to aggravate the pain. Patients may describe noticing a limp and may have resolved to using crutches or other assistive devices to avoid weight-bearing on the affected side. Popping, catching, locking, and other mechanical symptoms are atypical and, if described, suggest alternative explanations for hip pain.

Physical Examination Patients may demonstrate an antalgic gait. A full range of motion of the hip is typically present, with pain only observed at extremes of internal and/or external rotation of the hip. Crepitus and mechanical symptoms are typically not observed during range of motion testing.

Diagnostic Workup Radiographs of the hip may be normal in early stages but may reveal demineralization of the femoral head and neck if symptoms have been present for several weeks. There is a notable lack of joint space narrowing, subchondral cysts, and osteophyte formation, which are typical of osteoarthritis. Bone scintigraphy has largely been replaced by MRI as the diagnostic modality of choice, but it can show increased radionuclide uptake in the femoral head prior to the development of changes on x-rays, owing to the increased capillary permeability and osteoblast activity. MRI shows low signal intensity on T1-weighted images and high signal intensity on T2-weighted images. While other causes of hip pain, such as osteonecrosis or septic arthritis, may show similar findings on MRI, osteonecrosis may demonstrate areas of low signal intensity alternating with high signal intensity on T2-weighted images, while septic arthritis typically shows synovial enhancement, large joint effusion, and periarticular soft tissue involvement.

Treatment Transient osteoporosis of the hip typically resolves with time, but fracture secondary to reduced bone mineral density can rarely occur. To reduce this risk, patients are treated with partial weight-bearing precautions, often with the use of crutches. Oral medications such as acetaminophen and nonsteroidal anti-inflammatory drugs can help manage pain. Resolution of symptoms can take 3–6 months and sometimes longer. Treatment with bisphosphonates and calcitonin may increase the rate of recovery, with some studies showing resolution in 1–2 months. However, it must be noted that bisphosphonate treatment during pregnancy can affect fetal skeletal mineralization and cause other hazardous effects; conversely, calcitonin does not cross the placenta and is considered safe during pregnancy. Calcium and vitamin D supplementation is also recommended, particularly when a deficiency is present. Surgery is not indicated for transient osteoporosis of the hip.

References [64–68]

Hip Pointer

Description Hip pointers are iliac crest contusions, commonly due to blunt trauma during sporting activities. Subperiosteal edema and hematoma in surrounding soft tissue may be associated findings. Contact sports such as American football, hockey, and lacrosse are more likely to precipitate this injury. Hip pointers can be exquisitely painful and may lead to missed training time or games.

Clinical Presentation Symptoms are typically preceded by a direct blow to the iliac crest, such as a tackle or a fall to the ground. Pain and tenderness are often described in the iliac crest and lateral hip region, and patients may describe an inability to bear weight on the ipsilateral extremity.

Physical Examination Patients may demonstrate an antalgic gait. Bruising and tenderness to palpation of the iliac crest are often present. Active and passive range of motion of the hip, as well as flexion, extension, and rotation of the lumbar spine, may reproduce pain.

Diagnostic Workup Radiographs of the hip are normal, but may be obtained to rule out other injuries such as fractures. Ultrasound may show subperiosteal fluid and/or hematoma in the surrounding gluteal musculature. MRI is typically unnecessary, particularly in cases with a clear mechanism of injury, consistent physical exam, and unremarkable radiographs.

Treatment Compressive wrapping and cryotherapy should be initiated immediately to help reduce the risk of swelling at the affected area. If there is concern for a substantial hematoma, an ultrasound-guided aspiration of the hematoma may be considered to help improve pain and reduce the risk of heterotopic ossification, although this is typically unnecessary. An injection containing corticosteroid and local anesthetic may be used at the iliac crest to facilitate recovery and return to play. If return to play and normalization of gait does not return quickly, crutches may be used for comfort. Physical therapy for hip strengthening and mobility may be initiated after the acute pain and swelling have sufficiently resolved. Adequate padding to the iliac crest in athletic uniforms may help to reduce the risk of hip pointers.

References [69–72]

Hip Fractures and Dislocations

Description Hip fractures are proximal femur fractures that can be categorized as intracapsular (femoral head and neck) or extracapsular based on location with respect to the hip joint capsule. Their incidence occurs in a bimodal distribution, with younger patients typically sustaining fractures due to high-energy trauma and older patients often experiencing low-energy mechanisms such as ground-level falls. Hip dislocations are dissociations of the femoral head from the acetabulum and are less common than fractures but may occur in conjunction with a fracture or in isolation. The urgent reduction of dislocations is vital to reduce the risk of osteonecrosis of the femoral head. Most dislocations are characterized by posterior positioning of the femoral head with respect to the acetabulum, although anterior dislocations also occur. Conversely, stress fractures of the femoral neck are not caused by acute trauma but are more insidious injuries caused by repetitive loading and microscopic fractures that accumulate over time. The blood supply to the femoral head and neck is intimately tied to the outcome of fractures in this location and, therefore, to the treatment options for these injuries. The primary blood supply of the adult hip is derived from the retinacular arteries branching from the medial femoral circumflex artery, which are more likely to be disrupted in more significantly displaced femoral neck fractures. Damage to the femoral head blood supply increases the risk of femoral head osteonecrosis. For both intracapsular and extracapsular fractures, treatment that allows early return to mobility is crucial for reducing the risk of morbidity and mortality.

Clinical Presentation Trauma in the form of a fall or motor vehicle collision often precedes pain in complete fractures. Hip dislocations are typically the result of high-energy trauma such as a motor vehicle collision, when dashboard impact to the knee can exert a posteriorly-directed force on the femoral head. Patients may complain of pain in the groin, the general hip region, the thigh, and/or the knee with both fractures and dislocations. Pain may be worse with weight-bearing or may preclude weight-bearing altogether. In contrast, stress fractures of the femoral neck may be associated with prior extensive running or other increases in physical training volume and are usually characterized by a more gradual onset of pain. In later stages, stress fracture pain may also occur at rest and/or at night. If completion of a stress fracture occurs, patients may describe a pop in the hip and subsequent increased pain.

Physical Examination Patients may be unable to place weight on the affected extremity or exhibit an antalgic gait. Many patients with fractures present without obvious deformity, but displaced fractures may result in the affected leg resting in a shortened and externally rotated position. Rotation and axial loading of the hip results in significant groin, thigh, and/or knee pain in the case of complete fractures, whereas less severe pain may be encountered with stress fractures. A neurovascular examination should be performed, although major nerve or blood vessel injury is uncommon in isolated proximal femur fractures. However, a thorough neurovascular exam is critical in patients with hip dislocations, which demonstrate higher rates of sciatic nerve injury. Patients with hip dislocations may present with the affected leg flexed, adducted, and internally rotated (posterior dislocation), or extended, abducted, and externally rotated (anterior dislocation).

Diagnostic Workup AP pelvis, AP hip, and lateral hip views should be obtained. A cross-table lateral can often easily be obtained even in patients with fractures and/or dislocations and can be performed by flexing the unaffected leg at the hip and knee to allow for an X-ray beam parallel to the table. Radiographs of the femur are helpful in ruling out more distal femur fractures. CT may be used for select fractures to better characterize morphology for treatment planning, such as in the case of femoral head fractures. Simple hip dislocations (without fracture) that are identified on radiographs do not require further imaging prior to hip reduction, and reduction should not be delayed for further imaging.

Stress fractures are typically associated with normal radiographs in the early stages, but a linear lucency with surrounding sclerosis may appear in later stages. If radiographs are unremarkable and there is suspicion of a stress fracture, an MRI should be obtained. MRI shows high signal intensity in the femoral neck on T2-weighted images, and the presence of a dark line perpendicular to the femoral cortex differentiates a stress fracture from a stress reaction. A hip effusion may also be present. Bone scintigraphy of stress fractures shows increased radioisotope uptake in the femoral neck but has largely been replaced by MRI as the recommended diagnostic study.

Treatment Nearly all complete and incomplete (not involving the entire width of the femoral neck) hip fractures require surgical treatment to restore mobility and reduce the risk of complications, with the exception of moribund patients and non-ambulatory patients with minimal pain. Femoral head fractures located inferior to the fovea and minimally displaced fractures superior to the fovea may be treated without surgery if loose osteochondral fragments within the joint are not present.

Surgery is recommended for displaced fractures, when intra-articular loose fragments are noted on imaging, and when associated femoral neck or acetabulum fractures are present. Complete and incomplete femoral neck fractures are treated either with fracture reduction and fixation or with hip arthroplasty, often depending on patient age. Extracapsular fractures in the intertrochanteric and subtrochanteric regions are treated with reduction and fixation. Most surgeons agree that surgery should proceed as soon as safely possible to facilitate early mobility and reduce the risk of medical complications, including mortality.

Simple hip dislocations should be treated with urgent closed reduction, ideally less than 6 h from the time of injury. Reduction entails sedation and traction of the hip in line with the deformity (flexion in posterior dislocations, extension in anterior dislocations), often performed in the emergency department. A CT of the hip should be obtained after reduction to assess for concentric reduction and rule out fractures and incarcerated fragments within the joint. Dislocations associated with an ipsilateral femoral neck fracture should not be treated with closed reduction and warrant operative fixation and reduction.

Femoral neck stress reactions (increased signal intensity on T2-weighted images) without distinct fracture on MRI may be treated with non-weight-bearing for 6 weeks, followed by progressive weight-bearing if symptoms improve. Stress fractures that occur on the compression side (inferior aspect) of the femoral neck and span less than 50% of the width of the neck may be treated similarly, but if symptoms persist or the fracture progresses on repeat imaging, surgical fixation is recommended. Patients with compression-sided fractures with a width of 50% or greater, patients with tension-sided (superior aspect of the neck) fractures, and patients with an associated hip effusion should undergo surgical fixation due to the risk of fracture progression.

References [73–78]

Tumors

Description Tumors of the hip can affect patients of all ages, with specific tumors occurring more commonly in certain age groups. Primary bone tumors, which are tumors that originate within the bone, can occur in both the pelvis and the femur. Bone is also one of the most common sites of metastatic disease, and the proximal femur is one of the most common locations of skeletal metastasis. Cancer cells metastasize via multiple mechanisms that facilitate immune system avoidance, tissue invasion, angiogenesis, and reduced cell death. Metastatic cells can cause lytic or blastic lesions by modulating the activity of osteoblasts and osteoclasts. Metastatic lesions most commonly originate from breast, lung, thyroid, kidney, or prostate cancer. The spectrum of oncologic disease that can occur in the hip region is broad, and a comprehensive review is beyond the scope of this chapter, but the practitioner evaluating hip pain should be aware of signs, symptoms, and imaging findings that may indicate the presence of metastasis or sarcoma. Definitive diagnosis typically requires a biopsy for histological examination.

Clinical Presentation Symptoms are dependent on the type, size, and location of the tumor. Some patients are asymptomatic and may present with only incidental findings on imaging. Others may complain of hip pain, which can be worse with weight-bearing and/or at night. Large pelvic tumors can result in symptoms of bowel and/or bladder obstruction. Some patients may describe constitutional symptoms such as fevers, night sweats, and weight loss. Pathologic fractures through weakened bone can occur even in the absence of trauma and often result in immediate pain and an inability to stand or walk.

Physical Examination An antalgic gait may be present, and in the case of a pathologic fracture, the patient may be unable to place weight on the affected area. Passive rotation and axial loading of the hip may aggravate pain. Swelling and tenderness to palpation are variably present. In patients with only incidental findings on imaging, physical examination may be unremarkable.

Diagnostic Workup Radiographs of the pelvis and/or hip should be obtained. Depending on the type of tumor present, lesions seen on an X-ray may be lytic, blastic, or mixed. Lytic lesions are regions of bone resorption that result in the appearance of thinned or absent bone. Blastic lesions are regions of increased bone formation that appear more dense on radiographs. Reactive cortical thickening or destruction of bone cortices may be present. In general, more aggressive lesions are characterized by ill-defined margins due to inadequate time for bone to remodel, whereas less aggressive lesions are associated with well-defined margins. Tumors derived from cartilage cells may demonstrate "popcorn calcifications," which describe amorphous calcifications in rings or arcs that resemble popcorn. A "sunburst" or "hair-on-end" appearance of bony spicules extending perpendicular to the bone, as well as raised periosteum known as "Codman's triangle," are often seen in osteosarcoma. An "onion skin" appearance of periosteum may be present in Ewing sarcoma. CT of the chest, abdomen, and pelvis to evaluate for the primary source is recommended for patients suspected of metastatic disease, such as those over the age of 50 with a bone lesion. MRI is often helpful in further characterizing the lesion and determining the extent of involvement. Lab work, including complete blood count, basic metabolic panel, electrolyte panel, and serum/urine protein electrophoresis, can contribute to the workup, and biopsy often provides a definitive diagnosis.

Treatment Treatment of tumors of the pelvis and proximal femur is dependent on tumor type and extent of bony destruction. Benign lesions such as osteoid osteoma and osteochondroma may be initially managed without surgery. Unicameral bone cysts and fibrous dysplasia are also benign entities, but may require surgical fixation if impending fracture is a concern. The Mirels classification can be used to help guide prophylactic treatment of impending fractures from benign and metastatic

Table 13.2 Mirels classification. Prophylactic fixation is typically considered for a cumulative score of 8 or greater

Score	1	2	3
Site	Upper extremity	Lower extremity	Peritrochanteric
Pain	Mild	Moderate	Functional
Appearance	Blastic	Mixed	Lytic
Size (proportion of bone diameter)	$< \frac{1}{3}$	$\frac{1}{3} - \frac{2}{3}$	$> \frac{2}{3}$

lesions and is based on lesion location, size, appearance (lytic, blastic, or mixed), and pain (Table 13.2). Importantly, biopsy to rule out primary neoplasm should precede prophylactic fixation of impending fractures, as fixation without biopsy can result in iatrogenic contamination of the bone with sarcoma. Pathologic fractures of the femoral head or neck are typically treated with arthroplasty, whereas peritrochanteric fractures are typically treated with intramedullary fixation. Sarcomas that occur most frequently in the proximal femur include chondrosarcoma, osteosarcoma, Ewing sarcoma, and fibrosarcoma; treatment entails surgery, often coupled with chemotherapy, except in most cases of chondrosarcoma.

References [79–86]

Takeaways

- Osteoarthritis of the hip is a degenerative condition that can result in debilitating pain. Initial treatment consists of nonsteroidal anti-inflammatory medications, physical therapy, and injections. If pain persists, total hip arthroplasty may be considered.
- Osteonecrosis of the hip is caused by an insult to the blood supply to the femoral head. Core decompression may help improve pain and slow disease progression in patients without femoral head collapse, but total hip arthroplasty is often preferred if collapse is present.
- Inflammatory arthropathies include multiple conditions, including rheumatoid arthritis, seronegative spondyloarthropathies, and crystal arthropathies. Treatment involves pharmacologic therapy aimed at the specific etiology.
- Septic arthritis is an orthopedic emergency that requires urgent surgical irrigation and debridement to maximize the likelihood of cartilage viability.
- Femoroacetabular impingement is caused by abnormal bony contact due to excess bone, whereas hip dysplasia is a lack of adequate bony coverage of the femoral head. Both diagnoses can predispose to labral tears and hip pain. Surgery aims to normalize bone contact, but if arthritis develops, arthroplasty may be recommended.
- Sports hernias are chronic overuse injuries to the inguinal region. Initial treatment is centered around physical therapy, but surgery may be considered for unremitting symptoms.

- Greater trochanteric pain syndrome includes abductor tendon pathology, trochanteric bursitis, and external coxa saltans. Anti-inflammatory medications, physical therapy, and injections are successful in treating most patients.
- Hamstring injuries can occur in both athletes and sedentary patients. Many can be treated nonsurgically, but patients with proximal avulsions or retracted, multiple-tendon tears are more likely to benefit from surgery.
- Iliopsoas syndrome includes iliopsoas tendinopathy, iliopsoas bursitis, and internal coxa saltans. Most patients improve with physical therapy.
- Meralgia paresthetica is caused by compression of the lateral femoral cutaneous nerve. Removing the cause of compression provides relief to most patients, but persistent symptoms may warrant neurolysis or neurectomy.
- Transient osteoporosis of the hip can cause significant pain, even in otherwise healthy patients, but is typically self-limiting.
- Hip pointers are iliac crest contusions caused by direct trauma. Ice, compression, and an injection can help facilitate recovery.
- Hip fractures occur most commonly in young patients due to high-energy trauma and in older patients due to falls. Stress fractures can occur due to repetitive excess loading, such as from physical training. Complete and incomplete proximal femur fractures should undergo surgical treatment in almost all patients. Stress fractures may warrant prophylactic fixation if certain radiologic criteria are met or if pain worsens or persists despite nonoperative treatment.
- Multiple benign and cancerous tumors can occur in the hip region. Lesions that are identified on radiographs warrant further workup, and a definitive diagnosis typically requires biopsy.

References

1. Bannuru RR, Osani MC, Vaysbrot EE, Arden NK, Bennell K, Bierma-Zeinstra SMA, Kraus VB, Lohmander LS, Abbott JH, Bhandari M, Blanco FJ, Espinosa R, Haugen IK, Lin J, Mandl LA, Moilanen E, Nakamura N, Snyder-Mackler L, Trojian T, Underwood M, McAlindon TE. OARSI guidelines for the non-surgical management of knee, hip, and polyarticular osteoarthritis. Osteoarthr Cartil. 2019;27(11):1578.
2. Ganz R, Leunig M, Leunig-Ganz K, Harris WH. The etiology of osteoarthritis of the hip: an integrated mechanical concept. Clin Orthop Relat Res. 2008;466(2):264.
3. Jeldi AJ, Deakin AH, Allen DJ, Granat MH, Grant M, Stansfield BW. Total hip arthroplasty improves pain and function but not physical activity. J Arthroplasty. 2017;32(7):2191.
4. Katz JN, Arant KR, Loeser RF. Diagnosis and treatment of hip and knee osteoarthritis: a review. JAMA. 2021;325(6):568.
5. Learmonth ID, Young C, Rorabeck C. The operation of the century: total hip replacement. Lancet. 2007;370(9597):1508.
6. Metcalfe D, Perry DC, Claireaux HA, Simel DL, Zogg CK, Costa ML. Does this patient have hip osteoarthritis?: the rational clinical examination systematic review. JAMA. 2019;322(23):2323.
7. Quinn RH, Murray J, Pezold R, Hall Q. Management of osteoarthritis of the hip. J Am Acad Orthop Surg. 2018;26(20):e434.
8. Cohen-Rosenblum A, Cui Q. Osteonecrosis of the femoral head. Orthop Clin North Am. 2019;50(2):139.

9. Issa K, Pivec R, Kapadia BH, Banerjee S, Mont MA. Osteonecrosis of the femoral head: the total hip replacement solution. Bone Joint J. 2013;95-B(11 Suppl A):46.
10. Mont MA, Salem HS, Piuzzi NS, Goodman SB, Jones LC. Nontraumatic osteonecrosis of the femoral head: where do we stand today?: a 5-year update. J Bone Joint Surg Am. 2020;102(12):1084.
11. Petek D, Hannouche D, Suva D. Osteonecrosis of the femoral head: pathophysiology and current concepts of treatment. EFORT Open Rev. 2019;4(3):85.
12. Petrigliano FA, Lieberman JR. Osteonecrosis of the hip: novel approaches to evaluation and treatment. Clin Orthop Relat Res. 2007;465:53.
13. Zalavras CG, Lieberman JR. Osteonecrosis of the femoral head: evaluation and treatment. J Am Acad Orthop Surg. 2014;22(7):455.
14. Aletaha D, Smolen JS. Diagnosis and management of rheumatoid arthritis: a review. JAMA. 2018;320(13):1360.
15. Duba AS, Mathew SD. The seronegative spondyloarthropathies. Prim Care. 2018;45(2):271.
16. Hainer BL, Matheson E, Wilkes RT. Diagnosis, treatment, and prevention of gout. Am Fam Physician. 2014;90(12):831.
17. Jubber A, Moorthy A. Reactive arthritis: a clinical review. J R Coll Physicians Edinb. 2021;51(3):288.
18. Liu JT, Yeh HM, Liu SY, Chen KT. Psoriatic arthritis: epidemiology, diagnosis, and treatment. World J Orthop. 2014;5(4):537.
19. Scott DL, Wolfe F, Huizinga TW. Rheumatoid arthritis. Lancet. 2010;376(9746):1094.
20. Sidari A, Hill E. Diagnosis and treatment of gout and pseudogout for everyday practice. Prim Care. 2018;45(2):213.
21. Zhu W, He X, Cheng K, Zhang L, Chen D, Wang X, Qiu G, Cao X, Weng X. Ankylosing spondylitis: etiology, pathogenesis, and treatments. Bone Res. 2019;7:22.
22. Balato G, de Matteo V, Ascione T, de Giovanni R, Marano E, Rizzo M, Mariconda M. Management of septic arthritis of the hip joint in adults. A systematic review of the literature. BMC Musculoskelet Disord. 2021;22(Suppl 2):1006.
23. D'Angelo F, Monestier L, Zagra L. Active septic arthritis of the hip in adults: what's new in the treatment? A systematic review. EFORT Open Rev. 2021;6(3):164.
24. Davis CM, Zamora RA. Surgical options and approaches for septic arthritis of the native hip and knee joint. J Arthroplasty. 2020;35(3S):S14.
25. de Darren SA, Cargnelli S, Catapano M, Peterson D, Simunovic N, Larson CM, Ayeni OR. Efficacy of hip arthroscopy for the management of septic arthritis: a systematic review. Arthroscopy. 2015;31(7):1358.
26. Margaretten ME, Kohlwes J, Moore D, Bent S. Does this adult patient have septic arthritis? JAMA. 2007;297(13):1478.
27. Amanatullah DF, Antkowiak T, Pillay K, Patel J, Refaat M, Toupadakis CA, Jamali AA. Femoroacetabular impingement: current concepts in diagnosis and treatment. Orthopedics. 2015;38(3):185.
28. Bedi A, Kelly BT. Femoroacetabular impingement. J Bone Joint Surg Am. 2013;95(1):82.
29. Gala L, Clohisy JC, Beaule PE. Hip dysplasia in the young adult. J Bone Joint Surg Am. 2016;98(1):63.
30. Ganz R, Parvizi J, Beck M, Leunig M, Notzli H, Siebenrock KA. Femoroacetabular impingement: a cause for osteoarthritis of the hip. Clin Orthop Relat Res. 2003;(417):112.
31. Harris JD, Lewis BD, Park KJ. Hip Dysplasia. Clin Sports Med. 2021;40(2):271.
32. Kirsch JM, Khan M, Bedi A. Does hip arthroscopy have a role in the treatment of developmental hip dysplasia? J Arthroplasty. 2017;32(9S):S28.
33. Reiman MP, Goode AP, Cook CE, Holmich P, Thorborg K. Diagnostic accuracy of clinical tests for the diagnosis of hip femoroacetabular impingement/labral tear: a systematic review with meta-analysis. Br J Sports Med. 2015;49(12):811.
34. Drager J, Rasio J, Newhouse A. Athletic Pubalgia (Sports Hernia): presentation and treatment. Arthroscopy. 2020;36(12):2952.

35. Farber AJ, Wilckens JH. Sports hernia: diagnosis and therapeutic approach. J Am Acad Orthop Surg. 2007;15(8):507.
36. Hopkins JN, Brown W, Lee CA. Sports hernia: definition, evaluation, and treatment. JBJS Rev. 2017;5(9):e6.
37. Kraeutler MJ, Mei-Dan O, Belk JW, Larson CM, Talishinskiy T, Scillia AJ. A systematic review shows high variation in terminology, surgical techniques, preoperative diagnostic measures, and geographic differences in the treatment of athletic pubalgia/sports hernia/core muscle injury/inguinal disruption. Arthroscopy. 2021;37(7):2377.
38. Minnich JM, Hanks JB, Muschaweck U, Brunt LM, Diduch DR. Sports hernia: diagnosis and treatment highlighting a minimal repair surgical technique. Am J Sports Med. 2011;39(6):1341.
39. Zuckerbraun BS, Cyr AR, Mauro CS. Groin pain syndrome known as sports hernia: a review. JAMA Surg. 2020;155(4):340.
40. Barratt PA, Brookes N, Newson A. Conservative treatments for greater trochanteric pain syndrome: a systematic review. Br J Sports Med. 2017;51(2):97.
41. Gazendam A, Ekhtiari S, Axelrod D, Gouveia K, Gyemi L, Ayeni O, Bhandari M. Comparative efficacy of nonoperative treatments for greater trochanteric pain syndrome: a systematic review and network meta-analysis of randomized controlled trials. Clin J Sport Med. 2022;32(4):427.
42. Heaver C, Pinches M, Kuiper JH, Thomas G, Lewthwaite S, Burston BJ, Banerjee RD. Greater trochanteric pain syndrome: focused shockwave therapy versus an ultrasound guided injection: a randomised control trial. Hip Int. 2023;33(3):490.
43. Lustenberger DP, Ng VY, Best TM, Ellis TJ. Efficacy of treatment of trochanteric bursitis: a systematic review. Clin J Sport Med. 2011;21(5):447.
44. Mallow M, Nazarian LN. Greater trochanteric pain syndrome diagnosis and treatment. Phys Med Rehabil Clin N Am. 2014;25(2):279.
45. Redmond JM, Chen AW, Domb BG. Greater trochanteric pain syndrome. J Am Acad Orthop Surg. 2016;24(4):231.
46. Reid D. The management of greater trochanteric pain syndrome: a systematic literature review. J Orthop. 2016;13(1):15.
47. Chang JS, Kayani B, Plastow R, Singh S, Magan A, Haddad FS. Management of hamstring injuries: current concepts review. Bone Joint J. 2020;102-B(10):1281.
48. Fletcher AN, Cheah JW, Nho SJ, Mather RC 3rd. Proximal hamstring injuries. Clin Sports Med. 2021;40(2):339.
49. Goom TS, Malliaras P, Reiman MP, Purdam CR. Proximal hamstring tendinopathy: clinical aspects of assessment and management. J Orthop Sports Phys Ther. 2016;46(6):483.
50. Marigi EM, Cummings PE, Marigi IM, Burgos W, Gillett J, Camp CL, Krych AJ, Okoroha KR. Hamstring injuries: critical analysis review of current nonoperative treatments. JBJS Rev. 2022;10(11):Article e22.00095.
51. Pietrzak JR, Kayani B, Tahmassebi J, Haddad FS. Proximal hamstring tendinopathy: pathophysiology, diagnosis and treatment. Br J Hosp Med (Lond). 2018;79(7):389.
52. Thompson SM, Fung S, Wood DG. The prevalence of proximal hamstring pathology on MRI in the asymptomatic population. Knee Surg Sports Traumatol Arthrosc. 2017;25(1):108.
53. Anderson CN. Iliopsoas: pathology, diagnosis, and treatment. Clin Sports Med. 2016;35(3):419.
54. Capogna BM, Shenoy K, Youm T, Stuchin SA. Tendon disorders after total hip arthroplasty: evaluation and management. J Arthroplasty. 2017;32(10):3249.
55. Johnston CA, Wiley JP, Lindsay DM, Wiseman DA. Iliopsoas bursitis and tendinitis. A review. Sports Med. 1998;25(4):271.
56. Lifshitz L, Bar Sela S, Gal N, Martin R, Fleitman KM. Iliopsoas the hidden muscle: anatomy, diagnosis, and treatment. Curr Sports Med Rep. 2020;19(6):235.
57. Sugranes J, Jackson GR, Warrier AA, Allahabadi S, Chahla J. Snapping hip syndrome: pathoanatomy, diagnosis, nonoperative therapy, and current concepts in operative management. JBJS Rev. 2023;11(6)
58. Yen YM, Lewis CL, Kim YJ. Understanding and treating the snapping hip. Sports Med Arthrosc Rev. 2015;23(4):194.
59. Grossman MG, Ducey SA, Nadler SS, Levy AS. Meralgia paresthetica: diagnosis and treatment. J Am Acad Orthop Surg. 2001;9(5):336.

60. Gurbuz H, Gultekin A. Medical and surgical treatment of meralgia paresthetica. Pain Manag. 2021;11(4):389.
61. Harney D, Patijn J. Meralgia paresthetica: diagnosis and management strategies. Pain Med. 2007;8(8):669.
62. Khalil N, Nicotra A, Rakowicz W. Treatment for meralgia paraesthetica. Cochrane Database Syst Rev. 2012;12(12):CD004159.
63. Tagliafico A, Serafini G, Lacelli F, Perrone N, Valsania V, Martinoli C. Ultrasound-guided treatment of meralgia paresthetica (lateral femoral cutaneous neuropathy): technical description and results of treatment in 20 consecutive patients. J Ultrasound Med. 2011;30(10):1341.
64. Asadipooya K, Graves L, Greene LW. Transient osteoporosis of the hip: review of the literature. Osteoporos Int. 1805;28(6):2017.
65. Emad Y, Ragab Y, El-Shaarawy N, Rasker JJ. Transient osteoporosis of the hip, complete resolution after treatment with alendronate as observed by MRI description of eight cases and review of the literature. Clin Rheumatol. 2012;31(11):1641.
66. Korompilias AV, Karantanas AH, Lykissas MG, Beris AE. Transient osteoporosis. J Am Acad Orthop Surg. 2008;16(8):480.
67. Stathopoulos IP, Liakou CG, Katsalira A, Trovas G, Lyritis GG, Papaioannou NA, Tournis S. The use of bisphosphonates in women prior to or during pregnancy and lactation. Hormones (Athens). 2011;10(4):280.
68. Vaishya R, Agarwal AK, Kumar V, Vijay V, Vaish A. Transient osteoporosis of the hip: a mysterious cause of hip pain in adults. Indian J Orthop. 2017;51(4):455.
69. Hall M, Anderson J. Hip pointers. Clin Sports Med. 2013;32(2):325.
70. Kuhn AW, Noonan BC, Kelly BT, Larson CM, Bedi A. The hip in ice hockey: a current concepts review. Arthroscopy. 1928;32(9):2016.
71. Varacallo M, Bordoni B. Hip pointer injuries. Treasure Island (FL): StatPearls; 2023.
72. Bernstein EM, Kelsey TJ, Cochran GK, Deafenbaugh BK, Kuhn KM. Femoral neck stress fractures: an updated review. J Am Acad Orthop Surg. 2022;30(7):302.
73. Bhandari M, Swiontkowski M. Management of acute hip fracture. N Engl J Med. 2017;377(21):2053.
74. Chang SM, Hou ZY, Hu SJ, Du SC. Intertrochanteric femur fracture treatment in Asia: what we know and what the world can learn. Orthop Clin North Am. 2020;51(2):189.
75. Florschutz AV, Langford JR, Haidukewych GJ, Koval KJ. Femoral neck fractures: current management. J Orthop Trauma. 2015;29(3):121.
76. Foulk DM, Mullis BH. Hip dislocation: evaluation and management. J Am Acad Orthop Surg. 2010;18(4):199.
77. Medda S, Snoap T, Carroll EA. Treatment of young femoral neck fractures. J Orthop Trauma. 2019;33(Suppl 1):S1.
78. Shaw KA, Moreland CM, Hunt TJ, Barkley C, O'Brien F, Jackson KL. Femoral neck stress fractures in athletes and the military. J Bone Joint Surg Am. 2022;104(5):473.
79. Afonso PD, Weber MA, Isaac A, Bloem JL. Hip and pelvis bone tumors: can you make it simple? Semin Musculoskelet Radiol. 2019;23(3):e37.
80. Balamuth NJ, Womer RB. Ewing's sarcoma. Lancet Oncol. 2010;11(2):184.
81. Bancroft LW, Peterson JJ, Kransdorf MJ. MR imaging of tumors and tumor-like lesions of the hip. Magn Reson Imaging Clin N Am. 2005;13(4):757.
82. Bloem JL, Reidsma II. Bone and soft tissue tumors of hip and pelvis. Eur J Radiol. 2012;81(12):3793.
83. Meltzer PS, Helman LJ. New horizons in the treatment of osteosarcoma. N Engl J Med. 2021;385(22):2066.
84. Mirels H. Metastatic disease in long bones. A proposed scoring system for diagnosing impending pathologic fractures. Clin Orthop Relat Res. 1989;(249):256.
85. O'Sullivan GJ, Carty FL, Cronin CG. Imaging of bone metastasis: an update. World J Radiol. 2015;7(8):202.
86. Whelan JS, Davis LE. Osteosarcoma, chondrosarcoma, and chordoma. J Clin Oncol. 2018;36(2):188.

Knee Pain and Leg Pain

14

Alison Cabrera and Juhno Ahn

Pain in the native knee is commonly observed and evaluated given the ubiquitous presentation in nearly every patient population from the young athlete to the octogenarian. However, with the standard of care shifting more toward surgical management of knee pathology, knee pain following surgery can be a challenging problem, particularly when the treating physician is not the original surgeon. With the growing population of patients undergoing knee surgery, there is a need for understanding the pathophysiology as well as the factors that predispose patients to postoperative knee pain [1, 2]. In addition to direct causes of knee pain, pathology as well as surgical management of other areas outside of the knee joint have also been linked with postoperative knee pain [3]. The purpose of this chapter is to describe the etiology of knee and lower extremity pain in the native knee as well as in the postoperative knee and the challenges with clinical evaluation. In addition, this chapter discusses the surgical and non-surgical management as well as the factors that may predispose patients to postoperative knee pain.

ACL Tear and PCL Tear

The dramatic rise in sports participation in the United States from adolescents to younger adults has resulted in increased rates of internal knee derangements, often involving the anterior cruciate ligament (ACL) and less often the posterior cruciate ligament (PCL). The spike in ACL rupture rates has led to a significant increase in arthroscopic knee surgeries for ACL reconstruction [4]. There has subsequently been an emphasis on understanding ACL injuries.

A. Cabrera (✉) · J. Ahn
UT Southwestern Medical Center, Dallas, TX, USA
e-mail: alison.cabrera@utsouthwestern.edu

C. E. Noe (ed.), *Musculoskeletal Pain*,
https://doi.org/10.1007/978-3-031-86057-7_14

The ACL is an intra-articular ligament within the knee joint originating from the posteromedial side of the lateral femoral condyle and attaches at the anterior intercondylar area of the proximal tibia. The ACL is comprised of two "bundles," the anteromedial and posterolateral bundles. The anteromedial bundle primarily functions to prevent the femur from translating posteriorly relative to the tibia, and the posterolateral bundle is more important for rotational stability. Understanding the anatomic relationship of these two bundles and their functions gives insight into the mechanism through which ACL tears occur in high-level athletes and recreational weekend warriors.

On initial evaluation, possible ACL injuries should be evaluated with a focused history and physical examination. In cases of ACL tears, individuals will typically recall the moment the injury happened. They will often describe a sudden "pop" and a feeling of hyperextension followed by significant knee swelling and pain. It is also common for this injury to occur during a pivoting maneuver to quickly change directions [4]. Forceful contact with an object or athlete may also be a contributing factor. Other activities, such as downhill skiing, that involve a similar action are associated with ACL injuries. Female athletes are also more prone to ACL injury, particularly with participation in soccer, due to the increased valgus moment during pivoting and jumping [5].

Physical examination of a suspected ACL injury begins with inspection. Knee swelling may persist, and depending on the level of effusion, the knee may be held in a slightly flexed position. The anterior drawer, Lachman, and pivot shift maneuvers are specific to evaluating the ACL. The anterior drawer test is performed by flexing the hip to 45° and the knee to 90° and anteriorly translating the proximal tibia relative to the femur while stabilizing the patient's foot. The Lachman test is similar to the anterior drawer, but the knee is flexed to 30°, while the examiner uses one hand to anteriorly translate the tibia, while using the other hand to stabilize the distal femur. The knee is evaluated on whether a firm or soft endpoint is felt in addition to the amount of translation. The pivot shift test is performed, while the patient is supine. The leg is held by the examiner with the knee in full extension and internal rotation. The knee is then brought slowly into flexion while applying a valgus force by pushing on the lateral knee. The test is positive when the anteriorly translated tibia is noted to reduce spontaneously during flexion. Prior studies have demonstrated that the Lachman test is the most sensitive with a positive predictive value of >10 and the pivot shift test is highly specific with a specificity of 98% [6].

In patients who elect for nonoperative management of their ACL tear, the knee kinematics are significantly affected and can result in changes in neuromuscular firing [7]. Following the immediate injury period, some patients do not report instability even after returning to sports involving cutting or pivoting. It has been postulated that these patients are able to compensate with dynamic stabilization through activation of the quadriceps muscles [8]. However, patients that continue to experience knee instability and laxity may compensate gait mechanics by limiting knee flexion and exaggerating hip flexion, leading to a thrust-like gait. Interestingly, quadriceps function is also correlated with postoperative functional recovery following ACL reconstructive surgery [9].

The evaluation of knee pain following ACL reconstruction can be challenging, but this presentation is becoming increasingly common. The first step is to differentiate patients who have a remote or recent history of surgery. In recent surgical patients, clinicians should have a high index of suspicion for infection as a possible cause. Although rare, septic knee arthritis can have devastating consequences [10]. These patients present with pain, swelling, incisional drainage, redness, and limited range of motion. They may also present with fever and have elevated inflammatory markers. If suspected, septic knee arthritis requires an immediate surgical consult. Minor infections of the soft tissue such as incisional cellulitis can also occur but have a less dramatic presentation than septic knee arthritis. If surgery was recent, plain radiographs should be obtained to evaluate for possible fracture. Fracture of the patella is uncommon, but is a described complication after use of bone-patellar tendon-bone autograft [11]. If plain radiographs are equivocal, advanced imaging studies such as computed tomography (CT) scan or magnetic resonance imaging (MRI) may be required.

The most common mechanisms for PCL injury include sports participation and direct trauma. Injuries to the PCL can occur in isolation or combined with other ligaments such as the ACL or the collateral ligaments. Overall, sports-related injuries are the most common mechanism of injury in isolated PCL ruptures but are still outweighed by isolated ACL ruptures. Injuries sustained during traffic accidents have a much higher ratio of PCL to ACL ruptures [12]. The presentation of PCL injuries is highly variable. After the initial acute injury phase, patients may not experience significant instability in the setting of low-grade tears, particularly with low activity demands, as the secondary stabilizers of the knee may adequately compensate. However, surgical reconstruction is often required in athletes or those with higher grade tears since the lack of restraint to posterior tibial translation can cause significant laxity [13].

Nonoperative rehabilitation for PCL ruptures is similar to those for operative management. The initial phase of management often involves bracing to prevent activation of the hamstring muscles, which act to posteriorly translate the tibia. Range of motion exercises are performed throughout the first several weeks with progressive increase in flexion to greater than 90°. Strengthening the quadriceps muscles is critical to counteract the posterior translation of the tibia. This is often achieved through isometric, concentric, and eccentric exercises. Afterward, activity is advanced to higher flexion open and closed chain exercises, such as cycling.

Injuries to the ACL and PCL are common in athletes and the recreational "weekend warriors." It is important for providers caring for patients presenting with ligamentous knee injuries to be aware of the clinical and examination findings. This includes prompt evaluation through advanced imaging as well as referral for surgical management.

Articular Cartilage Defects of the Knee

The articular cartilage in the knee joint is almost constantly under pressure during weight-bearing. Despite this, there is a limit to the amount of pressure that the articular surface can have before damage occurs. This can be the result of abnormal distribution of pressure over the knee joint from trauma or mechanical malalignment. Given the variety of cartilage defects, a detailed history and physical examination is key to clinical decision-making and treatment planning. Patients may present with pain during activity, mechanical symptoms, or clicking or catching of the knee with motion. External findings such as swelling, bruising, and lower extremity alignment should be noted. Routine physical examination of the knee should be performed with particular attention to areas of focal tenderness to palpation and pressure followed by plain radiographs. Multiple views, including anteroposterior, lateral, notch, and patellofemoral, should be obtained. MRI is more sensitive and specific than plain radiographs for osteochondral lesions. Early-stage osteochondral lesions may not be visible on plain radiographs if they are in the prefragmentation phase. MRI can identify areas of bony edema and beginning of subchondral bone involvement and can further determine the extent of involvement of the joint surface [14].

Cartilage is relatively avascular, and chondrocytes receive nutrients via diffusion. As a result, cartilage has poor regenerative potential. With acute trauma or chronic repetitive load, cartilage can soften and fissure, form flaps, or completely delaminate. The underlying subchondral bone may also be involved. Over time, focal osteochondral lesions can progress to degenerative osteoarthritis [15]. The following two sections will go into more depth on specific osteochondral lesions: osteochondritis dissecans (OCD) and osteoarthritis.

Osteochondritis Dissecans

Osteochondritis dissecans was described more than a hundred years ago. Loose bodies within the knee joint were initially described by Paget in 1870, but in 1888 König suggested the three ways in which these loose bodies could form: (1) direct trauma with osteochondral fracture, (2) minimal trauma with subsequent osteonecrosis and fragmentation, or (3) no specific incidence of trauma with spontaneous loose body formation. He coined this third description as osteochondritis dissecans (OCD) [16]. Despite the following hundred years of study of this process, it is still unclear how OCD lesions form or occur. In patients who present with symptomatic knees after OCD lesions form, the natural history of formation of these lesions is not fully understood. In this chapter, we will focus primarily on the clinical presentation, subsequent evaluation, and treatment algorithm of OCD lesions.

Relative to knee osteoarthritis, OCD lesions of the knee are uncommon. Linden et al. studied a population of adolescents in Sweden and found an incidence of 29 cases per 100,000 in boys and 19 per 100,000 in girls [17]. These lesions typically present on the posterolateral aspect of the medial femoral condyle, but may be present on the patella or lateral femoral condyle as well [18]. It is also possible to have an OCD lesion in the contralateral knee which may or may not be symptomatic.

Patients with OCD lesions can present with complaints of knee pain during activity, but may also present for an unrelated issue with incidental finding of OCD on imaging. The symptoms can range from knee effusion, mild pain with activity to severe pain with or without mechanical symptoms of locking, popping, and catching during knee motion. In these patients, the examiner should perform a thorough knee examination going through knee range of motion, competency of the knee stabilizers, and mechanical alignment. Wilson described a maneuver to diagnose OCD lesions by flexing the knee to 90° and externally rotating the tibia as the knee is extended to 30° of flexion. The test is positive if the patient feels pain over the anteromedial knee at the 30° of flexion that is relieved once the tibia is rotated from external to internal rotation [19]. However, this test is nonspecific and of limited diagnostic value. OCD lesions are truly a radiographic diagnosis.

Because the clinical presentation of OCD lesions can be similar to that of meniscal tears, it is not unusual to discover these lesions initially on MRI. However, most lesions can be seen on plain radiographs. The appearance of the OCD lesions on imaging varies with regards to the subchondral bone and articular cartilage. Classification systems are based on the description of these two components [20]. Low-grade lesions are characterized by a depression type fracture of the subchondral bone without separation from the surrounding bone. Higher-grade lesions involve complete detachment of the fragment but are separated by whether the fragment is displaced or not displaced from its origin. This staging system helps to categorize stable (low-grade) and unstable (high-grade) lesions to guide treatment. Patients with stable, low-grade lesions can be initially managed nonoperatively through bracing, activity modification (avoiding high-impact activities), and protected weight-bearing with crutches with or without a period of immobilization. Repeat imaging is used to assess healing over a period of 3–6 months. Evidence of incomplete or absent healing on radiographs or MRI is a relative indication for surgical management. When lesions fail to heal with nonoperative management or if unstable lesions are suspected, surgical treatment can range from arthroscopic surgery to osteochondral autograft transfer or allograft transplant [21].

Knee Osteoarthritis

Osteoarthritis is the most common joint disease with the knee being the most involved joint [22]. Given its ubiquity, knee osteoarthritis is one of the most common reasons to see a physician, and the prevalence of knee osteoarthritis is projected to increase with an aging population. In general, knee osteoarthritis is a "wear and tear" problem. However, symptoms can be quite variable. Routine imaging of knees of patients above the age of 50 without knee symptoms would likely demonstrate varying grades of knee osteoarthritis. Radiographic appearance of knee osteoarthritis does not always correlate with knee pain or mechanical symptoms. Risk factors that predispose to the development of knee osteoarthritis include high body mass index (BMI), female gender, family history, prior trauma, occupation, and reduced muscle strength [23].

Initial evaluation of knee osteoarthritis is driven by the patient's experience and complaints. Early-stage knee osteoarthritis presents with weeks to months of symptoms including but not limited to stiffness, pain, locking, and catching, particularly at the end of the day and after a period of activity [23]. Initial radiographs of early-stage knee osteoarthritis may demonstrate normal or near-normal findings. As it progresses, more signs of degenerative changes such as joint space narrowing, subchondral sclerosis, and osteophyte formation can be observed. The Kellgren–Lawrence grading system was designed to describe these findings with increasing severity of osteoarthritis.

Management of knee osteoarthritis requires a multidisciplinary approach and careful consideration of patient factors. The American Academy of Orthopaedic Surgery in conjunction with societies, including those in physical therapy, family medicine, and pain management, release clinical practice guidelines regarding non-arthroplasty means of managing knee osteoarthritis [24]. Following review of hundreds of peer-reviewed literature, 27 recommendations were released. Non-pharmacological interventions include activity modifications, orthotics, and physical therapy.

Regarding orthotics, there is moderate evidence in support of knee braces and use of canes. Lateral wedge insoles designed to off-load the medial compartment of the knee joint have not been shown to significantly improve pain or function. Physical therapy, neuromuscular training, and weight loss with supervised exercise are supported by moderate to strong level of evidence for improvement of pain, function, balance, and coordination. Massage therapy and acupuncture have not shown significant improvement in pain and functional scores in studies with a high-level of evidence. Although their benefits are unclear from the existing literature, practitioners should rely on their clinical judgment to pursue these methods as they carry low-risk of morbidity.

Oral medications such as nonsteroidal anti-inflammatory drugs (NSAIDs) and acetaminophen as well as topical drugs like topical NSAIDs and lidocaine all have strong level recommendations for their routine use in knee osteoarthritis when not contraindicated. In contrast, oral narcotics including tramadol have been strongly associated with adverse events and higher mortality [25]. The evidence for dietary supplements including turmeric, glucosamine, chondroitin, and vitamin D is limited, and there is not a clear consensus on their benefits.

More invasive methods such as intra-articular injection with corticosteroids, hyaluronic acid, platelet-rich plasma (PRP) are often performed in the clinic. Although corticosteroid injection has moderate level of support from the literature in their routine use, the results of hyaluronic acid injection have been inconsistent when demonstrating significant benefits. The current guidelines recommend against routine use of hyaluronic acid. However, given its relatively low-risk profile, practitioners may consider it as an option. Platelet-rich plasma (PRP) has been gaining popularity. Recent studies have shown reduction in pain and improved functional scores after PRP injection with increasing efficacy with subsequent injections [26, 27].

Surgical management relies on a variety of patient factors. In younger patients with early unicompartmental medial knee osteoarthritis, high tibial osteotomies can correct the mechanical alignment of the joint to evenly distribute pressure on the joint surface and improve the cartilage structure [28]. However, the indication for high tibial osteotomy is limited as it is contraindicated in patients with more severe osteoarthritis, multicompartmental osteoarthritis, or limited knee range of motion. In patients above the age of 50 who present with knee osteoarthritis, the benefits of arthroscopic surgery have been investigated. In a double-blinded, randomized-controlled trial comparing arthroscopic partial meniscectomy versus sham surgery in patients with primary knee osteoarthritis, no significant differences in pain or functional scores were noted [29]. Subsequent studies have investigated the effects of arthroscopic partial meniscectomy, but the general conclusion has remained unchanged. More recent trials have shown greater radiographic progression of knee osteoarthritis following partial meniscectomy and have shown non-inferiority of physical therapy compared to partial meniscectomy [30, 31]. However, arthroscopic partial meniscectomy may help certain patients with mild to moderate knee arthritis who have failed therapy and other conservative measures, but are not ready for consideration of a total knee arthroplasty. Patients with osteoarthritis considering arthroscopic partial meniscectomy should be counseled that they may not get any benefit from this surgery or may only notice temporary pain relief. Total knee replacement is considered in patients who fail conservative management and have significant joint degeneration. Joint replacement surgery has advanced considerably since the first iterations in the mid-1950s. Advancements in the understanding of knee kinematics, materials science, and robotics have improved outcomes and survivorship of knee arthroplasty [32]. In addition, with an aging population, more total knee arthroplasties are being performed overtime with decreasing length of stay [33]. However, outcomes have generally not improved. Readmission, revision, and infection rates have significantly increased between 1991 and 2010 [33]. Most patients are satisfied with their total knee replacement but with satisfaction rates ranging from about 75% to 85% [34]. Total knee replacement is a major surgery with significant associated risks. As such, efforts to preserve joints with conservative measures should be pursued as much as possible with arthroplasty reserved as a last resort.

Patellar Instability

Patellar instability is a broad term to describe conditions that affect the position of the patella relative to the femur, which includes dislocation, subluxation, and recurrent instability [35]. This condition is commonly seen in patients during adolescence and into the second and third decades of their life. Patellar instability accounts for approximately 11% of clinic visits associated with musculoskeletal issues. As such, careful examination of patient biomechanics and risk factors is critical in determining effective treatment.

The stability of the patellofemoral joint relies on the combination of bony anatomy, integrity of surrounding soft-tissue structures, and the overall alignment of the lower extremity. In full knee extension, the patella does not engage the trochlea of the femur. At this position, the medial patellofemoral ligament (MPFL) is the primary stabilizer of the patella. Between 10° and 30° of knee flexion, the patella engages the femur and glides along the sulcus [36]. The depth of the trochlea acts as a valley for which the patella can glide, which provides stability in the coronal plane. With increasing flexion, the vastus medialis obliquus (VMO) muscle of the quadriceps, helps pull the patella medially. This muscle is also the most important dynamic stabilizer. The position of the patella may also differ between patients. An abnormally proximal position of the patella is termed patella alta as opposed to patella baja, which describes an abnormally distal position of the patella. Finally, the overall alignment of the lower extremity plays a significant role in patellar stability. The angle between the vector of pull from the quadriceps muscles relative to the direction of the patella tendon or "q angle", has been suggested as a potential risk factor as increasing this angle places a greater laterally directed force on the patella during quadricep activation. Coronal deviation of knee alignment into valgus also creates additional force in this direction [36]. Further, excessive femoral anteversion and external tibial torsion also lead to lateral shift of the patella. The combination of both is often termed "miserable malalignment" [37]. Assessment of these factors provides diagnostic and prognostic insight into patellar instability, which is critical in guiding management.

Evaluation of possible patellar instability begins with a thorough history. The inciting traumatic event that led to the initial dislocation is often noncontact related [38]. The number of subsequent dislocation events should also be noted as with any lingering symptoms of instability, pain, and swelling. Physical examination is focused on static and dynamic patellar motion. In full extension, the mobility of the patella in lateral and medial direction is assessed by the amount of translation that can be achieved with direct manipulation. This is measured in the number of quadrants of the patella that can be translated in either direction. The knee should then be ranged in full extension and maximal flexion, noting the position of the patella. A laterally shifting patella, while moving from a flexed to an extended position, is referred to as a "J sign" which signifies insufficiency of the medial soft tissue restraints including the MPFL. The patella may also frankly dislocate with range of motion. However, patients with grossly unstable patellofemoral joints may exhibit apprehension with increasing knee flexion and stop their motion. In these patients, a relocation test should be performed by placing a medially directed pressure on the lateral patella through knee flexion. The test is positive if the patient reports less apprehension and better stability. Radiographic evaluation is performed to evaluate knee alignment, rotational profile, and bony structure as described in the previous paragraph. Plain radiographs in the anteroposterior, lateral, and sunrise views can identify deviation of the mechanical axis of the knee, patella alta and baja, and trochlear dysplasia, respectively. Rotational profile of the femur and tibia requires advanced imaging in the form of MRI and computed tomography (CT) scan.

Prognosis after an initial event of patellar instability depends on several patient factors. Previous studies have proposed scoring systems for recurrence risk [39–41]. Among the most commonly used scoring systems, patient age less than 25 years at time of dislocation, presence of trochlear dysplasia, and presence of patella alta are the most cited risk factors. Patients with at least two of these risk factors have approximately a 30–60% risk of recurrence. This risk is halved when only one risk factor is present and is nearly 0% when none are present. As such, these scoring systems are valuable tools in guiding treatment. Patients who have a low-risk of recurrence are almost always managed conservatively with knee bracing, physical therapy, and symptomatic management. Patients with a 50% chance of recurrence may elect for surgical treatment through MPFL reconstruction, growth modulation if open growth physes are present, and corrective osteotomies. However, close observation with bracing and therapy is also a reasonable option in the absence of recurrent instability or pain.

Quadriceps Tendon Rupture, Exertional Compartment Syndrome, and Prepatellar Bursitis

The quadriceps are made up of four muscles, the rectus femoris, vastus lateralis, vastus medialis, and the vastus intermedius. During knee extension, force is generated by the quadriceps and is transmitted to the patella and subsequently to the tibial tubercle via the patellar tendon. Quadriceps ruptures are relatively uncommon injuries of the knee extensor mechanism that particularly affect older males with chronic conditions such as diabetes, gout, and chronic kidney disease [42]. A previous study evaluating the causes of quadriceps tears found that most (61.5%) were caused by simple falls followed by falling down stairs (23.4%), sports (6%), and other less common mechanisms [43]. It is thought that patients with underlying chronic illnesses lead to degenerative changes of the quadriceps tendon leading to fatty infiltration and diminished vascularity [42].

The presentation of quadriceps ruptures can vary depending on the degree of involvement of the tendon. In partial ruptures, patients may present after feeling a pop around the knee and having swelling and pain around the proximal portion of the anterior knee. However, patients with partial ruptures can perform a straight leg raise as the extensor mechanism remains intact, opposed to those with complete ruptures. However, physical examination can be limited by significant pain with any maneuvers by the examiner or the patient. Plain radiographic evaluation may also assist in differentiating partial and complete ruptures as complete ruptures may show low-lying patella (patella baja) on lateral projection radiographs. Ultrasound imaging of the quadriceps may also be helpful to identify tears. However, it is user-dependent and is sensitive but less specific [44]. MRI is the most sensitive and specific examination and can help direct management. As such, patients with suspected quadriceps ruptures should be referred for immediate MRI following plain radiograph or ultrasound imaging to reduce false negative results and for treatment planning purposes [45].

Treatment of quadriceps ruptures varies by the severity of the tear. Partial ruptures can be treated conservatively with knee immobilization in full extension. Knee aspiration of the hematoma in the office setting can also aid in pain control and improve stress on the quadriceps tendon. Compressive dressings following aspiration can help to prevent recurrent knee effusion. This can be followed by a period of rest, ice, elevation, and NSAIDs for pain control. However, NSAIDs should be used sparingly as they can cause impaired tendon healing [46]. After a period of 6–8 weeks of knee immobilization, patients may progress passive range of motion steadily over the following months in a hinged knee brace until a 90° arc of motion is reached. Afterwards, active motion against light resistance can be advanced as tolerated. In patients with complete ruptures, prompt surgical treatment is recommended. Delay in surgical management increases the technical difficulty of the repair and leads to worse functional outcomes [47]. Although there is not a clear consensus on timing of surgery, it is generally recommended that patients receive surgical treatment within a month at the latest [48]. However, studies have demonstrated that surgical treatment within a week of injury improves functional outcomes [49].

Unlike acute compartment syndrome, exertional compartment syndrome is characterized by a more chronic clinical presentation associated with pain and moderately elevated compartment pressures usually affecting the anterior and lateral compartments of the lower leg. There is often a lack of a traumatic event and can normalize with rest. Despite the name, exertional compartment syndrome does not pose the same limb-threatening risk as acute compartment syndrome. However, a more acute presentation of exertional compartment syndrome has been described [50]. The presentation can be misleading as there is often no history of trauma but there is often anterior leg pain with associated swelling and redness. Neuropathies with weakness and numbness may also be present. However, the classic pain out of proportion with passive stretch in acute compartment syndrome may not be present. As such, the diagnosis of exertional compartment syndrome is commonly missed. More specific findings may include elevated creatinine kinase, elevated liver enzymes, and increased signal on MRI. Treatment for acute exertional compartment syndrome is immediate emergent fasciotomies to relieve compartment pressures [51]. A high index of suspicion is required to diagnose acute exertional compartment syndrome as prompt fasciotomies can prevent chronic weakness, particularly with ankle dorsiflexion. In contrast, chronic presentations with symptoms over a period of months may be treated with a period of rest, ice, and elevation with fasciotomy being performed on an elective basis [52].

Prepatellar bursitis is a common cause of anterior knee pain and swelling from inflammation of the bursa, a fluid-filled sac of synovial membrane that functions to decrease friction between tissue layers. Inflammation can occur due to septic and aseptic causes. Aseptic bursitis is a sterile inflammation of the bursa due to mechanical irritation or systemic inflammatory conditions. In comparison, septic bursitis is a bacterial infection of the bursal tissue often secondary to local spread from a more superficial lesion such as cellulitis [53]. The classic presentation for prepatellar bursitis involves anterior knee pain, pain with flexion, and anterior knee swelling. This is differentiated from septic arthritis of the knee, which presents with diffuse knee swelling, pain circumferentially along the joint line, flexion posturing, and pain with flexion and extension. Aspiration has been recommended in the past for prepatellar bursitis [54]. However, a study of patients treated empirically with antibiotics without aspiration compared to those who did undergo aspiration found no difference in resolution of symptoms or recurrence [55]. As such, the vast majority of aseptic and septic bursitis can be treated nonsurgically. There has not been any strong evidence supporting more than a week of antibiotics or operative versus nonoperative treatment [56]. In most cases, rest, ice, compression, NSAIDs, and in the case of septic bursitis, antibiotics are sufficient for the treatment for prepatellar bursitis. Surgery should be reserved for patients with severe presentations such as those with sepsis and those with bursitis that is refractory to nonoperative management.

Meniscus Tear

Meniscal pathology is an extensive topic and is the cause of one of the most commonly performed orthopedic surgeries in the United States [57]. The menisci are "C" shaped fibrocartilaginous structures that act as shock absorbers around the knee. They provide stability with load-bearing through hoop stresses around the femoral condyles when a compressive force is applied. In younger, active patients, meniscus tears are usually a result of an acute traumatic event causing excessive stress on the meniscus. This can be accompanied by other injuries in the knee including the ACL, PCL, and other structures as mentioned in prior sections. In older, less active patients, meniscus tears are often degenerative and do not have a history of a traumatic event.

The menisci are attached to the periphery of the tibia and capsule via the coronary ligaments as well as the posterior roots. As a result, the blood flow to the meniscus is primarily around the peripheral portions of the meniscus [58]. The most perfused area is the outer one-third portion described as the "red-red" zone. This is followed by the middle portion, the "red-white" zone, and the inner portion, the "white-white" zone. Injuries to the meniscus in the red-red zone have a high chance of healing, whereas white-white zone injuries have a relatively low chance. The crescent shape of the menisci allows compressive forces to be translated to concentric force around the meniscus to provide stability around the femoral condyles. The medial meniscus has more of a cup shape than the lateral meniscus. This allows for greater contact with the femoral condyle through range of motion and provides stability to anteroposterior translation. Biomechanical studies have demonstrated that reduction in meniscus volume leads to decreased joint contact surface area and increases the pressure on a smaller contact area [59]. A study of knees following total meniscectomy showed an increase in joint space narrowing and femoral condyle flattening [60]. Absence or dysfunction of the menisci carries significant repercussions on knee function and subsequent degenerative changes over time.

Given the increase in sports participation in pediatric and adolescent age groups, knee injuries are becoming more prevalent each year [61]. Consequently, the majority of meniscal injuries in the pediatric population occur during sports participation [62]. Patients often describe feeling a pop during a pivoting maneuver as well as swelling and pain. They may report initial inability to bear weight despite negative plain radiographic evaluation. Once the swelling has improved after the immediate acute injury period, patients may report difficulty navigating stairs, sensation of locking, catching, and intermittent pain with weight-bearing and range of motion. However, the quality and frequency of symptoms can vary depending on the morphology of the meniscus tear. Initial evaluation should begin with careful history and physical examination. Joint line tenderness and pain or crepitus with range of motion are common but nonspecific findings. Several physical examination maneuvers specific for meniscus injuries have been described, including the McMurray, Thessaly, and Apley maneuvers, which involve stressing the menisci to illicit pain or a clicking sensation [63]. However, the examination findings are variable and a wide-range of sensitivities and specificities have been reported [64, 65]. Plain radiographic imaging should be routinely performed to rule out potential osteochondral injuries with views of anteroposterior, lateral, and sunrise views to evaluate each articular surface. Suspected meniscal injuries should then be evaluated with MRI followed by a referral to an orthopedic sports surgeon.

Although acute traumatic tears do occur in adults, degenerative meniscus tears are much more commonly encountered in the outpatient settings [66]. The medial meniscus is typically affected, and the tear pattern is often complex with edge fraying and multiple orientations of tears. Degenerative meniscal tears are highly prevalent in patients older than 50 years of age. Imaging studies have demonstrated that 35% of those over the age of 50 have meniscal tears [67]. Of these, two-thirds of these tears are asymptomatic. Osteoarthritis is also a common concurrent finding with degenerative meniscal tears. These tears are frequently treated with arthroscopic partial meniscectomy. However, studies have suggested that outcomes are equivocal with or without surgical treatment [29, 68]. Initial treatment of degenerative meniscal tears in the setting of knee osteoarthritis should involve physical therapy, NSAIDs, and intra-articular steroid injections for symptom relief. Arthroscopic partial meniscectomy should be reserved for patients who fail conservative management [69].

Tibial Tubercle Apophysitis & Tibial Stress Syndrome

Tibial tubercle apophysitis and tibial stress syndrome ("shin splints") are overuse injuries commonly seen in adolescent athletes. With tibial tubercle apophysitis, also commonly known as Osgood–Schlatter disease (OSD), young athletes with open growth plates experience irritation at the insertion of the patellar tendon from repetitive strain with active knee extension [70]. Adolescents are particularly susceptible to OSD during the period of accelerated growth [71]. Risk factors for OSD include higher BMI, quadriceps tightness, hamstring tightness, and reduced flexibility [72]. Healthcare providers assessing anterior knee pain about the tibial tubercle in young athletes should counsel patients on the importance of stretching, balance training, and cross-training, in order to prevent overloading the area. Initial treatment of OSD includes an initial period of rest, ice, NSAIDs, bracing, and physical therapy. Cast immobilization can also be attempted to keep the knee in extension to reduce the stress on the extensor mechanism of the knee. However, certain patients may experience continued pain despite conservative management over several months. A prior study comparing surgical treatments for patients with OSD found that patients who present with an ossicle within the patellar tendon have a higher frequency of excellent or good results with ossicle excision [73]. However, the vast majority of patients with OSD can be treated successfully without surgery.

Tibial stress syndrome is a common overuse injury that presents as posteromedial lower leg pain along the distal two-thirds of the tibia. There may be tenderness to palpation in this area as well. It is believed that repetitive stress along the posteromedial tibia with impact activities causes an imbalance in osteoclast and osteoblast activities leading to relative osteopenia in the area and formation of microfractures [74]. Treatment for tibial stress syndrome includes rest, ice, and NSAIDs. A review of treatment options involving various therapies did not reveal any significant differences with specialized treatments, such as ultrasound therapy, bracing, pulsed electromagnetic field, and extracorporeal shockwave therapy compared to standard therapy protocols involving rest and home exercises [75].

Knee Pain and Leg Pain

- Knee pain is common, but management is evolving.
- A wide variety of knee pathologies requires a systematic approach.

ACL Tear & PCL Tear

- Ligamentous knee injuries are becoming increasingly common with increased sports participation.
- The anterior and posterior cruciate ligaments are key structures for knee stability.
- Females are more likely to injure their ACL.
- ACL injuries are more common than PCL injuries.
- Surgical reconstruction is recommended for ACL injury while isolated PCL injuries can be treated conservatively.
- Quadriceps functioning can determine knee stability after injury and correlates with postoperative recovery.

Articular Cartilage Defects of the Knee

- Articular cartilage allows near frictionless motion of joints.
- Damage to articular cartilage may be difficult to identify as plain radiographs may be normal.
- Articular cartilage has poor regenerative potential.

Osteochondritis Dissecans

- Osteochondritis dissecans is an alteration of articular cartilage and subchondral bone.
- Osteochondritis dissecans may be asymptomatic and found incidentally.
- Medial femoral condyle is the most common location.
- Treatment depends on symptoms, patient factors, and lesion characteristics.

Knee Osteoarthritis

- Knee osteoarthritis is the most common joint pathology.
- Osteoarthritis is a result of "wear and tear."
- Clinical Practice Guidelines can help guide nonoperative treatments.
- Arthroscopic surgery may not be of any more benefit than physical therapy.
- Knee replacement surgery is recommended for advanced knee arthritis that has failed conservative treatment.

Patellar Instability

- The patella is critical for mechanical advantage during knee extension.
- Instability can be a consequence of anatomic variation and dynamic neuromuscular control.
- Patient risk factors can predict recurrence of instability.
- Most patients can be managed conservatively after initial instability event.
- Those at high-risk for recurrent instability may consider surgery.

Quadriceps Tendon Rupture, Exertional Compartment Syndrome, and Prepatellar Bursitis

- Quadriceps ruptures require prompt recognition and treatment for optimal outcomes.
- Exertional compartment syndrome is subacute to chronic in presentation.
- Prepatellar bursitis presents as anterior knee pain and rarely requires surgery.

Meniscus Tear

- The meniscus aids in distribution of force around the knee.
- Meniscus injuries are commonly associated with other knee injuries.
- Acute tears in younger patients may require surgery and therefore prompt referral to orthopedic surgeon.
- Degenerative meniscus injuries may not be reparable.
- Outcomes are equivocal for operative and nonoperative management of degenerative meniscal tears.

Tibial Tubercle Apophysitis & Tibial Stress Syndrome

- Adolescent athletes experience repetitive stress of the lower extremities.
- Tibial tubercle apophysis is part of the distal insertion of the knee extensor mechanism.
- Tibial stress syndrome is caused by imbalance of osteoclast and osteoblast activity leading to relative osteopenia and microfracture.
- Mainstay of treatment for both is conservative.

References

1. Severino FR, de Oliveira VM, de Paula Leite Cury R, Severino NR, de Moraes Barros Fucs PM. Causes of knee pain evaluated by arthroscopy after knee arthroplasty: a case series. Int Orthop. 2022;46(4):697–703. https://doi.org/10.1007/s00264-021-05048-8.
2. Niki Y, Hakozaki A, Iwamoto W, et al. Factors affecting anterior knee pain following anatomic double-bundle anterior cruciate ligament reconstruction. Knee Surg Sports Traumatol Arthrosc. 2012;20(8):1543–9. https://doi.org/10.1007/s00167-011-1746-z.
3. Rowan FE, O'Malley N, Poynton A. RhBMP-2 use in lumbar fusion surgery is associated with transient immediate post-operative leg pain. Eur Spine J. 2012;21(7):1331–7. https://doi.org/10.1007/s00586-011-2113-y.
4. Kaeding CC, Léger-St-Jean B, Magnussen RA. Epidemiology and diagnosis of anterior cruciate ligament injuries. Clin Sports Med. 2017;36(1):1–8. https://doi.org/10.1016/j.csm.2016.08.001.
5. Hewett TE, Myer GD, Ford KR, et al. Biomechanical measures of neuromuscular control and valgus loading of the knee predict anterior cruciate ligament injury risk in female athletes: a prospective study. Am J Sports Med. 2005;33(4):492–501. https://doi.org/10.1177/0363546504269591.
6. Benjaminse A, Gokeler A, van der Schans CP. Clinical diagnosis of an anterior cruciate ligament rupture: a meta-analysis. J Orthop Sports Phys Ther. 2006;36(5):267–88. https://doi.org/10.2519/jospt.2006.2011.
7. Lindström M, Felländer-Tsai L, Wredmark T, Henriksson M. Adaptations of gait and muscle activation in chronic ACL deficiency. Knee Surg Sports Traumatol Arthrosc. 2010;18(1):106–14. https://doi.org/10.1007/s00167-009-0886-x.
8. Rudolph KS, Axe MJ, Buchanan TS, Scholz JP, Snyder-Mackler L. Dynamic stability in the anterior cruciate ligament deficient knee. Knee Surg Sports Traumatol Arthrosc. 2001;9(2):62–71. https://doi.org/10.1007/s001670000166.

9. Snyder-Mackler L, Delitto A, Bailey SL, Stralka SW. Strength of the quadriceps femoris muscle and functional recovery after reconstruction of the anterior cruciate ligament. A prospective, randomized clinical trial of electrical stimulation. J Bone Joint Surg Am. 1995;77(8):1166–73. https://doi.org/10.2106/00004623-199508000-00004.
10. Mouzopoulos G, Fotopoulos VC, Tzurbakis M. Septic knee arthritis following ACL reconstruction: a systematic review. Knee Surg Sports Traumatol Arthrosc. 2009;17(9):1033–42. https://doi.org/10.1007/s00167-009-0793-1.
11. Stein DA, Hunt SA, Rosen JE, Sherman OH. The incidence and outcome of patella fractures after anterior cruciate ligament reconstruction. Arthroscopy. 2002;18(6):578–83. https://doi.org/10.1053/jars.2002.30658.
12. Zsidai B, Horvath A, Winkler PW, et al. Different injury patterns exist among patients undergoing operative treatment of isolated PCL, combined PCL/ACL, and isolated ACL injuries: a study from the Swedish National Knee Ligament Registry. Knee Surg Sports Traumatol Arthrosc. 2022;30(10):3451–60. https://doi.org/10.1007/s00167-022-06948-x.
13. Kew ME, Cavanaugh JT, Elnemer WG, Marx RG. Return to play after posterior cruciate ligament injuries. Curr Rev Musculoskelet Med. 2022;15(6):606–15. https://doi.org/10.1007/s12178-022-09794-z.
14. Baker H, Dickherber J, Reddy M, Rizzi A, Kahn A, Athiviraham A. Diagnostic value of MRI and radiographs of the knee to identify osteochondral lesions in acute patellar instability. J Knee Surg. 2022;35(14):1604–9. https://doi.org/10.1055/s-0041-1729551.
15. Guettler JH, Demetropoulos CK, Yang KH, Jurist KA. Osteochondral defects in the human knee: influence of defect size on cartilage rim stress and load redistribution to surrounding cartilage. Am J Sports Med. 2004;32(6):1451–8. https://doi.org/10.1177/0363546504263234.
16. Edmonds EW, Polousky J. A review of knowledge in osteochondritis dissecans: 123 years of minimal evolution from König to the ROCK study group. Clin Orthop Relat Res. 2013;471(4):1118–26. https://doi.org/10.1007/s11999-012-2290-y.
17. Linden B. Osteochondritis dissecans of the femoral condyles: a long-term follow-up study. J Bone Joint Surg Am. 1977;59(6):769–76.
18. Kessler JI, Nikizad H, Shea KG, Jacobs JC, Bebchuk JD, Weiss JM. The demographics and epidemiology of osteochondritis dissecans of the knee in children and adolescents. Am J Sports Med. 2014;42(2):320–6. https://doi.org/10.1177/0363546513510390.
19. Wilson JN. A diagnostic sign in osteochondritis DISSECANS OF THE KNEE. J Bone Joint Surg Am. 1967;49(3):477–80.
20. Clanton TO, DeLee JC. Osteochondritis dissecans. History, pathophysiology and current treatment concepts. Clin Orthop Relat Res. 1982;(167):50–64.
21. Waters T, Gowd AK, Waterman BR. Management of symptomatic osteochondritis dissecans of the knee. Arthroscopy. 2020;36(7):1803–4. https://doi.org/10.1016/j.arthro.2020.04.002.
22. Mahmoudian A, Lohmander LS, Mobasheri A, Englund M, Luyten FP. Early-stage symptomatic osteoarthritis of the knee – time for action. Nat Rev Rheumatol. 2021;17(10):621–32. https://doi.org/10.1038/s41584-021-00673-4.
23. O'Neill TW, McCabe PS, McBeth J. Update on the epidemiology, risk factors and disease outcomes of osteoarthritis. Best Pract Res Clin Rheumatol. 2018;32(2):312–26. https://doi.org/10.1016/j.berh.2018.10.007.
24. Brophy RH, Fillingham YA. AAOS clinical practice guideline summary: management of osteoarthritis of the knee (nonarthroplasty), third edition. J Am Acad Orthop Surg. 2022;30(9):e721–9. https://doi.org/10.5435/JAAOS-D-21-01233.
25. Zeng C, Dubreuil M, LaRochelle MR, et al. Association of tramadol with all-cause mortality among patients with osteoarthritis. JAMA. 2019;321(10):969–82. https://doi.org/10.1001/jama.2019.1347.
26. Simental-Mendía M, Ortega-Mata D, Tamez-Mata Y, Olivo CAA, Vilchez-Cavazos F. Comparison of the clinical effectiveness of activated and non-activated platelet-rich plasma in the treatment of knee osteoarthritis: a systematic review and meta-analysis. Clin Rheumatol. 2022. https://doi.org/10.1007/s10067-022-06463-x.

27. Filardo G, Previtali D, Napoli F, Candrian C, Zaffagnini S, Grassi A. PRP injections for the treatment of knee osteoarthritis: a meta-analysis of randomized controlled trials. Cartilage. 2021;13(1_suppl):364S–75S. https://doi.org/10.1177/1947603520931170.
28. Atkinson HF, Birmingham TB, Schulz JM, et al. High tibial osteotomy to neutral alignment improves medial knee articular cartilage composition. Knee Surg Sports Traumatol Arthrosc. 2022;30(3):1065–74. https://doi.org/10.1007/s00167-021-06516-9.
29. Sihvonen R, Paavola M, Malmivaara A, et al. Arthroscopic partial meniscectomy versus sham surgery for a degenerative meniscal tear. N Engl J Med. 2013;369(26):2515–24. https://doi.org/10.1056/NEJMoa1305189.
30. Sihvonen R, Paavola M, Malmivaara A, et al. Arthroscopic partial meniscectomy for a degenerative meniscus tear: a 5 year follow-up of the placebo-surgery controlled FIDELITY (Finnish Degenerative Meniscus Lesion Study) trial. Br J Sports Med. 2020;54(22):1332–9. https://doi.org/10.1136/bjsports-2020-102813.
31. Noorduyn JCA, van de Graaf VA, Willigenburg NW, et al. Effect of physical therapy vs arthroscopic partial meniscectomy in people with degenerative meniscal tears: five-year follow-up of the ESCAPE Randomized Clinical Trial. JAMA Netw Open. 2022;5(7):e2220394. https://doi.org/10.1001/jamanetworkopen.2022.20394.
32. Nagira K, Hagino H, Enokida M, et al. Total knee arthroplasty in the past three decades: trends in patient characteristics and implant survivorship. Mod Rheumatol. 2022;32(2):432–7. https://doi.org/10.1080/14397595.2021.1913823.
33. Cram P, Lu X, Kates SL, Singh JA, Li Y, Wolf BR. Total knee arthroplasty volume, utilization, and outcomes among Medicare beneficiaries, 1991–2010. JAMA. 2012;308(12):1227–36. https://doi.org/10.1001/2012.jama.11153.
34. Bourne RB, Chesworth BM, Davis AM, Mahomed NN, Charron KD. Patient satisfaction after total knee arthroplasty: who is satisfied and who is not? Clin Orthop Relat Res. 2010;468(1):57–63. https://doi.org/10.1007/s11999-009-1119-9.
35. Aglietti P, Buzzi R, Insall J. Disorders of the patellofemoral joint. In: Surgery of the knee. 3rd ed. New York: Churchill Livingstone; 2001. p. 913–1043.
36. Tecklenburg K, Dejour D, Hoser C, Fink C. Bony and cartilaginous anatomy of the patellofemoral joint. Knee Surg Sports Traumatol Arthrosc. 2006;14(3):235–40. https://doi.org/10.1007/s00167-005-0683-0.
37. Bruce WD, Stevens PM. Surgical correction of miserable malalignment syndrome. J Pediatr Orthop. 2004;24(4):392–6. https://doi.org/10.1097/00004694-200407000-00009.
38. Hawkins RJ, Bell RH, Anisette G. Acute patellar dislocations. The natural history. Am J Sports Med. 1986;14(2):117–20.
39. Lewallen LW, McIntosh AL, Dahm DL. Predictors of recurrent instability after acute patellofemoral dislocation in pediatric and adolescent patients. Am J Sports Med. 2013;41(3):575–81. https://doi.org/10.1177/0363546512472873.
40. Hevesi M, Heidenreich MJ, Camp CL, et al. The recurrent instability of the patella score: a statistically based model for prediction of long-term recurrence risk after first-time dislocation. Arthroscopy. 2019;35(2):537–43. https://doi.org/10.1016/j.arthro.2018.09.017.
41. Jaquith BP, Parikh SN. Predictors of recurrent patellar instability in children and adolescents after first-time dislocation. J Pediatr Orthop. 2017;37(7):484–90. https://doi.org/10.1097/BPO.0000000000000674.
42. Ilan DI, Tejwani N, Keschner M, Leibman M. Quadriceps tendon rupture. J Am Acad Orthop Surg. 2003;11(3):192–200. https://doi.org/10.5435/00124635-200305000-00006.
43. Ciriello V, Gudipati S, Tosounidis T, Soucacos PN, Giannoudis PV. Clinical outcomes after repair of quadriceps tendon rupture: a systematic review. Injury. 2012;43(11):1931–8. https://doi.org/10.1016/j.injury.2012.08.044.
44. Nelson M, Jersey A, Okumura Y, Stankard B. Bedside ultrasound diagnosis of quadriceps tendon rupture and avulsed patella. Curr Sports Med Rep. 2017;16(3):153–5. https://doi.org/10.1249/JSR.0000000000000354.

45. Perfitt JS, Petrie MJ, Blundell CM, Davies MB. Acute quadriceps tendon rupture: a pragmatic approach to diagnostic imaging. Eur J Orthop Surg Traumatol. 2014;24(7):1237–41. https://doi.org/10.1007/s00590-013-1307-x.
46. Connizzo BK, Yannascoli SM, Tucker JJ, et al. The detrimental effects of systemic Ibuprofen delivery on tendon healing are time-dependent. Clin Orthop Relat Res. 2014;472(8):2433–9. https://doi.org/10.1007/s11999-013-3258-2.
47. Rasul AT, Fischer DA. Primary repair of quadriceps tendon ruptures. Results of treatment. Clin Orthop Relat Res. 1993;(289):205–7.
48. Konrath GA, Chen D, Lock T, et al. Outcomes following repair of quadriceps tendon ruptures. J Orthop Trauma. 1998;12(4):273–9. https://doi.org/10.1097/00005131-199805000-00010.
49. Rougraff BT, Reeck CC, Essenmacher J. Complete quadriceps tendon ruptures. Orthopedics. 1996;19(6):509–14.
50. McKinney B, Gaunder C, Schumer R. Acute exertional compartment syndrome with rhabdomyolysis: case report and review of literature. Am J Case Rep. 2018;19:145–9. https://doi.org/10.12659/ajcr.907304.
51. Keeling LE, Chang ES. Acute exertional compartment syndrome of the leg following brief activity: a case report. JBJS Case Connect. 2020;10(3):e1900498. https://doi.org/10.2106/JBJS.CC.19.00498.
52. Livingston KS, Meehan WP, Hresko MT, Matheney TH, Shore BJ. Acute exertional compartment syndrome in young athletes: a descriptive case series and review of the literature. Pediatr Emerg Care. 2018;34(2):76–80. https://doi.org/10.1097/PEC.0000000000000647.
53. Cea-Pereiro JC, Garcia-Meijide J, Mera-Varela A, Gomez-Reino JJ. A comparison between septic bursitis caused by Staphylococcus aureus and those caused by other organisms. Clin Rheumatol. 2001;20(1):10–4. https://doi.org/10.1007/s100670170096.
54. Baumbach SF, Lobo CM, Badyine I, Mutschler W, Kanz KG. Prepatellar and olecranon bursitis: literature review and development of a treatment algorithm. Arch Orthop Trauma Surg. 2014;134(3):359–70. https://doi.org/10.1007/s00402-013-1882-7.
55. Thomas AL, Beyde A, Sandefur BJ, et al. Efficacy of empiric antibiotic therapy without aspiration for septic prepatellar bursitis in emergency department patients. Acad Emerg Med. 2022;29(8):1027–32. https://doi.org/10.1111/acem.14499.
56. Brown OS, Smith TO, Parsons T, Benjamin M, Hing CB. Management of septic and aseptic prepatellar bursitis: a systematic review. Arch Orthop Trauma Surg. 2022;142(10):2445–57. https://doi.org/10.1007/s00402-021-03853-9.
57. Kim S, Bosque J, Meehan JP, Jamali A, Marder R. Increase in outpatient knee arthroscopy in the United States: a comparison of National Surveys of Ambulatory Surgery, 1996 and 2006. J Bone Joint Surg Am. 2011;93(11):994–1000. https://doi.org/10.2106/JBJS.I.01618.
58. Arnoczky SP, Warren RF. Microvasculature of the human meniscus. Am J Sports Med. 1982;10(2):90–5. https://doi.org/10.1177/036354658201000205.
59. Ahmed AM, Burke DL. In-vitro measurement of static pressure distribution in synovial joints—Part I: tibial surface of the knee. J Biomech Eng. 1983;105(3):216–25. https://doi.org/10.1115/1.3138409.
60. Fairbank TJ. Knee joint changes after meniscectomy. J Bone Joint Surg Br. 1948;30B(4):664–70.
61. Bellisari G, Samora W, Klingele K. Meniscus tears in children. Sports Med Arthrosc Rev. 2011;19(1):50–5. https://doi.org/10.1097/JSA.0b013e318204d01a.
62. Andrish JT. Meniscal injuries in children and adolescents: diagnosis and management. J Am Acad Orthop Surg. 1996;4(5):231–7. https://doi.org/10.5435/00124635-199609000-00001.
63. Bronstein RD, Schaffer JC. Physical examination of the knee: meniscus, cartilage, and patellofemoral conditions. J Am Acad Orthop Surg. 2017;25(5):365–74. https://doi.org/10.5435/JAAOS-D-15-00464.
64. Solomon DH, Simel DL, Bates DW, Katz JN, Schaffer JL. The rational clinical examination. Does this patient have a torn meniscus or ligament of the knee? Value of the physical examination. JAMA. 2001;286(13):1610–20. https://doi.org/10.1001/jama.286.13.1610.

65. Hegedus EJ, Cook C, Hasselblad V, Goode A, McCrory DC. Physical examination tests for assessing a torn meniscus in the knee: a systematic review with meta-analysis. J Orthop Sports Phys Ther. 2007;37(9):541–50. https://doi.org/10.2519/jospt.2007.2560.
66. Hohmann E. Treatment of degenerative meniscus tears. Arthroscopy. 2023;39(4):911–2. https://doi.org/10.1016/j.arthro.2022.12.002.
67. Englund M, Guermazi A, Gale D, et al. Incidental meniscal findings on knee MRI in middle-aged and elderly persons. N Engl J Med. 2008;359(11):1108–15. https://doi.org/10.1056/NEJMoa0800777.
68. Katz JN, Brophy RH, Chaisson CE, et al. Surgery versus physical therapy for a meniscal tear and osteoarthritis. N Engl J Med. 2013;368(18):1675–84. https://doi.org/10.1056/NEJMoa1301408.
69. Katz JN, Wright J, Spindler KP, et al. Predictors and outcomes of crossover to surgery from physical therapy for meniscal tear and osteoarthritis: a randomized trial comparing physical therapy and surgery. J Bone Joint Surg Am. 2016;98(22):1890–6. https://doi.org/10.2106/JBJS.15.01466.
70. Ladenhauf HN, Seitlinger G, Green DW. Osgood-Schlatter disease: a 2020 update of a common knee condition in children. Curr Opin Pediatr. 2020;32(1):107–12. https://doi.org/10.1097/MOP.0000000000000842.
71. de Lucena GL, dos Santos GC, Guerra RO. Prevalence and associated factors of Osgood-Schlatter syndrome in a population-based sample of Brazilian adolescents. Am J Sports Med. 2011;39(2):415–20. https://doi.org/10.1177/0363546510383835.
72. Nakase J, Goshima K, Numata H, Oshima T, Takata Y, Tsuchiya H. Precise risk factors for Osgood-Schlatter disease. Arch Orthop Trauma Surg. 2015;135(9):1277–81. https://doi.org/10.1007/s00402-015-2270-2.
73. Glynn MK, Regan BF. Surgical treatment of Osgood-Schlatter's disease. J Pediatr Orthop. 1983;3(2):216–9. https://doi.org/10.1097/01241398-198305000-00012.
74. Frost HM. From Wolff's law to the Utah paradigm: insights about bone physiology and its clinical applications. Anat Rec. 2001;262(4):398–419. https://doi.org/10.1002/ar.1049.
75. Winters M, Eskes M, Weir A, Moen MH, Backx FJ, Bakker EW. Treatment of medial tibial stress syndrome: a systematic review. Sports Med. 2013;43(12):1315–33. https://doi.org/10.1007/s40279-013-0087-0.

Foot and Ankle Pain

15

Suganthi Kandasamy and Dane K. Wukich

Introduction

Foot pain and ankle pain are common among adults in the general population. Literature has shown that 90% of individuals have pain in more than one region of the foot and ankle [1]. Foot and ankle pain can contribute to functional impairment and hinder the undertaking of daily activities, especially in individuals over 55 years of age [2].

Common foot and ankle conditions addressed in this chapter include:

- Hallux valgus
- Hallux rigidus
- Morton's neuroma
- Plantar fasciitis
- Tarsal tunnel syndrome
- Achilles tendinopathy

Hallux Valgus

Overview

Hallux valgus is a common painful and disabling forefoot deformity that affects 23% of adults aged 18–65 years of age and 36% of adults over 65 years [3]. Hallux valgus can be characterized as a malpositioning of the first ray caused by a medial

S. Kandasamy · D. K. Wukich (✉)
Department of Orthopaedic Surgery, University of Texas Southwestern Medical Center, Dallas, TX, USA
e-mail: suganthi.kandasamy@utsouthwestern.edu; dane.wukich@utsouthwestern.edu

C. E. Noe (ed.), *Musculoskeletal Pain*,
https://doi.org/10.1007/978-3-031-86057-7_15

deviation of the first metatarsal bone, lateral deviation of the hallux, and pronation of the hallux [4, 5]. The development and progression of hallux valgus is multifactorial. Many factors have been identified that predispose individuals to develop hallux valgus including genetics, constricting footwear, female gender, and age [6]. Pes planus, metatarsus adductus, 1st ray hypermobility, 1st metatarsal length, hammertoe deformity, and equinus contracture [5, 7, 8] are other risk factors that can contribute to the development of hallux valgus.

Clinical Presentation and Physical Examination

Patients with hallux valgus often complain of pain in the medial aspect of the forefoot. Patients may have a prominent medial eminence at the 1st metatarsophalangeal joint (MPJ), which is tender to palpation, especially with certain shoes [6]. Patients often characterize their pain as aching and constant [9]. Patients may also endorse tingling and burning at the dorsal 1st MPJ, secondary to medial dorsal cutaneous nerve neuritis [10]. On clinical examination, the feet should be inspected in both a non-weightbearing seated position and a weight-bearing position. The 1st ray should be evaluated for range of motion, ligamentous laxity, and reducibility of the deformity. Limited motion of the 1st MPJ can indicate degenerative changes in the joint [6, 11]. Patients with hallux valgus often endorse pain with 1st MPJ range of motion, pain at the medial eminence, or the sesamoid bones. Patients may also report pain to the lesser toes or lesser metatarsal heads, secondary to transfer metatarsalgia [6].

Diagnosis

On radiographic examination, weight-bearing anteroposterior (AP), lateral, oblique, and sesamoid axial views should be obtained of the affected foot. On the AP view, the intermetatarsal angle (IMA: the angle between the shaft axis of the 1st and 2nd metatarsals), the hallux valgus angle (HVA: the angle between the shaft axis of the 1st metatarsal and the proximal phalanx of the hallux), the distal metatarsal articular angle (DMAA: measured between the distal articular surface and the perpendicular line of the 1st metatarsal), and the hallux interphalangeus angle (HIA: formed between the metaphyseal and diaphyseal axis of the proximal phalanx) are all measured. The sesamoid axial view can be used to evaluate the position of the sesamoids in relation to the cristae of the 1st metatarsal and to identify any subluxation of the sesamoids [6, 11]. Normal values are defined as HVA $< 15^\circ$, IMA $< 9^\circ$, and DMAA $<10^\circ$. Mild hallux valgus deformity is characterized as HVA $< 20^\circ$ and IMA $< 11^\circ$. Moderate hallux valgus deformity is characterized as HVA of 20–40° and IMA of 11–16°. Severe hallux valgus deformity is characterized as HVA $> 40^\circ$ and IMA $> 16^\circ$ [6]. Hallux valgus has traditionally been viewed as a biplanar deformity affecting the transverse and sagittal planes. However, over the past two decades, hallux valgus has been more recognized as a triplanar deformity, taking into account the frontal component [12].

Treatment

To treat hallux valgus conservatively, patients are counseled to use supportive shoes with a wide toe box to accommodate the bunion deformity and to mitigate pain at the medial eminence [13]. Nonsteroidal inflammatory medications are often prescribed to decrease pain and inflammation at the 1st MPJ [9]. Bunion shields and toe spacers are further recommended to provide cushioning in shoes and to further reduce pain. Orthoses also can help control abnormal forces acting on the first ray [14]. These accommodations and shoe gear modifications can help reduce pain in individuals, but will not correct the underlying deformity.

If conservative treatment fails and patients have continued pain, surgery is indicated. The surgical procedure is chosen based on the severity of the hallux valgus deformity. There is considerable variability in surgical treatment options. Soft tissue rebalancing procedures and distal metatarsal osteotomies are used for milder deformities, whereas proximal metatarsal osteotomies and 1st MPJ arthrodesis or 1st TMT arthrodesis are used for moderate to severe deformities [6].

Hallux Rigidus

Overview

Hallux rigidus is the most common arthritic condition in the foot and affects 2.5% of patients over the age of 50 [15] and has a higher predilection for females [16]. This condition refers to degenerative arthritis at the 1st metatarsophalangeal joint (MPJ). Various etiologies have been proposed for hallux rigidus. Trauma or damage to the articular cartilage of the 1st MPJ is the most reported cause of hallux rigidus [17]. Biomechanical and structural factors like hallux valgus interphalangeus, metatarsus adductus, long first metatarsal, and metatarsus elevatus can also lead to the development of hallux rigidus [18, 19].

Clinical Presentation and Examination

Patients with hallux rigidus often complain of pain and restriction of motion at the 1st MPJ [20]. Individuals often may note difficulty wearing particular shoes due to the dorsal osteophytes that may be present at the first metatarsal head or proximal phalanx of the hallux. On clinical examination, the 1st MPJ is often tender dorsally along the osteophytes. Dorsal osteophytes may compress the dorsal medial cutaneous nerve, which can cause sensation deficits. It is important to evaluate the range of motion at the 1st MPJ, which can shed light on the severity of the condition [21]. The Coughlin and Shurnas classification is most commonly used to grade hallux rigidus as described below [22].

- Grade 0
  - Clinical findings: No pain on the exam, only stiffness seen
  - Dorsiflexion of the 1st MPJ: 40–60° and/or 10–20% loss compared with normal side
  - Radiographic findings: Normal
- Grade 1
  - Clinical findings: Occasional pain and stiffness; pain with extreme dorsiflexion and/or plantarflexion
  - Dorsiflexion of the 1st MPJ: 30–40° and/or 20–50% loss compared with normal side
  - Radiographic findings: Dorsal osteophyte, minimal joint space narrowing, minimal periarticular sclerosis, and minimal flattening of the metatarsal head.
- Grade 2
  - Clinical findings: Moderate to severe pain and stiffness that may be constant; pain occurs just before maximum dorsiflexion and maximum plantarflexion
  - Dorsiflexion of the 1st MPJ: 10–30° and/or 50–75% loss compared with normal side
  - Radiographic findings: Dorsal, lateral, and possibly medial osteophytes, flattened metatarsal head, no more than ¼ of dorsal joint space involved on lateral radiograph, mild-to-moderate joint space narrowing and sclerosis, no sesamoid involvement
- Grade 3
  - Clinical findings: Constant pain and stiffness at extreme ranges of motion, but not at mid-range
  - Dorsiflexion of the 1st MPJ: <10° and/or 75–100% loss compared with normal side. Often will see a loss of MPJ plantarflexion (less than 10°)
  - Radiographic findings: Same as in Grade 2, but with substantial narrowing and possible periarticular cystic changes, more than ¼ dorsal joint space involved on lateral radiograph, sesamoids enlarged and/or cystic and/or irregular
- Grade 4
  - Clinical findings: Constant pain and stiffness at extreme ranges of motion and mid-range of motion
  - Dorsiflexion of the 1st MPJ: <10° and/or 75–100% loss compared with normal side. Often will see a loss of MPJ plantarflexion (less than 10°).
  - Radiographic findings: Same as in Grade 3

Imaging

Standing AP, lateral and oblique radiographs should be obtained. The amount of joint space narrowing, the presence of dorsal osteophytes, and the shape of the metatarsal head can all be noted. As hallux rigidus progresses, increased joint space narrowing is seen along with flattening of the metatarsal head, osteophytosis, cystic changes at the joint, and sesamoid involvement [21, 22]. Magnetic resonance imaging (MRI) and computed tomography (CT) scans are not necessary to diagnose hallux rigidus.

Treatment

Nonoperative treatment is initially considered for hallux rigidus. Nonsteroidal anti-inflammatory drugs may help to reduce swelling and pain at the 1st MPJ [15, 23]. Patients are advised to modify their activities and avoid extreme dorsiflexion of the 1st MPJ like climbing stairs or running [15]. Physical therapy with the incorporation of sesamoid mobilization, flexor hallucis strengthening, and gait training has been shown to decrease pain in the early stages of hallux rigidus [24]. Shoes with a wide toe box can also help prevent compression of prominent osteophytes. Shoes with a rocker bottom sole and the use of Morton's extension carbon fiber insole can further aid in reducing dorsiflexion at the 1st MPJ [15, 25]. Additionally, intra-articular injections with corticosteroid and local anesthetic have been shown to provide symptomatic relief in patients with Grade 1 or Grade 2 of hallux rigidus [26]. Nonoperative treatment can be successful in many patients. Grady et al. reported a 55% success rate with nonoperative treatment including shoe modifications, orthotics, and corticosteroid injections [27].

When conservative management fails, surgical correction of hallux rigidus is considered based on the severity of the condition and the patient's goals and expectations. The surgical options include either preservation or destruction of the articular cartilage at the 1st MPJ. In mild-to-moderate stages, joint-preserving procedures are considered including cheilectomy, proximal phalangeal osteotomy, and decompressive osteotomy. In more advanced stages, joint-altering procedures are selected including hemiarthroplasty, total joint arthroplasty, Keller resection arthroplasty, and 1st MPJ arthrodesis [19].

Morton's Neuroma

Overview

Morton's neuroma is a common cause of forefoot pain. It is characterized as a fibrosis of the interdigital nerve, which is caused by repetitive irritation or pressure leading to the thickening of the nerve. Morton's neuroma is most commonly seen in the third intermetatarsal space, followed by the second intermetatarsal space [28], and has a higher predilection for females versus males [29]. Literature suggests that compression of the interdigital nerve beneath the deep transverse metatarsal ligament (e.g., secondary to shoes with a narrow toe box) plays a role in contributing to the formation of an interdigital neuroma [30, 31].

Clinical Presentation and Examination

Patients describe their pain to be localized to the plantar surface of the forefoot at the level of the metatarsal heads. Patients often describe their pain as burning and associated with paresthesias radiating to the toes [32]. The symptoms worsen with weight-bearing or by wearing tight shoes [28]. Patients may complain of having a lump in the bottom of their foot and report they are walking on a pebble [33].

On clinical examination, one sensitive test that can be performed is the thumb index finger squeeze test, which is performed by applying pressure to the intermetatarsal space, which produces pain [28]. The webspace compression test is another provocative maneuver that can be performed. Pain is elicited when compressing the metatarsal heads together and simultaneously palpating the affected web space with the opposite hand [30]. Additionally, with compression of the metatarsals and concomitantly applying pressure to the affected interspace, a Mulder's click can be produced [34].

Role of Imaging

Imaging can be used to further aid in the diagnosis of a Morton's neuroma. Radiographs are often normal. On occasion, radiographs may show divergence of adjacent digits known as the Sullivan's sign [35]. Magnetic resonance imaging (MRI) and ultrasonography are widely used to confirm the clinical diagnosis of a Morton's neuroma. They can also help to exclude other pathologies like bursitis, synovitis, or arthritis [36].

Treatment

Many nonoperative treatments are utilized to treat Morton's neuroma. These strive to minimize nerve irritation and pressure in the affected web space. Initial treatment includes avoidance of narrow-toed shoes and use of nonsteroidal anti-inflammatory medications (NSAIDs) [9]. Additionally, the use of metatarsal pads proximal to the metatarsal head has been shown to reduce pressure at the metatarsal head [37]. Customized insoles with a built-in metatarsal and arch support are also effective for pain relief in patients with a Morton's neuroma [38]. Localized injections with local anesthesia and corticosteroid into the affected web space are often utilized for pain relief [39, 40]. Ultrasound-guided corticosteroid injections have been shown to be more accurate in locating and appropriately injecting the neuroma [41]. When conservative treatment measures fail to provide adequate pain relief, operative management is then considered. Surgical excision of the neuroma and release of the deep transverse intermetatarsal ligament often provides good clinical results and relief of pain in patients [42].

Plantar Fasciitis

Overview

Plantar fasciitis is one of the most common causes of foot pain in adults and affects approximately one million individuals every year [43]. It is estimated that one in ten people will develop this condition during their lifetime [44]. A higher prevalence of plantar fasciitis is seen in women and middle-aged adults [9, 43].

Plantar fasciitis is characterized by pain and inflammation on the plantar surface of the calcaneus, particularly at the medial tuberosity of the calcaneus. The plantar fascia is a thick fibrous aponeurosis that extends from the calcaneus to the base of the toes. The function of the plantar fascia is to provide support for the medial longitudinal arch and shock absorption [45]. Plantar fasciitis is most commonly caused by biomechanical overuse due to prolonged standing or activity, which creates microtears at the calcaneus enthesis [46]. More recently, the term plantar fasciosis fasciitis has been advocated to emphasize that the etiology is due to a chronic degenerative process rather than an acute inflammation [46, 47]. Common intrinsic risk factors for developing plantar fasciitis include biomechanical overuse, standing for prolonged periods of time, increased body mass index, individuals with pes planus or pes cavus foot types, and limited ankle dorsiflexion. Common extrinsic risk factors include walking on hard surfaces, barefoot walking, and poor footwear [45, 48].

Signs and Symptoms

Classic symptoms include severe pain with the first steps in the morning or after a period of rest and is aggravated by extended periods of weight-bearing [9, 49]. On physical examination, tenderness to palpation over the medial calcaneal tubercle is seen. When activating the windless mechanism by dorsiflexing the toes and making the plantar fascia taut, pain may also be elicited along the plantar fascia [50].

Testing and Differential Diagnoses

Plantar fasciitis is often diagnosed based on the medical history and clinical examination. Imaging, including radiographs, magnetic resonance imaging, and ultrasound, is not necessary to make a diagnosis but can be helpful in ruling out other causes for heel pain [48]. Other differential diagnoses of heel pain include calcaneal stress or acute calcaneal fractures, systemic arthritides like rheumatoid arthritis, calcaneal apophysitis, tarsal tunnel syndrome, fat pad atrophy, Achilles tendinitis, retrocalcaneal bursitis, or posterior tibial tendonitis [45].

Treatment

Initial treatment of plantar fasciitis often includes a combination of rest, activity modification [49, 51], use of nonsteroidal anti-inflammatory medications [52], icing [49], padding and strapping [53, 54], and stretching [55]. Supportive shoes [56] and use of over-the-counter or custom orthotics [57, 58] are also suggested to patients. Night splints have also been shown to be another effective conservative treatment option [59]. If symptoms do not improve after 6–8 weeks, formal physical therapy is recommended. Physical therapy incorporates stretching and strengthening programs which can address risk factors like tightness of the gastrocsoleus complex or weakness of the intrinsic foot muscles [45]. For patients who do not respond to physical therapy, corticosteroid injection with local anesthetic is offered [60, 61]. Ultrasound-guided corticosteroid injections have been shown to improve the accuracy of needle placement and avoidance of injury to surrounding soft tissues [62]. Extracorporeal shock wave therapy [63, 64] and the platelet-rich plasma injections [65] also have favorable outcomes in patients. Plantar fasciitis pain in most patients will resolve with time and conservative treatment alone. In patients who do not respond to conservative treatment, surgical release of the plantar fascia is considered. Plantar fasciotomy can be performed using open or endoscopic techniques [66]. Radiofrequency coblation also has been effective in the treatment of recalcitrant plantar fasciitis [67].

Tarsal Tunnel Syndrome

Overview

Tarsal tunnel syndrome is caused by compression of the posterior tibial nerve in the tarsal tunnel. The tarsal tunnel is a fibrous osseous space that runs posterior and inferior to the medial malleolus. The tarsal tunnel is bounded by the medial malleolus, talus, calcaneus, and flexor retinaculum. In addition to the posterior tibial nerve, the tarsal tunnel is occupied by the posterior tibial artery, posterior tibial vein, flexor digitorum longus and hallucis tendons, and the posterior tibial tendon [68]. The tibial nerve is one of the two terminal branches of the sciatic nerve. At the ankle, it runs posterior and inferior to the medial malleolus, passing through the tarsal tunnel bounded by the flexor retinaculum. Distal to the tunnel, the posterior tibial nerve divides into calcaneal sensory branches and two plantar nerves (medial and lateral) that supply the muscles of the plantar foot and the sensation of the plantar skin and the toes [69]. Compression of the tibial nerve at the level of the tarsal tunnel can lead to sensory and motor disturbances [70].

This condition is most frequently caused by extrinsic factors including ill-fitting shoes, trauma, biomechanical abnormalities (tarsal coalition, hindfoot varus or valgus) systemic inflammatory arthropathies, diabetes mellitus, postsurgical scarring, tendinopathy, tenosynovitis, or intrinsic factors like space-occupying lesion (enlarged veins, lipoma, ganglion cyst, neoplasm), hypertrophic retinaculum, or perineural fibrosis [71–73]. There is also a higher incidence of tarsal tunnel syndrome in females versus males [74].

Symptoms and Clinical Examination

Patients often complain of sharp shooting pain, numbness on the plantar surface of the foot, and radiation of paresthesias along the distribution of the posterior tibial nerve [9]. In some patients, these symptoms are worse at night or with extended periods of walking or standing. Patients may also complain of weakness in the muscles in their foot [71, 75]. On clinical examination, patients often have pain with deep palpation of the tarsal tunnel [74]. Pain is also elicited at the tarsal tunnel with the dorsiflexion-eversion test, which entails dorsiflexing and everting the foot with the extension of the metatarsophalangeal joints [76]. Biomechanical abnormalities like pes planus or increased pronation or supination during gait may also be noted in patients [71]. Additionally, light touch and two-point discrimination can show decreased plantar sensation along the posterior tibial nerve branches [71]. Furthermore, the Tinel's test can be performed by lightly tapping over the tarsal tunnel; a positive Tinel's sign is confirmed if paresthesias or pain are elicited with this maneuver [9, 76]. Proximal radiation of the tingling and numbness can also be seen and is known as the Valleix phenomenon [77].

Testing and Diagnosis

Plain radiographs of the foot and ankle are performed to evaluate for any osseous abnormalities including tarsal coalition, abnormal hindfoot position, or osteophytes [71]. Ultrasound and magnetic resonance imaging can evaluate for any soft tissue abnormalities in the tarsal tunnel including lipoma, ganglion cyst, varicosities, or tendinopathy [78–80]. Electromyography and nerve conduction studies can further be helpful in the diagnosis of tarsal tunnel syndrome [69].

Treatment

Many patients improve with conservative treatment measures. Rest, activity modification, use of nonsteroidal anti-inflammatory medications (NSAIDs), or use of neuropathic pain medications like gabapentin or pregabalin can be helpful in treating tarsal tunnel syndrome [71]. Physical therapy modalities like ultrasound, iontophoresis, E-Stim, or posterior tibial tendon strengthening can further help manage symptoms [71]. Orthotics can also be used to help correct overpronation of the foot and provide support for the medial and lateral longitudinal arches of the foot [81].

Patients with persistent symptoms who fail conservative treatment can undergo tarsal tunnel release surgery to decompress the tibial nerve and its branches [81]. Studies have shown improvement in symptom relief and quality of life after tarsal tunnel release surgery [82, 83].

Achilles Tendinopathy

Overview

Achilles tendinopathy is a common cause of ankle pain and disability in both the general population and athletes [84, 85]. Achilles tendinopathy can be described as a degenerative process caused by overuse and repetitive microtrauma [86]. The etiology of this condition is multifactorial and associated with both intrinsic and extrinsic factors. The intrinsic factors include age, gender, family history, increased body weight, systemic and metabolic diseases, abnormal ankle joint and subtalar joint range of motion, increased foot pronation, decreased ankle plantarflexion strength, and abnormal tendon structure [87–89]. Extrinsic factors that may contribute to Achilles tendinopathy include changes in training pattern, footwear, environmental factors (e.g., training on hard or slanted surfaces), inadequate stretching, physical activity/sports participation, and use of fluoroquinolones [88–91].

Achilles tendinopathy is classified based on its anatomic location: insertional or non-insertional (midportion) tendinopathy. Insertional Achilles tendinopathy occurs at the insertion site of the Achilles tendon on the calcaneus and is found to be more common in active patients. Non-insertional Achilles tendinopathy occurs 2–6 cm proximal to the insertion and is more common in the general population [86].

Symptoms and Clinical Examination

Patients with Achilles tendinopathy often complain of morning stiffness or stiffness after a period of inactivity, pain with activity, and impaired function [92]. Patients note their pain is exacerbated by exercise or climbing stairs [93]. In patients with insertional Achilles tendinopathy, pain is seen within the distal 2 cm of the Achilles tendon, whereas, in patients with non-insertional Achilles tendinopathy, pain is seen 2–6 cm proximal to the insertion of the Achilles at the calcaneus. On clinical examination, redness and swelling may also be visible and a bony spur may be palpable [94, 95]. In all patients, it is also important to examine the ankle range of motion to identify limited ankle dorsiflexion and assess any weakness in ankle plantarflexion [94].

Imaging

Lateral weight-bearing radiographs can be used to evaluate for any retrocalcaneal osteophytes or intratendinous calcifications within the Achilles tendon. It has been shown that the size of the osteophyte formation at the Achilles insertion can contribute to the development of symptoms in patients with insertional Achilles tendinopathy [94]. Ultrasound and magnetic resonance imaging can further be used to evaluate for any soft tissue pathology including tendon degeneration, bursitis, paratendinitis, or neovascularization [86, 94].

Treatment

Rest, ice, compression, bracing, nonsteroidal anti-inflammatory medications, and activity modification are all included in the initial treatment of Achilles tendinopathy [86, 96]. The mainstay of treatment for Achilles tendinopathy is physical therapy and exercise rehabilitation to help restore the tendon's ability to withstand the load. Most beneficial are programs that incorporate eccentric exercises [86, 97–99]. Extracorporeal shockwave therapy in conjunction with eccentric exercises has shown significant improvement in comparison to eccentric exercises alone [100]. In addition, ultrasound-guided high-volume injection with local anesthetic and corticosteroid is a newer technique that has shown favorable results in decreasing pain and improving function in patients who have failed other conservative treatment options [101, 102]. These conservative treatment measures often are successful in treating patients with Achilles tendinopathy. For patients with recalcitrant Achilles tendinopathy, surgical treatment is considered. Depending on the degree of Achilles tendinopathy, surgical options that are considered include a percutaneous longitudinal tenotomy, open tendon debridement, gastrocnemius recession, and flexor hallucis longus tendon transfer [86, 94, 103].

References

1. Chean CS, Lingham A, Rathod-Mistry T, Thomas MJ, Marshall M, Menz HB, et al. Identification of patterns of foot and ankle pain in the community: cross-sectional findings from the clinical assessment study of the foot. Musculoskeletal Care. 2021;19(1):9–19.
2. Keenan AM, Drake C, Conaghan PG, Tennant A. The prevalence and impact of self-reported foot and ankle pain in the over 55 age group: a secondary data analysis from a large community sample. J Foot Ankle Res. 2019;12:53.
3. Nix S, Smith M, Vicenzino B. Prevalence of hallux valgus in the general population: a systematic review and meta-analysis. J Foot Ankle Res. 2010;3:21.
4. Mann RA, Coughlin MJ. Hallux valgus—etiology, anatomy, treatment and surgical considerations. Clin Orthop Relat Res. 1981;157:31–41.

5. Easley ME, Trnka HJ. Current concepts review: hallux valgus part 1: pathomechanics, clinical assessment, and nonoperative management. Foot Ankle Int. 2007;28(5):654–9.
6. Ray JJ, Friedmann AJ, Hanselman AE, Vaida J, Dayton PD, Hatch DJ, et al. Hallux valgus. Foot Ankle Orthop. 2019;4(2):2473011419838500.
7. Perera AM, Mason L, Stephens MM. The pathogenesis of hallux valgus. J Bone Joint Surg Am. 2011;93(17):1650–61.
8. Coughlin MJ, Jones CP. Hallux valgus: demographics, etiology, and radiographic assessment. Foot Ankle Int. 2007;28(7):759–77.
9. Waldman SD. Atlas of common pain syndromes. 4th ed. Philadelphia: Elsevier Inc.; 2019.
10. Kuhn J, Alvi F. Hallux valgus. Treasure Island (FL): StatPearls Publishing; 2022.
11. Fraissler L, Konrads C, Hoberg M, Rudert M, Walcher M. Treatment of hallux valgus deformity. EFORT Open Rev. 2016;1(8):295–302.
12. Do DH, Sun JJ, Wukich DK. Modified lapidus procedure and hallux valgus: a systematic review and update on triplanar correction. Orthop Clin North Am. 2022;53(4):499–508.
13. Donley BG, Tisdel CL, Sferra JJ, Hall JO. Diagnosing and treating hallux valgus: a conservative approach for a common problem. Cleve Clin J Med. 1997;64(9):469–74.
14. Ying J, Xu Y, István B, Ren F. Adjusted indirect and mixed comparisons of conservative treatments for hallux valgus: a systematic review and network meta-analysis. Int J Environ Res Public Health. 2021;18(7):3841.
15. Ho B, Baumhauer J. Hallux rigidus. EFORT Open Rev. 2017;2(1):13–20.
16. Razik A, Sott AH. Cheilectomy for hallux rigidus. Foot Ankle Clin. 2016;21(3):451–7.
17. Yee G, Lau J. Current concepts review: hallux rigidus. Foot Ankle Int. 2008;29(6):637–46.
18. Coughlin MJ, Shurnas PS. Hallux rigidus: demographics, etiology, and radiographic assessment. Foot Ankle Int. 2003;24(10):731–43.
19. Hamid KS, Parekh SG. Clinical presentation and management of hallux rigidus. Foot Ankle Clin. 2015;20(3):391–9.
20. Migues A, Slullitel G. Joint-preserving procedure for moderate hallux rigidus. Foot Ankle Clin. 2012;17(3):459–71.
21. Lam A, Chan JJ, Surace MF, Vulcano E. Hallux rigidus: how do I approach it? World J Orthop. 2017;8(5):364–71.
22. Coughlin MJ, Shurnas PS, Hallux rigidus. Grading and long-term results of operative treatment. J Bone Joint Surg Am. 2003;85(11):2072–88.
23. Nawoczenski DA. Nonoperative and operative intervention for hallux rigidus. J Orthop Sports Phys Ther. 1999;29(12):727–35.
24. Shamus J, Shamus E, Gugel RN, Brucker BS, Skaruppa C. The effect of sesamoid mobilization, flexor hallucis strengthening, and gait training on reducing pain and restoring function in individuals with hallux limitus: a clinical trial. J Orthop Sports Phys Ther. 2004;34(7):368–76.
25. Deland JT, Williams BR. Surgical management of hallux rigidus. J Am Acad Orthop Surg. 2012;20(6):347–58.
26. Solan MC, Calder JD, Bendall SP. Manipulation and injection for hallux rigidus. Is it worthwhile? J Bone Joint Surg Br. 2001;83(5):706–8.
27. Grady JF, Axe TM, Zager EJ, Sheldon LA. A retrospective analysis of 772 patients with hallux limitus. J Am Podiatr Med Assoc. 2002;92(2):102–8.
28. Bhatia M, Thomson L. Morton's neuroma – current concepts review. J Clin Orthop Trauma. 2020;11(3):406–9.
29. Peters PG, Adams SB, Schon LC. Interdigital neuralgia. Foot Ankle Clin. 2011;16(2):305–15.
30. Wu KK. Morton's interdigital neuroma: a clinical review of its etiology, treatment, and results. J Foot Ankle Surg. 1996;35(2):112–9; discussion 87–8.
31. Coughlin MJ, Pinsonneault T. Operative treatment of interdigital neuroma. A long-term follow-up study. J Bone Joint Surg Am. 2001;83(9):1321–8.
32. Di Caprio F, Meringolo R, Shehab Eddine M, Ponziani L. Morton's interdigital neuroma of the foot: a literature review. Foot Ankle Surg. 2018;24(2):92–8.
33. Ganguly A, Warner J, Aniq H. Central metatarsalgia and walking on pebbles: beyond morton neuroma. AJR Am J Roentgenol. 2018;210(4):821–33.

34. Mulder JD. The causative mechanism in Morton's metatarsalgia. J Bone Joint Surg Br. 1951;33-B(1):94–5.
35. Sobiesk GA, Wertheimer SJ, Schulz R, Dalfovo M. Sonographic evaluation of interdigital neuromas. J Foot Ankle Surg. 1997;36(5):364–6.
36. Bignotti B, Signori A, Sormani MP, Molfetta L, Martinoli C, Tagliafico A. Ultrasound versus magnetic resonance imaging for Morton neuroma: systematic review and meta-analysis. Eur Radiol. 2015;25(8):2254–62.
37. Hsi WL, Kang JH, Lee XX. Optimum position of metatarsal pad in metatarsalgia for pressure relief. Am J Phys Med Rehabil. 2005;84(7):514–20.
38. de Oliveira HAV, Natour J, Vassalli M, Rosenfeld A, Jennings F, Jones A. Effectiveness of customized insoles in patients with Morton's neuroma: a randomized, controlled, double-blind clinical trial. Clin Rehabil. 2019;33(12):1898–907.
39. Choi JY, Lee HI, Hong WH, Suh JS, Hur JW. Corticosteroid injection for Morton's interdigital neuroma: a systematic review. Clin Orthop Surg. 2021;13(2):266–77.
40. Saygi B, Yildirim Y, Saygi EK, Kara H, Esemenli T. Morton neuroma: comparative results of two conservative methods. Foot Ankle Int. 2005;26(7):556–9.
41. Sofka CM, Adler RS, Ciavarra GA, Pavlov H. Ultrasound-guided interdigital neuroma injections: short-term clinical outcomes after a single percutaneous injection—preliminary results. HSS J. 2007;3(1):44–9.
42. Bauer T, Gaumetou E, Klouche S, Hardy P, Maffulli N. Metatarsalgia and Morton's disease: comparison of outcomes between open procedure and neurectomy versus percutaneous metatarsal osteotomies and ligament release with a minimum of 2 years of follow-up. J Foot Ankle Surg. 2015;54(3):373–7.
43. Riddle DL, Schappert SM. Volume of ambulatory care visits and patterns of care for patients diagnosed with plantar fasciitis: a national study of medical doctors. Foot Ankle Int. 2004;25(5):303–10.
44. Riddle DL, Pulisic M, Pidcoe P, Johnson RE. Risk factors for Plantar fasciitis: a matched case-control study. J Bone Joint Surg Am. 2003;85(5):872–7.
45. Schwartz EN, Su J. Plantar fasciitis: a concise review. Perm J. 2014;18(1):e105–7.
46. Thomas JL, Christensen JC, Kravitz SR, Mendicino RW, Schuberth JM, Vanore JV, et al. The diagnosis and treatment of heel pain: a clinical practice guideline-revision 2010. J Foot Ankle Surg. 2010;49(3 Suppl):S1–19.
47. Lemont H, Ammirati KM, Usen N. Plantar fasciitis: a degenerative process (fasciosis) without inflammation. J Am Podiatr Med Assoc. 2003;93(3):234–7.
48. Goff JD, Crawford R. Diagnosis and treatment of plantar fasciitis. Am Fam Physician. 2011;84(6):676–82.
49. Gill LH. Plantar fasciitis: diagnosis and conservative management. J Am Acad Orthop Surg. 1997;5(2):109–17.
50. Neufeld SK, Cerrato R. Plantar fasciitis: evaluation and treatment. J Am Acad Orthop Surg. 2008;16(6):338–46.
51. Thompson JV, Saini SS, Reb CW, Daniel JN. Diagnosis and management of plantar fasciitis. J Am Osteopath Assoc. 2014;114(12):900–6.
52. Donley BG, Moore T, Sferra J, Gozdanovic J, Smith R. The efficacy of oral nonsteroidal anti-inflammatory medication (NSAID) in the treatment of plantar fasciitis: a randomized, prospective, placebo-controlled study. Foot Ankle Int. 2007;28(1):20–3.
53. Schuitema D, Greve C, Postema K, Dekker R, Hijmans JM. Effectiveness of mechanical treatment for plantar fasciitis: a systematic review. J Sport Rehabil. 2020;29(5):657–74.
54. Landorf KB, Radford JA, Keenan AM, Redmond AC. Effectiveness of low-Dye taping for the short-term management of plantar fasciitis. J Am Podiatr Med Assoc. 2005;95(6):525–30.
55. Latt LD, Jaffe DE, Tang Y, Taljanovic MS. Evaluation and treatment of chronic plantar fasciitis. Foot Ankle Orthop. 2020;5(1):2473011419896763.
56. Wolgin M, Cook C, Graham C, Mauldin D. Conservative treatment of plantar heel pain: long-term follow-up. Foot Ankle Int. 1994;15(3):97–102.

57. Landorf KB, Keenan AM, Herbert RD. Effectiveness of different types of foot orthoses for the treatment of plantar fasciitis. J Am Podiatr Med Assoc. 2004;94(6):542–9.
58. Roos E, Engström M, Söderberg B. Foot orthoses for the treatment of plantar fasciitis. Foot Ankle Int. 2006;27(8):606–11.
59. Barry LD, Barry AN, Chen Y. A retrospective study of standing gastrocnemius-soleus stretching versus night splinting in the treatment of plantar fasciitis. J Foot Ankle Surg. 2002;41(4):221–7.
60. Pribut SM. Current approaches to the management of plantar heel pain syndrome, including the role of injectable corticosteroids. J Am Podiatr Med Assoc. 2007;97(1):68–74.
61. Crawford F, Atkins D, Young P, Edwards J. Steroid injection for heel pain: evidence of short-term effectiveness. A randomized controlled trial. Rheumatology (Oxford). 1999;38(10):974–7.
62. Nair AS, Sahoo RK. Ultrasound-guided injection for plantar fasciitis: a brief review. Saudi J Anaesth. 2016;10(4):440–3.
63. Weil LS, Roukis TS, Borrelli AH. Extracorporeal shock wave therapy for the treatment of chronic plantar fasciitis: indications, protocol, intermediate results, and a comparison of results to fasciotomy. J Foot Ankle Surg. 2002;41(3):166–72.
64. Sun K, Zhou H, Jiang W. Extracorporeal shock wave therapy versus other therapeutic methods for chronic plantar fasciitis. Foot Ankle Surg. 2020;26(1):33–8.
65. Jain SK, Suprashant K, Kumar S, Yadav A, Kearns SR. Comparison of plantar fasciitis injected with platelet-rich plasma vs corticosteroids. Foot Ankle Int. 2018;39(7):780–6.
66. Luffy L, Grosel J, Thomas R, So E. Plantar fasciitis: a review of treatments. JAAPA. 2018;31(1):20–4.
67. Tay KS, Ng YC, Singh IR, Chong KW. Open technique is more effective than percutaneous technique for TOPAZ radiofrequency coblation for plantar fasciitis. Foot Ankle Surg. 2012;18(4):287–92.
68. Ahmad M, Tsang K, Mackenney PJ, Adedapo AO. Tarsal tunnel syndrome: a literature review. Foot Ankle Surg. 2012;18(3):149–52.
69. Scura D, Garcia-Lopez B. Electrodiagnostic evaluation of tarsal tunnel neuropathy. Treasure Island (FL): StatPearls Publishing; 2022.
70. Bailie DS, Kelikian AS. Tarsal tunnel syndrome: diagnosis, surgical technique, and functional outcome. Foot Ankle Int. 1998;19(2):65–72.
71. Kiel J, Kaiser K. Tarsal tunnel syndrome. In: StatPearls (Internet). Treasure Island (FL): StatPearls Publishing; 2022.
72. Hudes K. Conservative management of a case of tarsal tunnel syndrome. J Can Chiropr Assoc. 2010;54(2):100–6.
73. Rodríguez-Merchán EC, Moracia-Ochagavía I. Tarsal tunnel syndrome: current rationale, indications and results. EFORT Open Rev. 2021;6(12):1140–7.
74. Lau JT, Daniels TR. Tarsal tunnel syndrome: a review of the literature. Foot Ankle Int. 1999;20(3):201–9.
75. Mondelli M, Morana P, Padua L. An electrophysiological severity scale in tarsal tunnel syndrome. Acta Neurol Scand. 2004;109(4):284–9.
76. Antoniadis G, Scheglmann K. Posterior tarsal tunnel syndrome: diagnosis and treatment. Dtsch Arztebl Int. 2008;105(45):776–81.
77. Cimino WR. Tarsal tunnel syndrome: review of the literature. Foot Ankle. 1990;11(1):47–52.
78. McSweeney SC, Cichero M. Tarsal tunnel syndrome-A narrative literature review. Foot (Edinb). 2015;25(4):244–50.
79. Kim K, Kokubo R, Isu T, Nariai M, Morimoto D, Kawauchi M, et al. Magnetic resonance imaging findings in patients with tarsal tunnel syndrome. Neurol Med Chir (Tokyo). 2022;62(12):552–8.
80. Fantino O. Role of ultrasound in posteromedial tarsal tunnel syndrome: 81 cases. J Ultrasound. 2014;17(2):99–112.
81. Fortier LM, Leethy KN, Smith M, McCarron MM, Lee C, Sherman WF, et al. An update on posterior tarsal tunnel syndrome. Orthop Rev (Pavia). 2022;14(4):35444.

82. Gondring WH, Shields B, Wenger S. An outcomes analysis of surgical treatment of tarsal tunnel syndrome. Foot Ankle Int. 2003;24(7):545–50.
83. Sammarco GJ, Chang L. Outcome of surgical treatment of tarsal tunnel syndrome. Foot Ankle Int. 2003;24(2):125–31.
84. de Jonge S, van den Berg C, de Vos RJ, van der Heide HJ, Weir A, Verhaar JA, et al. Incidence of midportion Achilles tendinopathy in the general population. Br J Sports Med. 2011;45(13):1026–8.
85. Zafar MS, Mahmood A, Maffulli N. Basic science and clinical aspects of achilles tendinopathy. Sports Med Arthrosc Rev. 2009;17(3):190–7.
86. von Rickenbach KJ, Borgstrom H, Tenforde A, Borg-Stein J, McInnis KC. Achilles tendinopathy: evaluation, rehabilitation, and prevention. Curr Sports Med Rep. 2021;20(6):327–34.
87. Martin RL, Chimenti R, Cuddeford T, Houck J, Matheson JW, McDonough CM, et al. Achilles pain, stiffness, and muscle power deficits: midportion achilles tendinopathy revision 2018. J Orthop Sports Phys Ther. 2018;48(5):A1–A38.
88. Magnan B, Bondi M, Pierantoni S, Samaila E. The pathogenesis of Achilles tendinopathy: a systematic review. Foot Ankle Surg. 2014;20(3):154–9.
89. Kraemer R, Wuerfel W, Lorenzen J, Busche M, Vogt PM, Knobloch K. Analysis of hereditary and medical risk factors in Achilles tendinopathy and Achilles tendon ruptures: a matched pair analysis. Arch Orthop Trauma Surg. 2012;132(6):847–53.
90. Vora AM, Myerson MS, Oliva F, Maffulli N. Tendinopathy of the main body of the Achilles tendon. Foot Ankle Clin. 2005;10(2):293–308.
91. Lewis T, Cook J. Fluoroquinolones and tendinopathy: a guide for athletes and sports clinicians and a systematic review of the literature. J Athl Train. 2014;49(3):422–7.
92. Maffulli N, Longo UG, Kadakia A, Spiezia F. Achilles tendinopathy. Foot Ankle Surg. 2020;26(3):240–9.
93. Krishna Sayana M, Maffulli N. Insertional Achilles tendinopathy. Foot Ankle Clin. 2005;10(2):309–20.
94. Chimenti RL, Cychosz CC, Hall MM, Phisitkul P. Current concepts review update: insertional achilles tendinopathy. Foot Ankle Int. 2017;38(10):1160–9.
95. van Dijk CN, van Sterkenburg MN, Wiegerinck JI, Karlsson J, Maffulli N. Terminology for Achilles tendon related disorders. Knee Surg Sports Traumatol Arthrosc. 2011;19(5):835–41.
96. Irwin TA. Current concepts review: insertional achilles tendinopathy. Foot Ankle Int. 2010;31(10):933–9.
97. Mafi N, Lorentzon R, Alfredson H. Superior short-term results with eccentric calf muscle training compared to concentric training in a randomized prospective multicenter study on patients with chronic Achilles tendinosis. Knee Surg Sports Traumatol Arthrosc. 2001;9(1):42–7.
98. Pavone V, Vescio A, Mobilia G, Dimartino S, Di Stefano G, Culmone A, et al. Conservative treatment of chronic achilles tendinopathy: a systematic review. J Funct Morphol Kinesiol. 2019;4(3):46.
99. Sussmilch-Leitch SP, Collins NJ, Bialocerkowski AE, Warden SJ, Crossley KM. Physical therapies for Achilles tendinopathy: systematic review and meta-analysis. J Foot Ankle Res. 2012;5(1):15.
100. Rompe JD, Furia J, Maffulli N. Eccentric loading versus eccentric loading plus shock-wave treatment for midportion achilles tendinopathy: a randomized controlled trial. Am J Sports Med. 2009;37(3):463–70.
101. Kakkos GA, Klontzas ME, Koltsakis E, Karantanas AH. US-guided high-volume injection for Achilles tendinopathy. J Ultrason. 2021;21(85):e127–e33.
102. Boesen AP, Langberg H, Hansen R, Malliaras P, Boesen MI. High volume injection with and without corticosteroid in chronic midportion achilles tendinopathy. Scand J Med Sci Sports. 2019;29(8):1223–31.
103. Singh A, Calafi A, Diefenbach C, Kreulen C, Giza E. Noninsertional tendinopathy of the achilles. Foot Ankle Clin. 2017;22(4):745–60.

Chest Wall Pain

16

Jessica Ibañez, Matthew Vassaur, Margret Zorc,
Matthew Weinstein, Frances Walson,
and Robert S. Ackerman

Introduction

Chest wall pain disorders are common, with both benign and serious etiologies. Adult and pediatric patients often present in the ambulatory and emergency settings with chest pain and all clinicians should be adept at diagnosis and management strategies for both familiar and life-threatening conditions [1, 2].

Serious causes are often cardiopulmonary in nature, including myocardial infarction, aortic dissection, and pneumothorax. Thankfully, these are rare compared to more common causes of chest wall pain, such as costochondritis, intercostal neuralgia, and fibromyalgia. A systemic approach to diagnostic evaluation with appropriate ordering of testing and imaging is key to establishing a diagnosis and formulating a thorough and effective treatment plan [3]. Even the postsurgical pain with expected incisional and postoperative pain may present a challenge to the clinician in the recovery period [4].

In this chapter, we review the features, diagnostic evaluation, and treatment options for many chest wall pain disorders, with an emphasis on the formulation of a differential diagnosis (as summarized in Fig. 16.1) and a staged or tiered treatment plan.

J. Ibañez · R. S. Ackerman (✉)
Division of Interventional Pain Medicine, Department of Anesthesiology, Moffitt Cancer Center and Research Institute, Tampa, FL, USA

Department of Oncologic Sciences, Morsani College of Medicine, University of South Florida, Tampa, FL, USA
e-mail: rackerman@usf.edu

M. Vassaur · M. Zorc · M. Weinstein
Morsani College of Medicine, University of South Florida, Tampa, FL, USA

F. Walson
Physical Medicine and Rehabilitation, Cleveland, OH, USA

C. E. Noe (ed.), *Musculoskeletal Pain*,
https://doi.org/10.1007/978-3-031-86057-7_16

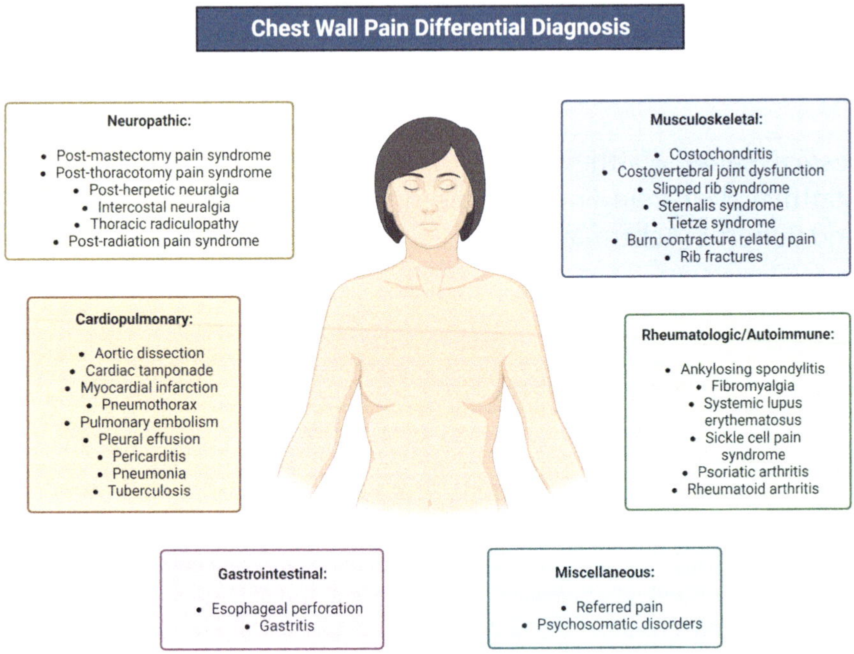

Fig. 16.1 Chest wall pain differential diagnosis. Common and rare diagnoses are listed, organized by organ system. (Created with BioRender.com)

Evaluation of Chest Wall Pain

Musculoskeletal Disorders

Costochondritis

Costochondritis is one of the most common causes of musculoskeletal chest wall pain. Costochondritis presents as acute anterior chest wall pain due to inflammation at the costochondral or chondrosternal articulations. The epidemiology of costochondritis is not well-documented; however, a small prospective study in 1994 demonstrated that 30% of the patients presenting to the emergency department with chest pain not due to trauma, malignancy, or fever were diagnosed with costochondritis. The study also found the diagnosis to be more common in females and Hispanics [5].

After the exclusion of other underlying causes, the diagnosis of costochondritis is made by history and physical exam. Laboratory evaluation, chest X-ray, and electrocardiogram are often obtained to rule out cardiac and pulmonary causes for chest wall pain and should be normal in the setting of costochondritis [6]. Patients may report a history of recent upper respiratory illness with coughing, recent vigorous exercise, or activity stressing the upper body [7]. The pain can be exacerbated by certain upper body movements, deep inhalations, or strenuous activity. Pain is typically reproducible with palpation along one or more rib segments at the costochondral junction and can radiate along the chest wall [6]. Multiple rib segments are affected in more than 90% of cases. Any of the costochondral joints can be involved, however the second to fifth are the most common sites of pain. In contrast to Tietze syndrome, no swelling at the costochondral junction should be appreciated [8].

Costochondritis is a self-limited condition that usually lasts for weeks to months. First-line therapies include oral analgesics, such as acetaminophen and/or NSAIDs, and local application of heat or ice. Patients should also be instructed to minimize activities that aggravate the pain [7]. Physical therapy (PT) and gentle mobilization have been shown to have some benefit in prolonged cases [9, 10]. Corticosteroid or local anesthetic injections into the costochondral joint can be considered in severe, refractory cases [11].

Costovertebral Joint Dysfunction

Chest wall pain due to costovertebral joint dysfunction is often referenced in manual medicine textbooks; however, the condition is often overlooked in traditional health care settings. Costovertebral joint dysfunction is due to abnormal movement or posterior subluxation of the rib at the costovertebral articulation [12]. The costovertebral ligaments are innervated by the lateral branches of the dorsal rami of spinal nerves C8-T11, with each joint receiving fibers from the spinal nerve exiting directly above and below [13]. Excessive movement or trauma at these articulations can produce localized or radiating thoracic pain along the associated dermatome.

Extensive and costly diagnostic workup is often performed on patients presenting with this atypical chest pain to rule out the cardiac or pulmonary origin; however, diagnosis of costovertebral dysfunction is based primarily on clinical examination [12]. Patients will often present with a recent history of minor trauma to the chest wall, prolonged abnormal positioning, or pain after a sudden movement such as twisting, bending, or overextension. The affected rib segment may be tender to touch, and symptoms are typically exacerbated with coughing, deep inhalation, lateral bending, or rotational movements of the torso [13]. Pain is often unilateral and can radiate to the chest or scapula. Localized skin hyperalgesia or dysesthesia may also be appreciated [12].

Treatment of costovertebral joint dysfunction can include activity modification, anti-inflammatory medications, manual therapy with soft tissue or joint mobilization at the affected rib, stretching, postural improvement, or injections. A case series demonstrated complete resolution of costovertebral joint dysfunction pain following intercostal nerve blockade in four out of five patients and spontaneous resolution of pain in another patient following clinical examination ("manipulation-like" effect) [12].

Slipped Rib Syndrome

Slipped rib syndrome (SRS) is a rare cause of lower anterior chest wall pain due to hypermobility of the costal cartilage of the false ribs (ribs eight through ten). The tip of the rib slips or clicks superiorly and abuts the above rib, leading to irritation of the surrounding soft tissue and traversing intercostal nerve [14]. Risk factors for developing SRS include hypermobility, congenital deformity, or disruption of the fibrous articulation due to direct trauma or overuse. SRS can occur at any age with studies citing cases in patients ranging from 7 to 86 years old. It is more commonly seen in females and female athletes which is hypothesized to be due to increased joint laxity and hormonal fluctuations [15, 16].

The pain with SRS can be felt as a localized somatic pain or a diffuse visceral pain, which can lead clinicians to a broad differential for chest and abdominal pain. However, patients typically present with sharp or stabbing pain at the costal margin that transitions to dull, aching pain caused by movements such as twisting, side bending, coughing, or sneezing [14]. The pain is most commonly unilateral but there are case studies describing bilateral SRS [16]. Patients occasionally report a clicking or grinding sensation with certain movements. Symptoms may be relieved by lying down, stretching the affected side, or applying pressure to the area [14]. The hook maneuver is a provocative test that can be used for diagnosis. The practitioner slides their fingers under the costal margin and applies an anterior and superior force to the ribs. A click or reproduction of the pain indicates a positive test. Imaging studies including X-ray, computed tomography (CT) scan, MRI, and static ultrasound are of limited use as the costal cartilage is poorly visualized. Dynamic ultrasound may be useful to demonstrate mobility of the affected rib as the patient performs movements such as coughing, crunching, or pressure applied directly to the rib. A retrospective review study of suspected SRS patients demonstrated that dynamic ultrasound can identify SRS in ~90% of cases with 100% specificity [17].

Once SRS is diagnosed, the patient should be reassured that it is a benign, treatable condition. A study revealed on average patients experienced pain for 15.4 months prior to the diagnosis of SRS [16]. Initial treatment consists of limiting aggravating activity, ice, topical anti-inflammatories, and oral nonsteroidal antiinflammatory drugs (NSAIDs). Osteopathic manipulative treatment, physical therapy, heat, and massage are other conservative treatments that can be utilized [15]. In refractory cases, intercostal nerve blocks with steroid and/or local anesthetic can provide long-lasting relief [18]. The most definitive treatment, which should be reserved as a last option, is surgical resection of the costal cartilage [15].

Sternalis Syndrome

The sternalis muscle is an accessory muscle found in approximately 7.8% of the population [19]. It is hypothesized to originate from adjacent musculature as cadaveric studies have found that it is most commonly innervated by the pectoral and intercostal nerves [19]. The presence of a sternalis muscle has been well-documented for its ability to skew routine mammograms, alter electrocardiograms, and impact breast or thoracic surgeries. There are few case studies describing clinical symptoms due to the sternalis muscle which can likely be attributed to its relatively small size and no apparent physiological function [20]. When inflammation of the sternalis muscle does occur, patients may experience pain and tenderness in the sternal region [21]. These symptoms can mimic those of other conditions such as angina or musculoskeletal injuries, therefore a thorough physical exam and diagnostic workup should be performed for an accurate diagnosis. Sternalis syndrome is characterized by tenderness to palpation along the sternalis muscles which can radiate into the neck or arms [22]. Ultrasound can be a useful tool to identify the presence of an accessory sternalis muscle, and sonopalpation can be used to confirm the source of the pain. MRI can also be used to identify the presence of a sternalis muscle; however, edema or abnormalities within the tissue may not be appreciated in either of these studies [21].

Sternalis syndrome is a self-limited condition that rarely progresses to persistent pain [22]. Initial treatment includes conservative measures, such as rest, ice, anti-inflammatory medications, and physical therapy. In refractory cases, trigger point injections with local anesthetic can be considered.

Tietze Syndrome

Tietze syndrome is a benign, painful arthropathy characterized by inflammation of a single costochondral, sternocostal, or sternoclavicular joint. It is often confused with costochondritis but can be differentiated by the presence of swelling at the affected joint [23]. It is believed to be caused by microtrauma or respiratory infections and patients may present with a history of recent coughing, vomiting, or chest impact. The unilateral, anterior chest wall pain may radiate along the chest wall and to the ipsilateral arm. Pain is exacerbated by movement of the arm, coughing, sneezing, or deep inhalation [23, 24]. The affected joint will be tender to palpation and swollen, with ribs two and three being the common segments involved [8].

Diagnosis is made based on the history and clinical exam after the exclusion of other costochondral conditions such as rheumatoid arthritis (RA), costochondritis, and coronary syndromes. Laboratory workup may reveal elevated erythrocyte sedimentation rate (ESR) or C-reactive protein (CRP). Imaging studies should be performed to help differentiate Tietze syndrome as it is a relatively rare condition. Ultrasound is one of the most effective modalities and will demonstrate soft tissue swelling at the affected segment. Nuclear magnetic resonance (NMR) may show inflammatory changes in the surrounding fat tissue and bone marrow edema [24]. Skeletal scintigraphy and PET/CT scan can demonstrate increased radioactive uptake and increased metabolic activity, respectively, at the symptomatic joint [25]. Early biopsy of the lesion should be considered in cases with increasing swelling to rule out primary chest wall tumor [26].

Tietze syndrome is a self-limited condition that can be treated with conservative therapies. Oral and topical analgesics and anti-inflammatories are first-line treatments. Local application of heat can also be utilized. Corticosteroid medication and/or lidocaine injection can be considered for refractory cases. On average, the pain may resolve within 1–2 weeks with conservative care. However, in some cases, the pain may become chronic [24].

Burn Contracture Related Pain

Burn contractures are a major cause of pain and functional limitations following a burn injury. A large, multicenter study of ~1800 burn patients found that 33% demonstrated at least one contracture at hospital discharge. However, contracture of the thoracic region was rare, comprising only 0.4% of the ~2100 total contractures in the study [27]. Contractures are defined as shortening or distortion of tissue leading to reduced mobility or impaired function of a joint. Pain, disfigurement, and itching from burn contracture are common and can strongly impact a patient's quality of life [27, 28]. In chest wall burns specifically, respiratory muscle contracture can result in impaired respiratory function due to impaired mobility of the rib cage, further limiting the patient's functional capacity [29].

Although 18–35% of burn survivors report persistent burn-related pain, there is sparse literature on the treatment of chronic burn contracture-related pain [30]. The mainstay treatments for burn scar pain include the use of silicone, compression garments, scar massage, and oral analgesics [28, 31]. If neuropathic pain is present, antiepileptic drugs such as gabapentin or pregabalin can be used [32]. Non-pharmacologic approaches such as hypnosis, cognitive behavioral techniques, and virtual reality have also been utilized in burn patients but there is limited research supporting the efficacy [32]. In chest wall burn contracture specifically, yoga with pranayama breathing exercise and arm cycling exercises have both been shown to have some positive benefits on quality of life and pulmonary function; however, neither study noted the presence or impact on chest wall pain [33, 34].

Rib Fractures

Rib fractures are one of the most common thoracic traumas and have been associated with significant morbidity and mortality, especially in the elderly [35]. The severity of trauma can be correlated with the number of rib fractures as more than 90% of patients with multiple rib fractures have associated head, abdominal, and/or extremity injuries [36]. Rib fractures can cause debilitating chest wall pain that is particularly worse during breathing and coughing. When pain is not well-controlled, respiratory complications such as pneumonia, atelectasis, and impaired ventilatory function can occur. While the majority of rib fractures are not life-threatening and can be treated nonoperatively, prompt management with pain control, respiratory support, and pulmonary hygiene is critical to prevent further complications [37].

Radiographic imaging is required for the diagnosis of rib fractures as clinical symptoms do not reliably predict the presence of a rib fracture [38]. Chest radiographs and chest computed tomography (CT) scans should be obtained in patients presenting with chest pain after blunt trauma or a fall. A study of over 2000 patients diagnosed with rib fractures who had both chest radiographs and chest CT scans demonstrated that 66% of rib fractures were observed on chest CT scans only [39]. CT imaging also provides a more accurate assessment of the number of ribs fractured, the location of injury, and associated pulmonary contusions or visceral injuries that may need further treatment.

Effective and continuous pain control is one of the key components of rib fracture management. A multimodal approach with both pharmacological and non-pharmacological modalities is recommended. Pharmacological modalities include analgesics such as opioids (intravenous and oral), NSAIDS, and acetaminophen, as well as adjuvant medications such as gabapentin and pregabalin [37, 40]. Transdermal lidocaine patches are effective in some cases and may be a useful adjunct given the excellent safety profile. Opioids are very effective for treating the acute pain associated with rib fractures but carry a significant risk of respiratory depression, decreased cough reflex, sedation, and falls [40]. Hence, non-pharmacological modalities such as thoracic epidural analgesia or regional nerve blocks are often used in conjunction with pharmacological treatments.

Thoracic epidural analgesia is considered the "gold standard" of pain control for rib fractures. A meta-analysis demonstrated thoracic epidurals provide better pain reduction compared with other modalities (intravenous analgesia, paravertebral blocks, and intercostal blocks), but there was no difference found in the secondary outcomes such as ICU stay, length of mechanical ventilation, or pulmonary complications [41]. Epidural analgesia is contraindicated in thoracic vertebral fractures, spinal cord injury, ongoing coagulopathy, bacteremia, and severe head injury which may limit its use in many trauma patients [42]. Paravertebral blocks can be considered in unilateral rib fractures when epidurals are not recommended. The utilization of landmark-based and ultrasound-guided techniques can improve their accuracy and safety. Body habitus, pneumothorax, transverse process fractures, or surgical emphysema may make guidance with ultrasound more challenging [43]. While thoracic paravertebral blocks have a lower risk of complications such as hypotension, motor block, or epidural hematoma, they still carry a high-risk in anticoagulated patients, which should be considered with the potential benefits [40]. Intercostal nerve blocks and serratus anterior plane blocks are also effective for immediate pain control; however, they may be repeated, which can be logistically difficult in both the hospital and outpatient setting [44, 45]. An ultrasound-guided serratus anterior plane blocks can be considered in cases with multiple rib fractures when the patient is restricted to lying supine. The catheter-based technique can allow for continuous infusion of local anesthetic over several days and is considered a lower risk in the anticoagulated patient [45].

Effective pain control is critical in the management of rib fractures to improve respiratory function and prevent associated complications. The choice of pain control modality should be individualized based on the patient's specific needs and risk profile.

Neuropathic Disorders

Postmastectomy Pain Syndrome

Postmastectomy pain syndrome (PMPS) is a chronic neuropathic pain condition defined as pain located in the anterior surface of the chest axilla, shoulder, or upper half of the arm persisting for at least 3 months after breast cancer-related surgery [46, 47]. However, it is important to keep in mind that despite its name, PMPS is likely not limited to just mastectomy procedures and could be a result of any other surgical procedure involving the breast parenchyma or underlying muscle [48]. PMPS has generally been thought of as being due to intercostobrachial nerve damage during surgery but other nerves, including the medial pectoral, lateral pectoral, thoracodorsal, and long thoracic nerves, can also be injured from surgery [48–50].

PMPS has been estimated to affect as many as 20–50% of postmastectomy patients [47, 49]. Risk factors for the development of PMPS include psychological factors (anxiety, mood, and sleep disorders), younger age, minority race/ethnicity, preexisting pain, and genetic polymorphisms [49, 51]. Axillary lymph node dissection is a well-known intraoperative risk factor for PMPS. The presence of acute postoperative pain is also strongly associated with PMPS development. Additionally, administration of radiation therapy in conjunction with surgery can increase the risk of PMPS [49].

Its presentation can vary based on which nerves are affected; however, the classic characteristics include a shooting, stabbing, pulling, tight, burning, and/or aching pain often with palpable allodynia located at the axilla, breast/chest wall, and/or medial upper extremity [49, 51]. PMPS pain is typically worsened with movement, straining, overhead activity, and/or cold weather [49].

There is no gold standard treatment guideline for PMPS, and interventions vary from conservative to more invasive modalities. As with all chronic pain, a multimodal, multidisciplinary approach is essential [46, 49].

Numerous psychological interventions have been studied given breast cancer survivors often cope with a complex combination of physical, psychological, and social comorbidities. Of those techniques, cognitive-behavioral therapy has consistently shown the greatest benefits [46, 47, 49].

Physical therapy (PT) interventions, especially exercise therapy with stretching and active exercises, have shown to be of great benefit to PMPS patients [49, 52]. There may also be utility for laser therapy combined with PT for the treatment of PMPS. A study on the combination of pulsed high-intensity laser therapy with PT showed this combination to be more effective than PT alone in improving both quality of life and pain in PMPS patients [53]. Aquatic therapy, massage, myofascial release, and acupuncture are other modalities that may be beneficial as well [46, 52].

Medications with the strongest recommendation for use in PMPS include gabapentin, pregabalin, serotonin-norepinephrine reuptake inhibitors (SNRIs, i.e., duloxetine), and tricyclic antidepressants (TCAs, i.e., amitriptyline). Topical medication may also provide benefits, with capsaicin being the most promising of those studied [46, 49].

A variety of nonsurgical interventional procedures have been studied in the treatment of PMPS. Trigger point injections for postmastectomy patients with identified trigger points along the inframammary fold can provide significant relief [54]. Intercostal nerve blocks are another effective intervention for pain from PMPS [55, 56]. Thoracic paravertebral blocks have been shown to achieve immediate but short-term pain relief (<1 month). Pulsed radiofrequency ablation (RFA) with steroid injection targeting the T2–T3 dorsal root ganglia for intercostal brachial neuralgia post-mastectomy can provide longer-lasting (6 months) relief [46]. Studies have also shown that blockade or neurolysis of C7-T4 stellate ganglions could be successful in treating PMPS [46, 57].

Surgical procedures may also be of benefit in certain situations. For patients with peripheral nerve injury and subsequent neuroma formation, neuroma excision, and implantation can provide long-term relief. Fat grafting for patients at high-risk of scar contracture has shown promising results, as has laser therapy to help with the release of scar contractures. There is also potential for the use of lymph node transplantation for the treatment of chronic pain and lymphedema after breast cancer surgery [46].

Post-thoracotomy Pain Syndrome

Thoracic surgery, and especially thoracotomy, is associated with severe postoperative pain which can lead to not only respiratory complications but also chronic, persistent pain [58]. Post-thoracotomy pain syndrome (PTPS) is defined as pain that recurs or persists along a thoracotomy scar for at least 2 months following the surgery [59]. PTPS affects approximately 50% of post-thoracotomy patients and is most likely due to a combination of neuropathic and myofascial pain related to intercostal nerve trauma [60–62].

The clinical presentation of PTPS is most consistent with neuropathic pain as symptoms of lancinating pain, dysesthesias, aching sensations, and allodynia have been described. Symptoms can be intermittent, constant, or related to activity, and are often localized around the incision scar but can also radiate to the back, shoulder, or other chest wall locations [61].

There is no true gold standard for the treatment of PTPS. For acute post-thoracotomy pain, thoracic epidural analgesia is generally considered the first-line option, although paravertebral blocks have shown similar effectiveness [58, 61]. Studies observing ultrasound-guided blocks, including erector spinae and serratus anterior plane blocks, have yielded promising results as well for controlling early post-thoracotomy pain.

Multimodal pain control targeting different pain receptors is essential for the treatment of PTPS. Medications commonly utilized include NSAIDs, acetaminophen, and gabapentin or pregabalin. TCAs and SNRIs can also be used for the neuropathic pain component. PTPS has also been treated with NMDA receptor antagonists i.e., ketamine; however, recent research has shown that while ketamine is helpful in the immediate postoperative period, it may not be effective for chronic pain after 2 months [61, 63, 64].

Minimally invasive interventional techniques can be performed as well for PTPS. The use of diagnostic intercostal nerve blocks followed by radiofrequency ablation is supported by multiple case reports [61, 65, 66]. Peripheral nerve stimulation and dorsal root ganglion stimulation have had encouraging results in treating PTPS [61]. Spinal cord stimulation (SCS) has been shown to be an effective treatment option for persistent, intractable PTPS [61, 67–69]. A retrospective study examining percutaneous computed tomography (CT)-guided intercostal nerve cryoablation for refractory PTPS found of the 13 patients included in the study, 69% experienced significant improvement, making this a potentially effective option to consider in the future [62].

There may be an opportunity for the prevention of PTPS through a newer surgical technique known as “integrated” thoracotomy, which minimizes nerve damage during thoracotomy via retractor-free exposure and neurovascular exclusion sutures. One prospective study found that this technique is effective at reducing post-thoracotomy pain by up to 6 months postoperatively, but further research is needed [61, 70].

Postherpetic Neuralgia

Herpes zoster (HZ), or shingles, is a common disease in the elderly that usually presents as a vesicular rash in a unilateral, dermatomal distribution with concurrent or subsequent pain. The rash is often located in the mid- to low thoracic region. When the pain persists and is prolonged, a diagnosis of postherpetic neuralgia (PHN) can be made [71].

According to Johnson et al., "postherpetic neuralgia (PHN) is a neuropathic pain syndrome, resulting from a combination of inflammatory and viral damage to primary afferent fibers of sensory nerves and the corresponding levels of the spinal cord, as well as peripheral and central sensitization" [72]. There have been multiple definitions proposed throughout the years for what constitutes PHN; however, none of them are universally agreed upon. Generally, PHN is described as pain that persists for 3–4 months following the onset of zoster rash [71–75].

The proportion of HZ patients who go on to develop PHN varies. Multiple risk factors have been identified, including older age, prodromal pain, greater acute pain, severe rash, ophthalmic location, psychosocial distress, immunocompromised state, and, potentially, female sex [71, 72].

Clinically, patients with PHN present with pain that is usually localized to the dermatome affected by the rash. Characteristics are that of a typical neuropathic pain syndrome and include burning, throbbing, sharp, shooting, stabbing, lancinating, and/or aching pains. Allodynia is also common in PHN and is usually the most distressing and debilitating component of PHN [72, 74].

PHN can be challenging to treat, but a wide range of options do exist [71, 74]. Starting with the more conservative measures first, wearing natural fiber clothing is preferable to artificial fibers to reduce peripheral stimulation and decrease allodynia. Along the same lines, a protective layer between the skin and provoking stimuli may also help. The application of cold packs can provide short-term relief [74]. Transcutaneous electrical nerve stimulation (TENS) could be helpful; however, the results from studies have been mixed [74, 76]. Acupuncture may be beneficial during the early course of PHN, while ultrasound has not been found to have any benefit [74]. A recent study found that low-level laser therapy, which is noninvasive, painless, and safe, is effective for the treatment of PHN, and could reduce the use of medications [77].

With regards to topical medications, lidocaine may have the strongest evidence for use in PHN. In a study by Binder et al., 5% lidocaine medicated plaster provided more than half of the 265 patients included in the study with at least moderate pain relief. It was also associated with improvements in allodynia, quality of life, and sleep [73]. Another study found that 5% lidocaine medicated plaster for PHN was a more cost-effective treatment than gabapentin and was both more effective and less costly than 300 and 600 mg/day of pregabalin [75]. Other studies have found that both lidocaine gel and patch are effective in treating PHN [74, 78, 79]. Capsaicin may provide a small benefit but is often difficult to tolerate due to the intense burning after application. Evidence is inconclusive for the use of NSAID creams in PHN [74].

In terms of oral medications, TCAs have long been the first-line treatment for PHN. Amitriptyline is the most commonly used TCA for PHN; however, nortriptyline has been found to provide similar analgesia and have fewer side effects compared to amitriptyline [74, 80]. Desipramine can be used if sedation is an issue and has similar effectiveness to amitriptyline [74]. SNRIs like duloxetine are another class of antidepressants that can be considered given their effectiveness in other neuropathic pain conditions [72]. Of the anticonvulsants, gabapentin should also be considered first-line for treating PHN and appears to be at least equally as effective and safe as TCAs [74, 81]. Pregabalin acts similarly to gabapentin and has also been approved for the treatment of PHN [71]. Regarding analgesics, the opioids oxycodone and tramadol have evidence for use in PHN [71, 72, 74, 82, 83]. Oral NSAIDs have little role in the treatment of PHN [74, 84].

Minimally invasive procedures including intrathecal and epidural corticosteroids and sympathetic blockade may have a role in treatment of refractory PHN. The study by Kikuchi et al. (1999) found intrathecal administration of methylprednisolone to be more effective than epidural [71, 85]. However, intrathecal administration of corticosteroids has been associated with risks of arachnoiditis, meningitis, cauda equina syndrome, and cerebral vein thrombosis [71]. Sympathetic blockade with local anesthetics has also been studied for use in PHN; however, this technique seems to have more of a benefit in acute HZ as it has not provided sustained relief in PHN patients [71, 86]. Spinal cord stimulation is another consideration as it has been shown to provide satisfactory pain relief over a ~2–4 years interval for intractable PHN [71, 87, 88].

Surgical treatments that have been studied for severe intractable PHN include skin excision, sympathectomy, dorsal root entry zone (DREZ) lesions, cordotomy, thalamotomy, cingulumotomy, and deep brain stimulation. All other options should be exhausted prior to consideration of any of these neurosurgical procedures [71, 74].

Methods of prevention against PHN include vaccination against *Varicella zoster* virus and treatment of acute HZ with antiviral drugs [72, 74].

Intercostal Neuralgia

Intercostal neuralgia is characterized by neuropathic pain in the distribution of affected intercostal nerve(s) along the ribs, chest, or abdomen. A variety of causes have been described in the literature, with the two most common being tissue and nerve injury from thoracotomy (acute and chronic i.e., PTPS) and HZ infection (acute and chronic i.e., PHN) [89, 90]. Other less common etiologies include iatrogenic from chest tube placement or surgery, trauma, pregnancy, anatomical compression, inflammatory/reactive neoplastic, or infectious [89, 91].

The diagnosis of intercostal neuralgia is based solely on history and physical exam [89]. Presenting symptoms are those of typical neuropathic pain syndromes and are usually sensory in nature, with severe cases affecting motor function. Pain can be constant or intermittent and is described as radiating, sharp, burning, stabbing, and/or aching, sometimes occurring with associated paresthesias like numbness or tingling [89, 90]. The pain wraps around in a band-like fashion along the chest and back or in a thoracic dermatomal pattern and can be worsened with physical activity or unexpected movements such as jumping, sneezing, coughing, etc.

Patients may endorse allodynia on physical exam, and palpation or stretching of the affected nerve(s) can reproduce the pain. Additional signs of nerve damage on physical exam include involuntary muscle contractions and skin color changes above the affected area along with loss of sensitivity over the affected dermatome. An exam finding known as Schepelmann's sign may also be positive in intercostal neuralgia. With this exam maneuver, the patient will report increased pain with lateral lumbar–thoracic bending toward the side of pain, which compresses the intercostal structures. Increased pain with bending away from the side of pain may represent pleuritic pain.

A diagnostic intercostal nerve block can also assist in diagnosis. Depending on the cause, additional diagnostic and/or imaging studies may be necessary such as X-ray, CT, or MRI for trauma or cancer, or PCR or skin biopsy for cases of suspected HZ [89]. Electromyography (EMG) may be helpful in some cases for evaluating intercostal nerve function [89, 92]. One recent study also showed promising results for the use of magnetic resonance neurography (MRN) as part of the diagnostic workup for intercostal neuralgia. MRN could help with treatment planning too as the study found that MRN-positive cases of intercostal neuralgia show favorable treatment outcomes with perineural injections and subsequent surgical management [93].

There are multiple treatment options for intercostal neuralgia, ranging from conservative to more invasive. The underlying cause of intercostal neuralgia should obviously be addressed first. For chronic pain control, oral medications that have been shown to be helpful are NSAIDs, gabapentin, pregabalin, TCAs, SNRIs, bupropion, and opioids. Topical medications such as capsaicin and lidocaine can also provide relief.

In addition to aiding in diagnosis, interventional techniques such as intercostal nerve blocks can be used in the treatment of intercostal neuralgia [89]. Neurolytic intercostal nerve block with phenol or alcohol can be performed if long-term relief was not achieved with intercostal nerve block using local anesthetic plus or minus steroid after discussion of risk and benefits [89, 94]. Image-guided intercostal nerve radiofrequency ablation has also been shown to provide long-term relief that can sometimes even last for >1 year [65, 66, 89].

More invasive treatments can be used for refractory intercostal neuralgia once more conservative measures have been tried and failed. Options that can be considered include dorsal rhizotomy, surgical neurectomy, endoscopic intercostal neurotomy, and sensory ganglionectomy of corresponding intercostal nerves [89, 90, 95, 96].

Since deconditioning can result from the pain of intercostal neuralgia, modalities like PT, psychotherapy, and acupuncture should always be considered as additions to the above treatments [89]. While its efficacy is debatable, TENS could also be useful as an adjunct to therapy [89, 97]. Additionally, manipulation of the thoracic spine and manual release of the intervertebral and costovertebral joints can remove impingement in some cases [89, 98].

Thoracic Radiculopathy

Thoracic radiculopathy is a relatively rare spinal disorder that is often overlooked when evaluating a patient with back pain. There are a wide variety of etiologies of thoracic radiculopathy and differentiating other causes of pain from thoracic radiculopathy is essential. For example, coronary artery disease must be ruled out in any patient presenting with left-sided chest pain that worsens with activity. Other conditions that can cause or present similarly to thoracic radiculopathy include compression fractures, infection, congenital or acquired lesions (i.e., arachnoid cysts or epidermoid inclusion tumors), metastatic cancer, renal lithiasis, hepatobiliary disease, myofascial pain, fibromyalgia, and costochondritis.

Ultimately, two of the most common causes of thoracic radiculopathy are thoracic disc disease and diabetes mellitus [99]. While thoracic disc herniations can occur at any level in the thoracic spine, most occur in the lower thoracic spine between the T8 and T12 levels, with T11–T12 being the most common level overall [99–101]. Depending on which nerve root(s) are affected, thoracic disc herniation symptoms radiate in a segmental distribution across the anterior chest, thorax, and/or abdomen. As with radiculopathies in the cervical and lumbar spine, these radicular symptoms include variable pain, paresthesias, dysesthesias, allodynia, and/or loss of sensation [99]. There have also been case reports on lower-level thoracic disc herniations (T11, T12) causing atypical symptoms of lower extremity leg pain and/or weakness, i.e., foot drop, that mimic lumbosacral pathology [99, 102, 103]. Diabetic radiculopathy is a non-compressive source of pain and presents similarly to discogenic thoracic radiculopathy [99]. Cases of thoracic radiculopathy following spinal cord stimulation (SCS) implantation have also been reported [104].

A physical exam is unreliable in the diagnosis of thoracic radiculopathy since the presenting symptoms are not universal. Additionally, isolated muscle testing of the likely affected muscles (paraspinal, intercostal, and abdominal muscles) is difficult. Thus, there is no dependable way to test for muscle weakness in a myotomal pattern like there is for cervical or lumbosacral radiculopathies. A physical exam in this case is more useful for ruling out other causes of chest pain. Imaging studies can obviously be of use in the evaluation of thoracic radiculopathy. Electrodiagnostic studies with needle electromyography (EMG) of the thoracic paraspinal muscles plus or minus the intercostal and abdominal musculature can also be utilized for thoracic radiculopathy diagnosis in the appropriate clinical setting.

Treatments for thoracic radiculopathy are like those of radiculopathies in the other regions of the spine, with conservative measures usually being tried first. Short-term symptomatic relief may be achieved with the use of ice, heat, ultrasound, and/or electrical stimulation. For subacute and chronic symptoms, orthotics and spinal extension exercises can be helpful [99]. Regarding spinal manipulation or mobilization, there is little evidence for its use in treating thoracic radiculopathy

[105]. Medications that can be used for symptomatic relief include anticonvulsants (i.e., gabapentin, pregabalin), SNRIs (i.e., duloxetine), NSAIDs, acetaminophen, muscle relaxants, opiates, and sleep medications.

While minimally invasive procedures are gaining more and more popularity for the diagnosis and treatment of spinal pain syndromes, there are not as many studies on their efficacy at the thoracic level [99]. Epidural steroid injections can be utilized. One high-quality randomized controlled trial provided level II evidence with moderate to strong recommendations for the long-term effectiveness of thoracic epidural injection in treating thoracic disc herniation [106]. In addition to their use in some other chest wall pain syndromes, selective spinal nerve root and intercostal nerve blocks can also be beneficial in treating thoracic radiculopathy and discogenic pain [99]. There may also be utility for nerve root blocks and ablations in the treatment of thoracic radiculopathy. One study looked at the efficacy of CT-guided nerve root block and ablation on patients with identified disc herniation or foraminal stenosis on imaging at a variety of spinal levels. The nerve root blocks were performed with a diagnostic purpose to determine the clinical significance of the imaging findings, with a positive response being followed by nerve root ablation. At the thoracic level, significant relief was observed with nerve root ablation in 90% (nine of ten) patients [99, 107]. For patients with thoracic radicular pain secondary to vertebral body compression fractures, vertebroplasty can provide relief [99].

If more conservative options fail to provide significant relief, surgical intervention can be considered. Laminectomy and discectomy are a couple of the more studied surgical treatment options [99, 108–110]. Other open surgical correction procedures like fusions can be performed but are riskier at the thoracic level due to the proximity of major organs and neurovasculature. With any deeply invasive procedure, there is of course the additional risk of complications such as infection, blood loss, postoperative pain, and extended hospital stay. One study explored a less invasive procedure known as endoscopic thoracic lamino foraminoplasty (ELFP) in the treatment of thoracic radicular pain involving the lower thoracic levels, defined as at or below T6. Marked improvement in pain scores was seen in seven of the twelve patients [111].

Postradiation Pain Syndrome

While radiation therapy is a mainstay of cancer treatment, it can unfortunately harm exposed areas. The inflammatory reaction induced by radiation therapy can lead to fibrosis, atrophy, and ulceration of the related tissue, including vessels and nerves. This cascade can result in myelin destruction and axonal injury to the nerve(s), which are the main mechanisms behind radiation-induced neuropathic pain [112]. Nerve compression from radiation-induced fibrosis is another mechanism that can lead to postradiation neuropathic pain. The nerve damage from radiation is often progressive and irreversible and can sometimes present months or even years after receiving radiation therapy [113].

One presentation of postradiation pain syndrome is radiation-induced brachial plexus neuropathy (RIBPN), which can occur following radiation treatment for cancer in the neck, axilla, and chest wall. Symptoms vary and can include numbness, paresthesia, dysesthesia, lymphedema, and motor weakness, which may happen later in the disease course and can even lead to complete paralysis of the upper limb. Fibrosis of the scapulothoracic and glenohumeral joints can also occur in severe cases, resulting in a restricted range of motion at the shoulder joint [114].

Treatments for radiation-induced neuropathic pain are like those for other neuropathic pain syndromes. First-line treatment options include TCAs and gabapentin. If coexisting neurogenic inflammation is suspected, NSAIDs and steroids can be of benefit. Opioids can be trialed for refractory pain, although their use in neuropathic pain is limited. Second-line treatment options include lidocaine or ketamine. More invasive options can be considered as well for refractory pain and include SCS, spinal analgesia through epidural or intrathecal infusion, and dorsal root entry zone (DREZ) lesioning [115]. DREZ lesioning has especially been shown to be useful for treating RIBPN [115, 116]. Last, as with any chronic pain disorder, interdisciplinary management should be utilized to address physical and psychosocial factors as well. CBT and PT are a couple of options available to help address these components [115].

Rheumatologic/Autoimmune Disorders

Ankylosing Spondylitis

Ankylosing spondylitis (AS) is a chronic inflammatory disease that predominately affects the axial spine. The disease is characterized by progressive, debilitating arthritis that typically begins in the second to third decade of life and is seen predominantly in HLA-B27-positive white males [117, 118]. Involvement of the spine, bilateral sacroiliac joints, and entheses are hallmarks of the disease. Extra-axial manifestations are also commonly seen and include inflammatory bowel disease, peripheral joint arthritis, acute uveitis, and psoriasis [118]. AS is associated with aortitis and has a two-fold increased risk of ischemic heart disease; therefore, it is imperative to perform a thorough cardiac workup in AS patients presenting with acute chest pain [119].

Patients with AS typically present with back pain and significant stiffness, most notably in the morning and at night. Symptoms tend to worsen with rest and improve with activity. On physical exam, patients can have spinal stiffness seen on Schober's test and increased thoracic kyphosis. Imaging of the spine is important for both the diagnosis and monitoring of the disease progression. "Squaring" of the vertebral bodies is an early sign seen on lateral radiographs. Fusion of the facet joints of the spine, syndesmophytes, and calcification of the spinal ligaments occur as the disease progresses resulting in "bamboo spine," the classic radiographic finding seen in late-stage AS [118].

Chest wall pain is common in AS due to thoracic spine and costosternal involvement. Enthesopathy at the thoracic vertebral bodies, facet joints, costosternal, and manubriosternal joints results in rigidity and decreased chest expansion with associated pain which eventually leads to a restrictive pulmonary function impairment. Patients with active disease can experience significant muscle tension and increased chest wall pain with coughing, sneezing, or lying supine. Tender points and trigger points are often appreciated in the upper trapezius, sternocostal and costochondral junctions, and vertebral spinous processes [120].

The main goals of treatment for AS are relieving pain and stiffness to maintain spinal motion and prevent complications due to spinal rigidity. A similar treatment approach should be utilized in patients presenting with musculoskeletal chest wall pain. Pharmacological treatments aim to reduce systemic inflammation. Daily NSAIDs are first-line treatment with disease-modifying antirheumatic drugs (DMARDs) such as tumor necrosis factor (TNF) inhibitors, interleukin inhibitors, and Janus kinase (JAK) inhibitors used as second-line. Non-pharmacological treatments including physical therapy, regular exercise, and postural training are imperative to prevent deformities and maintain respiratory function [121]. Intra-articular corticosteroid injections are often used for sacroiliitis and extra-axial joint arthritis of AS and have proven effective [122]. However, there is a lack of literature on interventional pain procedures for thoracic back pain in these patients.

Fibromyalgia

Fibromyalgia is a syndrome characterized by widespread, chronic musculoskeletal pain. It is often accompanied by fatigue, sleep disturbances, gastrointestinal (GI) dysfunction, and mood disorders. Central pain sensitization is believed to be the underlying cause of fibromyalgia, but inflammatory, genetic, endocrine, and psychosocial factors have also been linked [123]. It affects an estimated 2–4% of the population and is more commonly seen in women. Fibromyalgia is typically diagnosed with the American College of Rheumatology (ACR) criteria when widespread pain has been present for at least 3 months and other similar diseases have been excluded [124].

As stated above, fibromyalgia pain is widespread and the chest wall is often involved. The original 18 tender points used for fibromyalgia diagnosis included the second rib, the trapezius, and the supraspinatus bilaterally (6 points total). ACR criteria now use the widespread pain index (WPI) which quantifies the number of areas a patient has had pain over the last week. There are 19 painful areas in total including the chest wall and upper back [124]. Chest wall pain in fibromyalgia can mimic angina, and a thorough workup is warranted to exclude cardiac, upper GI, or other potential causes of chest pain.

Once other causes have been excluded, treatment of chest wall pain in fibromyalgia should be multimodal. Various pharmacological and non-pharmacological treatments have been demonstrated to improve the central pain sensitization seen in fibromyalgia. Pregabalin, duloxetine, and milnacipran are the only FDA-approved pharmacological treatments for fibromyalgia and should be used first-line. However, studies have shown that tricyclic antidepressants (amitriptyline) and muscle relaxants (cyclobenzaprine) can also be helpful [125, 126]. NSAIDs are frequently taken by patients with fibromyalgia, but studies have not demonstrated their effectiveness. There is also no data supporting the use of opioids. Pharmacological treatment should be tailored to the individual patient and comorbid symptoms should also be targeted with each drug (e.g., amitriptyline or cyclobenzaprine for sleep disturbances).

Non-pharmacological therapies should be emphasized for all fibromyalgia patients. Cognitive behavioral therapy should be recommended to enhance effective coping and promote self-efficacy [127]. Aerobic exercise has also been shown to improve health-related quality of life, decrease pain intensity, and improve physical functioning. Land-based and aquatic exercise training are both effective [128]. The best type of exercise has not been established; therefore, patients should be encouraged to choose a form of exercise that is enjoyable and easy to adhere to [126]. Acupuncture, trigger point injections, meditation, massage, and biofeedback can also be recommended; however, there are varying degrees of evidence supporting their benefits [129].

Systemic Lupus Erythematosus

Systemic Lupus Erythematosus (SLE) is an autoimmune disease that affects nearly every organ in the body and relies on a variety of factors when it comes to its presentation and prognosis, including genetics, environmental triggers, and hormonal milieu. It is a worldwide disease that tends to affect women of childbearing age and is more prevalent in non-Caucasians [130].

The exact etiology of SLE remains obscure and multifactorial, in nature. However, it is important to note that many of the clinical manifestations of this condition are mediated by the formation of autoantibodies and the deposition of immune complexes in various organs [131]. Constitutional symptoms such as fatigue, fever, and myalgias are very common among patients with SLE, and also overlap in onset and duration with other common conditions, making it very difficult for providers to correctly diagnose SLE. Particular attention is also paid to symptoms such as malar rash, painless ulcers, Raynaud phenomenon, exposure to medications associated with drug-induced lupus, and joint pain [132].

One of the earliest manifestations of SLE is arthritis, which occurs in over 90% of patients [130]. Another painful manifestation of SLE is pericarditis, which occurs in about 25% of patients and can present with chest pain [133]. Pleuritic chest pain and dyspnea can also occur in SLE due to the inflammation of the serosa. Coronary artery disease should always be on the differential for patients with lupus that experience chest pain as cardiovascular mortality is approximately 2.7-fold higher in patients with SLE than in the general population [133].

There is also new evidence that chest pain in patients with SLE can also stem from ischemia with no obstructive coronary arteries (INOCA) [134], often due to microvascular coronary dysfunction (MCD). This is important because SLE patients, who present with chest pain similar to a myocardial infarction but do not have obstructive coronary artery disease may be experiencing this MCD. One more common etiology of chest pain for SLE patients is costochondritis, a common musculoskeletal manifestation of the condition that should be considered after excluding more severe and life-threatening causes and can account for up to 25% of chest pain visits for SLE patients [133].

Diagnosis of SLE relies on astute clinical judgment due to the variability of patients presenting with this condition. The 2019 European Alliance of Associations for Rheumatology (EULAR)/American College of Rheumatology (ACR) classification criteria for systemic lupus erythematosus denotes that patients must have an antinuclear antibody (ANA) at a titer of ≥1:80 and satisfy at least four of eleven criteria [135]. If patients do not fulfill the ACR criterion, they are still managed similarly to patients with SLE and treated based on predominant symptoms. This is because SLE evolves overtime and patients can eventually develop further symptoms and reach definite SLE.

Treating pain requires the same approach as treating any of the other aspects of SLE, it is individualized based on predominant symptoms. All patients with SLE are recommended to take hydroxychloroquine unless otherwise contraindicated because it relieves many of the constitutional, musculoskeletal, and mucocutaneous symptoms [132]. This medication is also shown to reduce the rates of lupus flares. If a patient is experiencing mild disease with joint arthralgia and skin involvement as well, they may require short-term prednisone [136]. From that point, if it is not resolved and patients require glucocorticoids longer than 2–4 weeks, then methotrexate is suggested [137]. If it is determined during workup, that a patient has concurrent fibromyalgia with their SLE, they may receive pharmacotherapy tailored to that condition, namely tricyclic antidepressants [138].

Chest wall pain in SLE can either be musculoskeletal or pleuritic, in nature, and in either case, it ultimately responds well to NSAIDs, local heat, and acetaminophen. However, if a workup reveals that chest pain is of cardiac origin, particularly because of myocarditis, first-line therapy should be systemic glucocorticoids, IV cyclophosphamide, or mycophenolate mofetil, usually with hydroxychloroquine [139].

If chest pain in SLE patients stems from coronary artery disease, then strategies tailored toward addressing risk factors for atherosclerosis in individuals can reduce the severity and frequency of pain [138]. This includes the following: quit smoking, encourage regular exercise, optimize lipid levels, control blood pressure in those with hypertension, and use prophylactic low-dose aspirin if not contraindicated. Hydroxychloroquine also has additional antithrombotic and antiatherogenic benefits, and therefore may be beneficial in the treatment of chest pain in SLE stemming from coronary artery disease [140].

Sickle Cell Pain Syndrome

Sickle cell disease is an autosomal recessive genetic condition, characterized by a genetic mutation in the hemoglobin beta chain that distorts the erythrocyte's shape and causes increased adherence to vascular endothelium in the setting of dehydration or hypoxia [141]. This abnormality leads to increased adhesion of erythrocytes, small vessel occlusion, and subsequent hypoxia that results in the clinical manifestations of this condition.

The hallmarks of this condition are related to vaso-occlusion and hemolytic anemia, which can vary in severity depending on the genotype of the patient. Clinical manifestations from sickle cell disease can be further broken down into acute and chronic complications. Acute complications include pain episodes due to vaso-occlusion, acute chest syndrome, infection, stroke, splenic sequestration crisis, avascular necrosis, myocardial infarction, and thromboembolism. Chronic complications include anemia, functional asplenia, osteomyelitis, heart failure, and chronic pain from tissue infarction [142].

Despite the variety of manifestations associated with sickle cell disease, the most common reason for individuals with sickle cell disease to seek medical attention is pain [143]. The three types of sickle cell pain include acute, chronic, and neuropathic, with acute pain being the most common cause of hospitalization and visits to the ER for patients with sickle cell disease. This is typically due to occlusion of micro and microvasculature. Evidence also suggests that vascular occlusion results in the creation of an inflammatory state, which generates an increased sensation of pain [144]. Common locations for acute vaso-occlusive pain include long bones, the abdomen, and the chest.

Therefore, when a patient presents to the hospital for a sickle cell pain episode, it is crucial to assess their pain and treat it promptly. Unfortunately, there are no known specific labs or findings associated with vaso-occlusive pain, but it is important to trust the patient's report of pain severity and how the current episode is compared to previous episodes of pain. Furthermore, clinicians must assess for other potential precipitating conditions, including pneumonia, acute chest syndrome, pulmonary embolism, and myocardial infarction. These other precipitating conditions should be treated accordingly and ruled out with necessary imaging and tests.

Vaso-occlusive pain is typically managed with pharmacologic analgesia. It is recommended to promptly provide patients with IV opioids, including either morphine or hydromorphone [145]. If patients have previously been treated for pain episodes, that treatment plan should be followed depending on the intensity of current pain compared to previous episodes. In patients with difficult IV access, intranasal fentanyl has also been used, particularly in pediatric populations [146]. Ketamine may also be used for pain that does not respond to opioids [147].

Following opioid administration, it is important to reassess pain shortly after. If pain relief is adequate with a single dose of opioids, it may be appropriate to discharge the individual home with a long-acting opioid and a short-acting medication for breakthrough pain [148]. Repeat dosing is used if pain relief is inadequate from the initial dose. Repeat dosing is typically at 20% of the initial dose (or up to 50% of the initial dose depending on the clinician's judgment) [149]. Reassessment should occur within 30 min and retreatment must be given, if needed. If pain is not relieved with three or more doses of morphine or hydromorphone, hospitalization for around-the-clock parenteral analgesics is generally indicated. Continuous infusion by patient-controlled analgesia (PCA) should be considered because it provides the most even pain control within the therapeutic window without side effects, along with the option for self-administration of additional doses for breakthrough pain [150]. Also, multiple studies point to decreased length of stay, increased satisfaction, and less opioid consumption associated with PCA use [151, 152].

Besides opioids, it is important to maintain adequate hydration for patients with sickle cell pain syndrome as many are hypovolemic during pain episodes. Fluid intake and output must be monitored closely if hospitalized [145]. With this in mind, many of these patients are at risk for acute tubular necrosis when dehydrated, so NSAID use in addition to opioid use is a conditional recommendation in outpatient settings and should not exceed 5 consecutive days [153]. Other adjuvants to consider include breathing exercises, and hydroxyurea at their regular dose (if they were taking it prior to admission) [149].

Psoriatic Arthritis

Psoriatic arthritis is a type of spondyloarthropathy associated with psoriasis. It is found in up to 30% of patients with psoriasis and shares many features with other spondyloarthropathies as well as rheumatoid arthritis, but it is usually seronegative [154]. It manifests heterogeneously and can present with nail changes, dactylitis, axial spondylarthritis, and enthesitis. It affects men and women equally and commonly affects patients between the ages of 30 and 50 years old [155].

Cutaneous manifestations of psoriasis typically precede this condition, and diagnosis should be considered based on the pattern of joint involvement, characteristic features, and radiographic findings. Criteria to classify patients as having psoriatic arthritis are based upon the international classification of psoriatic arthritis (CASPAR) study, which concluded that a patient with an inflammatory musculoskeletal disease (peripheral arthritis, spondylitis, or enthesitis) can be classified as having psoriatic arthritis, following list of features related to current psoriasis, a history of psoriasis and a family history of psoriasis [156].

Individuals who manifest with axial psoriatic arthritis tend to experience inflammatory back pain or sacroiliitis, with chest wall pain being far less common. However, if individuals with psoriatic arthritis develop chest pain, it is crucial that clinicians rule out cardiac etiology given that individuals with comorbid psoriatic arthritis have an increased prevalence of severe coronary calcification and increased risk of cardiovascular disease [157]. So if adequate workup rules out a cardiac event, it is important to consider costochondritis due to enthesitis, particularly at the costosternal, sternoclavicular, and manubriosternal joints [158, 159]. The diagnosis of chest wall pain in limited investigations was confirmed with bone scintigraphy.

However, there is limited literature regarding the management of anterior chest wall involvement in psoriatic arthritis. In limited case reports with chest wall pain in this condition, it appears that patients with this manifestation of pain with psoriatic arthritis do not respond to conventional disease-modifying antirheumatic drugs (DMARDs), but they responded very well with complete resolution of pain with biological drugs such as adalimumab and infliximab [158, 159]. With this in mind, it is a rare manifestation of psoriatic arthritis, but should still be considered.

Rheumatoid Arthritis

Rheumatoid arthritis (RA) is chronic, autoimmune inflammatory condition that involves synovial joints and is characterized by inflammatory arthritis along with extra-articular involvement. It is usually a symmetrical arthritis that can lead to joint destruction and permanent articular deformities through erosion of the bone and cartilage [160]. The pathogenesis of this condition is complex and a product of interactions between genes and the environment, but an environmental factor that is strongly associated with rheumatoid arthritis is cigarette smoking [161].

RA most typically presents as polyarticular disease with a gradual onset, but some patients can present with acute onset, with intermittent or migratory joint involvement, or with monoarticular disease. Systemic symptoms may also be present in these patients, particularly those with disease onset after age 60. The predominant symptoms during onset are pain, morning stiffness, and swelling of numerous joints. The most commonly affected joints include the metacarpophalangeal (MCP) and proximal interphalangeal (PIP) joints, the interphalangeal joints of the thumbs, the wrists, and the metatarsophalangeal (MTP) joints of the toes.

With regard to RA presentation within the chest wall, it is important to consider the articular and extra-articular manifestations. As with any patient presenting for chest pain, it is important to rule out cardiac etiology of pain given that rheumatoid arthritis is an independent risk factor for atherosclerotic coronary artery disease, the primary source of morbidity and mortality in this patient population [162]. In addition to cardiovascular disease, pericardial disease is another well-recognized extra-articular manifestation of rheumatoid arthritis. It is often asymptomatic in patients, but when it begins to present with severe or prolonged chest pain, infective pericarditis should be on the differential. Therefore, pericardiocentesis should be undertaken to exclude infection if a patient with RA who is receiving immunosuppressive treatment develops an effusion [163]. If that is the source of chest pain, appropriate antibiotic therapy should be administered to treat the underlying infection.

If cardiac etiology is ruled out with appropriate workup, other things to consider with chest pain in rheumatoid arthritis can include pleural involvement. Pleuritic chest pain and fever are more common in individuals with rheumatoid nodules that can be identified on computed tomography scans [164]. Thoracentesis should be performed for any effusion with >1 cm of layering on decubitus films, and one could expect sterile exudative fluid with low pH (<7.3), low glucose (<60 $mg \cdot dL^{-1}$), and elevated lactate dehydrogenase (may be >700 $IU \cdot L^{-1}$) [165]. Most cases of rheumatoid pleuritis improve with treatment of the underlying rheumatoid arthritis.

After ruling out extra-articular manifestations, which are the more common reasons for chest pain from rheumatoid arthritis, one should consider the primary pathology of the condition, joint inflammation. The costochondral joint is a synovial joint between the costal cartilage and sternum, so it is susceptible to inflammation and subsequent chest wall pain that presents as costochondritis. However, it is a rarer presentation of rheumatoid arthritis with very little literature on it, but it was reported to be the cause of 19% of patients with costochondritis, alongside other systemic diarthrodial joint disorders in one study [166]. With other cases of costochondritis, patients with this case can benefit from symptomatic care with anti-inflammatories and spontaneous resolution is seen in most patients within a year.

Cardiopulmonary Disorders

Properly diagnosing and triaging chest wall pain is of the utmost importance, particularly while distinguishing between serious and benign etiologies. Recognizing hallmark signs and discerning the gravity of a patient's presentation are crucial to responsibly assessing and treating these patients. The priority is always medical stabilization and urgent treatment by the appropriate medical specialists.

Aortic Dissection

Aortic dissection is the separation of layers of the aorta (intima and media), which results in blood flow between the intima and media layers causing further exacerbation of the tear [167]. It is critical to recognize this condition as the lethality rate increases 1–2% each hour after symptoms onset in untreated patients [168].

Patients with medical comorbidities, such as hypertension, atherosclerosis, connective tissue disorders, vasculitis, family history of aortic dissection, use of sympathomimetic agents (cocaine, ecstasy, energy drinks), and preexisting aortic aneurysm all contributed to increased risk of nontraumatic aortic dissection. Patients will often endorse a tearing sensation, pain radiating to the back or abdomen, and a high degree of pain severity [169].

Cardiac Tamponade

Cardiac tamponade is a potentially fatal condition that results after sudden and/or excessive accumulation of fluid in the pericardial space, which is a progression from pericardial effusion [170]. The end result is a restriction of appropriate filling of the chambers of the heart, which alters the hemodynamic state and ultimately leads to hypotension and, if untreated, cardiac arrest.

Risk factors are primarily comorbid pericarditis, pericardial effusion, or recent history of trauma. Patients most often experience anxiety, restlessness, hypotension, tachycardia, dyspnea, and severe chest pain that may radiate to the neck, shoulders, or back [171].

Myocardial Infarction

Myocardial infarction is the disruption of blood supply to the heart and resultant ischemia secondary to obstruction in the major arteries supplying blood to the heart.

Patients with medical comorbidities most often including hypertension, atherosclerosis, coronary artery disease, and diabetes mellitus (secondary to metabolic syndrome) are at an increased risk of myocardial infarction. The patients present with substernal chest pain, headache, arm/neck pain, nausea/vomiting, diaphoresis, and other symptoms. It is important to note that not all myocardial infarctions present with substernal chest pain, and special attention must also be given to pain radiating to the left upper extremity or neck in a patient demonstrating hemodynamic instability.

Pneumothorax

Pneumothorax is a collapsing of the lung that may be due to a number of different etiologies, such as penetrating chest trauma, chronic obstructive pulmonary disease, or the presence of pleural blebs.

Aside from trauma, a significant history of cigarette smoking is most often linked to pneumothorax. Patients typically present with pleuritic chest pain and dyspnea, but it should be noted that patients may present with epigastric abdominal pain rather than chest pain [171].

Pulmonary Embolism

Pulmonary embolism is a blockage of an artery in the lungs that can occur due to a number of risk factors.

Risk factors for pulmonary embolism include major trauma, surgery, lower limb fractures, joint replacements, spinal cord injury and resultant immobility, cancer, oral contraception use, and others [172]. A classic presentation of pulmonary embolism is marked by an acute onset of dyspnea, pleuritic chest pain, and unilateral leg swelling.

Malignant Pleural Effusion

Differing from pleural effusion with the presence of cancer cells in the pleural fluid, this condition is not acutely life-threatening, but quite serious. According to a recent study, survival of patients with malignant pleural effusions was 5.49 months [173].

Patients with a history of past/current malignancy are at risk of malignant pleural effusion, secondary to active neoplasm. The typical presentation is similar to other conditions, such as tuberculosis, in that the patient will typically exhibit dyspnea, night sweats, and weight loss. Older patients and those who use tobacco are at an increased risk.

Pericarditis

Pericarditis is the inflammation of the pericardium, which may be the result of infectious or noninfectious etiologies, though is most often idiopathic, in nature [174].

Infectious agents that may lead to pericarditis include mycobacterium tuberculosis (the most frequent cause of acute pericarditis in developing countries), *Borrelia burgdorferi*, parvovirus B19, and Epstein-Barr virus. Noninfectious etiologies include autoimmune diseases, hypothyroidism, cancer (metastasis or secondary to radiotherapy for chest cancers), and secondary to cardiac procedure [175, 176]. Once pericarditis occurs it often recurs in the future. In fact, recurrent episodes of acute pericarditis occur in 20–30% of patients, and up to 50% of those with recurrent episodes will experience further recurrences in the future [177]. Patients typically present with pleuritic chest pain that improves with leaning forward, a friction rub may be discernible at the left lower sternal border, and various changes are notable on electrocardiogram (EKG) (ST segment elevation acutely that may normalize and over time develop into T-wave inversion).

Pneumonia

Pneumonia is a common respiratory infection, which accounts for more than 800,000 hospitalizations in the United States each year [178].

Pneumonia is a respiratory illness that preferentially affects the elderly and disabled due to decreased immune function and mechanical impairments leading to reduced respiratory function. Etiologies vary including post-viral and community versus hospital-associated pneumonia. Due to the infectious etiology, patients will typically present with fever, dyspnea, pleuritic chest pain, productive cough, fatigue, and loss of appetite.

Tuberculosis

Tuberculosis is an illness caused by mycobacterium tuberculosis, which typically affects the respiratory system, but can also attack other organs/systems, such as the kidneys, spine, and brain. It is also the leading cause of pericarditis in Africa and other areas where tuberculosis is common [179].

Exposure to tuberculosis, which typically occurs in less developed countries, is the primary risk factor for developing the illness. Patients present with fever, night sweats, pleuritic chest pain, weight loss, and hemoptysis.

Gastrointestinal Disorders

Esophageal Perforation

Esophageal perforation is rupture of the esophageal wall and is a rare and life-threatening emergency that presents with a diversity of clinical symptoms and signs that mirror other medical emergencies, including myocardial infarction, perforated peptic ulcers, and acute pancreatitis [180, 181]. However, the rarity of this condition makes it difficult for physicians to obtain clinical experience to identify it, leading to delayed diagnostic workup and negative patient outcomes [182].

Iatrogenic perforation accounts for about 70% of esophageal perforations, with the most common culprits being endoscopic procedures, nasogastric tube insertion, difficult intubations, or transesophageal echocardiograms [183]. Perforation may also occur due to trauma to the chest or upper abdomen as well as penetrating injuries, foreign bodies, and caustic agents.

The cardinal symptom of esophageal perforation is chest pain. It is reported to be the primary symptom in about 70% of patients who were diagnosed with a full-thickness esophageal rupture [182]. The pain associated with esophageal perforation is usually acute with sudden onset, characterized by radiation to the back or left shoulder [184]. It is important to note that the pain usually refers directly to the site of perforation. In the case of thoracic perforations, severe chest pain with features of mediastinitis is common. However, with cervical perforations, the pain localizes more to the neck with concomitant neck stiffness. Subcutaneous emphysema is also present in up to 60% of perforations [185].

As it pertains to diagnosis, clinicians must always consider esophageal perforation in the setting of pain following esophageal instrumentation, chest trauma, or forceful vomiting. The gold standard for diagnosis is a contrast-enhanced esophagogram, which will reveal a contrast leak in most cases of perforation [181]. If suspicion is high despite a negative study result, the study should be repeated within 4–6 h with a chest radiograph or computer tomography (CT) scan of the chest and upper abdomen [182]. Other findings indicative of esophageal perforation include pleural effusions, pneumoperitoneum, and pneumopericardium. Aortic dissection or pulmonary embolism can also be ruled out via MRI or CT scan of the lungs, respectively [186].

Management of suspected esophageal perforation is very time-sensitive, with overall mortality approaching 20%. A delay in treatment of more than 24 h after rupture can result in doubling of the mortality [187]. Surgical intervention is the main treatment for this condition, with primary closure being performed in healthier esophageal tissue and esophagectomy with reconstruction being performed in diseased esophagus. Note that there is no gold standard surgical procedure described in the literature but is dependent on the surgeon's experience, the etiology of the perforation, and various factors unique to each case [184].

Nonoperative measures are also increasingly common, especially for patients with well-defined small tears. These procedures include endoscopic placement of esophageal stents, fibrin sealant, and metallic clips. These methods have been described with excellent results and should be considered in select patients with small ($\leq$1.5 cm) clean perforations and minimal symptoms of infection. With nonoperative management, it is important to provide adequate narcotic analgesia to control pain [188, 189].

Gastritis

Gastritis is a broad term used to characterize inflammation associated with any form of gastric mucosa injury. It is usually caused by infection or immune-mediated inflammation, but many cases of gastritis have idiopathic etiology [190]. Although there are various proposed classifications for gastritis, they all center on time course and histological features. The most common causes of gastritis are *Helicobacter pylori* infection, autoimmune etiology, bile acid reflux, and infection with other organisms such as *Mycobacterium avium*, *Herpes simplex*, and *Cytomegalovirus* [191].

Although there is a wide variety of clinical presentations of gastritis, patients with gastritis typically experience burning epigastric pain accompanied by nausea or vomiting. Evidence in the literature has also pointed out that chest pain may also be a manifestation of gastritis, particularly in the pediatric population [192]. Other unique manifestations of gastritis may originate from suppurative gastritis, a rare and often fatal form of gastritis caused by diffuse infection of the stomach wall that can cause thoracic pain [193]. With this in mind, it is important to consider that gastritis is associated with risk factors such as a history of autoimmune conditions (i.e., Crohn's disease), smoking, long-term alcohol consumption, routine use of NSAIDs or steroids, and gallbladder disorders [191].

Biopsy is the gold standard in diagnosing gastritis in conjunction with clinical history [190]. If a provider has high clinical suspicion for *H. pylori* infection, urea breath and stool antigen tests can also be performed [194]. If a patient has possible autoimmune mediated gastritis, diagnosis can be supported with antibodies to intrinsic factor or parietal cells plus elevated fasting serum gastrin levels [195].

Management of gastritis depends on the underlying cause. A triple therapy of clarithromycin, proton-pump inhibitor, and amoxicillin for 2–3 weeks is recommended if the patient has gastritis due to *H. pylori* infection [196]. In areas where there may be clarithromycin resistance, metronidazole is the antibiotic of choice with quadruple bismuth-containing therapy [197].

With regard to the management of pain, treating the underlying cause typically results in improvement and/or resolution of symptoms. Mucosal coating agents such as antacids and sucralfate or short-term histamine-2 antagonists can provide adequate analgesia. Last, in patients with risk factors, long-term cessation of routine NSAID and/or steroid use, smoking, or alcohol consumption is associated with greater reduction of gastritis symptoms [198].

Miscellaneous Disorders

Aside from all of the many other etiologies listed previously, there are other causes of chest wall pain that still must be considered. Radiation of pain from adjacent regions or structures may present as chest wall pain. Additionally, psychosomatic symptoms of chest wall pain may affect patients of all ages and demographics. In the aforementioned scenarios, it remains of the utmost importance to identify the underlying cause and treat it appropriately, rather than focusing on purely symptom management.

Summary

1. Chest wall pain disorders are common, often presenting after surgical treatment, trauma, and other injuries. They can be neuropathic or musculoskeletal in etiology, though may present from autoimmune, cardiopulmonary, gastrointestinal, or other sources.
2. Diagnosis and evaluation are focused on identifying the most likely etiology, while ruling out potentially serious, life-threatening causes. A focused history and physical examination are often most helpful compared to diagnostic testing and imaging.
3. Treatment and management rely on an accurate diagnosis with escalation of therapeutics from physical therapy, cognitive behavioral therapy, and oral analgesics to interventional pain procedures to invasive surgical options.

Box 16.1 Evidence-based diagnosis and evaluation of chest wall pain

- Initial evaluation starts with a focused history taking, interview, and physical examination with particular attention to pain features, chronology, and past medical and surgical history
- Many common chest wall pain disorders are neurologic and musculoskeletal in etiology, though rarer and more life-threatening causes must be excluded
- Pain descriptors and features can give further clues to potential etiology, i.e., burning, lancinating, numbness, and tingling pain for neuropathic disorders, dull, achy, crampy pain for visceral pain sources, etc.
- Laboratory studies may be useful for specific pain disorders, i.e., ANA or specific autoimmune antibodies for rheumatologic sources, troponin and D-dimer for cardiopulmonary etiologies, but are not generally useful
- Imaging of the chest wall, either via chest X-ray, CT scan, MRI, ultrasound, etc. can be useful to identify structural causes as well as rule out potentially serious causes of chest wall pain. Angiography and color Doppler imaging may be useful for vascular sources
- Electromyography and nerve conduction studies can better elucidate neuropathic sources, such as thoracic radiculopathy or disc herniation
- Nerve blocks can serve both a diagnostic and therapeutic purpose, with a pain relief response suggesting the source of the pain symptoms

Box 16.2 Evidence-based management and treatment of chest wall pain

- Management of chest wall pain disorders starts with a thorough diagnostic evaluation, differential diagnoses list, and testing and imaging as deemed appropriate, ruling out serious or life-threatening causes
- Once a diagnosis is suspected, treatment specific to the disorder can be initiated. If no diagnosis is formally made, therapeutic modalities can also serve a diagnostic purpose
- Initial treatment often begins with physical therapy, cognitive behavioral therapy and psychological modalities, and oral analgesics
- For medications, application of analgesic class specific to suspected pain features is most appropriate (i.e., gabapentinoids and serotonin-norepinephrine reuptake inhibitors for neuropathic pain, anti-inflammatory drugs for musculoskeletal pain, etc.)
- If the patient responds poorly to first-line treatment, nerve blocks and interventional pain procedures may be warranted (i.e., intercostal nerve blocks and radiofrequency ablation for intercostal neuralgia, thoracic epidural steroid injection for thoracic radiculopathy, etc.)
- Surgical evaluation and management may be necessary for patients with refractory pain who respond poorly to first- or second-line treatments or have contraindications to such

References

Introduction

1. Expert Panel on Thoracic Imaging, Stowell JT, Walker CM, Chung JH, Bang TJ, Carter BW, Christensen JD, Donnelly EF, Hanna TN, Hobbs SB, Johnson BD, Kandathil A, Lo BM, Madan R, Majercik S, Moore WH, Kanne JP. ACR appropriateness criteria® nontraumatic chest wall pain. J Am Coll Radiol. 2021;18(11S):S394–405. https://doi.org/10.1016/j.jacr.2021.08.004. PMID: 34794596.
2. Gokhale J, Selbst SM. Chest pain and chest wall deformity. Pediatr Clin N Am. 2009;56(1):49–65, x. https://doi.org/10.1016/j.pcl.2008.10.001. PMID: 19135581.
3. Winzenberg T, Jones G, Callisaya M. Musculoskeletal chest wall pain. Aust Fam Physician. 2015;44(8):540–4. PMID: 26510139.
4. Bessoff KE, Ko A, Forrester JD. Chest wall analgesia-where do we go from here? JAMA Netw Open. 2021;4(11):e2133839. https://doi.org/10.1001/jamanetworkopen.2021.33839. PMID: 34779854.

Musculoskeletal

5. Disla E, et al. Costochondritis. A prospective analysis in an emergency department setting. Arch Intern Med. 1994;154(21):2466–9.
6. Schumann JA, Sood T, Parente JJ. Costochondritis. In: StatPearls. Treasure Island (FL): StatPearls Publishing; 2022.
7. Proulx AM, Zryd TW. Costochondritis: diagnosis and treatment. Am Fam Physician. 2009;80(6):617–20.
8. Fam AG, Smythe HA. Musculoskeletal chest wall pain. CMAJ. 1985;133(5):379–89.
9. Barranco-Trabi J, et al. Atypical costochondritis: complete resolution of symptoms after rib manipulation and soft tissue mobilization. Cureus. 2021;13(4):e14369.
10. Zaruba RA, Wilson E. Impairment based examination and treatment of costochondritis: a case series. Int J Sports Phys Ther. 2017;12(3):458–67.
11. Mott T, Jones G, Roman K. Costochondritis: rapid evidence review. Am Fam Physician. 2021;104(1):73–8.
12. Arroyo JF, Jolliet P, Junod AF. Costovertebral joint dysfunction: another misdiagnosed cause of atypical chest pain. Postgrad Med J. 1992;68(802):655–9.
13. Saker E, et al. Ligaments of the costovertebral joints including biomechanics, innervations, and clinical applications: a comprehensive review with application to approaches to the thoracic spine. Cureus. 2016;8(11):e874.
14. McMahon LE. Slipping rib syndrome: a review of evaluation, diagnosis and treatment. Semin Pediatr Surg. 2018;27(3):183–8.
15. Gress K, et al. A comprehensive review of slipping rib syndrome: treatment and management. Psychopharmacol Bull. 2020;50(4 Suppl 1):189–96.
16. Foley CM, et al. Diagnosis and treatment of slipping rib syndrome. Clin J Sport Med. 2019;29(1):18–23.
17. Van Tassel D, et al. Dynamic ultrasound in the evaluation of patients with suspected slipping rib syndrome. Skeletal Radiol. 2019;48(5):741–51.
18. Wright JT. Slipping-rib syndrome. Lancet. 1980;2(8195 pt 1):632–4.
19. Snosek M, Tubbs RS, Loukas M. Sternalis muscle, what every anatomist and clinician should know. Clin Anat. 2014;27(6):866–84.
20. Raikos A, et al. Sternalis muscle: an underestimated anterior chest wall anatomical variant. J Cardiothorac Surg. 2011;6:73.

21. Gruber L, et al. A rare case of a symptomatic sternalis muscle: ultrasonograpy and MRI correlation. Ultrasound Int Open. 2016;2(4):E140–1.
22. Winzenberg T, Jones G, Callisaya M. Musculoskeletal chest wall pain. Aust Fam Physician. 2015;44(8):540–4.
23. Rokicki W, Rokicki M, Rydel M. What do we know about Tietze's syndrome? Kardiochir Torakochirurgia Pol. 2018;15(3):180–2.
24. Rosenberg M, Conermann T. Tietze syndrome. In: StatPearls. Treasure Island (FL): StatPearls Publishing; 2022.
25. Oh JH, Park SB, Oh HC. 18F-FDG PET/CT and bone scintigraphy findings in Tietze syndrome. Clin Nucl Med. 2018;43(11):832–4.
26. Kaplan T, et al. Painful chest wall swellings: Tietze syndrome or chest wall tumor? Thorac Cardiovasc Surg. 2016;64(3):239–44.
27. Goverman J, et al. Adult contractures in burn injury: a burn model system national database study. J Burn Care Res. 2017;38(1):e328–36.
28. Young AW, Dewey WS, King BT. Rehabilitation of burn injuries: an update. Phys Med Rehabil Clin N Am. 2019;30(1):111–32.
29. Sulli D, Dhopte A, Agrawal K. Impact of burn contractures of chest wall and their surgical release on pulmonary function. Burns. 2019;45(4):929–35.
30. Browne AL, et al. Persistent pain outcomes and patient satisfaction with pain management after burn injury. Clin J Pain. 2011;27(2):136–45.
31. Ashouri S. An introduction to burns. Phys Med Rehabil Clin N Am. 2022;33(4):871–83.
32. Griggs C, et al. Sedation and pain management in burn patients. Clin Plast Surg. 2017;44(3):535–40.
33. Nambi G, et al. Yoga in burn: role of pranayama breathing exercise on pulmonary function, respiratory muscle activity and exercise tolerance in full-thickness circumferential burns of the chest. Burns. 2021;47(1):206–14.
34. Abdelbasset WK, et al. Optimization of pulmonary function, functional capacity, and quality of life in adolescents with thoracic burns after a 2-month arm cycling exercise programme: a randomized controlled study. Burns. 2022;48(1):78–84.
35. Kerr-Valentic MA, et al. Rib fracture pain and disability: can we do better? J Trauma. 2003;54(6):1058–63; discussion 1063–4.
36. Ziegler DW, Agarwal NN. The morbidity and mortality of rib fractures. J Trauma. 1994;37(6):975–9.
37. Martin TJ, et al. Clinical management of rib fractures and methods for prevention of pulmonary complications: a review. Injury. 2019;50(6):1159–65.
38. Dubinsky I, Low A. Non-life-threatening blunt chest trauma: appropriate investigation and treatment. Am J Emerg Med. 1997;15(3):240–3.
39. Murphy CEt, et al. Rib fracture diagnosis in the Panscan era. Ann Emerg Med. 2017;70(6):904–9.
40. Coary R, et al. New horizons in rib fracture management in the older adult. Age Ageing. 2020;49(2):161–7.
41. Peek J, et al. Comparison of analgesic interventions for traumatic rib fractures: a systematic review and meta-analysis. Eur J Trauma Emerg Surg. 2019;45(4):597–622.
42. Bulger EM, et al. Rib fractures in the elderly. J Trauma. 2000;48(6):1040–6; discussion 1046–7.
43. Wardhan R, Kantamneni S. The challenges of ultrasound-guided thoracic paravertebral blocks in rib fracture patients. Cureus. 2020;12(4):e7626.
44. Hwang EG, Lee Y. Effectiveness of intercostal nerve block for management of pain in rib fracture patients. J Exerc Rehabil. 2014;10(4):241–4.
45. Nair A, Diwan S. Efficacy of ultrasound-guided serratus anterior plane block for managing pain due to multiple rib fractures: a scoping review. Cureus. 2022;14(1):e21322.

Neuropathic

46. Chappell AG, et al. Post-mastectomy pain syndrome: an up-to-date review of treatment outcomes. JPRAS Open. 2021;30:97–109.
47. Yuksel SS, et al. Post mastectomy pain syndrome: a systematic review of prevention modalities. JPRAS Open. 2022;31:32–49.
48. Waltho D, Rockwell G. Post-breast surgery pain syndrome: establishing a consensus for the definition of post-mastectomy pain syndrome to provide a standardized clinical and research approach – a review of the literature and discussion. Can J Surg. 2016;59(5):342–50.
49. Tait RC, et al. Persistent post-mastectomy pain: risk factors and current approaches to treatment. J Pain. 2018;19(12):1367–83.
50. Brackstone M. A review of the literature and discussion: establishing a consensus for the definition of post-mastectomy pain syndrome to provide a standardized clinical and research approach. Can J Surg. 2016;59(5):294–5.
51. Calapai M, et al. Post-mastectomy pain: an updated overview on risk factors, predictors, and markers. Life (Basel). 2021;11(10):1026.
52. Kannan P, et al. Efficacy of physical therapy interventions on quality of life and upper quadrant pain severity in women with post-mastectomy pain syndrome: a systematic review and meta-analysis. Qual Life Res. 2022;31(4):951–73.
53. Ebid AA, El-Sodany AM. Long-term effect of pulsed high-intensity laser therapy in the treatment of post-mastectomy pain syndrome: a double blind, placebo-control, randomized study. Lasers Med Sci. 2015;30(6):1747–55.
54. Khoury AL, et al. Trigger point injection for post-mastectomy pain: a simple intervention with high rate of long-term relief. NPJ Breast Cancer. 2021;7(1):123.
55. Elkhashab Y, Wang D. Correction to: a review of techniques of intercostal nerve blocks. Curr Pain Headache Rep. 2021;25(10):74.
56. Rokhtabnak F, et al. Pain control after mastectomy in transgender patients: ultrasound-guided pectoral nerve block II versus conventional intercostal nerve block: a randomized clinical trial. Anesth Pain Med. 2021;11(5):e119440.
57. Abbas DN, Reyad RM. Thermal versus super voltage pulsed radiofrequency of stellate ganglion in post-mastectomy neuropathic pain syndrome: a prospective randomized trial. Pain Physician. 2018;21(4):351–62.
58. Kelsheimer B, Williams C, Kelsheimer C. New emerging modalities to treat post-thoracotomy pain syndrome: a review. Mo Med. 2019;116(1):41–4.
59. Hetmann F, et al. Post-thoracotomy pain syndrome and sensory disturbances following thoracotomy at 6- and 12-month follow-ups. J Pain Res. 2017;10:663–8.
60. Hopkins KG, Rosenzweig M. Post-thoracotomy pain syndrome: assessment and intervention. Clin J Oncol Nurs. 2012;16(4):365–70.
61. Maloney J, et al. Post-thoracotomy pain syndrome. Curr Pain Headache Rep. 2022;26(9):677–81.
62. Yasin J, et al. CT-guided cryoablation for post-thoracotomy pain syndrome: a retrospective analysis. Diagn Interv Radiol. 2020;26(1):53–7.
63. Israel JE, et al. Ketamine for the treatment of chronic pain: a comprehensive review. Health Psychol Res. 2021;9(1):25535.
64. Mendola C, et al. S(+)-ketamine for control of perioperative pain and prevention of post thoracotomy pain syndrome: a randomized, double-blind study. Minerva Anestesiol. 2012;78(7):757–66.
65. Abd-Elsayed A, Lee S, Jackson M. Radiofrequency ablation for treating resistant intercostal neuralgia. Ochsner J. 2018;18(1):91–3.
66. Engel AJ. Utility of intercostal nerve conventional thermal radiofrequency ablations in the injured worker after blunt trauma. Pain Physician. 2012;15(5):E711–8.
67. Graybill J, et al. Spinal cord stimulation for treatment of pain in a patient with post thoracotomy pain syndrome. Pain Physician. 2011;14(5):441–5.
68. Lee HK, et al. Spinal cord stimulation for intractable post-thoracotomy pain syndrome: a case report. Korean J Anesthesiol. 2009;57(5):678–81.

69. Wininger KL, Bester ML, Deshpande KK. Spinal cord stimulation to treat postthoracotomy neuralgia: non-small-cell lung cancer: a case report. Pain Manag Nurs. 2012;13(1):52–9.
70. El-Hag-Aly MA, Hagag MG, Allam HK. If post-thoracotomy pain is the target, Integrated thoracotomy is the choice. Gen Thorac Cardiovasc Surg. 2019;67(11):955–61.
71. Christo PJ, Hobelmann G, Maine DN. Post-herpetic neuralgia in older adults: evidence-based approaches to clinical management. Drugs Aging. 2007;24(1):1–19.
72. Johnson RW, et al. Herpes zoster and postherpetic neuralgia: optimizing management in the elderly patient. Drugs Aging. 2008;25(12):991–1006.
73. Binder A, et al. Topical 5% lidocaine (lignocaine) medicated plaster treatment for post-herpetic neuralgia: results of a double-blind, placebo-controlled, multinational efficacy and safety trial. Clin Drug Investig. 2009;29(6):393–408.
74. Kanazi GE, Johnson RW, Dworkin RH. Treatment of postherpetic neuralgia: an update. Drugs. 2000;59(5):1113–26.
75. Liedgens H, et al. Cost-effectiveness analysis of a lidocaine 5% medicated plaster compared with gabapentin and pregabalin for treating postherpetic neuralgia: a German perspective. Clin Drug Investig. 2008;28(9):583–601.
76. Nathan PW, Wall PD. Treatment of post-herpetic neuralgia by prolonged electric stimulation. Br Med J. 1974;3(5932):645–7.
77. Mukhtar R, et al. Role of low-level laser therapy in post-herpetic neuralgia: a pilot study. Lasers Med Sci. 2020;35(8):1759–64.
78. Rowbotham MC, Davies PS, Fields HL. Topical lidocaine gel relieves postherpetic neuralgia. Ann Neurol. 1995;37(2):246–53.
79. Rowbotham MC, et al. Lidocaine patch: double-blind controlled study of a new treatment method for post-herpetic neuralgia. Pain. 1996;65(1):39–44.
80. Watson CP, et al. Nortriptyline versus amitriptyline in postherpetic neuralgia: a randomized trial. Neurology. 1998;51(4):1166–71.
81. Rowbotham M, et al. Gabapentin for the treatment of postherpetic neuralgia: a randomized controlled trial. JAMA. 1998;280(21):1837–42.
82. Boureau F, Legallicier P, Kabir-Ahmadi M. Tramadol in post-herpetic neuralgia: a randomized, double-blind, placebo-controlled trial. Pain. 2003;104(1–2):323–31.
83. Watson CP, Babul N. Efficacy of oxycodone in neuropathic pain: a randomized trial in postherpetic neuralgia. Neurology. 1998;50(6):1837–41.
84. Max MB, et al. Association of pain relief with drug side effects in postherpetic neuralgia: a single-dose study of clonidine, codeine, ibuprofen, and placebo. Clin Pharmacol Ther. 1988;43(4):363–71.
85. Kikuchi A, et al. Comparative therapeutic evaluation of intrathecal versus epidural methylprednisolone for long-term analgesia in patients with intractable postherpetic neuralgia. Reg Anesth Pain Med. 1999;24(4):287–93.
86. Wu CL, Marsh A, Dworkin RH. The role of sympathetic nerve blocks in herpes zoster and postherpetic neuralgia. Pain. 2000;87(2):121–9.
87. Harke H, et al. Spinal cord stimulation in postherpetic neuralgia and in acute herpes zoster pain. Anesth Analg. 2002;94(3):694–700; table of contents.
88. Meglio M, et al. Spinal cord stimulation (SCS) in the treatment of postherpetic pain. Acta Neurochir Suppl (Wien). 1989;46:65–6.
89. Fazekas D, Doroshenko M, Horn DB. Intercostal neuralgia. In: StatPearls. Treasure Island (FL): StatPearls Publishing; 2022.
90. Williams EH, et al. Neurectomy for treatment of intercostal neuralgia. Ann Thorac Surg. 2008;85(5):1766–70.
91. Samlaska S, Dews TE. Long-term epidural analgesia for pregnancy-induced intercostal neuralgia. Pain. 1995;62(2):245–8.
92. Santos PS, et al. Intercostal nerve mononeuropathy: study of 14 cases. Arq Neuropsiquiatr. 2005;63(3B):776–8.
93. Chalian M, et al. Role of magnetic resonance neurography in intercostal neuralgia; diagnostic utility and efficacy. Br J Radiol. 2021;94(1122):20200603.

94. Weksler N, et al. Phenol neurolysis for severe chronic nonmalignant pain: is the old also obsolete? Pain Med. 2007;8(4):332–7.
95. Dorsi MJ, et al. Dorsal rhizotomy for treatment of bilateral intercostal neuralgia following augmentation mammaplasty: case report and review of the literature. Microsurgery. 2011;31(1):41–4.
96. Wei J, et al. Percutaneous endoscopic intercostal neurectomy for refractory intercostal neuralgia. Pain Physician. 2021;24(7):E1147–53.
97. Gibson W, Wand BM, O'Connell NE. Transcutaneous electrical nerve stimulation (TENS) for neuropathic pain in adults. Cochrane Database Syst Rev. 2017;9(9):CD011976.
98. Schenk R, et al. Effectiveness of cervicothoracic and thoracic manual physical therapy in managing upper quarter disorders – a systematic review. J Man Manip Ther. 2022;30(1):46–55.
99. O'Connor RC, et al. Thoracic radiculopathy. Phys Med Rehabil Clin N Am. 2002;13(3):623–44, viii.
100. Gille O, et al. Analysis of hard thoracic herniated discs: review of 18 cases operated by thoracoscopy. Eur Spine J. 2006;15(5):537–42.
101. Rahimizadeh A, et al. T1–T2 disc herniation: report of four cases and review of the literature. Surg Neurol Int. 2019;10:56.
102. Cong M, et al. Foot drop as the initial symptom caused by thoracic disc herniation. Eur Spine J. 2022;31(7):1795–801.
103. Lyu RK, et al. Thoracic disc herniation mimicking acute lumbar disc disease. Spine (Phila Pa 1976). 1999;24(4):416–8.
104. Ghosh R, Holland R, Mammis A. Thoracic radiculopathy following spinal cord stimulator implantation treated with corticosteroids. World Neurosurg. 2017;100:712.e1–4.
105. Leininger B, et al. Spinal manipulation or mobilization for radiculopathy: a systematic review. Phys Med Rehabil Clin N Am. 2011;22(1):105–25.
106. Manchikanti L, et al. Epidural interventions in the management of chronic spinal pain: American Society of Interventional Pain Physicians (ASIPP) comprehensive evidence-based guidelines. Pain Physician. 2021;24(S1):S27–S208.
107. Quinn SF, et al. CT-guided nerve root block and ablation. AJR Am J Roentgenol. 1988;151(6):1213–6.
108. Chen TC. Surgical outcome for thoracic disc surgery in the postlaminectomy era. Neurosurg Focus. 2000;9(4):e12.
109. Kalfas IH. Laminectomy for thoracic spinal canal stenosis. Neurosurg Focus. 2000;9(4):e2.
110. Oskouian RJ, Johnson JP. Endoscopic thoracic microdiscectomy. J Neurosurg Spine. 2005;3(6):459–64.
111. Haufe SM, Baker RA, Pyne ML. Endoscopic thoracic laminoforaminoplasty for the treatment of thoracic radiculopathy: report of 12 cases. Int J Med Sci. 2009;6(4):224–6.
112. Doo AR, et al. Radiation-induced neuropathic pain successfully treated with systemic lidocaine administration. J Pain Res. 2018;11:545–8.
113. Edwards HL, Mulvey MR, Bennett MI. Cancer-related neuropathic pain. Cancers (Basel). 2019;11(3):373.
114. Warade AC, et al. Radiation-induced brachial plexus neuropathy: a review. Neurol India. 2019;67(Supplement):S47–52.
115. Clubb B. Management of neuropathic pain following treatment for breast cancer in the absence of recurrence: a challenge for the radiation oncologist. Australas Radiol. 2004;48(4):459–65.
116. Zeidman SM, Rossitch EJ, Nashold BS Jr. Dorsal root entry zone lesions in the treatment of pain related to radiation-induced brachial plexopathy. J Spinal Disord. 1993;6(1):44–7.

Rheum/Autoimmune

117. Smith JA. Update on ankylosing spondylitis: current concepts in pathogenesis. Curr Allergy Asthma Rep. 2015;15(1):489.

118. Wenker KJ, Quint JM. Ankylosing spondylitis. In: StatPearls. Treasure Island (FL): StatPearls Publishing; 2023.
119. Atzeni F, et al. Cardiovascular risk in ankylosing spondylitis and the effect of anti-TNF drugs: a narrative review. Expert Opin Biol Ther. 2020;20(5):517–24.
120. Gyurcsik Z, et al. Treatment of ankylosing spondylitis with biologics and targeted physical therapy: positive effect on chest pain, diminished chest mobility, and respiratory function. Z Rheumatol. 2013;72(10):997–1004.
121. Dougados M, et al. Conventional treatments for ankylosing spondylitis. Ann Rheum Dis. 2002;61 Suppl 3(Suppl 3):iii40–50.
122. Dhir V, Mishra D, Samanta J. Glucocorticoids in spondyloarthritis-systematic review and real-world analysis. Rheumatology (Oxford). 2021;60(10):4463–75.
123. Siracusa R, et al. Fibromyalgia: pathogenesis, mechanisms, diagnosis and treatment options update. Int J Mol Sci. 2021;22(8):3891.
124. Galvez-Sanchez CM, Reyes Del Paso GA. Diagnostic criteria for fibromyalgia: critical review and future perspectives. J Clin Med. 2020;9(4):1219.
125. Hauser W, et al. The role of antidepressants in the management of fibromyalgia syndrome: a systematic review and meta-analysis. CNS Drugs. 2012;26(4):297–307.
126. Tofferi JK, Jackson JL, O'Malley PG. Treatment of fibromyalgia with cyclobenzaprine: a meta-analysis. Arthritis Rheum. 2004;51(1):9–13.
127. Borchers AT, Gershwin ME. Fibromyalgia: a critical and comprehensive review. Clin Rev Allergy Immunol. 2015;49(2):100–51.
128. Bidonde J, et al. Aquatic exercise training for fibromyalgia. Cochrane Database Syst Rev. 2014;(10):CD011336.
129. Hauser W, et al. Management of fibromyalgia: practical guides from recent evidence-based guidelines. Pol Arch Intern Med. 2017;127(1):47–56.
130. Pons-Estel GJ, et al. Understanding the epidemiology and progression of systemic lupus erythematosus. Semin Arthritis Rheum. 2010;39(4):257–68.
131. Kaul A, et al. Systemic lupus erythematosus. Nat Rev Dis Primers. 2016;2:16039.
132. Fava A, Petri M. Systemic lupus erythematosus: diagnosis and clinical management. J Autoimmun. 2019;96:1–13.
133. Modi M, et al. Chest pain in lupus patients: the emergency department experience. Clin Rheumatol. 2015;34(11):1969–73.
134. Manchanda AS, et al. Coronary microvascular dysfunction in patients with systemic lupus erythematosus and chest pain. Front Cardiovasc Med. 2022;9:867155.
135. Aringer M, et al. 2019 European League against rheumatism/American College of Rheumatology classification criteria for systemic lupus erythematosus. Arthritis Rheumatol. 2019;71(9):1400–12.
136. Waldheim E, et al. Variation in pain related to systemic lupus erythematosus (SLE): a 7-year follow-up study. Clin Rheumatol. 2018;37(7):1825–34.
137. Islam MN, et al. Efficacy and safety of methotrexate in articular and cutaneous manifestations of systemic lupus erythematosus. Int J Rheum Dis. 2012;15(1):62–8.
138. Di Franco M, et al. Pain and systemic lupus erythematosus. Reumatismo. 2014;66(1):33–8.
139. Al-Nokhatha SA, et al. Myocarditis as a lupus challenge: two case reports. J Med Case Rep. 2019;13(1):343.
140. Misra DP, Gasparyan AY, Zimba O. Benefits and adverse effects of hydroxychloroquine, methotrexate and colchicine: searching for repurposable drug candidates. Rheumatol Int. 2020;40(11):1741–51.
141. Bunn HF. Pathogenesis and treatment of sickle cell disease. N Engl J Med. 1997;337(11):762–9.
142. Schnog JB, et al. Sickle cell disease; a general overview. Neth J Med. 2004;62(10):364–74.
143. Ballas SK. Pain management of sickle cell disease. Hematol Oncol Clin North Am. 2005;19(5):785–802, v.
144. Conran N, Belcher JD. Inflammation in sickle cell disease. Clin Hemorheol Microcirc. 2018;68(2–3):263–99.

145. Yawn BP, et al. Management of sickle cell disease: summary of the 2014 evidence-based report by expert panel members. JAMA. 2014;312(10):1033–48.
146. Kavanagh PL, et al. Improving the management of vaso-occlusive episodes in the pediatric emergency department. Pediatrics. 2015;136(4):e1016–25.
147. Alshahrani MS, et al. Ketamine administration for acute painful sickle cell crisis: a randomized controlled trial. Acad Emerg Med. 2022;29(2):150–8.
148. Raphael JL, Oyeku SO. Sickle cell disease pain management and the medical home. Hematology Am Soc Hematol Educ Program. 2013;2013:433–8.
149. Miller ST, et al. Inpatient management of sickle cell pain: a 'snapshot' of current practice. Am J Hematol. 2012;87(3):333–6.
150. van Beers EJ, et al. Patient-controlled analgesia versus continuous infusion of morphine during vaso-occlusive crisis in sickle cell disease, a randomized controlled trial. Am J Hematol. 2007;82(11):955–60.
151. Gonzalez ER, et al. Intermittent injection vs patient-controlled analgesia for sickle cell crisis pain. Comparison in patients in the emergency department. Arch Intern Med. 1991;151(7):1373–8.
152. Melzer-Lange MD, et al. Patient-controlled analgesia for sickle cell pain crisis in a pediatric emergency department. Pediatr Emerg Care. 2004;20(1):2–4.
153. Schneider V, et al. Association of selective and conventional nonsteroidal antiinflammatory drugs with acute renal failure: a population-based, nested case-control analysis. Am J Epidemiol. 2006;164(9):881–9.
154. Tiwari V, Brent LH. Psoriatic arthritis. In: StatPearls. Treasure Island (FL): StatPearls Publishing; 2022. Copyright © 2022, StatPearls Publishing LLC.
155. Gottlieb AB, Merola JF. Axial psoriatic arthritis: an update for dermatologists. J Am Acad Dermatol. 2021;84(1):92–101.
156. Taylor W, et al. Classification criteria for psoriatic arthritis: development of new criteria from a large international study. Arthritis Rheum. 2006;54(8):2665–73.
157. Tinggaard AB, et al. Prevalence and severity of coronary artery disease linked to prognosis in psoriasis and psoriatic arthritis patients: a multi-centre cohort study. J Intern Med. 2021;290(3):693–703.
158. Fournié B, et al. Prospective study of anterior chest wall involvement in ankylosing spondylitis and psoriatic arthritis. Rev Rhum Engl Ed. 1997;64(1):22–5.
159. Fragoulis GE, et al. Anterior chest wall involvement in psoriatic arthritis: a forgotten entity? Rheumatology. 2020;59(10):3113–4.
160. Sparks JA. Rheumatoid arthritis. Ann Intern Med. 2019;170(1):Itc1–itc16.
161. Smolen JS, Aletaha D, McInnes IB. Rheumatoid arthritis. Lancet. 2016;388(10055):2023–38.
162. Groner LK, et al. Thoracic manifestations of rheumatoid arthritis. Radiographics. 2021;41(1):32–55.
163. Martin JC, Harvey J, Dixey J. Chest pain in patients with rheumatoid arthritis. Ann Rheum Dis. 1996;55(3):152–3.
164. Shaw M, et al. Rheumatoid arthritis-associated lung disease. Eur Respir Rev. 2015;24(135):1–16.
165. Balbir-Gurman A, et al. Rheumatoid pleural effusion. Semin Arthritis Rheum. 2006;35(6):368–78.
166. Disla E, et al. Costochondritis. A prospective analysis in an emergency department setting. Arch Intern Med. 1994;154(21):2466–9.

Cardiopulmonary

167. Levy D, Goyal A, Grigorova Y, Farci F, Le JK. Aortic dissection. In: StatPearls; 2022. https://www.ncbi.nlm.nih.gov/pubmed/28722992.

168. Gawinecka J, Schonrath F, von Eckardstein A. Acute aortic dissection: pathogenesis, risk factors and diagnosis. Swiss Med Wkly. 2017;147:w14489. https://doi.org/10.4414/smw.2017.14489.
169. Reamy BV, Williams PM, Odom MR. Pleuritic chest pain: sorting through the differential diagnosis. Am Fam Physician. 2017;96(5):306–12. https://www.ncbi.nlm.nih.gov/pubmed/28925655.
170. Sharma NK, Waymack JR. Acute cardiac tamponade. In: StatPearls; 2022. https://www.ncbi.nlm.nih.gov/pubmed/30521227.
171. Mizumoto J. Pneumothorax presenting as epigastric pain. J Gen Fam Med. 2021;22(5):291–2. https://doi.org/10.1002/jgf2.447.
172. Konstantinides SV, Torbicki A, Agnelli G, Danchin N, Fitzmaurice D, Galie N, Gibbs JS, Huisman MV, Humbert M, Kucher N, Lang I, Lankeit M, Lekakis J, Maack C, Mayer E, Meneveau N, Perrier A, Pruszczyk P, Rasmussen LH, Schindler TH, Svitil P, Vonk Noordegraaf A, Zamorano JL, Zompatori M, Task Force for the, D, Management of Acute Pulmonary Embolism of the European Society of, C. 2014 ESC guidelines on the diagnosis and management of acute pulmonary embolism. Eur Heart J. 2014;35(43):3033–69, 3069a–3069k. https://doi.org/10.1093/eurheartj/ehu283.
173. Porcel JM, Gasol A, Bielsa S, Civit C, Light RW, Salud A. Clinical features and survival of lung cancer patients with pleural effusions. Respirology. 2015;20(4):654–9. https://doi.org/10.1111/resp.12496.
174. Brucato A, Imazio M, Cremer PC, Adler Y, Maisch B, Lazaros G, Gattorno M, Caforio ALP, Marcolongo R, Emmi G, Martini A, Klein AL. Recurrent pericarditis: still idiopathic? The pros and cons of a well-honoured term. Intern Emerg Med. 2018;13(6):839–44. https://doi.org/10.1007/s11739-018-1907-x.
175. Ghosh AK, Crake T, Manisty C, Westwood M. Pericardial disease in cancer patients. Curr Treat Options Cardiovasc Med. 2018;20(7):60. https://doi.org/10.1007/s11936-018-0654-7.
176. Altan M, Toki MI, Gettinger SN, Carvajal-Hausdorf DE, Zugazagoitia J, Sinard JH, Herbst RS, Rimm DL. Immune checkpoint inhibitor-associated pericarditis. J Thorac Oncol. 2019;14(6):1102–8. https://doi.org/10.1016/j.jtho.2019.02.026.
177. Imazio M, Brucato A, Cemin R, Ferrua S, Maggiolini S, Beqaraj F, Demarie D, Forno D, Ferro S, Maestroni S, Belli R, Trinchero R, Spodick DH, Adler Y, Investigators I. A randomized trial of colchicine for acute pericarditis. N Engl J Med. 2013;369(16):1522–8. https://doi.org/10.1056/NEJMoa1208536.
178. Grief SN, Loza JK. Guidelines for the evaluation and treatment of pneumonia. Prim Care. 2018;45(3):485–503. https://doi.org/10.1016/j.pop.2018.04.001.
179. Mayosi BM, Burgess LJ, Doubell AF. Tuberculous pericarditis. Circulation. 2005;112(23):3608–16. https://doi.org/10.1161/CIRCULATIONAHA.105.543066.

GI

180. Noda K, et al. We should pay attention to "referred pain" – a case of acute myocardial infarction that masked and delayed the diagnosis of esophageal perforation. Intern Med. 2022;61(8):1295–8.
181. Razi E, Davoodabadi A, Razi A. Spontaneous esophageal perforation presenting as a right-sided pleural effusion: a case report. Tanaffos. 2013;12(4):53–7.
182. Søreide JA, Viste A. Esophageal perforation: diagnostic work-up and clinical decision-making in the first 24 hours. Scand J Trauma Resusc Emerg Med. 2011;19:66.
183. Kallmeyer IJ, et al. The safety of intraoperative transesophageal echocardiography: a case series of 7200 cardiac surgical patients. Anesth Analg. 2001;92(5):1126–30.
184. Khaitan PG, Famiglietti A, Watson TJ. The etiology, diagnosis, and management of esophageal perforation. J Gastrointest Surg. 2022;26(12):2606–15.

185. Kaman L, et al. Management of esophageal perforation in adults. Gastroenterology Res. 2010;3(6):235–44.
186. Rubesin SE, Levine MS. Radiologic diagnosis of gastrointestinal perforation. Radiol Clin North Am. 2003;41(6):1095–115, v.
187. Brinster CJ, et al. Evolving options in the management of esophageal perforation. Ann Thorac Surg. 2004;77(4):1475–83.
188. Freeman RK, Van Woerkom JM, Ascioti AJ. Esophageal stent placement for the treatment of iatrogenic intrathoracic esophageal perforation. Ann Thorac Surg. 2007;83(6):2003–7; discussion 2007–8.
189. Tuebergen D, et al. Treatment of thoracic esophageal anastomotic leaks and esophageal perforations with endoluminal stents: efficacy and current limitations. J Gastrointest Surg. 2008;12(7):1168–76.
190. Sepulveda AR, Patil M. Practical approach to the pathologic diagnosis of gastritis. Arch Pathol Lab Med. 2008;132(10):1586–93.
191. Feyisa ZT, Woldeamanuel BT. Prevalence and associated risk factors of gastritis among patients visiting Saint Paul Hospital Millennium Medical College, Addis Ababa, Ethiopia. PLoS One. 2021;16(2):e0246619.
192. Berezin S, et al. Chest pain of gastrointestinal origin. Arch Dis Child. 1988;63(12):1457–60.
193. Alonso JV, et al. Gastric wall abscess presenting as thoracic pain: rare presentation of an old disease. Ann Gastroenterol. 2013;26(4):360–2.
194. Ricci C, Holton J, Vaira D. Diagnosis of Helicobacter pylori: invasive and non-invasive tests. Best Pract Res Clin Gastroenterol. 2007;21(2):299–313.
195. Manger K, Kalden JR. Gastritis and thoracic pain. Churg-Strauss vasculitis. Med Klin (Munich). 1998;93(3):190.
196. Fischbach W, Malfertheiner P. Helicobacter pylori infection. Dtsch Arztebl Int. 2018;115(25):429–36.
197. Yang JC, Lu CW, Lin CJ. Treatment of Helicobacter pylori infection: current status and future concepts. World J Gastroenterol. 2014;20(18):5283–93.
198. Neumann WL, et al. Autoimmune atrophic gastritis—pathogenesis, pathology and management. Nat Rev Gastroenterol Hepatol. 2013;10(9):529–41.

Abdominal Wall Pain

17

Alejandro J. Carruyo, Peter Y. Yi, and Robert S. Ackerman

Diagnostic Evaluation

When evaluating patients with chronic abdominal wall pain, a thorough diagnostic approach is essential to identify the underlying cause. In the case of post-herniorrhaphy neuralgia (PHN), the diagnosis is based on the characteristic clinical presentation of moderate to severe groin pain lasting more than 3 months and affecting activities of daily living (ADLs). However, it is important to consider non-neuropathic causes, such as mesh migration or infection, hernia recurrence, fluid collection, or local inflammatory reactions. Imaging studies, such as magnetic resonance imaging (MRI) or ultrasound, can be valuable in identifying these potential causes.

In anterior cutaneous nerve entrapment syndrome (ACNES), the diagnosis can be challenging due to its nonspecific symptoms, which may overlap with other abdominal pathologies. Healthcare professionals should be aware of this condition and its potential prevalence of 12–30% among patients with chronic abdominal pain. A thorough clinical assessment should be conducted to differentiate ACNES from other conditions. Local anesthetic injections targeting the suspected entrapment sites can be used to confirm the diagnosis, although their diagnostic accuracy is variable.

A. J. Carruyo
School of Medicine, Duke University, Durham, NC, USA

P. Y. Yi
Division of Pain Medicine, Department of Anesthesiology, Duke University Medical Center, Durham, NC, USA

R. S. Ackerman (✉)
Morsani College of Medicine, University of South Florida, Tampa, FL, USA

Division of Interventional Pain Medicine, Department of Anesthesiology, Moffitt Cancer Center and Research Institute, Tampa, FL, USA
e-mail: rackerman@usf.edu

C. E. Noe (ed.), *Musculoskeletal Pain*,
https://doi.org/10.1007/978-3-031-86057-7_17

In the case of xiphodynia, the diagnosis is primarily based on the characteristic clinical presentation of localized pain at the xiphoid process. However, it is crucial to differentiate xiphodynia from other potential causes, such as costochondritis, gastroesophageal reflux disease (GERD), or anginal pain. Adequate workup, including physical examination and potentially imaging studies, should be conducted to exclude other conditions before considering xiphodynia as the diagnosis.

Rectus sheath hematoma (RSH) presents as acute abdominal pain and can mimic other sources of abdominal pain, making diagnosis challenging. A careful clinical evaluation, including a detailed history and physical examination, is crucial. Imaging studies, such as computed tomography (CT) scans, can help confirm the diagnosis by visualizing the hematoma. Serial monitoring of hemoglobin and hematocrit levels is essential to assess for potential bleeding and monitor hemodynamic changes.

When evaluating slipping rib syndrome (SRS), the diagnosis is primarily based on the clinical presentation of localized pain in the lower chest or upper abdomen, exacerbated by certain movements or pressure on the affected area. The diagnosis can be challenging due to the lack of specific diagnostic tests. A thorough clinical assessment should be conducted to differentiate slipping rib syndrome from other potential causes of abdominal or chest pain.

Overall, a comprehensive diagnostic evaluation for these conditions involves a combination of clinical assessment, imaging studies, and in some cases, diagnostic injections. It is crucial to consider both neuropathic and non-neuropathic causes, exclude other potential diagnoses, and tailor the diagnostic approach based on the individual patient's presentation. Collaboration among healthcare professionals from various specialties may be necessary to reach an accurate diagnosis and develop an appropriate treatment plan for these chronic pain conditions.

Post-herniorrhaphy Neuralgia

Chronic groin pain (CGP) following the laparoscopic or open repair of hernias is a potential long-term complication that should be communicated to patients poised to undergo repair. Chronic pain is a result of surgical injury to surrounding nerves, and the ilioinguinal, iliohypogastric, genitofemoral, and lateral femoral cutaneous nerves are most frequently injured [1]. Injury to these nerves is thought to be due to their anatomical course and the presence of innervating branches where incision and mesh placement are established [2]. In most recent definitions, CGP is characterized by moderate to severe groin pain lasting greater than 3 months while affecting activities of daily living (ADLs), and meeting this criterion establishes the diagnosis of post-herniorrhaphy neuralgia (PHN). While postoperative groin pain is common in the short course, only about 0.5–6.0% of patients develop PHN [3]. Rates of PHN are higher in open hernial repair as opposed to laparoscopic total extraperitoneal (TEP) repair, although this trend is not seen in patients that experience pain for more than 5 years [1].

Historical factors aligning with post-herniorrhaphy neuralgia detail burning or stabbing in the skin or deep to the skin along the injured nerve distribution [4]. Hyperextension of the hip joint can potentially aggravate symptoms, along with manipulation of the skin overlying the site of the incision. Flexion of the hip and recumbency can alleviate symptoms [5]. Radiation of pain can occur in the hemiscrotum or back, highlighting genitofemoral nerve injury. Men can also have painful ejaculations [6]. Noting the kind of hernia and the presence of any procedural complications can direct diagnostic evaluation.

Diagnostic considerations of patients with persistent groin pain for 2 months or more should include non-neuropathic causes, like mesh migration or infection, recurrence of hernia, fluid collection, or local inflammatory reactions within soft tissue or bone (meshoma or periosteal reactions) [7]. As such, imaging with MRI or ultrasound should be carried out, although MRI is preferred because its sensitivity is not user-dependent. While the treatment of postsurgical groin pain is done with NSAIDs and other analgesics, a multimodal approach to pain relief should be carried out with patients with post-herniorrhaphy neuralgia. A groin nerve block can be both diagnostic and therapeutic, although a lack of improvement does not rule out diagnosis [2]. Patients with refractory pain to nerve block can receive radiofrequency ablation or nerve stimulation as an alternate treatment modality, while surgery and neurectomy are the final interventional options [8].

Anterior Cutaneous Nerve Entrapment Syndrome

Anterior cutaneous entrapment syndrome (ACNES), also known as abdominal cutaneous nerve entrapment syndrome (ACNES), is a condition characterized by chronic abdominal pain resulting from the entrapment of cutaneous nerves within the abdominal wall. Innervation to the abdominal wall is provided by anterior branches of the intercostal nerves (T7–T12) and the subcostal nerve (T12). In ACNES, cutaneous nerves become entrapped or compressed within the abdominal musculature or fibrous bands, leading to chronic abdominal pain [9]. ACNES has been underdiagnosed or misdiagnosed in many cases. This is partly due to its nonspecific symptoms, which may overlap with other abdominal pathologies, such as appendicitis, irritable bowel syndrome, or musculoskeletal disorders. The lack of awareness among healthcare professionals and the absence of specific diagnostic tests further contribute to the diagnostic challenges associated with ACNES [10, 11].

Exact prevalence rates remain uncertain due to the underdiagnosis and misdiagnosis of the condition, although research conducted among patients with chronic abdominal pain highlights ACNES can account for a significant proportion of cases, with a prevalence of 12–30%. Of note, ACNES may be underdiagnosed in certain patient populations, such as those presenting with atypical symptoms, leading to an underestimation of its true prevalence. Risk factors for ACNES include obesity, as increased adiposity can contribute to pressure and entrapment, previous abdominal surgery, connective tissue disorders like that of Ehlers–Danlos and Marfan syndromes, and female sex and OCP use [12].

The pain in ACNES is usually localized to specific areas of the abdominal wall, often described as focal or well-demarcated. The most common sites include the midline (around the rectus abdominis) and the lateral aspects of the abdomen. The pain may be unilateral or bilateral and can involve multiple dermatomes. The precise location of pain can vary among individuals and may correspond to the entrapment site of the cutaneous nerves [9, 10, 13]. Pain is often described as a dull, aching, or burning sensation. It is often persistent and may have paroxysmal exacerbations. The intensity of pain can range from mild to severe, and it may be associated with sensory disturbances such as numbness, tingling, or hypersensitivity in the affected area. The pain is usually superficial and does not penetrate deeply into the abdomen. Aggravating factors include coughing, sneezing, or deep breathing. The pain may also be aggravated by direct pressure on the affected area or by wearing tight clothing. ACNES is not associated with visceral symptoms such as nausea, vomiting, changes in bowel habits, or weight loss. The absence of these symptoms, along with a normal physical examination of the abdomen, can aid in differentiating ACNES from other conditions [9].

Local anesthetic injections targeting the suspected entrapment sites can be used to confirm the diagnosis of ACNES. However, the diagnostic accuracy of nerve blocks is variable, and false-positive or false-negative results can occur. Factors such as technical expertise, patient variability in response to injections, and the potential for transient symptom relief can impact the interpretation of diagnostic injections [11, 14]. Conservative medical treatments include the use of NSAIDs, gabapentinoids, or tricyclic antidepressants, while interventional treatment options include radiofrequency ablation, peripheral nerve stimulation, and surgical release of entrapped nerves as a last resort [15, 16].

Xiphodynia

Xiphodynia, or xiphoidalgia, is characterized by localized pain in the xiphoid process. While xiphodynia is considered relatively uncommon, it can cause significant discomfort and impact an individual's activities of daily living (ADLs). The exact etiology of xiphodynia remains unclear, while various factors are potential contributors to the development of the condition including direct injury or repetitive strain to the xiphoid process, such as from physical activities or poor posture. Similarly, activities that may contribute to long-standing micro-irritation or mechanical stress can contribute to the condition. In some cases, underlying musculoskeletal conditions, such as costochondritis or Tietze syndrome, may be associated, while psychosomatic influences have been suggested as potential contributing factors to the development or exacerbation of xiphodynia symptoms [17, 18].

The clinical presentation of xiphodynia is notable for being localized to the xiphoid process, while pain at the attachment site of the xiphoid process is common. The pain may vary in intensity, ranging from mild to severe, and can be described as aching, sharp, or stabbing in nature. Pain may be exacerbated by certain movements, palpation, deep breathing, or pressure on the area. While the clinical presentation of xiphodynia is crucial to accurate diagnosis, the condition should be differentiated from other potential diagnoses that can manifest with similar symptoms. The differential diagnosis for xiphodynia includes costochondritis, gastroesophageal reflux disease (GERD), anginal pain, or musculoskeletal related pain, although the list is not exhaustive. Adequate workup to exclude other conditions should be done, and xiphodynia can be regarded after exclusion [17, 18].

Treatments of xiphodynia are scantly reviewed in the current body of literature, while medications utilized in a small number of case series mentioned include the use of NSAIDs, topical anesthetics/analgesics, gabapentinoids, and muscle relaxers. Interventional options are available, although extreme caution should be taken due to the proximity of the xiphoid process to structures such as the pericardium, liver, stomach, and lungs. Interventional options include local anesthetic/glucocorticoid injection, and surgery has been documented as a final resort [17, 18].

Rectus Sheath Hematoma

Rectus sheath hematoma (RSH) is a relatively uncommon but serious presentation of acute abdominal pain. The rectus sheath is a fibrous space that contains the rectus abdominis muscle and is composed of aponeurotic segments from the external oblique, internal oblique, and transversus abdominis muscles. Internal epigastric vasculature, emanating from the mammary arteries and external iliac vessels, runs posteriorly to the rectus abdominis muscle. At the level superior to the arcuate line, the rectus abdominis muscle is enclosed entirely by the internal oblique aponeurosis, while the transversus abdominis aponeurosis and external oblique aponeurosis run posteriorly and anteriorly, respectively. Below the arcuate line—located at one-third of the distance from the umbilicus to the physis in a superomedial fashion—all aponeurotic segments run anteriorly to the rectus abdominis muscle, while the inferior epigastric artery perforates the rectus abdominis muscles. This perforation of epigastric vessels predisposes to stress from shearing forces to fenestrating branches, which is thought to contribute to the predominant incidence of RSH in the lower abdomen [19–21].

Several predisposing factors for RSH have been identified and include trauma, anticoagulant use or coagulopathies, prior abdominal or vascular surgery, pregnancy, and childbirth. Trauma directed to the abdominal wall can provide shearing forces to the branches of the epigastric vessels. Similarly, pregnancy and childbirth can contribute to increased abdominal wall pressure with the potential to tear small branches. RSH can have a wide array of presentations, varying due to the size of the hematoma and location. Thus, the presentations can pose diagnostic challenges given the overlap with other sources of acute abdominal pain. Symptoms often experienced include sharp or tearing abdominal pain with ecchymoses. Palpable abdominal swelling may be examined, and the mass typically does not cross the midline or change in location with the movement of the lower extremities or bearing down (Fothergill's sign). Diagnosis can be made with computed tomography scans of the abdomen and pelvis using iodinated contrast when available. For pregnant women and children, an ultrasound may be performed. The collection of serial hemoglobin and hematocrit is crucial to monitor hemodynamic changes in the setting of a potential bleed and inadequate RSH tamponade. Depending on the size of the hematoma, hemorrhagic shock or abdominal compartment syndrome are potential complications [21–23].

The management of RSH is best done with a multidisciplinary approach and includes potential medical and interventional approaches. Ensuring the differentiation of active bleeding from non-active bleeding is crucial, while vital signs, serial abdominal examinations, imaging, and blood values can be utilized to aid in determination. Medical therapy can be implemented to reverse anticoagulation, coagulopathies, or bleeding if appropriate. Blood pressure support with vasopressors and fluid resuscitation may be required. Interventional escalation may be needed, while angiography or even surgical exploration may be required for ligation and cessation of bleeding [20, 21, 24].

Slipping Rib Syndrome

Slipping rib syndrome (SRS), also known by an array of other names including twelfth-rib syndrome and rib-tip syndrome, is characterized by a stabbing or sharp pain that emanates from the costochondral junctions, typically in the lower eighth to tenth ribs (false ribs). Pain can last for minutes to hours and can be exacerbated by activities that elicit truncal movement, while lying down and resting can alleviate symptoms. Radiation of pain can occur in the anterior chest or back in concordance with the costal nerve involved and is often described as burning, shooting, or tingling. The pathogenesis of the condition has been attributed to aberrations in fibrocartilage in the costochondral junctions, particularly in the lower ribs. Whether due to trauma, muscular imbalance, or connective tissue disorders, this aberration in the cartilaginous attachment leads to hypermobility and slipping of the false ribs. Patients with this condition tend to also have highly arched 11th and 12th ribs, contributing to traction of the superior ribs and impingement of costal nerves at the above levels. A hooking maneuver may elicit symptoms and can aid in diagnosis; the hooking maneuver entails the grasping (hooking) of fingers inferiorly to the ribs in question while providing anterior and superior traction [25–27].

SRS is considered a relatively rare condition, and its exact prevalence is not well-established due to underdiagnosis and a lack of population-based studies. The condition has been reported to occur more frequently in women than in men and is often observed in athletes involved in sports requiring repetitive truncal movements, such as rowing, golf, tennis, or cricket. SRS remains underdiagnosed and may be mistaken for other conditions presenting with similar symptoms, such as musculoskeletal pain, gastrointestinal disorders, or respiratory conditions, due to the lack of awareness and familiarity with SRS among healthcare professionals [26–29].

The diagnosis of SRS can be clinical, although some diligence should be taken to rule out other causes of thoracic or upper abdominal pain. The afferent sensory nerves for the costal nerves mix with visceral sympathetic afferents, which may mimic visceral pathologies like that of appendicitis, cholecystitis, or gastritis. Careful physical examination along with the use of plain films can aid in diagnosis. Diagnostic considerations include costochondritis, intercostal muscle strain, gallbladder or liver pathologies, and pleurisy. Intercostal nerve blocks can aid in both diagnosis and treatment, along with topical analgesic creams or lidocaine patches. Refrainment from offending activities, like sports or daily movements that contribute to pain, should be trialed. Poor posture can also be a contributing factor, while proper posture education and training can improve symptoms [25–28].

Last, physical therapy and rehabilitation play a crucial role in the management of SRS while improving muscle strength, flexibility, and overall postural stability. Individualized exercise programs that target the muscles supporting the rib cage, enhance rib stability, and reduce the risk of further subluxation can have the most potential to alleviate pain. Surgery or cryoablations have been performed as last-resort measures, although not enough evidence is available to allow overarching recommendations on these measures [25, 30, 31].

References

1. Sekhon Inderjit Singh HK, Massey LH, Arulampalam T, Motson RW, Pawa N. Chronic groin pain following inguinal hernia repair in the laparoscopic era: systematic review and meta-analysis. Am J Surg. 2022;224(4):1135–49.
2. Alfieri S, Amid PK, Campanelli G, Izard G, Kehlet H, Wijsmuller AR, et al. International guidelines for prevention and management of post-operative chronic pain following inguinal hernia surgery. Hernia. 2011;15(3):239–49.
3. HerniaSurge G. International guidelines for groin hernia management. Hernia. 2018;22(1):1–165.
4. Hakeem A, Shanmugam V. Current trends in the diagnosis and management of post-herniorraphy chronic groin pain. World J Gastrointest Surg. 2011;3(6):73–81.
5. Kehlet H, Jensen TS, Woolf CJ. Persistent postsurgical pain: risk factors and prevention. Lancet. 2006;367(9522):1618–25.
6. Aasvang EK, Mohl B, Kehlet H. Ejaculatory pain: a specific postherniotomy pain syndrome? Anesthesiology. 2007;107(2):298–304.
7. Amid PK. Radiologic images of meshoma: a new phenomenon causing chronic pain after prosthetic repair of abdominal wall hernias. Arch Surg. 2004;139(12):1297–8.
8. Lee CH, Dellon AL. Surgical management of groin pain of neural origin. J Am Coll Surg. 2000;191(2):137–42.
9. Applegate WV. Abdominal cutaneous nerve entrapment syndrome. Am Fam Physician. 1973;8(3):132–3.
10. Hershfield NB. The abdominal wall. A frequently overlooked source of abdominal pain. J Clin Gastroenterol. 1992;14(3):199–202.
11. Srinivasan R, Greenbaum DS. Chronic abdominal wall pain: a frequently overlooked problem – practical approach to diagnosis and management. Am J Gastroenterol. 2002;97(4):824–30.
12. van Assen T, Brouns JAGM, Scheltinga MR, Roumen RM. Incidence of abdominal pain due to the anterior cutaneous nerve entrapment syndrome in an emergency department. Scand J Trauma Resusc Emerg Med. 2015;23:19.

13. Greenbaum DS, Greenbaum RB, Joseph JG, Natale JE. Chronic abdominal wall pain. Diagnostic validity and costs. Dig Dis Sci. 1994;39(9):1935–41.
14. Jacobs M, van den Dungen-Roelofsen R, Heemskerk J, Scheltinga MRM, Roumen RMH. Ultrasound-guided abdominal wall infiltration versus freehand technique in anterior cutaneous nerve entrapment syndrome (ACNES): randomized clinical trial. BJS Open. 2021;5(6):zrab124.
15. Boelens OB, van Assen T, Houterman S, Scheltinga MR, Roumen RM. A double-blind, randomized, controlled trial on surgery for chronic abdominal pain due to anterior cutaneous nerve entrapment syndrome. Ann Surg. 2013;257(5):845–9.
16. Mol FMU, Jansen CH, van Dijk W, van Eerten P, Scheltinga MR, Roumen RM. Factors predicting outcome after anterior neurectomy in patients with chronic abdominal pain due to anterior cutaneous nerve entrapment syndrome (ACNES). Surgery. 2019;165(2):417–22.
17. Howell JM. Xiphodynia: a report of three cases. J Emerg Med. 1992;10(4):435–8.
18. Lipkin M, Fulton LA, Wolfson EA. The syndrome of the hypersensitive xiphoid. N Engl J Med. 1955;253(14):591–7.
19. Carr C, Rhyne R. Diagnosis of rectus sheath hematoma by point-of-care ultrasound. J Emerg Med. 2019;56(6):680–3.
20. Salemis NS, Gourgiotis S, Karalis G. Diagnostic evaluation and management of patients with rectus sheath hematoma. A retrospective study. Int J Surg. 2010;8(4):290–3.
21. Sunga KL, Bellolio MF, Gilmore RM, Cabrera D. Spontaneous retroperitoneal hematoma: etiology, characteristics, management, and outcome. J Emerg Med. 2012;43(2):e157–61.
22. Gocke JE, MacCarty RL, Foulk WT. Rectus sheath hematoma: diagnosis by computed tomography scanning. Mayo Clin Proc. 1981;56(12):757–61.
23. Lewiss RE, Wu S. Ultrasound diagnosis of rectus sheath hematoma. J Emerg Med. 2012;43(5):e337–8.
24. Rimola J, Perendreu J, Falco J, Fortuno JR, Massuet A, Branera J. Percutaneous arterial embolization in the management of rectus sheath hematoma. AJR Am J Roentgenol. 2007;188(6):W497–502.
25. McMahon LE. Slipping Rib Syndrome: a review of evaluation, diagnosis and treatment. Semin Pediatr Surg. 2018;27(3):183–8.
26. Mekhail FG, Montgomery JR, Spicer PJ. Slipping rib syndrome presentation in a young woman. Radiol Case Rep. 2022;17(11):4376–8.
27. Vincent FM. Abdominal pain and slipping-rib syndrome. Ann Intern Med. 1978;88(1):129–30.
28. Foley CM, Sugimoto D, Mooney DP, Meehan WP 3rd, Stracciolini A. Diagnosis and treatment of slipping rib syndrome. Clin J Sport Med. 2019;29(1):18–23.
29. MacGregor RM, Schulte LJ, Merritt TC, Keller MS, Aubuchon JD, Abarbanell AM. Slipping rib syndrome in children: natural history and outcomes following costal cartilage excision. J Surg Res. 2022;280:204–8.
30. Mazzella A, Fournel L, Bobbio A, Janet-Vendroux A, Lococo F, Hamelin EC, et al. Costal cartilage resection for the treatment of slipping rib syndrome (Cyriax syndrome) in adults. J Thorac Dis. 2020;12(1):10–6.
31. Ninad N, Christie DB. Minimally invasive realignment for slipping rib syndrome. Am Surg. 2023;89(7):3246–7. https://doi.org/10.1177/00031348231157893.

18 Non-pharmacologic Treatment for Musculoskeletal Conditions

Timothy Olivier and G. Sunny Sharma

Introduction

The non-pharmacologic treatment of musculoskeletal pain spans a wide variety of treatments, including both conventional and complementary medicine modalities. Given the breadth of potential treatments, we have divided this chapter into large categories for easier review, including integrative medicine, psychological interventions, external devices, and manual treatments.

Within each of these broad groups, we chose to describe and give an overview of the treatments available. We have also presented potential conditions treated, available evidence, and contraindications/adverse effects of these treatments. A summary of the available evidence is included in Tables 18.1, 18.2, 18.3, and 18.4 at the end of this chapter. The summary tables are not an exhaustive list of appropriate indications, but rather a list of pathologies for which evidence was found, for or against, in the literature examined.

Table 18.1 Integrative medicine treatments and evidence

Treatment	Recommendation	Level of evidence
Acupuncture	Supported for low back pain, neck pain, fibromyalgia, lateral epicondylitis, knee osteoarthritis, and generalized shoulder pain	CPG, SR
Tai chi/qi gong	Supported for low back pain, knee osteoarthritis, and general chronic pain	SR, RCT
Yoga	Supported for low back pain, knee osteoarthritis, and fibromyalgia (in women)	CPG, SR, RCT

CPG clinical practice guideline, *SR* systematic review, *RCT* randomized control trial

T. Olivier · G. S. Sharma (✉)
University of Texas Southwestern Medical Center, Dallas, TX, USA
e-mail: gaurav.sharma3@utsouthwestern.edu

C. E. Noe (ed.), *Musculoskeletal Pain*,
https://doi.org/10.1007/978-3-031-86057-7_18

Table 18.2 Psychological interventions and evidence

Treatment	Recommendation	Level of evidence
Cognitive behavioral therapy	Supported for general chronic pain, low back pain, and neck pain	CPG, SR
Mindfulness-based stress reduction	Supported for low back pain, knee osteoarthritis, and fibromyalgia	SR, RCT
Biofeedback	Supported for low back pain, acute postoperative knee pain Not supported for chronic knee pain syndromes	SR
Hypnosis	Supported for chronic pain, non-specific low back pain (when combined with pain education)	RCTs
Guided imagery	Supported for various arthritic and rheumatic diseases	RCTs

CPG clinical practice guideline, *SR* systematic review, *RCT* randomized control trial

Table 18.3 External device treatments and evidence

Treatment	Recommendation	Level of evidence
Iontophoresis	Supported for diseases such as tendinitis, bursitis, tenosynovitis, and epicondylitis	RCTs
Phonophoresis	Supported for carpal tunnel syndrome (with ketoprofen), knee osteoarthritis and myofascial pain syndrome (with topical steroids or NSAID creams), in addition to diseases such as tendinitis, bursitis, tenosynovitis, and epicondylitis	CPG, RCTs
Superficial heat	Supported for low back pain, hand osteoarthritis (with paraffin)	SR
Diathermy	Supported for low back pain, knee osteoarthritis, pelvic floor disorders	SR, RCT
Therapeutic Ultrasound	Supported for carpal tunnel syndrome	CPG
Laser Therapy	Supported for low back pain, neck pain, knee osteoarthritis, hand and wrist pain, carpal tunnel syndrome, rheumatoid arthritis, fibromyalgia	CPG, SR
TENS	Supported generally for acute and chronic musculoskeletal pain, chronic neurogenic pain Conflicting recommendations for knee and hip osteoarthritis Not enough data to support for low back pain	CPG
Extracorporeal Shockwave Therapy	Supported for myofascial pain syndrome, plantar fasciitis, calcified rotator cuff tendinopathy, Achilles tendonitis, lateral epicondylitis, greater trochanteric pain syndrome	CPG, RCTs
Cryotherapy	Supported for arthritis, acute and chronic myofascial pain, and other soft tissue injuries	Review, case-control, RCT
Magnetic Therapy	Supported for knee osteoarthritis (pulsed electromagnetic) Not supported for carpal tunnel syndrome	CPG

CPG clinical practice guideline, *SR* systematic review, *RCT* randomized control trial

Table 18.4 Manual Medicine Treatments and Evidence

Treatment	Recommendation	Level of evidence
Spinal Manipulation Therapy	Supported for lumbar disc herniation with radiculopathy	CPG, SR
Physical Therapy	Supported for hip osteoarthritis, other types of osteoarthritis, small/medium/full thickness rotator cuff tears	CPG
McKenzie Method	Supported for chronic low back pain	CPG
Traction	Supported for neck pain Not supported for subacute or chronic low back pain	CPG, SR, review
Massage	Supported for chronic pain, chronic low back pain, neck pain Not supported for knee osteoarthritis, hip osteoarthritis	CPG, SR
Manual Therapy	Supported for low back pain	CPG
Exercise	Supported for knee osteoarthritis, hip osteoarthritis, hand osteoarthritis, chronic low back pain, fibromyalgia	CPG, SR

CPG clinical practice guideline, *SR* systematic review, *RCT* randomized control trial

Integrative Medicine

Integrative medicine uses therapeutic approaches from conventional and alternative medicine with the goal of providing patient-centered, healing-oriented care, emphasizing the whole person. Integrative medicine has historically been known by different names, such as complementary and alternative medicine (CAM) and holistic medicine. As support has increased over the years for their safety and effectiveness, these treatments have begun to be seen more as additions to treatment, as opposed to mutually exclusive alternatives. Depending on the organization or discipline, certain modalities are considered complementary versus conventional. Some modalities are considered complementary by consensus including acupuncture, tai chi, and yoga [1, 2]. There are many subcategories of integrative medicine, such as traditional Chinese medicine (TCM), which includes acupuncture and tai chi [3]. The use of integrative medicine has been growing overtime in the United States, therefore understanding its place in the treatment of pain is important [4]. In this section, we specifically discuss acupuncture, tai chi/qigong, and yoga.

Acupuncture

Acupuncture is a procedure by which filiform needles are inserted and/or manipulated at various points on the body. This can be done for pain relief as well as other purposes. This modality was developed more than 2500 years ago in China, with the idea being to restore the normal flow of energy (Qi, sometimes written as Chi, and pronounced "Chee") through the body [5, 6]. Qi is thought to flow through channels called "meridians" that exist through the body and connect this energy to organs and functions. Disease is thought to occur when the flow of qi is blocked or unbalanced [7].

Acupuncture has been shown to be beneficial in the treatment of low back pain, neck pain, and fibromyalgia among other musculoskeletal pathologies [8–14]. It has also been shown to be beneficial in the treatment of peripheral joint and tendon pain, such as lateral epicondylitis, knee osteoarthritis, and generalized shoulder pain [10, 12, 15, 16]. Although the included collection of nine trials on acupuncture for the treatment of fibromyalgia showed improvement in pain with acupuncture treatment compared to no acupuncture, no improvement was seen when compared to sham acupuncture [14]. This was also true for one of the examined clinical practice guidelines (CPGs), which showed that acupuncture led to improvement in chronic low back pain when compared to usual care, but not when compared to sham treatment [8]. There are several inherent difficulties when comparing true acupuncture to sham acupuncture in studies [17]. A possible area of focus to create more clarity in future studies could be to better define the physiologic effects of acupuncture, which then researchers can actively avoid in sham treatments [17].

Deep needling should not be performed close to the lungs, heart, or liver to avoid damage to these organs [4]. Some possible adverse effects of acupuncture, depending on the location of treatment, include fainting, hematoma, pneumothorax, infection, and injury to nerves or the spinal cord [4]. There is also the possibility of a needle being left in the body [4].

Tai Chi/Qigong

Qigong is a mindfulness practice that utilizes slow movements with coordinated breathing. The practice promotes circulation, strength, health, and spirituality. Like acupuncture, it focuses on the flow of "qi" throughout the body. Tai chi is a subset of qigong and involves a series of consecutive motions, whereas qigong can be just one motion repeated over and over. Tai chi promotes the balance between yin and yang by keeping both in flux and is an exercise of constant motion [18].

Tai chi is supported for the treatment of low back pain, knee osteoarthritis, and general chronic pain among other pathologies [11, 16, 19–21]. One analyzed collection of 18 randomized control trials (RCTs) stated that relief of pain for patients with osteoarthritis and low back pain was immediate and that a course of at least 5 weeks of tai chi was recommended for these conditions [19]. A separate set of seven RCTs recommended 12 weeks as the appropriate course of tai chi in the treatment of osteoarthritis-related pain [21]. Whether longer or shorter treatment times, at least a month is likely appropriate as long as the patient is seeing benefits.

Contraindications to tai chi and qigong are similar to other forms of aerobic activity. If a patient has limitations to how much physical activity they can tolerate, due to pulmonary or cardiac disease, for example, this might preclude them from fully participating in tai chi or qi gong.

Yoga

Yoga is a popular mind and body practice originating in India, which combines physical postures, breathing techniques, meditation, and relaxation. Modern yoga has evolved with a greater emphasis on exercise, strength, and flexibility. There are many different subsets including Vinyasa, Bikram, and Hatha [22]. Whereas tai chi involves constant motion, yoga focuses more on holding poses and postures [23].

The areas in which yoga has the most supporting evidence are for low back pain and knee osteoarthritis [8, 11, 24–28]. Some analyzed literature specifically comments on the benefits for women, with one RCT commenting on knee osteoarthritis and another commenting on fibromyalgia [29, 30]. Two analyzed RCTs commented on the Hatha and Iyengar subtypes of yoga, which showed improvement in knee osteoarthritis and low back pain, respectively. Most of the literature discusses yoga in general [11, 26].

In the examined literature, yoga was not seen to be associated with any serious adverse events [25]. Like tai chi, activity restrictions might preclude the patient from participating in this treatment modality. Even if cleared to participate, a patient's medical status may make some positions unsafe. For example, pregnant patients should not perform poses that lead to compression of their abdomen.

Psychological Interventions

The sensation of pain can lead to psychological distress, including depression and anxiety among other manifestations. Comorbid psychological history can also exacerbate a patient's sensation of pain. Psychological interventions are used to alter a patient's emotions, behaviors, or feelings, to decrease the adverse role pain has on their life. Psychological interventions can lead to improvement in disability level, quality of life, and activity level among other measures. There are a wide variety of psychological interventions available for the treatment of pain, most performed by psychologists, psychiatrists, or other providers with behavioral health training. The psychological interventions discussed in this section include cognitive behavioral therapy (CBT), mindfulness-based stress reduction (MBSR), biofeedback, hypnosis, meditation, and guided imagery. For all psychological interventions, if there are signs of severe mental illness or acute psychiatric illness, medical intervention will likely be more appropriate.

Cognitive Behavioral Therapy

Cognitive behavioral therapy (CBT) is a type of psychotherapy that focuses on addressing inaccurate or unhelpful negative thought processes and changing them. The goal of CBT is to think through overwhelming problems in a more positive and constructive way [31, 32]. This is usually done in a clinical setting with a behavioral health provider.

CBT for the treatment of chronic pain in general is supported by a large Cochrane review of 59 studies, though the effect was noted as small [33]. There is stronger support for the treatment of back pain than for neck pain with CBT in the analyzed literature. One CPG has a strong recommendation for CBT in combination with physical therapy (PT) for low back pain [8]. An analysis of three studies found both CBT and MBSR to be effective for the treatment of low back pain, with no statistical difference between the treatments [11].

There are no absolute contraindications to CBT, though comorbid severe personality disorders might make it difficult to treat patients with CBT. Providers with special training may be needed to adequately treat these patients [34]. If a patient does not have a positive response to the treatment, a different psychological modality might be more effective.

Mindfulness-Based Stress Reduction

Mindfulness is a type of meditation that focuses on staying aware of your surroundings and feelings without interpretation or judgment. Mindfulness utilizes guided imagery and breathing techniques in addition to other methods. The goal of mindfulness is to spend more time engaging in the present moment and less time on negative or random thoughts [35]. MBSR uses the mindfulness method to specifically target a patient's mental distress. MBSR was developed in the 1970s at the University of Massachusetts Medical Center, primarily by Dr Kabat–Zinn, and utilizes mindfulness meditation, yoga, group sessions, and other psychological methodologies [36]. The program developed by Dr. Kabat–Zinn takes place over 8 weeks [37].

The strongest evidence for the use of MBSR for the treatment of musculoskeletal pain is for low back pain [10, 11]. Other conditions, such as knee osteoarthritis or fibromyalgia, have weaker bases of support but do show potential [10, 36, 38–41]. Improvement in other variables, such as function or psychological factors like depression are seen for these conditions, but the evidence base needs to be augmented with future studies to further define the effect on pain specifically.

There are no strict contraindications regarding the use of MBSR, though certainly a patient's psychiatric history should be reviewed to ascertain if another treatment is necessary. There are no consistently documented adverse events documented in the literature [37].

Biofeedback

Biofeedback is a modality that uses auditory and visual physiologic monitoring to teach patients how to modify physiologic functions that are not normally under conscious control. This could include heart rate, blood pressure, temperature, or muscle tension [31]. When compared to no psychological therapy at all, electromyography (EMG) biofeedback was found to be beneficial in the treatment of chronic lower back pain by a set of three RCTs [11]. A set of four studies also analyzing EMG-based biofeedback did not recommend this modality in the treatment of chronic knee pain syndromes, such as patellofemoral pain syndrome and knee osteoarthritis but did remark that EMG biofeedback can be helpful acutely after knee surgeries such as ACL reconstruction and arthroscopic meniscectomy [42]. Biofeedback does not have any absolute contraindications. Biofeedback using electromyography, if using intramuscular needles, can have some rare adverse effects such as infection or bleeding [43].

Hypnosis

Hypnosis is a trance-like state in which a person becomes more aware and focused on particular thoughts, feelings, or behaviors. During this treatment, patients feel calm, relaxed, and more open to suggestions. Hypnosis was found to be beneficial for the treatment of chronic pain by a collection of nine RCTs [44]. There is also a single RCT that states hypnosis in combination with pain education is beneficial for patients with chronic non-specific low back pain [45]. Otherwise, the literature is sparse on the clinical efficacy of hypnosis. There are no absolute contraindications to hypnosis. Adverse effects are rare and usually short-lived but can include symptoms such as headaches, dizziness, and drowsiness among others [46].

Guided Imagery

Guided imagery is a method through which a patient visualizes positive scenarios and images. This is to relax the body and relieve stress, anxiety, and depression, among other symptoms [47]. Guided imagery was found to be beneficial for a variety of arthritic and other rheumatic diseases by a set of seven RCTs [48]. There are no absolute contraindications to the use of guided imagery.

External Devices

In this section, we will be discussing common external devices and technologies that can be used to address pain. All the discussed modalities apply energy to the outside of the patient's body to achieve pain relief. These treatments use different forms of energy to achieve pain relief including thermal, sound, light, magnetic, and electrical energies. Some modalities, such as iontophoresis and phonophoresis, use these energy forms to deliver a therapeutic substance into the body through the skin, such as corticosteroids or local anesthetics. Others use the energy form itself as the treatment. In this section, the modalities discussed include iontophoresis, phonophoresis, superficial heat, diathermy, therapeutic ultrasound, laser therapy, transcutaneous electrical nerve stimulation (TENS), extracorporeal shockwave therapy (ESWT), cryotherapy, and magnetic therapy including low-level laser therapy (LLLT).

Iontophoresis and Phonophoresis

Iontophoresis uses the charges of ions and particles to drive substances across tissues and membranes by passing a weak electrical current through the skin. The solution to be administered is placed on the electrode of the same polarity, electrodes are placed on the skin, and then a current is applied to drive the solution into the tissues. In contrast, phonophoresis is the use of ultrasound to increase the permeability of the skin which in turn increases percutaneous drug absorption and drives substances across tissues [49]. Similar to therapeutic ultrasound, it can be used in continuous or pulsed mode. Low frequency (typically 20–100 kHz) is most commonly utilized. Both modalities are used to administer medications percutaneously to a specific location [50]. This includes corticosteroids and local anesthetics [51].

Both iontophoresis and phonophoresis can deliver anti-inflammatory medications to inflamed tissues to treat diseases such as tendinitis, bursitis, tenosynovitis, and epicondylitis [52]. Phonophoresis with ketoprofen is specifically supported for the treatment of carpal tunnel syndrome, and phonophoresis with topical steroids or non-steroidal anti-inflammatory creams has been found to be useful for pain related to knee osteoarthritis and myofascial pain syndrome [4, 53]. It is important to keep in mind the specific mechanism of the applied solution when assessing change in the level of pain, duration of effect, and other variables. Deciding whether iontophoresis or phonophoresis is more appropriate can be based on provider training, or whether the patient has contraindications to electrical or ultrasound modalities.

Contraindications to iontophoresis can either be those related to direct electrical stimulation or those related to the therapeutic agent involved. Iontophoresis near implanted wires such as pacemakers, or other hardware should be avoided. Iontophoresis in regions of skin with impaired sensation should be used with caution [54]. Iontophoresis is usually well-tolerated but can have some minor temporary symptoms such as itching or redness of the skin [4]. Contraindications to phonophoresis can either be related to the ultrasound technology or those related to the therapeutic agent involved. If the patient has a history of hypersensitivity or adverse reactions associated with the delivered drug, iontophoresis or phonophoresis with that drug should be avoided.

Heating Modalities (Superficial Heat, Diathermy, and Therapeutic Ultrasound)

Superficial heat is typically used for tissue as deep as 1 cm. Diathermy is heat therapy that is applied deep into the tissues, at a level of 3–5 cm. Diathermy is not used to heat superficial tissues. Deep heat can be applied through ultrasound, shortwave, or microwave. Shortwave and microwave diathermy create heat by converting electromagnetic energy to thermal energy, with microwave diathermy using higher frequency waves [4]. Wavelengths used in shortwave diathermy are typically 1–100 MHz, whereas wavelengths used in microwave diathermy are typically 915–2450 MHz. Heat leads to pain relief through increased local blood flow, the gate control mechanism of pain control, and relaxed skeletal muscle [55]. Shortwave diathermy in particular heats skeletal muscle, blood, and synovial fluid, making it a good choice for deep muscle heating [52]. Some examples of ways to apply superficial heat include hot packs, heating pads, paraffin baths, heated hydrotherapy, and infrared lamps [52]. Therapeutic ultrasound can be considered a subset of diathermy because of its thermal effects. Compared to shortwave diathermy and microwave diathermy, it has the greatest depth of penetration, sometimes heating as deep as 8 cm [52]. Ultrasound itself can be used for both diagnostic and therapeutic purposes. Therapeutic ultrasound uses sound waves targeted at tissues in the body to treat pathology in the tissues and reduce pain. The sound waves work through both thermal and non-thermal pathways [56]. The ultrasound can be utilized as either continuous sound or pulsed sound waves [52]. Also in comparison to shortwave and microwave diathermy, therapeutic ultrasound is thought to be the only type of diathermy that can be applied in areas with surgical metal implants [4].

Heating modalities are most beneficial in the subacute and chronic time frames [4]. For the treatment of low back pain, superficial heat has been shown to have benefits in the short-term, and shortwave diathermy has shown benefits but with a limited base of support [57–61]. In regard to peripheral joint disease and peripheral nerve disorders, diathermy has been shown to be beneficial for knee osteoarthritis and therapeutic ultrasound has limited evidence for the treatment of carpal tunnel syndrome [4, 53, 61–63]. Superficial heat specifically using paraffin has been shown to have benefits in the treatment of hand osteoarthritis pain [64]. The use of diathermy has been shown to be helpful in a 15-study set for the treatment of pelvic floor disorders and can be used for refractory pelvic inflammatory disease as well [52, 65]. In general, these modalities tend to have a short duration of benefits [64].

The use of heat is contraindicated near areas of ischemia (i.e., peripheral vascular disease), areas of impaired sensation, areas of malignancy, areas of scarring, areas of infection, areas with open wounds, areas of edema, and areas of acute trauma and inflammation. It should also be avoided in patients that have the inability to communicate or respond to pain [52, 66]. Superficial heat should be avoided in the acute time frame as it can worsen acute inflammation [4]. Contraindications to diathermy and therapeutic ultrasound also include pacemakers, use near epiphyses, and use near areas with implants with plastic material. Diathermy and therapeutic ultrasound should also not be used near reproductive organs or a pregnant uterus. It should also not be used near nerves, the brain, or the eyes. Diathermy and therapeutic ultrasound are also contraindicated near the spine or laminectomy sites as they can cause spinal cord heating. Diathermy and therapeutic ultrasound should not be used near metal items such as jewelry, or implanted devices that contain metal. Diathermy and therapeutic ultrasound should not be used near fluid-filled areas which include the eyes, but also joints with effusion for example [4].

Laser Therapy

Laser is an acronym for light amplification of stimulated emissions of radiation. It is essentially an amplified and focused light. Low-level laser therapy (LLLT) is the common form of these treatments, and results in photochemical changes in the targeted cells themselves, which include effects that decrease pain and inflammation, stimulate collagen metabolism and wound healing, and promote fracture healing [67]. Laser therapy has supportive literature for the treatment of many pathologies including low back pain, neck pain, knee osteoarthritis, hand and wrist pain, carpal tunnel syndrome, rheumatoid arthritis, and fibromyalgia [4, 8, 13, 15, 53, 68]. LLLT has been shown to be better for low back pain in combination with exercise as posited by one clinical practice guideline [8]. The literature mostly demonstrates short-term improvement if the time frame is mentioned [8, 13]. Laser therapy should be avoided near areas of malignancy. It can also cause damage if the beam directly hits the eye or hits it off a reflection [69].

Transcutaneous Electrical Nerve Stimulation

Transcutaneous Electrical Nerve Stimulation (TENS) is a procedure where mild electric currents are applied to the skin through electrodes. The mechanism of pain relief is thought to be through gate control and/or the production of endorphins [70, 71]. The device is small and sends the electrical stimulation through wires to the electrodes on the patient's skin. TENS sessions are usually half an hour to an hour at a time with a maximum of 2 h per session and 8 h per day. These treatments are usually done for 3 weeks and then are gradually reduced over 8–12 weeks [52]. High frequency, low intensity stimulation is the most effective type of stimulation and is particularly useful for neuropathic pain [52].

TENS can be used for acute and chronic musculoskeletal pain, and chronic neurogenic pain [52]. However, the literature as it pertains to specific musculoskeletal pathologies is quite variable. One clinical practice guideline strongly recommends against the use of TENS for knee and hip osteoarthritis pain, and another weakly recommends its use for these diagnoses [15, 64]. Both CPGs state that higher-quality studies need to be done with larger sample sizes [15, 64]. Similarly, there is a lack of data to support the use of TENS for low back pain. Higher-quality studies with larger sample sizes are needed [4, 8]. There are several individual RCTs that indicate benefits from TENS, which shows promise if more research is able to be conducted on this modality [8, 15, 64].

TENS should be avoided near implanted devices such as pacemakers as well as near areas of malignancy, infection, active wounds, the abdomen or pelvis if the patient is pregnant, the head and neck if the patient has a history of seizures, directly over the spine, and near the chest if the patient has a history of heart disease [72]. TENS should also be avoided in someone who has a deep venous thrombosis (DVT) or thrombophlebitis, and in those with bleeding disorders [72]. TENS should also be avoided in the areas of decreased sensation, and in those who have trouble communicating potential adverse effects [72]. Use should also be avoided near the sympathetic ganglia or the carotid sinus due to the risk of abnormal vascular effects. Minor burns can be a possible complication of improperly applied electrodes [72].

Extracorporeal Shockwave Therapy

Extracorporeal shockwave therapy (ESWT) is a treatment involving the delivery of high-energy sound waves to injured tissues to promote the natural healing process and decrease pain. ESWT can take many different forms, including high-energy, low-energy, focused, and radial among others [73–75]. Thermal effects are negligible [76]. There is no consensus as to the best number of sessions or the most effective intensity of the shockwaves [77].

ESWT is supported for the treatment of pain due to a number of pathologies, including myofascial pain syndrome, plantar fasciitis, calcified rotator cuff tendinopathy, Achilles tendonitis, lateral epicondylitis, and greater trochanteric pain syndrome among many others [4, 78–83]. Benefits can be seen from ESWT rapidly and are most effective for long-term function and healing when used in combination with other treatment modalities [84].

ESWT is contraindicated in patients with bleeding disorders as well as in patients who are pregnant. Adverse effects are usually minor and temporary but can include swelling, hematoma, skin redness, or erosion. Humeral head osteonecrosis is a rare adverse event specifically when treating shoulder pathology such as rotator cuff tendinopathy. This is thought to be due to the effect on the blood supply to the humeral head during this procedure [83].

Cryotherapy

Cryotherapy is the use of cold to achieve pain relief. Cryotherapy utilizes cold to induce vasoconstriction and decrease inflammation and local metabolic demand. By decreasing tissue temperature, cryotherapy also leads to increased nerve pain threshold. Some examples of devices used are cold packs, chemical cool sprays, and cold baths [85]. Fifteen minutes is the usual minimum amount of time for application to achieve analgesic effect [4]. Cryotherapy can be used for inflammatory states such as arthritis, acute or chronic myofascial pain states, and other soft tissue injuries. It is most useful in the acute period when inflammation is greatest [4, 52]. Cryotherapy is contraindicated in those that have cold intolerance such as patients with Raynaud's disease. It is also contraindicated in areas with sensation deficits or arterial insufficiency. It should also be avoided in patients that have an inability to communicate or respond to pain [86]. Baths should be avoided in patients with open wounds and areas with local infection [4].

Magnetic, Electromagnetic, and Pulsed Electromagnetic Therapy

Magnetic therapy is a treatment involving the application of a magnetic field from a static or permanent magnet to an area of the body. It is electromagnetic therapy if the magnetic field is being created from an electric-powered device. The mechanisms of action of static magnets are more theoretical than those of the other external devices, but some hypotheses include an increase in blood flow or oxygenation, though these hypotheses are not supported in the literature. Pulsed electromagnetic field therapy (PEMF) has been used to treat delayed or non-union fractures, depression, and other non-pain-related illnesses.

The strongest evidence for the use of magnetic therapy is pulsed electromagnetic field therapy for the treatment of pain related to knee osteoarthritis, though the literature to support this is still limited [15]. Alternatively, there is strong evidence against the use of magnetic therapy for some pathologies, such as a strong recommendation against the use for carpal tunnel syndrome from a CPG [87]. Overall, most of the literature is of insufficient quality to comment on utility, including for pathologies such as neck pain. There is a need for more studies with greater sample sizes and treatment standardization [88, 89].

Though these devices are generally safe, caution should be taken if the patient has implanted devices that could be affected by the presence of electromagnetic fields, such as pacemakers, spinal cord stimulators, or intrathecal pumps. These therapies should also not be used in pregnant patients. Application of metal magnets to patients with allergies to certain metals should also be avoided.

Manual Medicine

Manual medicine is a collection of hands-on treatment modalities that involve a practitioner manipulating the patient physically to achieve a therapeutic effect. Possible mechanisms of action include improving restrictions in movement, vasodilation, and the gate control theory. The practitioners of these modalities can be physical therapists, chiropractors, osteopathic physicians, or others depending on the specific modality. The treatments discussed in this section include spinal manipulation therapy (SMT), physical therapy (PT), the McKenzie method, traction, massage, manual therapy, and exercise.

Spinal Manipulation Therapy

Spinal manipulation therapy (SMT) is a treatment in which practitioners apply a controlled thrust to the spine. This type of therapy is usually applied by chiropractors but can also be applied by osteopathic physicians or physical therapists with the proper training [90].

The greatest support for the use of SMT is for the treatment of lumbar disc herniation with radiculopathy, though the evidence is still limited [11, 91]. For the treatment of acute and chronic low back pain, CPGs stated SMT can be used as one of many treatment options although the clinical significance compared to no treatment, medication, or modalities is still unclear [8]. Additional research would help strengthen the use of SMT with specific diagnoses. One CPG recommends conducting studies comparing SMT to other treatments using validated outcome measures [92].

SMT may be associated with adverse events, such as headaches, dizziness, aches, and stiffness. Adverse events and complications from spinal manipulation therapy have the potential to be serious. The most common serious adverse effects are due to vertebral artery dissection, some of which have rarely resulted in death in the past [93]. Damage to other blood vessels or nerves in the head and neck region can also occur, depending on what maneuver is specifically being performed.

Physical Therapy

Physical therapy is a treatment modality and discipline that uses exercise, manual modalities, and passive techniques to help restore strength and movement, reduce pain, and prevent disability [94, 95]. This modality is provided by trained physical therapists. Treatment will include examination, diagnosis, intervention, preventive measures, and education. Interventions will include exercises, manual therapies, and the use of external devices. Physical therapy subspecialties include sports, wound management, cardiopulmonary, neurologic, and orthopedic among others. For the purpose of this section, the focus was put on physical therapy without the specific use of an external device or other treatment modality used elsewhere.

Physical therapy is strongly recommended for many different pathologies, such as pain related to hip osteoarthritis and pain related to small, medium, and full-thickness rotator cuff tears [96, 97]. It is also recommended with a call for further research on pathologies such as fibromyalgia [98]. As mentioned above, physical therapy can also include many of the other modalities mentioned in this chapter.

In terms of contraindications, if a patient has limitations to how much physical activity they can tolerate, due to pulmonary or cardiac disease for example, this might preclude them from taking part in physical therapy.

McKenzie Method

The McKenzie method is a specific type of therapy. It is also known as the Mechanical Diagnosis and Therapy method. It is a widely accepted program for back pain specifically, though can be used for extremity or neck pain as well. The McKenzie method focuses on the identification and classification of non-specific spine pain into subgroups (postural syndrome, dysfunction syndrome, derangement syndrome, or other). This method also focuses on the centralization concept of pain, through which the goal is to move lower extremity pain into the back [99]. Though the relevant CPG did not find the McKenzie method to be more beneficial than dynamic strengthening or back school for the treatment of chronic low back pain, it was still shown to be beneficial with limited evidence [8]. Anecdotally, many patients find benefits with the McKenzie method for back pain. Contraindications and adverse events related to McKenzie treatment are similar to those from therapeutic exercise and physical therapy.

Traction

Traction is the application of a force that stretches soft tissues and draws two adjacent bones apart to increase the shared joint space. The term spinal decompression refers to the relief of pressure on the spinal cord or nerve roots, whereas traction refers to the pulling apart of tissues [4]. There are different modalities of traction, including manual, gravitational, and mechanical [100]. It can also be applied in an intermittent, sustained, or continuous fashion. Sustained traction is with more applied force and a lesser amount of time, whereas continuous traction is with less applied force over a longer period. It is usually a modality targeted at the spine but can be targeted at other areas as well. Traction uses equipment such as a head or chin sling, or a traction table.

A CPG pertaining to the treatment of low back pain strongly recommends against traction for subacute or chronic low back pain [8]. Traction has stronger, though limited, evidence with other pathologies, such as neck pain [4].

Contraindications to traction include malignancy, infection, osteoporosis, fracture, or severe arthritis with instability in the region being treated. Contraindications also include severe cord compression, congenital spinal deformity, pregnancy, uncontrolled heart disease, uncontrolled hypertension, and carotid or vertebral artery disease. Specific cervical contraindications include ligamentous instability, atlantoaxial instability, and vertebrobasilar insufficiency. Specific lumbar contraindications include cauda equina syndrome and aortic aneurysms. Potential adverse events include worsened pain, worsened disc protrusion if concentrated on the back, or fracture.

Massage

Massage is a treatment where the soft tissues are kneaded, rubbed, stroked, tapped, and otherwise manipulated in a rhythm to help the patient decrease musculoskeletal pain among other effects [101]. There are many different types of massage, with different cultural origins and philosophies. Possible mechanisms of action for pain control include gate control theory, vasodilation, and skeletal muscle remodeling. Medical massage is any massage or massage modality used to treat a specific medical condition. Specific techniques include myofascial release and soft tissue mobilization.

Massage is generally recommended for the treatment of chronic pain [4]. However, a CPG pertaining to the management of osteoarthritis recommends against the use of massage for knee and hip osteoarthritis, with limited evidence [64]. Evidence is more supportive for the treatment of chronic low back pain, with improvement in the short-term found by a collection of four studies, though a CPG on low back pain stated that exercise alone is more effective than exercise with massage [8, 13]. For the treatment of neck pain, massage is similarly beneficial in the short-term [37].

Common contraindications include treatment over areas with open wounds, burns, bruises, malignancy, recent trauma, or fractures. Treatment should also be avoided in patients with active infection, pregnancy, uncontrolled hypertension, severe bleeding disorders, or other acute medical illnesses. Gentler manipulation should be used with people on anticoagulation. Possible adverse effects of massage are usually mild and temporary but can include headache, nausea, bruising, and increased pain.

Manual Therapy

Manual therapy is a physical treatment applied to patients to directly or indirectly target the tissues of the body and lead to decreased pain. These can be targeted at joints, muscles, connective tissues, or the neurovascular system. This encompasses many other specific therapies, including traction, osteopathy, and massage among others [100]. It is a manual force directed at a specific area of the body to decrease pain and increase mobility. These treatments can be applied by a number of different trained providers. This section focuses on literature that mentioned manual therapy as a whole, not one of its specific subsets.

Manual therapy can be used for any number of musculoskeletal complaints. However, there is conflicting evidence on whether manual therapy with exercise is better than exercise alone for the treatment of knee and hip osteoarthritis, with one CPG supporting its use and one not [15]. There is support in the literature for manual therapy for the treatment of low back pain [64].

For manual therapy in general, there are no absolute contraindications, but some relative contraindications include use over areas of active infection or acute inflammation. Treatment over the spine is relatively contraindicated for those with malignancy of the spine, myelopathy, or inflammatory disease of the spine. Adverse events after manual therapy are normally transient and mild and can include increased pain, headache, nausea, or stiffness.

Exercise

Exercise is a physical activity that is planned, structured, and repetitive with the goal of improving or maintaining physical fitness [102]. There are different types of exercises, including aerobic, anaerobic, balance, and flexibility among others. Aerobic exercise has a focus on increasing cardiovascular endurance. Anaerobic exercise has a focus on increasing strength and muscle mass.

The strongest evidence for exercise is in the treatment of osteoarthritis pain at the knee, hip, and hand [64]. Exercise for the treatment of low back pain has a variable evidence base, with more support for the treatment of chronic low back pain than acute, and more support for short-term improvements than long-term improvements [8, 13]. Exercise and aquatic exercise are recommended with limited evidence for the treatment of pain related to fibromyalgia [103]. Exercise is many a times analyzed in the context of other therapies, either in comparison or in addition to. For baseline physical activity for all adults, the recommendation from the American Heart Association is for 150 min per week of moderate-intensity aerobic activity or 75 min a week of vigorous aerobic activity, usually spread throughout the week [104]. Moderate-intensity activities can include walking at least 2.5 miles per hour, gardening, and biking slower than 10 miles per hour among others. Vigorous activities include running, swimming, and doing heavy yard work among others [104]. Even greater benefits are seen if 5 h of physical activity can be obtained [104]. Additionally, at least 2 days of moderate to high-intensity muscle strengthening is recommended [104].

Adverse events from therapeutic exercise are possible, and the specific types of adverse events would depend on factors related to the exercise. For instance, aerobic exercise through long-distance running could lead to strains, sprains, or tendinopathies of the lower extremities. Per the American College of Sports Medicine and the American Heart Association, absolute contraindications to aerobic and resistance exercise include recent myocardial infarction or ECG changes, complete heart block, acute heart failure, unstable angina, uncontrolled diabetes, uncontrolled arrhythmias, and uncontrolled hypertension [105]. Other contraindications include acute severe illnesses such as endocarditis, severe symptomatic aortic stenosis, and pulmonary embolism.

References

1. Integrative medicine – Mayo Clinic [Internet]. Mayoclinic.org. 2018. Available from: https://www.mayoclinic.org/tests-procedures/complementary-alternative-medicine/about/pac-20393581.
2. National Center for Complementary and Integrative Health. Complementary, alternative, or integrative health: what's in a name? [Internet]. NCCIH. 2021. Available from: https://www.nccih.nih.gov/health/complementary-alternative-or-integrative-health-whats-in-a-name.
3. NCCIH. Traditional Chinese medicine: what you need to know [Internet]. NCCIH. 2019. Available from: https://www.nccih.nih.gov/health/traditional-chinese-medicine-what-you-need-to-know.
4. Cifu DX, Kaelin DL, Kowalske KJ, Lew HL, Miller MA, Ragnarsson KT, et al. Braddom's physical medicine & rehabilitation. Philadelphia: Elsevier; 2016.
5. Acupuncture: what you need to know [Internet]. NCCIH. 2022. Available from: https://www.nccih.nih.gov/health/acupuncture-what-you-need-to-know.
6. Mayo Clinic. Acupuncture [Internet]. Mayoclinic.org. 2018. Available from: https://www.mayoclinic.org/tests-procedures/acupuncture/about/pac-20392763.
7. Langevin HM, Yandow JA. Relationship of acupuncture points and meridians to connective tissue planes. Anat Rec. 2002;269(6):257–65.
8. Evidence-based clinical guidelines for multidisciplinary spine care: diagnosis & treatment of low back pain [Internet]. Available from: https://www.spine.org/Portals/0/assets/downloads/ResearchClinicalCare/Guidelines/LowBackPain.pdf.
9. Furlan AD, van Tulder MW, Cherkin D, Tsukayama H, Lao L, Koes BW, Berman BM. Acupuncture and dry-needling for low back pain. Cochrane Database Syst Rev. 2005;(1):Art. No.: CD001351. https://doi.org/10.1002/14651858.CD001351.pub2.
10. Swedish Council on Health Technology Assessment. Methods of treating chronic pain: a systematic review [internet]. Stockholm: Swedish Council on Health Technology Assessment (SBU); 2006. SBU Yellow Report No. 177/1+2. PMID: 28876750.
11. Chou R, Deyo R, Friedly J, Skelly A, Hashimoto R, Weimer M, et al. Nonpharmacologic therapies for low back pain: a systematic review for an American College of Physicians Clinical Practice Guideline [Internet]. www.acpjournals.org. Ann Intern Med. 2017. Available from: https://www.acpjournals.org/doi/full/10.7326/M16-2459?rfr_dat=cr_pub++0pubmed&url_ver=Z39.88-2003&rfr_id=ori%3Arid%3Acrossref.org.
12. Ernst E, Lee MS. Acupuncture for rheumatic conditions: an overview of systematic reviews. Rheumatology. 2010;49(10):1957–61.
13. Skelly AC, Chou R, Dettori JR, Turner JA, Friedly JL, Rundell SD, et al. Noninvasive non-pharmacological treatment for chronic pain: a systematic review update [Internet]. PubMed. Rockville (MD): Agency for Healthcare Research and Quality (US); 2020. Available from: https://www.ncbi.nlm.nih.gov/books/NBK556229/.
14. Deare JC, Zheng Z, Xue CCL, Liu JP, Shang J, Scott SW, Littlejohn G. Acupuncture for treating fibromyalgia. Cochrane Database Syst Rev. 2013;(5):Art. No.: CD007070. https://doi.org/10.1002/14651858.CD007070.pub2.
15. Management of osteoarthritis of the knee (non-arthroplasty) [Internet]. Available from: https://www.aaos.org/globalassets/quality-and-practice-resources/osteoarthritis-of-the-knee/oak3cpg.pdf?trk=public_post_comment-text.
16. Shengelia R, Parker SJ, Ballin M, George T, Reid MC. Complementary therapies for osteoarthritis: are they effective? Pain Manag Nurs. 2013;14(4):e274–88. https://doi.org/10.1016/j.pmn.2012.01.001. Epub 2012 Mar 21. PMID: 24315281; PMCID: PMC3857560.

17. Langevin HM, Wayne PM, MacPherson H, Schnyer R, Milley RM, Napadow V, et al. Paradoxes in acupuncture research: strategies for moving forward. Evid Based Complement Alternat Med. 2011;2011:1–11.
18. Tai Chi: in depth [Internet]. NCCIH. 2022. Available from: https://www.nccih.nih.gov/health/tai-chi-what-you-need-to-know.
19. Kong LJ, Lauche R, Klose P, Bu JH, Yang XC, Guo CQ, Dobos G, Cheng YW. Tai Chi for chronic pain conditions: a systematic review and meta-analysis of randomized controlled trials. Sci Rep. 2016;6:25325. https://doi.org/10.1038/srep25325. PMID: 27125299; PMCID: PMC4850460.
20. Wang C, Schmid CH, Iversen MD, Harvey WF, Fielding RA, Driban JB, Price LL, Wong JB, Reid KF, Rones R, McAlindon T. Comparative effectiveness of tai chi versus physical therapy for knee osteoarthritis: a randomized trial. Ann Intern Med. 2016;165(2):77–86. https://doi.org/10.7326/M15-2143. Epub 2016 May 17. PMID: 27183035; PMCID: PMC4960454.
21. Yan J-H, Gu W-J, Sun J, Zhang W-X, Li B-W, Pan L. Efficacy of Tai Chi on pain, stiffness and function in patients with osteoarthritis: a meta-analysis. Milanese S, editor. PLoS ONE [Internet]. 2013 [cited 2019 Mar 6];8(4):e61672. Available from: https://www.ncbi.nlm.nih.gov/pmc/articles/PMC3631149/.
22. https://www.cancer.gov/publications/dictionaries/cancer-terms/def/yoga [Internet]. www.cancer.gov. 2011. Available from: https://www.cancer.gov/publications/dictionaries/cancer-terms/def/yoga.
23. Yoga vs. Tai Chi: which is better? [Internet]. wfaa.com. [cited 2023 Feb 17]. Available from: https://www.wfaa.com/article/news/national/yoga-vs-tai-chi-which-is-better/103-311318801#:~:text=The%20main%20difference%20is%20in.
24. Wieland LS, Skoetz N, Pilkington K, Vempati R, D'Adamo CR, Berman BM. Yoga treatment for chronic non-specific low back pain. Cochrane Database Syst Rev. 2017;1(1):CD010671.
25. Cramer H, Lauche R, Haller H, Dobos G. A systematic review and meta-analysis of yoga for low back pain. Clin J Pain. 2013;29(5):450–60.
26. Cheung C, Wyman JF, Bronas U, McCarthy T, Rudser K, Mathiason MA. Managing knee osteoarthritis with yoga or aerobic/strengthening exercise programs in older adults: a pilot randomized controlled trial. Rheumatol Int. 2017;37(3):389–98. https://doi.org/10.1007/s00296-016-3620-2. Epub 2016 Dec 2. PMID: 27913870; PMCID: PMC5569242.
27. Kan L, Zhang J, Yang Y, Wang P. The effects of yoga on pain, mobility, and quality of life in patients with knee osteoarthritis: a systematic review. Evid Based Complement Alternat Med. 2016;2016:6016532. https://doi.org/10.1155/2016/6016532. Epub 2016 Sep 29. PMID: 27777597; PMCID: PMC5061981.
28. Wang Y, Lu S, Wang R, Jiang P, Rao F, Wang B, Zhu Y, Hu Y, Zhu J. Integrative effect of yoga practice in patients with knee arthritis: a PRISMA-compliant meta-analysis. Medicine (Baltimore). 2018;97(31):e11742. https://doi.org/10.1097/MD.0000000000011742. PMID: 30075589; PMCID: PMC6081169.
29. Cheung C, Wyman JF, Resnick B, Savik K. Yoga for managing knee osteoarthritis in older women: a pilot randomized controlled trial. BMC Complement Altern Med. 2014;14:160. https://doi.org/10.1186/1472-6882-14-160. PMID: 24886638; PMCID: PMC4038088.
30. Carson JW, Carson KM, Jones KD, Bennett RM, Wright CL, Mist SD. A pilot randomized controlled trial of the Yoga of Awareness program in the management of fibromyalgia. Pain. 2010;151(2):530–9. https://doi.org/10.1016/j.pain.2010.08.020. PMID: 20946990; PMCID: PMC5568071.
31. Mayo Clinic. Cognitive behavioral therapy [Internet]. Mayoclinic.org. Mayo Clinic; 2019. Available from: https://www.mayoclinic.org/tests-procedures/cognitive-behavioral-therapy/about/pac-20384610.
32. NHS. Cognitive behavioural therapy (CBT) [Internet]. NHS. NHS; 2022. Available from: https://www.nhs.uk/mental-health/talking-therapies-medicine-treatments/talking-therapies-and-counselling/cognitive-behavioural-therapy-cbt/overview/.

33. Williams AC de C, Fisher E, Hearn L, Eccleston C. Psychological therapies for the management of chronic pain (excluding headache) in adults. Cochrane Database Syst Rev. 2020;8(8):Art. No.: CD007407. https://doi.org/10.1002/14651858.CD007407.pub4.
34. Gautam M, Tripathi A, Deshmukh D, Gaur M. Cognitive behavioral therapy for depression. Indian J Psychiatry [Internet]. 2020;62(8):223. Available from: https://www.ncbi.nlm.nih.gov/pmc/articles/PMC7001356/.
35. Mayo Clinic. Mindfulness exercises [Internet]. Mayo Clinic. 2020. Available from: https://www.mayoclinic.org/healthy-lifestyle/consumer-health/in-depth/mindfulness-exercises/art-20046356.
36. Marais C, Song Y, Ferreira R, et al. Evaluation of mindfulness based stress reduction in symptomatic knee or hip osteoarthritis patients: a pilot randomized controlled trial. BMC Rheumatol. 2022;6:46. https://doi.org/10.1186/s41927-022-00277-9.
37. Dobkin PL, Irving JA, Amar S. For whom may participation in a mindfulness-based stress reduction program be contraindicated? Mindfulness. 2011;3(1):44–50.
38. Lee AC, Harvey WF, Price LL, Morgan LPK, Morgan NL, Wang C. Mindfulness is associated with psychological health and moderates pain in knee osteoarthritis. Osteoarthritis Cartilage [Internet]. 2017;25(6):824–31. Available from: https://www.oarsijournal.com/article/S1063-4584(16)30153-4/fulltext.
39. Morgan NL, Ransford GL, Morgan LP, Driban JB, Wang C. Mindfulness is associated with psychological symptoms, self-efficacy, and quality of life among patients with symptomatic knee osteoarthritis. Osteoarthr Cartil. 2013;21:S257–8.
40. Marks R. Mindfulness and its application for older adults with chronically painful osteoarthritis [Internet]. researchgate.net. Int J Geriatr Gerontol. 2022. Available from: https://www.researchgate.net/profile/Ray-Marks/publication/361312230_Mindfulness_and_its_Application_for_Older_Adults_with_Chronically_Painful_Osteoarthritis/links/62aa00cf938bee3e3f36980d/Mindfulness-and-its-Application-for-Older-Adults-with-Chronically-Painful-Osteoarthritis.pdf.
41. Theadom A, Cropley M, Smith HE, Feigin VL, McPherson K. Mind and body therapy for fibromyalgia. Cochrane Database Syst Rev. 2015;(4):Art. No.: CD001980. https://doi.org/10.1002/14651858.CD001980.pub3.
42. Wasielewski NJ, Parker TM, Kotsko KM. Evaluation of electromyographic biofeedback for the quadriceps femoris: a systematic review. J Athl Train. 2011;46(5):543–54. https://doi.org/10.4085/1062-6050-46.5.543. PMID: 22488142; PMCID: PMC3418961.
43. Malik K, Dua A. Biofeedback [Internet]. PubMed. Treasure Island (FL): StatPearls Publishing; 2021. Available from: https://www.ncbi.nlm.nih.gov/books/NBK553075/.
44. Langlois P, Perrochon A, David R, Rainville P, Wood C, Vanhaudenhuyse A, et al. Hypnosis to manage musculoskeletal and neuropathic chronic pain: a systematic review and meta-analysis. Neurosci Biobehav Rev. 2022;135:104591.
45. Rizzo RRN, Medeiros FC, Pires LG, Pimenta RM, McAuley JH, Jensen MP, et al. Hypnosis enhances the effects of pain education in patients with chronic nonspecific low back pain: a randomized controlled trial. J Pain. 2018;19(10):1103.e1–9.
46. Gruzelier J. Unwanted effects of hypnosis: a review of the evidence and its implications. Contemp Hypn. 2000;17(4):163–93.
47. https://www.cancer.gov/publications/dictionaries/cancer-terms/def/guided-imagery [Internet]. www.cancer.gov. 2011. Available from: https://www.cancer.gov/publications/dictionaries/cancer-terms/def/guided-imagery.
48. Giacobbi PR Jr, Stabler ME, Stewart J, Jaeschke AM, Siebert JL, Kelley GA. Guided imagery for arthritis and other rheumatic diseases: a systematic review of randomized controlled trials. Pain Manag Nurs. 2015;16(5):792–803. https://doi.org/10.1016/j.pmn.2015.01.003. Epub 2015 Jul 11. PMID: 26174438; PMCID: PMC4605831.
49. Shiraz University of Medical Sciences. Effect of lidocaine phonophoresis on sensory blockade: pulsed or continuous mode of therapeutic ultrasound? [Internet]. clinicaltrials.gov. 2011. Available from: https://clinicaltrials.gov/ct2/show/NCT01404468.

50. Iontophoresis: MedlinePlus Medical Encyclopedia [Internet]. medlineplus.gov. Available from: https://medlineplus.gov/ency/article/007293.htm.
51. Karpiński T. Selected medicines used in iontophoresis. Pharmaceutics. 2018;10(4):204.
52. Cuccurullo S, Lee J. Physical medicine and rehabilitation board review. New York: Demos Medical; 2015.
53. Management of carpal tunnel syndrome evidence-based clinical practice guideline [Internet]. 2016. Available from: https://www.aaos.org/globalassets/quality-and-practice-resources/carpal-tunnel/cts_cpg_4-25-19.pdf.
54. Sheikh NK, Dua A. Iontophoresis analgesic medications [Internet]. PubMed. Treasure Island (FL): StatPearls Publishing; 2021. Available from: https://www.ncbi.nlm.nih.gov/books/NBK553090/.
55. Affairs O of R. Diathermy. FDA [Internet]. 2018. Available from: https://www.fda.gov/inspections-compliance-enforcement-and-criminal-investigations/inspection-guides/diathermy.
56. Haar G. Therapeutic applications of ultrasound. Prog Biophys Mol Biol. 2007;93(1–3):111–29.
57. French SD, Cameron M, Walker BF, Reggars JW, Esterman AJ. Superficial heat or cold for low back pain. Cochrane Database Syst Rev. 2006;(1):Art. No.: CD004750. https://doi.org/10.1002/14651858.CD004750.pub2. Accessed 5 Feb 2023.
58. Paladini LH, Almeida N, Korelo RIG, Macedo RMD, Guarita-Souza LC, Zotz TGG, et al. Short-wave diathermy in patients with chronic low back pain: a systematic review. Coluna/Columna. 2020;19(3):218–22.
59. Ahmed MS, Shakoor MA, Khan AA. Evaluation of the effects of shortwave diathermy in patients with chronic low back pain. Bangladesh Med Res Counc Bull. 2009;35(1):18–20.
60. Kerem M, Yigiter K. Effects of continuous and pulsed short-wave diathermy in low back pain. Pain Clinic. 2002;14(1):55–9.
61. Rabini A, Piazzini DB, Tancredi G, Foti C, Milano G, Ronconi G, Specchia A, Ferrara PE, Maggi L, Amabile E, Galli M, Bernabei R, Bertolini C, Marzetti E. Deep heating therapy via microwave diathermy relieves pain and improves physical function in patients with knee osteoarthritis: a double-blind randomized clinical trial. Eur J Phys Rehabil Med. 2012;48(4):549–59. Epub 2012 Jul 23. PMID: 22820824.
62. Berteau JP. Knee pain from osteoarthritis: pathogenesis, risk factors, and recent evidence on physical therapy interventions. J Clin Med. 2022;11(12):3252. https://doi.org/10.3390/jcm11123252. PMID: 35743322; PMCID: PMC9224572.
63. Laufer Y, Dar G. Effectiveness of thermal and athermal short-wave diathermy for the management of knee osteoarthritis: a systematic review and meta-analysis. Osteoarthr Cartil. 2012;20(9):957–66. https://doi.org/10.1016/j.joca.2012.05.005. Epub 2012 May 30. PMID: 22659070.
64. Kolasinski SL, Neogi T, Hochberg MC, Oatis C, Guyatt G, Block J, et al. 2019 American College of Rheumatology/Arthritis Foundation guideline for the management of osteoarthritis of the hand, hip, and knee. Arthritis Rheumatol. 2020;72(2):220–33.
65. González-Gutiérrez MD, López-Garrido Á, Cortés-Pérez I, Obrero-Gaitán E, León-Morillas F, Ibáñez-Vera AJ. Effects of non-invasive radiofrequency diathermy in pelvic floor disorders: a systematic review. Medicina (Kaunas). 2022;58(3):437. https://doi.org/10.3390/medicina58030437. PMID: 35334613; PMCID: PMC8951766.
66. Batavia M. Contraindications for superficial heat and therapeutic ultrasound: do sources agree? 11 No commercial party having a direct financial interest in the results of the research supporting this article has or will confer a benefit on the author(s) or on any organization with which the author(s) is/are associated. Arch Phys Med Rehabil. 2004;85(6):1006–12.
67. Cotler HB, Chow RT, Hamblin MR, Carroll J. The use of low level laser therapy (LLLT) for musculoskeletal pain. MOJ Orthop Rheumatol. 2015;2(5):00068. https://doi.org/10.15406/mojor.2015.02.00068. Epub 2015 Jun 9. PMID: 26858986; PMCID: PMC4743666.
68. Kuan Y-C. Low-level laser therapy for fibromyalgia: a systematic review and meta-analysis. Pain Physician. 2019;22(3):241–54.

69. Navratil L, Kymplova J. Contraindications in noninvasive laser therapy: truth and fiction. J Clin Laser Med Surg. 2002;20(6):341–3.
70. https://www.cancer.gov/publications/dictionaries/cancer-terms/def/tens [Internet]. www.cancer.gov. 2011. Available from: https://www.cancer.gov/publications/dictionaries/cancer-terms/def/tens.
71. Cleveland Clinic. Transcutaneous electrical nerve stimulation (TENS) [Internet]. Cleveland Clinic. 2015. Available from: https://my.clevelandclinic.org/health/treatments/15840-transcutaneous-electrical-nerve-stimulation-tens.
72. Jones I, Johnson MI. Transcutaneous electrical nerve stimulation. Contin Educ Anaesth Crit Care Pain [Internet]. 2009 [cited 2019 Nov 15];9(4):130–5. Available from: https://pdfs.semanticscholar.org/e7b0/221ed65efb26cea2b2d44ad9d4fe19169e6d.pdf.
73. Sports medicine practitioners embrace benefits of extracorporeal shock wave therapy – Mayo Clinic [Internet]. www.mayoclinic.org. 2019. Available from: https://www.mayoclinic.org/medical-professionals/physical-medicine-rehabilitation/news/sports-medicine-practitioners-embrace-benefits-of-extracorporeal-shock-wave-therapy/mac-20454275.
74. Dedes V, Stergioulas A, Kipreos G, Dede AM, Mitseas A, Panoutsopoulos GI. Effectiveness and safety of shockwave therapy in tendinopathies. Mater Sociomed. 2018;30(2):131–46. https://doi.org/10.5455/msm.2018.30.141-146. PMID: 30061805; PMCID: PMC6029898.
75. Shockwave therapy | Boston Children's Hospital [Internet]. www.childrenshospital.org. Available from: https://www.childrenshospital.org/treatments/shockwave-therapy.
76. Mcclure S, Vansickle D, White R. Extracorporeal shock wave therapy: what is it? what does it do to equine bone? ESWT-What is It? [Internet]. [cited 2023 Feb 25]. Available from: https://www.ivis.org/sites/default/files/library/aaep/2000/197.pdf.
77. Chung B, Wiley JP. Extracorporeal shockwave therapy. Sports Med. 2002;32(13):851–65.
78. Paoletta M, Moretti A, Liguori S, Toro G, Gimigliano F, Iolascon G. Efficacy and effectiveness of extracorporeal shockwave therapy in patients with myofascial pain or fibromyalgia: a scoping review. Medicina. 2022;58(8):1014.
79. Overview | Extracorporeal shockwave therapy for refractory greater trochanteric pain syndrome | Guidance | NICE [Internet]. Nice.org.uk. NICE; 2011. Available from: https://www.nice.org.uk/Guidance/IPG376.
80. Overview | Extracorporeal shockwave therapy for refractory tennis elbow | Guidance | NICE [Internet]. www.nice.org.uk. [cited 2023 Feb 17]. Available from: https://www.nice.org.uk/guidance/ipg313.
81. Thiele S, Thiele R, Gerdesmeyer L. Lateral epicondylitis: this is still a main indication for extracorporeal shockwave therapy. Int J Surg. 2015;24:165–70.
82. Extracorporeal shockwave therapy for refractory Achilles tendinopathy | Guidance | NICE [Internet]. www.nice.org.uk. [cited 2023 Feb 17]. Available from: https://www.nice.org.uk/guidance/ipg312.
83. DIGEST Guidelines for extracorporeal shock wave therapy [Internet]. 2019. Available from: https://www.shockwavetherapy.org/fileadmin/user_upload/ISMST_Guidelines.pdf.
84. Schroeder AN, Tenforde AS, Jelsing EJ. Extracorporeal shockwave therapy in the management of sports medicine injuries. Curr Sports Med Rep [Internet]. 2021;20(6):298–305. Available from: https://pubmed.ncbi.nlm.nih.gov/34099607/.
85. Swenson C, Swärd L, Karlsson J. Cryotherapy in sports medicine [Internet]. Scand J Med Sci Sports. 1996. Available from: https://pubmed.ncbi.nlm.nih.gov/8896090/.
86. Lesson 59: applying a cold, dry compress [Internet]. Available from: https://www.in.gov/health/files/l59.pdf.
87. Management of glenohumeral joint osteoarthritis evidence-based clinical practice guideline [Internet]. 2020. Available from: https://www.aaos.org/globalassets/quality-and-practice-resources/glenohumeral/gjo-cpg.pdf.
88. Kroeling P, Gross A, Graham N, Burnie SJ, Szeto G, Goldsmith CH, Haines T, Forget M. Electrotherapy for neck pain. Cochrane Database Syst Rev. 2013;(8):Art. No.: CD004251. https://doi.org/10.1002/14651858.CD004251.pub5.

89. Macfarlane GJ, et al. A systematic review of evidence for the effectiveness of practitioner-based complementary and alternative therapies in the management of rheumatic diseases: osteoarthritis. Rheumatology (Oxford). 2012;51(12):2224–33. https://doi.org/10.1093/rheumatology/kes200.
90. Spinal manipulation: what you need to know [Internet]. NCCIH. Available from: https://www.nccih.nih.gov/health/spinal-manipulation-what-you-need-to-know.
91. NASS – maintenance [Internet]. maintenance.spine.org. Available from: https://www.spine.org/Portals/0/assets/downloads/ResearchClinicalCare/Guidelines/LumbarDiscHerniation.pdf.
92. Diagnosis and treatment of degenerative lumbar stenosis [Internet]. North American Spine Society. Available from: https://www.spine.org/Portals/0/Assets/Downloads/ResearchClinicalCare/Guidelines/LumbarStenosis.pdf.
93. Ernst E. Adverse effects of spinal manipulation: a systematic review. J R Soc Med [Internet]. 2007;100(7):330–8. Available from: https://www.ncbi.nlm.nih.gov/pmc/articles/PMC1905885/.
94. https://www.cancer.gov/publications/dictionaries/cancer-terms/def/physical-therapy [Internet]. www.cancer.gov. 2011. Available from: https://www.cancer.gov/publications/dictionaries/cancer-terms/def/physical-therapy.
95. American Physical Therapy Association. Becoming a physical therapist [Internet]. APTA. 2021. Available from: https://www.apta.org/your-career/careers-in-physical-therapy/becoming-a-pt.
96. Management of osteoarthritis of the Hip – American Academy of … [Internet]. Available from: https://www.aaos.org/globalassets/quality-and-practice-resources/osteoarthritis-of-the-hip/oa-hip-auc.pdf.
97. Management of rotator cuff injuries evidence-based clinical practice guideline [Internet]. Available from: https://www.aaos.org/globalassets/quality-and-practice-resources/rotator-cuff/rotator-cuff-cpg-final-12-20-19.pdf.
98. Antunes MD, Marques AP. The role of physiotherapy in fibromyalgia: current and future perspectives. Front Physiol. 2022;13:968292. https://doi.org/10.3389/fphys.2022.968292. PMID: 36051912; PMCID: PMC9424756.
99. Mann SJ, Lam JC, Singh P. McKenzie back exercises [Internet]. PubMed. Treasure Island (FL): StatPearls Publishing; 2020. Available from: https://www.ncbi.nlm.nih.gov/books/NBK539720/.
100. Wegner I, Widyahening IS, van Tulder MW, Blomberg SE, de Vet HC, Brønfort G, Bouter LM, van der Heijden GJ. Traction for low-back pain with or without sciatica. Cochrane Database Syst Rev. 2013;2013(8):CD003010. https://doi.org/10.1002/14651858.CD003010.pub5. PMID: 23959683; PMCID: PMC6823219.
101. https://www.cancer.gov/publications/dictionaries/cancer-terms/def/massage-therapy [Internet]. www.cancer.gov. 2011. Available from: https://www.cancer.gov/publications/dictionaries/cancer-terms/def/massage-therapy.
102. Blair S, Jacobs D. Physical activity, exercise, and physical fitness: definitions and distinctions for health-related research [Internet]. 1985. Available from: https://www.ncbi.nlm.nih.gov/pmc/articles/PMC1424733/pdf/pubhealthrep00100-0016.pdf.
103. Bidonde J, Busch AJ, Webber SC, Schachter CL, Danyliw A, Overend TJ, Richards RS, Rader T. Aquatic exercise training for fibromyalgia. Cochrane Database Syst Rev. 2014;(10):Art. No.: CD011336. https://doi.org/10.1002/14651858.CD011336.
104. American Heart Association. American Heart Association recommendations for physical activity in adults and kids [Internet]. www.heart.org. 2018. Available from: https://www.heart.org/en/healthy-living/fitness/fitness-basics/aha-recs-for-physical-activity-in-adults.
105. Elsawy B, Higgins KE. Physical activity guidelines for older adults. Am Fam Physician [Internet]. 2010;81(1):55–9. Available from: https://www.aafp.org/pubs/afp/issues/2010/0101/p55.html#:~:text=Absolute%20contraindications%20to%20aerobic%20exercise.

Musculoskeletal Pain: Evidence-Based Clinical Evaluation and Management

19

Orthotics

David George Wilson

Introduction

Orthotics is the field that specializes in the design and application of orthoses. Orthoses are the devices that are used to aid an existing but functionally limited part of the body. The orthotist is the practitioner that is an integral member of the healthcare team, and who will evaluate and treat the patient's orthotic needs. Typically, orthoses are named by describing the part of the body they support or the joint that they cross. For example, foot orthosis (FO), ankle foot orthosis (AFO), knee orthosis (KO), lumbosacral orthosis (LSO), thoracolumbosacral (TLSO), etc. Each orthosis can be fabricated from a variety of materials, with some of the most common being thermoplastics, metals, composites, and foams.

When treating a patient with an orthosis, there are three main goals for each device: to control motion, to control deformity, and to control pain. For any one patient, these goals may be singular, or they may be combined or interconnected. Motion, or the position of a specific joint, can be controlled by stopping motion, resisting motion, or assisting motion. When controlling deformity, the orthosis can accommodate, resist, or correct the deformity. Accommodating the deformity will result in slowing the progression of the deformity; resisting will prevent the development or progression; and correcting will decrease or correct the existing deformity. Pain is typically controlled by limiting or stopping motion. Additionally, pain can also be controlled by reducing stress through a joint through support or shock-absorbing cushion.

In order to achieve these goals, orthoses work through three-point force systems (Fig. 19.1). The three-point force system works by applying a system of forces in the same plane that creates balanced moments about a joint to resist the angular

D. G. Wilson (✉)
The University of Texas Southwestern Medical Center, Dallas, TX, USA
e-mail: david.wilson2@utsouthwestern.edu

C. E. Noe (ed.), *Musculoskeletal Pain*,
https://doi.org/10.1007/978-3-031-86057-7_19

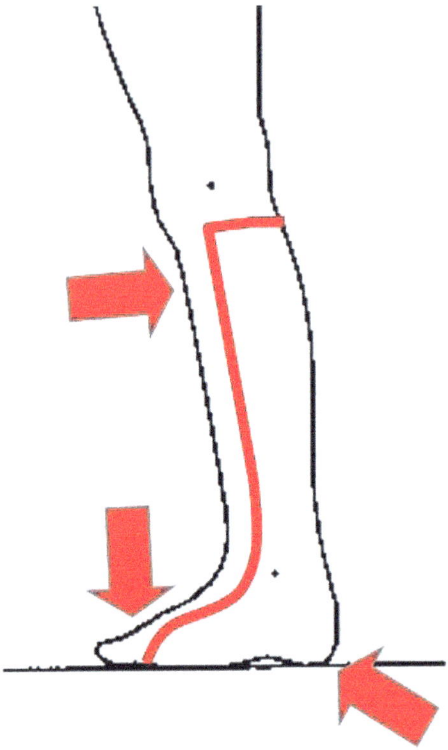

Fig. 19.1 Three-point force system example to prevent dorsiflexion

motion. Two of the forces create similar moments about the joint, while the third force provides an equal and opposite moment about the joint, to create a system in equilibrium. It is common to have multiple three-point force systems working in varying planes, as well as, overlapping across joints and the orthosis.

When evaluating a patient for an orthosis, it is important to identify what the goal of the orthosis will be. Assessing the patient's overall range of motion, range of motion limitations due to pain, manual muscle testing, gait, and posture will all contribute to making an appropriate prescription recommendation. Each component of the evaluation will provide insight into the overall goal of the orthosis: controlling motion, deformity, or pain. Ultimately, the patient's presentation should guide the prescription recommendation compared to their pathology alone.

- Orthotists specialize in designing and applying orthoses, devices used to aid a functionally limited part of the body.
- Orthoses are named by the part of the body or joint they support and can be made from various materials, including thermoplastics, metals, composites, and foams.
- The main goals of orthoses are to control motion, deformity, and pain, achieved through three-point force systems.

Foot Orthoses

Foot orthoses (FOs) are a common prescription recommendation for many musculoskeletal pain issues. With the foot being the foundation on which the rest of the body is connected to the ground, FOs have the potential to have a wide impact on pain up the kinetic chain of the body. This may include foot and ankle pain, knee pain, and back pain. An over-the-counter/off-the-shelf foot orthosis has the potential to be a cost-effective and simple conservative management option. When these devices are insufficient to control the patient's pain, a custom foot orthosis may be indicated. Custom foot orthoses can be characterized as accommodative, semi-rigid, or rigid in design. They typically consist of two to three layers of material of varying lengths and densities. When the patient presents with a flexible deformity, they will often tolerate partial to full correction of the deformity with a semi-rigid or rigid FO. Conversely, a rigid or fixed deformity should be treated with an accommodative design.

An accommodative FO is typically fabricated with three layers of material with the goal of the orthosis being to accommodate the natural foot position, reduce high points of pressure, and provide a soft interface for the plantar surface. The base layer of the orthosis is fabricated from a denser material (i.e., Pelite) with a middle layer of a shock-absorbing foam (i.e., PORON/PPT), and finally a top layer that provides pressure distribution (i.e., Plastazote/P-Cell). The combination of these materials allows the arches of the foot to be supported by the base layer and prevent a further progression of the deformity while reducing pain by supporting the foot and redistributing pressures across the entire plantar surface in combination with the top layer. The middle, shock-absorbing layer, will assist in reducing pain by decreasing stresses placed through the foot and joints.

Semi-rigid foot orthoses (Fig. 19.2) are similar in design to an accommodative foot orthosis but are typically constructed from denser materials, with a more significant goal to provide a corrective force to the foot. This corrective force can be accomplished by holding the foot in a corrected position during impression-taking, model modifications, or external wedges/additions. The firmer materials will be able to impart a greater force to the foot without being compressed by bodyweight. The semi-rigid FO will also have the goal of distributing pressure evenly across the plantar surface and supporting the arches of the foot.

A rigid foot orthosis is typically constructed from a thermoplastic or thermoset material that is very rigid and has reduced soft interfaces. These can be beneficial for high-activity individuals when maximum support and corrective forces are required, or when the shoe wear limits the thickness of the orthosis. The rigid foot

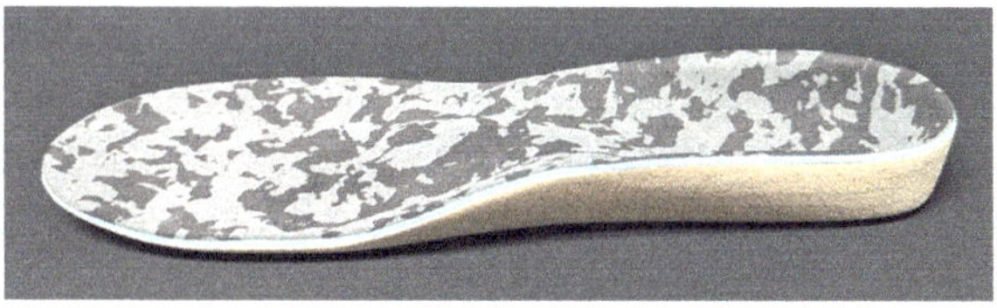

Fig. 19.2 Semi-rigid foot orthosis

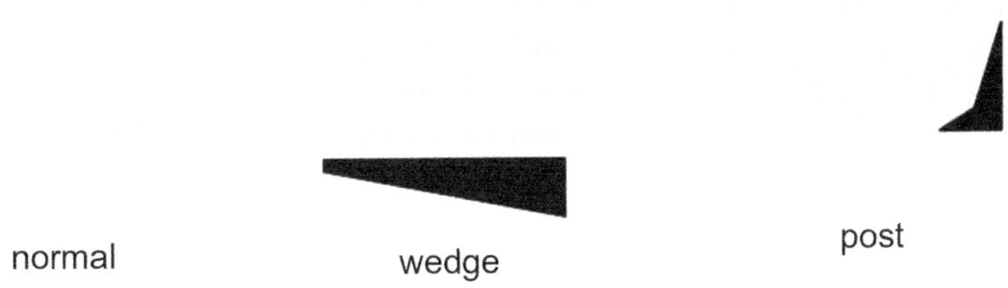

Fig. 19.3 Example of wedge vs post

orthosis is able to provide the maximum corrective control due to the material properties of the orthosis.

When applying a corrective force through the foot orthosis, this moment can be augmented by using wedges and posts (Fig. 19.3). A wedge or post is able to redirect the ground reaction forces. A wedge produces an angular change during weight bearing that impacts the subtalar joint. The wedge can be medial or lateral, depending on the change in ground reaction forces desired. A post will increase the surface area and stabilize the subtalar joint during weight bearing. These modifications can be applied to the full length of the FO, or isolated to the hindfoot or midfoot.

As foot orthoses have the potential to impact a wide array of underlying pathologies and pain, it is important to evaluate each patient as an individual. When isolating pain in the foot, evidence shows that FOs can be of benefit to patients in reducing their pain and increasing their function [1–3]. Custom foot orthoses are effective for painful pes cavus, rearfoot pain in rheumatoid arthritis, juvenile idiopathic arthritis, and hallux valgus [1]. Some of these benefits in rheumatoid arthritis can be attributed to the alterations in the ankle joint moments [2]. Perhaps, one of the most common painful foot pathologies where FOs are prescribed is for pes planus. Evidence supporting this intervention is varied and not clearly defined. There is some evidence that FOs do improve pain in patients with pes planus [4, 5].

When continuing up the kinetic chain, there exists a connection between a pes planus foot deformity and medial tibiofemoral knee osteoarthritis (OA) [6]. Additionally, there have been multiple studies to assess the impact of a lateral wedge or laterally wedged FO on the reduction of medial knee OA [6–8]. There is evidence to suggest a decrease in knee pain, but consideration for changes at the ankle joint should be considered and also balanced.

Foot orthoses are often prescribed for back pain and again there exists some limited, but positive evidence to show that FOs reduce back pain [4, 9, 10]. When evaluating for a leg length discrepancy and associated back pain, evidence reports decreased back pain when correcting the leg length discrepancy in the orthosis [11–13].

- Foot orthoses are a common prescription recommendation to reduce foot, ankle, knee, and back pain.
- Custom foot orthoses are typically characterized as accommodative, semi-rigid, and rigid designs.
- Additional corrective forces can be applied through wedges and posts to redirect the ground reaction force.

Ankle Foot Orthoses

Ankle foot orthoses (AFOs) are orthoses that begin distal to the malleoli and extend proximal to the malleoli but distal to the knee. These orthoses can be provided as custom fit or custom fabricated. Custom-fit orthoses are prefabricated and have limited adjustability options by the orthotist. They usually have limited sizing and are typically designed to provide limited control in a single plane. Custom-fabricated AFOs are fabricated from an impression of the patient's foot and leg. This allows for greater customization and fabrication options to meet the biomechanical needs of the patient. The overall height and length may vary between orthoses. In general, the longer the footplate and the taller the calf section, the more lever arm is available to control and distribute pressures.

AFOs can be fabricated from a wide variety of materials and are characterized as conventional, thermoplastic, composite, or hybrid orthoses. Conventional AFOs are fabricated with metal and leather and are attached to the outside of a patient's shoe. Thermoplastic AFOs are fabricated from thermoplastics such as polypropylene or copolymer (Fig. 19.4). Composite AFOs use thermoset composites, such as carbon fiber and fiberglass. These designs fit inside of a patient's shoe. Hybrid designs (Fig. 19.5) are a convergence of the conventional and thermoplastic or composite designs, with the ability to fit the orthosis in the patient's shoe.

By going proximal and distal to the ankle, AFOs have an extended lever arm and a three-point force system. This contributes to their ability to better control moments about the ankle. A conventional AFO has limited contact with the skin and leg, thus its ability to control moments in multiple planes is limited. Additional straps can be added to impart corrective forces at the ankle, but these may be incomplete. A thermoplastic AFO has increased surface area and contact with the leg and is able to provide increased corrective forces and better pressure distribution. When looking to maximize the corrective and tolerable forces, a thermoplastic AFO would be indicated. Composite AFOs can be designed similarly to thermoplastic AFOs and

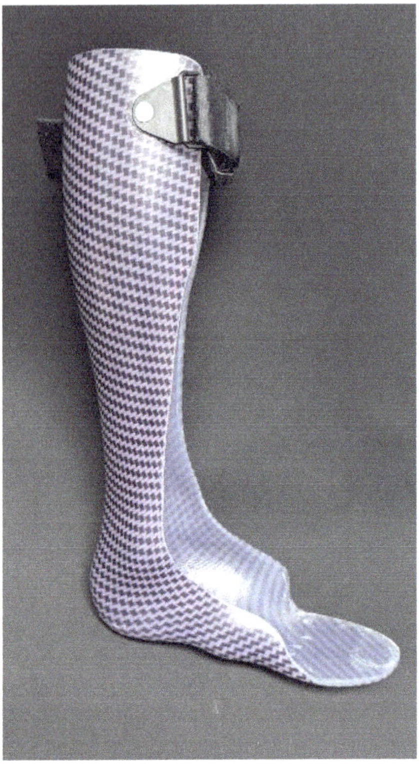

Fig. 19.4 Thermoplastic solid AFO

have increased surface area to provide control. However, due to their improved material properties, they can also provide increased rigidity in a lightweight design. They also have the potential to provide passive dynamics and energy return.

By crossing the ankle joint, AFOs are able to better control pain associated with pathologies of the ankle. Orthopedic issues can be stabilized, and abnormal joint and ligament movement can be reduced to control pain. To stabilize and prevent motion, the AFO must be fabricated from a rigid material with little flexibility, such as polypropylene. The trimlines of the AFO should be anterior to the malleoli, in order to limit motion in the foot and ankle. Generally speaking, the thicker the plastic and the more anterior the trimlines, the more rigid the AFO will be. The creation of a more rigid AFO will ultimately reduce the range of motion of the patient's ankle, with many studies showing that the ankle range of motion can be significantly limited with an orthosis [14].

A common pathology that an ankle foot orthosis can be prescribed for is posterior tibial tendon dysfunction. When a nonoperative approach is decided upon, custom AFOs [15, 16] or custom ankle gauntlet style AFOs (Fig. 19.6) may be indicated. While casting for this style of AFO, the foot and ankle are held in a corrected position. Once fabricated, this style of AFO extends a few inches proximal to the malleoli and maintains the corrected position of the foot and ankle. This corrected position attempts to allow the posterior tibial tendon to rest and has been shown to be the most effective in Stage I or II disease [17].

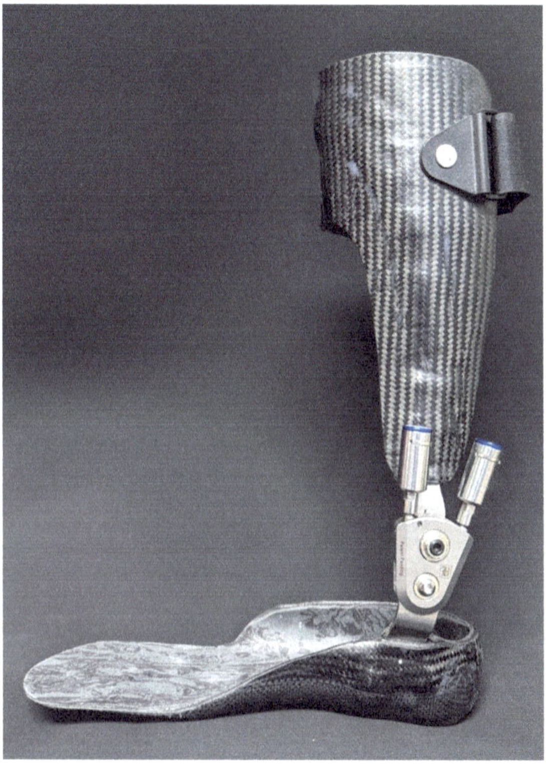

Fig. 19.5 Composite Hybrid AFO

With the greater use of composite materials and an understanding of their benefits, novel devices have been developed to improve function and reduce pain. A prime example of this is the intrepid dynamic exoskeletal orthosis (IDEO). The IDEO is a customized carbon fiber AFO that consists of a proximal patellar tendon bearing ground reaction cuff connected by carbon fiber posterior struts to a distal supramalleolar ankle foot orthosis [18]. It, along with a dedicated rehabilitation program, has been shown to decrease pain in service members with a wide range of diagnoses including lower extremity fractures, nerve and other soft tissue injuries, and post-traumatic or degenerative osteoarthritis [18]. This may be due to the proximal portion of the AFO having a patellar tendon bearing feature that allows enough off-loading of the lower leg to provide pain relief [18].

- Ankle foot orthoses can be fabricated from a wide range of materials and are categorized as conventional, thermoplastic, composite, or hybrid.
- Ankle foot orthoses have the advantage of longer lever arms to better control the lower extremity to reduce pain.
- Orthopedic dysfunctions respond well to AFOs in reducing pain.

Fig. 19.6 Ankle gauntlet AFO

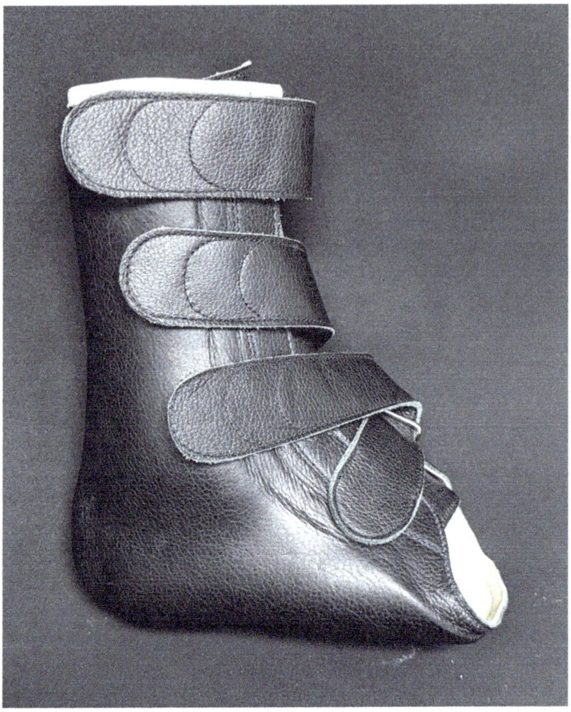

Knee Orthoses

Knee orthoses (KOs) come in a wide range of styles, designs, and materials, but all will extend proximal and distal to the knee joint in order to provide stability and control at the knee. These orthoses can be prefabricated, custom fit, or custom fabricated. They can be classified as support, prophylactic, or functional [19]. As prophylactic KOs are indicated to prevent injury, this section will focus on support and functional designs. Support KOs are knee sleeves that may or may not have the addition of knee joints. The addition of knee joints will provide additional medial–lateral and hyperextension stability. Due to support KOs being fabricated from fabrics and elastic materials, they provide a lower level of support when compared to functional designs. Functional KOs can have a single upright or double upright design and are fabricated from metal, composites, or rigid plastics in a frame design.

Most knee orthoses share the same difficulty of applying leverage through the soft tissue of the knee joint. This causes difficulty in controlling the skeletal anatomy, rotation, and distal orthosis migration. Because of these difficulties, it is important to properly diagnose and understand the cause of the underlying pain. In this manner, the appropriate style and design can be prescribed to achieve the best biomechanical control and effectively manage pain. For maximum effectiveness, KOs depend on proper placement on the leg and correct strap application.

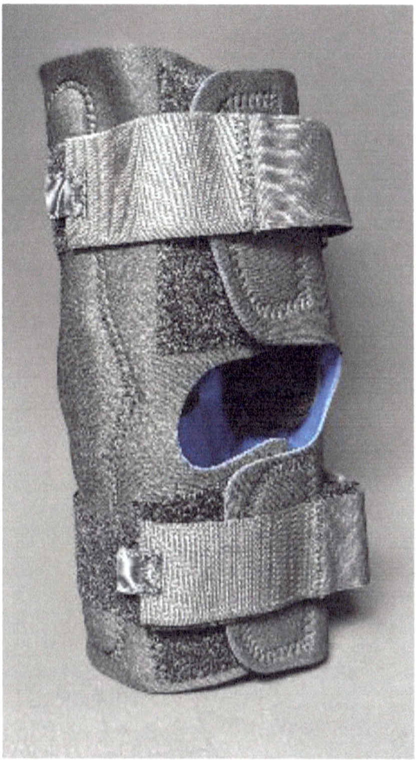

Fig. 19.7 Support knee orthosis

Support knee orthoses (Fig. 19.7), when used to treat anterior knee pain, are primarily designed to maintain patellar alignment. There is a lack of consensus in the literature on their efficacy due to an absence of well-controlled studies [20]. However, studies have shown their effectiveness and patients have reported subjective improvements in their pain [21].

Patients with unicompartmental knee osteoarthritis respond well to an unloader style knee orthosis [22]. The unloader style of knee orthosis (Fig. 19.8) is a functional design that maximizes the use of a three-point force system in the frontal plane to assist in better alignment of the knee joint. Most commonly, this is a valgus brace that is designed to reduce the load on the painful medial compartment by imparting a valgus moment at the knee and increasing the medial joint space [23].

- Knee orthoses can be classified as support or functional for the reduction of musculoskeletal pain.
- It can be difficult for knee orthoses to control the knee due to soft tissue, rotation, and orthosis migration.
- With a well-defined diagnosis, such as unicompartmental knee osteoarthritis, knee orthoses have been shown to reduce pain.

Fig. 19.8 Unloader KO

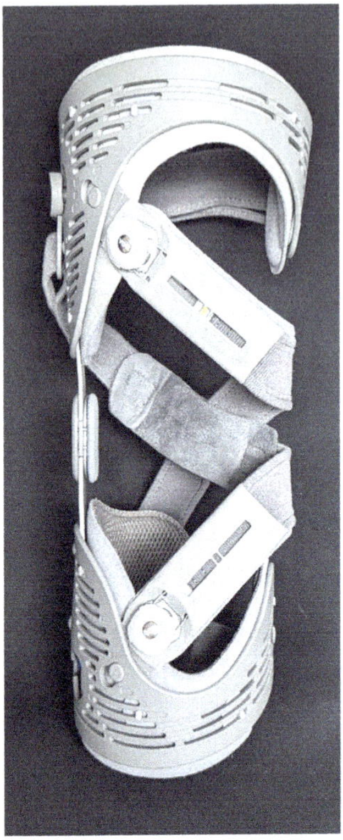

Spinal Orthoses

Spinal orthoses, like many of the orthoses previously discussed, come in a wide range of materials and varying designs to provide pain relief to different levels of the spine. Spinal orthoses use a common terminology to describe the spinal level they treat. The following list is not comprehensive and does not designate a particular orthosis; cervicothoracic lumbosacral orthosis (CTLSO), thoracolumbosacral orthosis (TLSO), and lumbosacral orthosis (LSO) (Fig. 19.9). Spinal orthoses are largely designed to impart biomechanical control to the spine, through three-point pressure systems, fluid compression, distraction, and as a kinesthetic reminder. Substantial difficulties exist in exerting complete control over the spine and axial musculature due to the significant soft tissue coverage surrounding the spinal column. Because of these difficulties, the impact of the kinesthetic reminder on the patient and their pain reduction is noteworthy.

Spinal orthoses also come in custom-fit and custom-fabricated designs. In both custom-fit and custom-fabricated spinal orthoses, the materials used can vary from flexible and elastic fabrics to rigid thermoplastic shells. Metal stays and compression straps are common additions to provide added support and allow for patient adjustability. There exists a large variety of custom-fit spinal orthoses available.

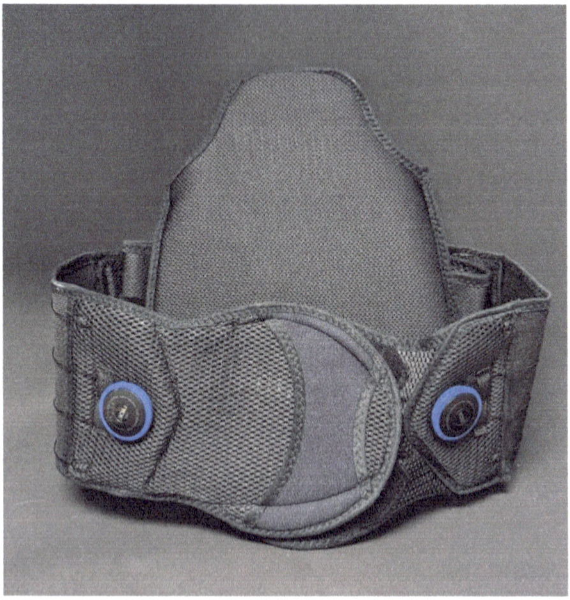

Fig. 19.9 Lumbosacral orthosis

Table 19.1 Guidelines for spinal orthosis control and orthosis type

Level	Control type	Orthosis
T6—L3	Minimum	TLSO corset
	Moderate	Conventional TLSO
		Hyperextension orthosis
	Maximum	Thermoplastic TLSO
L1—L3	Minimum	LSO corset
	Moderate	Conventional LSO
	Maximum	Thermoplastic LSO
L4—S1	Minimum	LSO corset
		Abdominal binder
	Moderate	Conventional LSO
		Thermoplastic LSO
		Conventional LSO w/hip spica
	Maximum	Thermoplastic LSO w/hip spica

Some general guidelines exist when determining the proper level and style of orthosis that is warranted based on the level of control desired (Table 19.1).

With low back pain being the leading cause of disability worldwide [24], it is critical to determine the level of injury and pain, as well as the underlying cause. For the reduction of muscle strain, spinal flexion is helpful, as it reduces spinal muscular activity. For the treatment of discogenic pathologies, spinal extension is indicated, as it shifts the axial load from the anterior disks to the posterior facet joints. The proper orthotic treatment and successful outcomes were shown when using Willner's instrument for spinal stabilization (WISS), an adjustable LSO [25].

Studies have also shown that more rigid and restrictive LSOs were more effective for low back pain, compared to elastic LSOs [26, 27]. Additional studies have shown a corset style LSO significantly improved patients' nonspecific acute low back pain [28]. The literature does not fully support the use of orthoses for low back pain, primarily due to inconsistencies in the cause of pain and the orthosis design. In literature with specific pain causes and orthosis design, there was a positive effect of using a spinal orthosis [29].

- Spinal orthoses use three-point pressure systems, fluid compression, and distraction, and are a kinesthetic reminder.
- Discogenic pathologies can be treated by placing the patient in increased spinal extension, while muscular strain is best treated with spinal flexion.
- For low back pain, with specific pain causes, orthoses can reduce pain.

Summary

- Orthoses have the goals of controlling motion, deformity, and pain.
- Orthoses achieve these goals through the use of multiple three-point force systems and material properties.
- Literature has shown that orthoses can be beneficial in reducing musculoskeletal pain.
- Orthoses should treat the biomechanical deficit and prescriptions should be individualized for each patient.

References

1. Hawke F, et al. Custom foot orthoses for the treatment of foot pain: a systematic review. J Foot Ankle Res. 2008;1(S1):O46.
2. Simonsen MB, et al. The effect of foot orthoses on gait biomechanics and pain among people with rheumatoid arthritis: a quasi-experimental study. Gait Posture. 2022;95:121–8.
3. Castro-Mendez A, Munuera PV, Albornoz-Cabello M. The short-term effect of custom-made foot orthoses in subjects with excessive foot pronation and lower back pain: a randomized, double-blinded, clinical trial. Prosthetics Orthot Int. 2013;37(5):384–90.
4. Castro-Mendez A, et al. Custom-made foot orthoses as non-specific chronic low back pain and pronated foot treatment. Int J Environ Res Public Health. 2021;18(13):6816.
5. Banwell HA, Mackintosh S, Thewlis D. Foot orthoses for adults with flexible pes planus: a systematic review. J Foot Ankle Res. 2014;7(1):23.
6. Hunt MA, et al. Lateral wedges with and without custom arch support for people with medial knee osteoarthritis and pronated feet: an exploratory randomized crossover study. J Foot Ankle Res. 2017;10:20.
7. Yeh H-C, et al. Immediate efficacy of laterally wedged insoles with arch support on walking in persons with bilateral medial knee osteoarthritis. Arch Phys Med Rehabil. 2014;95(12):2420–7.

8. Baert IA, et al. The effect of lateral wedge insoles in patients with medial compartment knee osteoarthritis: balancing biomechanics with pain neuroscience. Clin Rheumatol. 2014;33(11):1529–38.
9. Cambron JA, et al. Shoe orthotics for the treatment of chronic low back pain: a randomized controlled pilot study. J Manip Physiol Ther. 2011;34(4):254–60.
10. Dananberg HJ, Guiliano M. Chronic low-back pain and its response to custom-made foot orthoses. J Am Podiatr Med Assoc. 1999;89(3):109–17.
11. D'Amico M, Kinel E, Roncoletta P. Leg length discrepancy and nonspecific low Back pain: 3-D Stereophotogrammetric quantitative posture evaluation confirms positive effects of customized heel-lift orthotics. Front Bioeng Biotechnol. 2021;9:743132.
12. Menez C, L'Hermette M, Coquart J. Orthotic insoles improve gait symmetry and reduce immediate pain in subjects with mild leg length discrepancy. Front Sports Act Living. 2020;2:579152.
13. Rannisto S, et al. Correction of leg-length discrepancy among meat cutters with low back pain: a randomized controlled trial. BMC Musculoskelet Disord. 2019;20(1):105.
14. Hume PA, Gerrard DF. Effectiveness of external ankle support. Bracing and taping in rugby union. Sports Med. 1998;25(5):285–312.
15. Chao W, et al. Nonoperative management of posterior tibial tendon dysfunction. Foot Ankle Int. 1996;17(12):736–41.
16. Wapner KL, Chao W. Nonoperative treatment of posterior tibial tendon dysfunction. Clin Orthop Relat Res. 1999;365:39–45.
17. Augustin JF, et al. Nonoperative treatment of adult acquired flat foot with the Arizona brace. Foot Ankle Clin. 2003;8(3):491–502.
18. Bedigrew KM, et al. Can an integrated orthotic and rehabilitation program decrease pain and improve function after lower extremity trauma? Clin Orthop Relat Res. 2014;472(10):3017–25.
19. Fox JR, Lovegreen W. 22 – lower limb orthoses. In: Webster JB, Murphy DP, editors. Atlas of orthoses and assistive devices. 5th ed. Philadelphia: Elsevier; 2019. p. 239–246.e1.
20. Smith TO, et al. Knee orthoses for treating patellofemoral pain syndrome. Cochrane Database Syst Rev. 2015;2015(12):CD010513.
21. Paluska SA, McKeag DB. Knee braces: current evidence and clinical recommendations for their use. (0002-838X (Print)).
22. Mistry D, Chandratreya A, Lee P. An update on unloading knee braces in the treatment of unicompartmental knee osteoarthritis from the last 10 years: a literature review. Surg J. 2018;04(03):e110–8.
23. Raja K, Dewan N. Efficacy of knee braces and foot orthoses in conservative management of knee osteoarthritis: a systematic review. Am J Phys Med Rehabil. 2011;90(3):247–62.
24. Hartvigsen J, et al. What low back pain is and why we need to pay attention. Lancet. 2018;391(10137):2356–67.
25. Willner SW. Test instrument for predicting the effect of rigid braces in cases with low back pain. Prosthetics Orthot Int. 1990;14(1):22–6.
26. Morrisette DC, et al. A randomized clinical trial comparing extensible and inextensible lumbosacral orthoses and standard care alone in the management of lower back pain. Spine. 2014;39(21):1733–42.
27. Schott C, et al. Effectiveness of lumbar orthoses in low back pain: review of the literature and our results. Orthop Rev. 2018;10(4):7791.
28. Mwenda AS, et al. Lumbosacral corsets improve the outcome of patients with non-specific acute low back pain. Ann African Surg. 2017;14(1):33–7.
29. Landauer F, Trieb K. An indication-based concept for stepwise spinal orthosis in low back pain according to the current literature. J Clin Med. 2022;11(3):510.

Pharmacology and Opioid Minimization 20

Ivan Chew and Brianna Alvarado

Musculoskeletal pain is one of the most common concerns and chief complaints of patients worldwide. Chronic pain can affect every patient demographic and can have detrimental effects on quality of life, mental health, and functional capacity. It can be a very challenging condition. It is recognized that exercise, physical therapy, and stretching are vital in reducing musculoskeletal pain; however, pharmacological intervention may often be required. Musculoskeletal pain is primarily somatic and nociceptive in nature, but can often include neuropathic pain components. This chapter covers various pharmacological options for treating musculoskeletal pain, often as part of a multimodal, multidisciplinary approach to pain management.

Simple Analgesics

Acetaminophen has been used for pain relief across a wide range of indications because of its relative effectiveness in many pain conditions, high tolerability, and minimal adverse effects [1]. The exact mechanism of action is uncertain although it is thought to act predominantly on the central nervous system and have an effect on prostaglandin synthesis [2]. This produces an analgesic and antipyretic effect but does not reduce inflammation [3]. Acetaminophen may also act through cannabinoid systems [4].

Monitoring for hepatotoxicity is recommended for patients who receive acetaminophen on a regular basis and beyond the maximum dosage of 3 g daily. Acetaminophen is metabolized by the hepatic system with contraindications in the setting of severe active liver disease and/or impairment [5].

I. Chew · B. Alvarado (✉)
UT Southwestern Medical Center, Dallas, TX, USA
e-mail: ivan.chew@utsouthwestern.edu; Brianna.Alvarado@utsouthwestern.edu

C. E. Noe (ed.), *Musculoskeletal Pain*,
https://doi.org/10.1007/978-3-031-86057-7_20

While acetaminophen is not an effective sole analgesic for many patients, acetaminophen is an excellent coanalgesic with nonsteroidal anti-inflammatory drugs (NSAIDs) and opioids for acute pain [6].

Nonsteroidal anti-inflammatory drugs (NSAIDs) are indicated for nonspecific musculoskeletal pain and osteoarthritis [7]. The mechanism of action is focused on inhibition of COX which impairs the production of prostaglandin, prostacyclin, and thromboxane. Unlike acetaminophen, NSAIDs do provide anti-inflammatory and analgesic effects [8]. Contraindications include peptic ulcer disease or prior GI bleeding. Due to renal excretion, NSAIDs should also be avoided in glomerular disease, renal insufficiency, and hypercalcemia [9]. Prolonged use of NSAIDs is also associated with other adverse effects, including inhibition of platelet function as well as bronchospasm, following the administration of aspirin and other NSAIDs in some patients with asthma.

COX-2 selective inhibitors such as Celebrex are similar to NSAIDs in their impairment of cyclooxygenase. This again results in anti-inflammatory and analgesic effects [8]. COX-2 is constitutively expressed in the brain, kidneys, bone, and female reproductive system while COX-1 is expressed in most tissues. COX-2 selective inhibitors are reported to have fewer GI effects than NSAIDs, making peptic ulcer disease and prior GI bleeding less of a contraindication [10]. Selective COX-2 inhibitors do not affect platelet TXA_2 production and therefore do not directly impair platelet aggregation. Of note, long-term use of COX-2 inhibitors may be associated with an increased risk of cardiovascular side effects.

NSAIDs should be used in the lowest effective doses and, as with opioids, discontinued if clear benefit is not demonstrated [11].

NSAIDs may be more effective analgesics than opioids for many pain conditions including cancer pain [12].

Ketoprofen is a potent predominantly COX -1 NSAID and diclofenac is a potent predominantly COX -2 NSAID [13].

Gabapentinoids

Gabapentinoids were developed as antiseizure agents and act as inhibitors of voltage-gated calcium channels, which inhibit the release of excitatory neurotransmitters [14, 15]. Because of their ability to suppress neuronal excitability, they have been also used for pain [14]. *Gabapentin* and *pregabalin* bind to the voltage-gated calcium channels at the alpha 2-delta subunit in the central nervous system. Gabapentin is first-line and indicated for neuropathic pain conditions [16]. *Pregabalin* is similar to gabapentin in that it binds to voltage-gated calcium channels to decrease calcium influx and the release of excitatory neurotransmitters [17]. Common side effects are somnolence, dizziness, peripheral edema, and gait disturbance. Both drugs are excreted renally, with elimination half-lives of approximately 6 hours, and should be used with caution in patients with renal impairment or renal failure. The medications can accumulate with decreased renal function and dosage adjustments are recommended.

Gabapentin is FDA approved for postherpetic neuralgia (PHN), while pregabalin is FDA approved for fibromyalgia, diabetic neuropathy, postherpetic neuralgia, and spinal cord injury pain. The data for gabapentinoids in the treatment of musculoskeletal pain problems, other than fibromyalgia, is limited.

Antidepressants

While *tricyclic antidepressants (TCAs)* and *serotonin and norepinephrine reuptake inhibitors* (SNRIs) are traditionally used to treat depression, they have been shown to have analgesic effects and impact on pain. TCAs are indicated for chronic pain, especially neuropathic pain. TCAs work by blocking the reuptake of serotonin and norepinephrine which inhibits calcium channel release via alpha cholinergic inhibition. This reduces excitatory neurotransmission. Adverse effects are dose-related and include anticholinergic effects and cardiac effects such as conduction prolongation. Contraindications include QT prolongation, family or personal history of sudden cardiac death, concurrent monoamine oxidase inhibitor use, and selective serotonin reuptake inhibitors (SSRI) use. Similarly, SNRIs are also used for neuropathic pain, specifically fibromyalgia and diabetic neuropathy [18, 19]. They function similar to TCAs in that they block the reuptake of serotonin and norepinephrine [20]. The most common side effects include nausea, dry mouth, insomnia, drowsiness, constipation, fatigue, and dizziness. Serotonin syndrome is a serious drug reaction that can be caused by these medications as a result of a buildup of high levels of serotonin in the body. Signs and symptoms of serotonin syndrome include agitation or restlessness, confusion, muscle rigidity, rapid heart rate, and high blood pressure.

Duloxetine is FDA approved for chronic musculoskeletal pain, diabetic neuropathy, and fibromyalgia. These indications plus the lack of nephrotoxicity exhibited by NSAIDs and the lack of addiction potential associated with opioids, make duloxetine an attractive first-line drug for chronic musculoskeletal pain.

Musculoskeletal Agents

Baclofen is used as a skeletal muscle relaxant as well as used in the treatment of spasticity. It works by agonizing gamma-aminobutyric acid (GABA) which leads to skeletal muscle relaxation [21].

Tizanidine is indicated for neuropathic pain and myofascial pain [22]. Tizanidine functions by agonizing central a-2 adrenergic receptors, which inhibits presynaptic transmission and spasticity [23]. Contraindications include hepatic and renal impairment [24].

Cyclobenzaprine is indicated for back pain and myofascial pain [25, 26]. The mechanism of action is focused on the antagonism of the 5HT2 receptor on the brainstem, which results in decreased spasticity. Contraindications for cyclobenzaprine include hyperthyroidism, acute MI recovery, arrhythmias, heart failure, heart block, and MOAI administration within the last 14 days.

Topical Agents

Topical agents have several potential advantages over systemic drugs for pain. They can have more targeted delivery at the painful site of injury, lower initial rates of systemic absorption and thus fewer systemic effects, and lessen pill burden.

Topical *lidocaine* patches (4–5%) may be used for localized nociceptive and neuropathic pain. Lidocaine is a local anesthetic that works by binding to sodium channels. These are worn 12 h on and 12 h off. Few side effects have been reported however skin redness and irritation may occur.

Diclofenac gel and patches have become a popular option for patients. Diclofenac is indicated for osteoarthritis, specifically working best for knee and hand osteoarthritis [27, 28]. Studies also indicate that it may be effective in relieving neuropathic pain [29]. Diclofenac is considered an NSAID and thus functions by inhibiting COX enzymes [8]. Skin irritation can occur and may complicate dermatologic conditions [28].

Capsaicin is a topical agent that is FDA approved for the treatment of neuropathic pain conditions, such as peripheral diabetic neuropathy of the feet, and postherpetic neuralgia (PHN). It has also been used for osteoarthritis pain conditions [27]. Following application to the skin capsaicin causes enhanced sensitivity to noxious stimuli, followed by a period with reduced sensitivity [30]. Capsaicin worked by desensitizing nociceptor fibers by decreasing substance P. This causes a temporary loss of membrane potential that prevents nerve fiber transmission [31].

Opioids

Opioids refer to all substances (exogenous or endogenous) with morphine-like properties. Opioids produce analgesia by acting on central and peripheral mu, kappa, and delta opioid receptors to inhibit the transmission of pain signals and the perception of pain. These receptors are inhibitory through the closure of calcium channels and the opening of potassium channels, resulting in hyperpolarization and reduction of excitability [32]. Opioids can be classified based on their effects on the mu receptor and are often divided into pure agonists and agonist-antagonists. They can come in short and long-acting preparations and can be administered through a wide variety of routes with the most common routes of administration being oral or transdermal.

Opioid therapy for the treatment of musculoskeletal pain is controversial due to insufficient evidence of long-term efficacy and the risk of serious harm [33]. Opioids should be used when other potentially effective and safer therapies have not provided sufficient pain relief and pain is adversely affecting a patient's function and/or quality of life, and when the potential benefits of opioid therapy outweigh potential harms. When possible, opioids should be combined with non-opioid pharmacotherapy and non-pharmacological therapies as appropriate to achieve therapeutic goals with the lowest effective doses of all medications. If opioids are necessary, ongoing reassessment of the risks and benefits should continue as long as the patient is taking them [33].

Common side effects include constipation, nausea, vomiting, sedation, impaired psychomotor function, and urinary retention. Opioids are relatively contraindicated in individuals with a history of substance abuse, previous drug rehabilitation, and a history of untreated or uncontrolled major depression or anxiety.

Krebs reported better analgesia and similar function with non-opioid treatment of chronic musculoskeletal pain compared to opioids in one-year trial [34].

Whether or not opioids add benefit to non-opioid analgesics is an open question; however,

discontinuing opioids after long-term therapy does not seem to worsen pain [35, 36].

Buprenorphine may be a safer opioid to use compared to full opioid agonists [37].

Main Points

- Pharmacological treatment of musculoskeletal pain is an important part of a multimodal approach to pain. There are various classes of medications that have been shown to be helpful.
- Acetaminophen and NSAIDs are simple analgesics relatively effective for many pain conditions with high tolerability and minimal side effects.
- Gabapentinoids are anti-seizure medications that have the ability to suppress neuronal excitability and help with pain.
- Antidepressants such as tricyclic antidepressants and serotonin norepinephrine reuptake inhibitors have the ability to modulate pain and may be indicated in patients with mental health illnesses.
- Musculoskeletal agents are used for myofascial pain and spasticity. They may cause central nervous system (CNS) depression and have side effects such as drowsiness or dizziness.
- Opioids are medications with morphine-like properties. The evidence for the efficacy is controversial. Opioids should be used when other therapies have not provided sufficient relief. It is important to continually reassess the efficacy and side effects associated with opioids to avoid the risk of serious harm.

Evidence-based assessment for musculoskeletal pain before prescribing medication

1. Review the drug list for existing allergies
2. Review the drug list for potential interactions
3. History of renal disease
4. History of hepatic disease
5. History of GI distress, GI bleed, or peptic ulcer disease
6. History of cardiac disease and conduction abnormalities
7. History of substance abuse, untreated mental health disorder

Evidence-based medications for musculoskeletal pain
1. Non-opioid analgesics
   Acetaminophen
   NSAIDs
   Salicylates
2. Non-opioid adjuvants
   Gabapentinoids/anticonvulsants
   Muscle relaxants
   Antidepressants(TCAs, SNRIs)
3. Weak opioid analgesic + non-opioid analgesic + adjuvant
4. Strong opioid analgesic + non-opioid analgesic + adjuvant

References

1. da Costa BR, et al. Effectiveness of non-steroidal anti-inflammatory drugs for the treatment of pain in knee and hip osteoarthritis: a network meta-analysis. Lancet (London, England). 2017;390(10090):e21–33. https://doi.org/10.1016/S0140-6736(17)31744-0. https://link.springer.com/article/10.1007/s40122-021-00235-2#ref-CR41
2. Graham GG, et al. The modern pharmacology of paracetamol: therapeutic actions, mechanism of action, metabolism, toxicity and recent pharmacological findings. Inflammopharmacology. 2013;21(3):201–32. https://doi.org/10.1007/s10787-013-0172-x. https://pubmed.ncbi.nlm.nih.gov/23719833/
3. Chandrasekharan NV, Dai H, Roos KL, et al. COX-3, a cyclooxygenase-1 variant inhibited by acetaminophen and other analgesic/antipyretic drugs: cloning, structure, and expression. Proc Natl Acad Sci USA. 2002;99(21):13926–31. https://doi.org/10.1073/pnas.162468699. https://www.ncbi.nlm.nih.gov/books/NBK482369/
4. Klinger-Gratz PP, Ralvenius WT, Neumann E, Kato A, Nyilas R, Lele Z, Katona I, Zeilhofer HU. Acetaminophen relieves inflammatory pain through CB_1 Cannabinoid receptors in the rostral ventromedial medulla. J Neurosci. 2018;38(2):322–34. https://doi.org/10.1523/JNEUROSCI.1945-17.2017. Epub 2017 Nov 22. PMID: 29167401; PMCID: PMC6596108
5. Chandok N, Watt KDS. Pain management in the cirrhotic patient: the clinical challenge. Mayo Clin Proc. 2010;85(5):451–8. https://doi.org/10.4065/mcp.2009.0534. https://www-uptodate-com.foyer.swmed.edu/contents/acetaminophen-paracetamol-drug-information?search=acetaminophen&source=panel_search_result&selectedTitle=1~149&usage_type=panel&kp_tab=drug_general&display_rank=1#F129365
6. Derry CJ, Derry S, Moore RA. Single dose oral ibuprofen plus paracetamol (acetaminophen) for acute postoperative pain. Cochrane Database Syst Rev. 2013;6:CD010210. https://doi.org/10.1002/14651858.CD010210.pub2.
7. Practice Guidelines for Chronic Pain Management: An updated report by the American Society of Anesthesiologists Task Force on chronic pain management and the American Society of Regional Anesthesia and Pain Medicine. Anesthesiology. 2010;112:810–33. https://doi.org/10.1097/ALN.0b013e3181c43103. https://www.sign.ac.uk/assets/sign136.pdf; https://pubs.asahq.org/anesthesiology/article/112/4/810/10691/Practice-Guidelines-for-Chronic-Pain-ManagementAn
8. Vane J. Inhibition of prostaglandin synthesis as a mechanism of action for aspirin-like drugs. Nat New Biol. 1971;231:232–5. https://doi.org/10.1038/newbio231232a0.
9. Perazella MA, Tray K. Selective cyclooxygenase-2 inhibitors: a pattern of nephrotoxicity similar to traditional nonsteroidal anti-inflammatory drugs. Am J Med. 2001;111(1):64–7. https://doi.org/10.1016/s0002-9343(01)00757-4. https://www-uptodate-com.foyer.swmed.edu/contents/nonselective-nsaids-overview-of-adverse-effects?search=NSAID&source=search_result&selectedTitle=3~148&usage_type=default&display_rank=2#H4221767628

10. Hawkey CJ. COX-2 inhibitors. Lancet (London, England). 1999;353(9149):307–14. https://doi.org/10.1016/s0140-6736(98)12154-2. https://www-uptodate-com.foyer.swmed.edu/contents/nonselective-nsaids-overview-of-adverse-effects?search=NSAID&source=search_result&selectedTitle=3~148&usage_type=default&display_rank=2#H4221767628
11. Ho KY, Cardosa MS, Chaiamnuay S, Hidayat R, Ho HQT, Kamil O, Mokhtar SA, Nakata K, Navarra SV, Nguyen VH, Pinzon R, Tsuruoka S, Yim HB, Choy E. Practice advisory on the appropriate use of NSAIDs in primary care. J Pain Res. 2020;13:1925–39. https://doi.org/10.2147/JPR.S247781. PMID: 32821151; PMCID: PMC7422842
12. McNicol ED, Strassels S, Goudas L, Lau J, Carr DB. NSAIDS or paracetamol, alone or combined with opioids, for cancer pain. Cochrane Database Syst Rev. 2005;2:CD005180. https://doi.org/10.1002/14651858.CD005180.
13. Moore RA, Derry S, Aldington D, Wiffen PJ. Single dose oral analgesics for acute postoperative pain in adults – an overview of Cochrane reviews. Cochrane Database Syst Rev. 2015;9:CD008659. https://doi.org/10.1002/14651858.CD008659.pub3.
14. Chincholkar M. Gabapentinoids: pharmacokinetics, pharmacodynamics and considerations for clinical practice. Br J Pain. 2020;14(2):104–14. https://doi.org/10.1177/2049463720912496. https://www.ncbi.nlm.nih.gov/books/NBK493228/
15. Alles SRA, Cain SM, Snutch TP. Pregabalin as a pain therapeutic: beyond calcium channels. Front Cell Neurosci. 2020;14:83. https://doi.org/10.3389/fncel.2020.00083. PMID: 32351366; PMCID: PMC7174704
16. Viniol A, et al. Prescribing practice of pregabalin/gabapentin in pain therapy: an evaluation of German claim data. BMJ Open. 2019;9(3):e021535. https://doi.org/10.1136/bmjopen-2018-021535. https://www.ncbi.nlm.nih.gov/books/NBK493228/
17. Taylor CP, et al. Pharmacology and mechanism of action of pregabalin: the calcium channel alpha2-delta (alpha2-delta) subunit as a target for antiepileptic drug discovery. Epilepsy Res. 2007;73(2):137–50. https://doi.org/10.1016/j.eplepsyres.2006.09.008.
18. Goldenberg DL, Burckhardt C, Crofford L. Management of Fibromyalgia Syndrome. JAMA. 2004;292(19):2388–95. https://doi.org/10.1001/jama.292.19.2388. https://jamanetwork.com/journals/jama/article-abstract/199786
19. Kroenke K, et al. Pharmacotherapy of chronic pain: a synthesis of recommendations from systematic reviews. Gen Hosp Psychiatry. 2009;31(3):206–19. https://doi.org/10.1016/j.genhosppsych.2008.12.006. https://www.sciencedirect.com/science/article/pii/S0163834309000036?casa_token=Y9QtHvYkIp0AAAAA:y0qwx2Vb2vpICC5igZIqF-NA4E5P11XWlKWP4W1pWr8YlLWr6hg4CYrUDKG68ZD71dc9eSPQPXTA#bib86
20. Lu R-B, editor. Effects of antidepressants. InTech; 2012. https://books.google.com/books?hl=en&lr=&id=zOOZDwAAQBAJ&oi=fnd&pg=PA91&dq=snri+mode+of+action&ots=bQ4droKwF6&sig=A7n_K7q9rN8RD2xHRxXS-UNlLU4#v=onepage&q=snri%20mode%20of%20action&f=false
21. Witenko C, et al. Considerations for the appropriate use of skeletal muscle relaxants for the management of acute low back pain. P T. 2014;39(6):427–35. https://www.ncbi.nlm.nih.gov/pmc/articles/PMC4103716/
22. Berry H, Hutchinson DR. Tizanidine and ibuprofen in acute low-back pain: results of a double-blind multicentre study in general practice. J Int Med Res. 1988:83–91. https://doi.org/10.1177/030006058801600202. https://journals.sagepub.com/doi/abs/10.1177/030006058801600202
23. Malanga GA, et al. Tizanidine is effective in the treatment of myofascial pain syndrome. Pain Physician. 2002;5(4):422–32. https://www.researchgate.net/profile/Gerard-Malanga/publication/6900819_Tizanidine_is_effective_in_the_treatment_of_myofascial_pain_syndrome/links/00b7d52727d8b0800f000000/Tizanidine-is-effective-in-the-treatment-of-myofascial-pain-syndrome.pdf
24. Tizanidine. LiverTox: Clinical and Research Information on Drug-Induced Liver Injury, National Institute of Diabetes and Digestive and Kidney Diseases, 30 January 2017. https://www.ncbi.nlm.nih.gov/books/NBK519505/

25. Browning R, Jackson JL, O'Malley PG. Cyclobenzaprine and back pain: a meta-analysis. Arch Intern Med. 2001;161(13):1613–20. https://doi.org/10.1001/archinte.161.13.1613.
26. Leite FMG, Atallah ÁN, El Dib R, Grossmann E, Januzzi E, Andriolo RB, da Silva EMK. Cyclobenzaprine for the treatment of myofascial pain in adults. Cochrane Database Syst Rev. 2009;3:CD006830. https://doi.org/10.1002/14651858.CD006830.pub3. Accessed 20 June 2022. https://doi.org/10.1002/14651858.CD006830.pub3
27. Scottish Intercollegiate Guidelines Network (SIGN). Management of chronic pain. Edinburgh: SIGN; 2013, Revised 2019. (SIGN publication no. 136). https://www.sign.ac.uk/assets/sign136.pdf
28. Derry S, Moore RA, Rabbie R. Topical NSAIDs for chronic musculoskeletal pain in adults. Cochrane Database Syst Rev. 2012;9:CD007400. https://doi.org/10.1002/14651858.CD007400.pub2. Accessed 20 June 2022. https://www.cochranelibrary.com/cdsr/doi/10.1002/14651858.CD007400.pub2/full
29. Anand P, Bley K. Topical capsaicin for pain management: therapeutic potential and mechanisms of action of the new high-concentration capsaicin 8% patch. Br J Anaesth. 2011a;107(4):490–502. https://doi.org/10.1093/bja/aer260. https://www.ncbi.nlm.nih.gov/pmc/articles/PMC3169333/
30. Derry S, Moore RA. Topical capsaicin (low concentration) for chronic neuropathic pain in adults. Cochrane Database Syst Rev. 2012;12(9):CD010111. https://doi.org/10.1002/14651858.CD010111. PMID: 22972149; PMCID: PMC6540838
31. Anand P, Bley K. Topical capsaicin for pain management: therapeutic potential and mechanisms of action of the new high-concentration capsaicin 8% patch. Br J Anaesth. 2011b;107(4):490–502. https://doi.org/10.1093/bja/aer260. https://www.ncbi.nlm.nih.gov/pmc/articles/PMC3169333/
32. Bovill JG. Mechanisms of actions of opioids and non-steroidal anti-inflammatory drugs. Eur J Anaesthesiol Suppl. 1997;15:9–15. https://doi.org/10.1097/00003643-199705001-00003. PMID: 9202932
33. Dowell D, Haegerich TM, Chou R. CDC guideline for prescribing opioids for chronic pain – United States, 2016. MMWR Recomm Rep. 2016;65(1):1–49. https://doi.org/10.15585/mmwr.rr6501e1. Erratum in: MMWR Recomm Rep 2016;65(11):295. PMID: 26987082
34. Krebs EE, Gravely A, Nugent S, et al. Effect of opioid vs nonopioid medications on pain-related function in patients with chronic back pain or hip or knee osteoarthritis pain: the SPACE randomized clinical trial. JAMA. 2018;319(9):872–82. https://doi.org/10.1001/jama.2018.0899.
35. McPherson S, Lederhos Smith C, Dobscha SK, Morasco BJ, Demidenko MI, Meath THA, Lovejoy TI. Changes in pain intensity after discontinuation of long-term opioid therapy for chronic noncancer pain. Pain. 2018;159(10):2097–104. https://doi.org/10.1097/j.pain.0000000000001315. PMID: 29905648; PMCID: PMC6993952
36. Frank JW, Carey E, Nolan C, Hale A, Nugent S, Krebs EE. Association between opioid dose reduction against patients' wishes and change in pain severity. J Gen Intern Med. 2020;35(Suppl 3):910–7. https://doi.org/10.1007/s11606-020-06294-z.
37. VA/DoD Clinical Practice Guideline. Use of opioids in the Management of Chronic Pain Work Group. Washington, D.C.: U.S. Government Printing Office; 2022.

Procedural Therapy for Musculoskeletal Pain

21

Kevin Neal

The treatment of musculoskeletal pain is complex and multifaceted. Therapy includes not just interventional treatment but also lifestyle modification and strengthening including physical therapy, splinting, and medication management. For interventional pain specialists, injection therapy provides a treatment option to allow patients pain relief while they are making the underlying modifications necessary for long-term relief.

The first injectable therapy for musculoskeletal pain was likely the first intra-articular (IA) cortisol injection in 1948 [1]. Since that time, steroids have been the building block on which many other injection therapies have been built. Despite these advances, steroid injections remain a mainstay of procedural therapy for musculoskeletal pain. Inflammation remains the most common underlying etiology of musculoskeletal pain and having a procedural treatment with a strong anti-inflammatory mechanism of action is in-line with care paradigms. Despite its historic precedent of use, steroid injections have had mixed results in clinical efficacy. Recent studies have even called into question the effects of its long-term use as well as its contribution to disease progression within the joint.

In addition to the changing evidence around steroids, there has been increased interest in biological injectables as a treatment for musculoskeletal pain. Therapeutic time frames for many biological injectables are often longer. It is not uncommon for effects to take months for onset but with months to years of duration. There have been many barriers to improve access to nonsteroid injectables. Standardized formulas, improving evidence, and improved patient access may yield greater use for this category of treatment in the future.

The radiofrequency ablation of sensory nerves is another area that has gained increased attention in the last decade. Though this treatment modality has been

K. Neal (✉)
University of Texas Southwestern Medical Center, Dallas, TX, USA
e-mail: kevin.neal@utsouthwestern.edu

C. E. Noe (ed.), *Musculoskeletal Pain*,
https://doi.org/10.1007/978-3-031-86057-7_21

utilized for spine-related pain for many years, ablation of nerves innervating various peripheral joints is relatively new to the pain management algorithm.

After many years of limited changes in nonsurgical interventional treatment options, the advancements in injection/needle-based therapies are now providing many options for patients who do not qualify for or do not wish to have surgery for their musculoskeletal pain. Treatment options should always be discussed in the context of individual disease processes, prognosis, goals, expectations, and capabilities. Undoubtedly, the future of nonsurgical interventional therapy for musculoskeletal pain will bear little resemblance to the prior 70 years.

The focus of this chapter is on therapeutic choice and will outline the evidence behind the interventional therapies, most commonly in practice in the United States. Short introductions for each injectable will be provided, but specific procedural techniques will not be discussed. Side effect profile is a key determinant when choosing therapeutic options. Package insert should be reviewed for all therapeutics for a full list of side effects. Most studies focus on a single joint and the results have varied depending on which joint is being studied. The clinician's choice of therapy will vary depending on which joint they are treating. For this reason, this chapter will outline the options and evidence for therapeutics separately for each joint.

Injectates

Steroids

Steroids were first extracted from the adrenal cortex and injected as cortisone in 1948 for a patient with rheumatoid arthritis. This advancement, by Drs. Phillip Hench, Edward Kendall, and Tadeus Reichstein, was awarded the Nobel Prize for Physiology or Medicine in 1950. By 1958 six synthetic steroids were derived and intra-articular steroid injection therapy had gained increased popularity [1]. Since this time, steroid injections have continued to gain popularity for the treatment of musculoskeletal pain.

In pain management, steroid formulations are most often classified as particulate or non-particulate. Particulate steroids are those which, as the name suggests, have particles or particulate aggregates greater than the size of a red blood cell. The solubility of each particulate steroid medication is based on how it has been derived from its parent cortisone molecule. Non-particulate steroids do not have the ability to aggregate to that red blood cell size. This difference in size is relevant to a provider's steroid choice due to potential complications associated with particulate steroids. This topic will be covered in greater detail later in this chapter [2].

In addition to the particulate vs non-particulate classification, steroids are also classified as adrenal corticoids, glucocorticoids, or mineralocorticoids. Adrenal corticoids are not an injectable therapeutic for pain management and will not be covered here. Glucocorticoids traverse the target cell membranes, binding to the glucocorticoid receptors within the cytoplasm. The primary target cells for glucocorticoid steroids include T lymphocytes, neutrophils, basophils, eosinophils, fibroblasts, and macrophages [3]. The primary glucocorticoid synthesized in the human body is cortisol, with up to 5–10 mg/m^2 produced by the adrenal cortex each day. This is the equivalent of 20–30 mg of hydrocortisone or 5–7 mg of oral prednisone per day [4, 5].

Mineralocorticoids are a separate class of steroids and have a greater effect on renal physiology, fluid retention, and electrolyte homeostasis. Sodium resorption, potassium excretion, and water resorption are all affected by mineralocorticoid production. The primary natural mineralocorticoid steroid is aldosterone. Aldosterone also has effects on sweat glands, salivary glands, and the colon where sodium reabsorption subsequently increases water absorption. Cortisol, the primary glucocorticoid, does have weak mineralocorticoid activity as well [6].

The difference in efficacy of particulate versus non-particulate steroid injections has been studied extensively for multiple locations in the body. Though it was generally believed that particulate steroids provide reduced solubility and subsequently provide longer localized anti-inflammatory action, the scientific evidence has been mixed [7]. In fact, larger reviews have concluded there is no significant difference between these two classes. For epidurals, a 2017 systemic review of three cervical epidural steroid injection studies and six lumbar epidural steroid injection studies concluded there was no difference in pain reduction nor in functional outcome between particulate and non-particulate steroid use in the epidural space [8, 9]. When looking at peripheral joints, a double-blind randomized study of intra-articular knee injections came to a similar conclusion [10].

Without evidence for a significant difference in functional outcomes, the unique risks associated with particulate steroids are important to consider. Due to their size equal to or greater than a red blood cell, particulate steroids may have a reduced capacity to traverse arterioles and cause particulate aggregation. These have been theorized to lead to ischemic sequelae when incidentally injected intra-arterially [2]. Clinically, spinal infarcts have occurred in the setting of presumed intra-articular injection during attempted epidural injection with particulate steroids. No such complication has been documented in the literature for dexamethasone. Of the particulate steroids, methylprednisolone has the largest percentage of large particles followed by triamcinolone and then betamethasone [11].

Particulate and non-particulate steroids share many side effects. Though these are considered rare, they can be clinically significant when they do occur. The most common side effect is an elevation in blood glucose for 1 day after injection. For diabetic patients, preinjection glucose should be measured and counseled on postinjection glucose management. Brittle diabetics risk dangerously high glucose levels with just a single injection. In a 2020 study by Shin et al., patients with Hgb A1c <7% had an average increase of 47.6 mg/dL, whereas those with an A1c >7% increased their serum glucose by an average of 99.4 mg/dL for 1 day after steroid injection [12]. Average blood sugar returns to the preinjection range after that first day.

There are a number of soft tissue risks associated with steroid injection. Skin hypopigmentation occurs in 1.3–4% of patients due to melanocyte dysfunction. Soft tissue atrophy occurs in 1.5–40% of patients, primarily due to decreased collagen production along with reduced number and size of adipocytes [13]. Tendon rupture has been reported when steroids have been deposited directly into the tendon as opposed to around the tendon sheath. Osteomyelitis and necrotizing fasciitis have been reported but are considered very rare [14].

A commonly discussed concern with certain patient populations is long-term effects of steroids and their effects on bone health. In a retrospective study of 71 women receiving a steroid dose of less than 3 mg/kg triamcinolone per year via epidural steroid injection, bone density was shown to be lower in the steroid group compared to the nonsteroid treatment group [15]. It can take up to 1 year for bone mineral density to recover after epidural steroid injections cease [16]. High-risk populations for osteoporosis should be counseled on this risk and total yearly doses should be kept for all patients receiving regular steroid injections.

Systemic effects of steroids have been known for some time; however, there is recent evidence to suggest intra-articular steroid injections may affect long-term deleterious effects on joint health. In a 2017 retrospective study by McAlindon et al., regular intra-articular knee injections with triamcinolone led to a reduction in radiologic cartilage thickness at 2 years. Though this was radiologically evident, clinical significance is not clear as there was no difference in pain between groups [17].

Hyaluronic Acid

Hyaluronic acid is a large, high-molecular-weight polysaccharide that is naturally present in the extracellular matrix of connective tissue. With human aging, the concentration of hyaluronic acid, along with the size of individual hyaluronic acid molecules themselves, decreases in our joints. Subsequently, the viscosity of the synovial fluid also decreases, which can worsen degenerative osteoarthritis (OA). The mechanism of action of injected hyaluronic acid formulations is to provide a viscous supplementation to the joint. There is some evidence to suggest the presence of hyaluronic acid supplementation stimulates the production of natural hyaluronic acid as well as providing some anti-inflammatory and direct pain relief mechanisms [18]. The half-life of intra-articular hyaluronic acid supplementation is only between 17 h and 36 h; however, the secondary action of the injectate is felt to be the mechanism by which prolonged pain relief occurs [19]. In pain management, there are many forms of injectable hyaluronic acid available, including sodium hyaluronate, hylan polymers A and B, and hyaluronan.

Adverse events for intra-articular hyaluronic supplementations are rare. Pain, swelling, itching, and redness around the site of injection are possible. Increased pain after the procedure is also a potential side effect. Infection and hypersensitivity reactions are considered very rare [20]. Since there is no systemic activity, there are no known effects on other organ systems.

Platelet-Rich Plasma

Platelet-rich plasma (PRP) is obtained by removing a large volume of blood from the patient and centrifuging this until a small volume of plasma is obtained. This aliquot contains high concentrations of platelets, platelet-derived growth factors, transforming growth factor-β, vascular endothelial growth factor, epidermal growth factor, and adhesive proteins including fibrin, fibronectin, and vitronectin. From a volume of 20 cc of whole blood, the platelet-rich plasma comprises approximately 1–5 cc of this. PRP is utilized to treat many musculoskeletal pain generators. Mechanistically, the activation of the platelets and subsequent release of growth factors initiates the body's natural healing cascade. This creates a regenerative environment for normal tissue architecture to form [21]. There is no current standard method of preparation and no standard definition for what comprises platelet-rich plasma. Various centrifuge speeds and processing guidelines have been proposed for its preparation, but no consensus has been reached. One study demonstrated a difference in clinical response in patients based on the platelet count of the injected PRP. Injection responders had an average of 565 platelets/μL and nonresponders had a platelet concentration of 449 plt/μL [22].

Platelet-rich plasma can also be subdivided into leukocyte-rich and leukocyte-poor PRP. Leukocyte-rich PRP is defined as a leukocyte concentration greater than the baseline whole blood of the patient. Subsequently, leukocyte-poor PRP is defined by a leukocyte concentration equal to or less than the baseline whole blood [23]. Leukocyte involvement in PRP efficacy and side effects has been controversial. Leukocytes play various roles in the postinjection cascade, including both positive and negative effects. Leukocyte-rich PRP has been shown to have greater therapeutic outcomes, in some studies [23]. Despite these trends, there is no current consensus on the optimal composition of PRP injectate.

There have been very few adverse events described for PRP injection. Knee swelling after injection of PRP was greater in the leukocyte-rich PRP group versus the leukocyte-poor PRP group, though this was transient. Pain is also a reported side effect, which was higher in the leukocyte-rich PRP group [23]. There is no data available for the rate of intra-articular infection after PRP. Given the lack of systemic activity, there are no known effects on other organ systems.

Local Anesthetics

Local anesthetics were first discovered in the form of cocaine by Sigmund Freud. While utilizing the substance for psychological purposes, he incidentally discovered his mouth to have an insensate characteristic to it. He then encouraged his friend Karl Koller to explore its use in topical anesthesia for ocular surgery, which first occurred in 1884 [24]. Since then, many local anesthetics have been derived from this parent molecule.

Local anesthetics cause blockade of transmission of the neuronal action potential through inhibition of sodium ion channels. There are two major classes of local anesthetics, amides and esters. These are distinguished from one another by the character of the link present between the intermediate chain and the aromatic end. The injection of a local anesthetic around a nerve will cause paralysis of that nerve; however, local anesthetics have been utilized for muscular as well as intra-articular injection. Duration of action is dependent upon the local anesthetic chosen, with ropivacaine and bupivacaine being two of the most common long-acting local anesthetics utilized for musculoskeletal injections. Lidocaine remains the most common short-acting local anesthetic for this use. Though no clear mechanism has been elucidated, some patients appear to receive therapeutic benefits far beyond the anesthetic duration of action.

Local anesthetic side effects are significant, though not common. The side effect of the greatest consequence is local anesthetic systemic toxicity. This includes symptoms of a seizure, agitation, loss of consciousness, ECG alterations, and eventual cardiovascular collapse. Bupivacaine has a greater affinity for cardiac voltage-gated sodium channels compared to other local anesthetics (LAs) and is subsequently considered to have the highest cardiotoxic profile.

Bupivacaine, ropivacaine, and lidocaine have all been shown to be toxic to intra-articular cartilage, with continuous exposure through intra-articular infusions posing the greatest risk [25]. This is an independent risk with or without steroids in the solution. Mepivacaine was shown to have the least degree of toxicity when compared to bupivacaine and lidocaine. This effect appears to be dose-dependent [26, 27]. No cumulative toxic dose has been suggested, though intra-articular catheters are not recommended for postoperative pain control any longer.

Joint Specific Treatment

Large Joints

Knee

Indications and Contraindications

The most common indication for intra-articular (IA) knee injections is osteoarthritis (OA) of the joint. Of people older than 60, 10% of men and 13% of women will have symptomatic knee OA [28]. Given this high prevalence and significant burden to society, many procedures and therapies have been studied to provide pain control. In addition to osteoarthritis, rheumatoid arthritis, juvenile rheumatoid arthritis, and ligamental injury are all potential indications for interventional therapy.

Intra-articular infection, overlying infection, poor injection windows, and an allergy to injectate are all contraindications to IA injection. Edema is common in the various pathologies of the knee and is not, itself, a contraindication if it is not related to infection [29].

Evidence

Steroids

The knee is among the most frequently studied joints for injection-based pain relief. It was the first joint to be injected with steroids and IA steroids remain a leading first-line treatment regimen [1]. Interestingly, the initial studies of hydrocortisone indicated that intra-articular injections would only provide short-term relief (3 days to 3 weeks). More recent evidence continues to support the limited duration of relief for osteoarthritis, up to 1 week [30]. When compared to placebo, there is no difference between saline and steroid injections in long-term pain and function. For rheumatoid arthritis; however, evidence may suggest a prolonged improvement (up to 6 months) [10]. The presence of effusion, removal of fluid, severity of disease, absence of synovitis, use of ultrasound guidance, and increased symptoms prior to injection are all predictors of higher response to intra-articular steroid injection [29]. The dose of steroid injected does not appear to be linked to overall patient pain response. Given the side effect profile and possible toxic effect steroids may have on cartilage, mitigating the total steroid dose as much as possible is important. A 2023 randomized control double-blinded study demonstrated non-inferiority of 10 mg triamcinolone vs 40 mg at 12 weeks in patient with knee osteoarthritis [31].

Steroids are often injected into symptomatic OA knees in an attempt to delay surgery for those who may require a total knee arthroplasty. Some early studies raised a concern that steroid injection in close proximity to knee replacement surgery led to higher rates of infection postoperatively. More recent studies have demonstrated that this was not true and that higher postoperative complications were not related to steroid injection [32]. Multiple studies have brought up a concern for the reduction in cartilage thickness with chronic steroid exposure along with chondrocyte toxicity, particularly if local anesthetic is used. Though these results are concerning, the studies to date have been radiological surveillance studies and clinical effects on the patient were not reported [17, 33].

Given the current evidence, the use of steroids should continue to be considered an effective tool to assist in knee pain management. These benefits should not be expected to last past 1 week but may provide short-term relief to allow treatment of the underlying disease process and initiation or improved tolerance of muscular strengthening. Considering the recent evidence that patient response is not dose-dependent and that both short-and long-term exposure can have systemic and local side effects, providers should consider utilizing the lowest possible effective dose.

Hyaluronic Acid

Hyaluronic acid is a common injectate utilized for the treatment of knee osteoarthritis, particularly if steroid injections have failed. Evidence shows significant improvement in pain and function in patients with mild to moderate severity of osteoarthritis on x-rays; however, those with the most advanced radiographic disease had the lowest response rate [34]. When comparing intra-articular steroids to hyaluronic acid there have been many conflicting studies, a 2017 meta-analysis of 12 randomized controlled trials found that though steroids provided greater short-term pain relief (1 month), hyaluronic acid demonstrated greater pain relief long-term (6 months) [35]. Given this information, it is reasonable to consider hyaluronic acid injection earlier in the treatment regimen given its improved long-term outcomes compared to steroids.

Platelet-Rich Plasma (PRP)

The knee has been a commonly studied joint for PRP given the prevalence of knee osteoarthritis, ligamental injury, and pain. A 2021 meta-analysis demonstrated that both leukocyte-rich and leukocyte-poor PRP injections improved visual analog scale (VAS) scores above the minimally clinically important difference (MCID) for knee osteoarthritis, with no difference between the leukocyte-rich vs poor groups. This was seen at 3, 6, and 12-month follow-up. PRP injection also showed improvement above the MCID in the Western Ontario and McMaster University Osteoarthritis Index (WOMAC) and International Knee Documentation Committee (IKDC) functional scores [23]. A 2022 systematic review of ligamental injuries concluded there was too high a degree of heterogeneity of studies to draw any meaningful scientific conclusion on the role PRP can play in ligamental injury treatment [36].

PRP Plus Hyaluronic Acid

A meta-analysis of 941 patients published in 2020 by Zhao et al. looked at the efficacy of combining PRP and hyaluronic acid for knee osteoarthritis. The results demonstrated that this combination led to improved WOMAC total scores, improved WOMAC functional scores, lower VAS scores, and improved Lequesne index scores at 6 months compared to PRP alone. Adverse events were no different in the combination group versus the PRP or HA alone groups [37]. With improved long-term outcomes for PRP along with PRP plus HA, this biological therapy is likely to continue to grow in popularity. The low-risk of systemic side effects also lends itself to patients with multiple comorbidities along with those seeking long-term over short-term relief.

Local Anesthetic

The effect of local anesthetic on chondrocyte toxicity has been elucidated in multiple joints including the knee. A 2021 systemic review by Jayaram et al. demonstrated that all common local anesthetics, including lidocaine, bupivacaine, mepivacaine, and ropivacaine, had dose and time-dependent chondrocyte toxicity effects. These effects were made worse by the presence of corticosteroids. Of those studied, ropivacaine at a concentration of less than 0.5% was found to be the least toxic of the LAs [33]. Local anesthetic does not provide any known benefit beyond the analgesic duration of the LA chosen.

Radiofrequency Ablation

Radiofrequency ablation of the major sensory nerves of the knee, the genicular nerves, has increased in popularity over the past 10 years. Current evidence supports the ablation of the superior medial, superior lateral, and inferior medial genicular nerves for the treatment of chronic knee pain related to osteoarthritis with improvements in pain, function, quality of life, and composite scores [38]. Some randomized controlled trials support this treatment option over intra-articular steroid or hyaluronic acid. Unfortunately, many studies for this treatment have been industry-sponsored, particularly in relation to cooled radiofrequency ablation. This creates many questions on the biases present in these positive outcome studies.

Hip

Indications

1. The most common indication for intra-articular hip injection is osteoarthritis of the hip. Epidemiologically, hip osteoarthritis affects many people and is a common complaint to primary care and pain providers. Up to 27% of the people over the age of 45 have radiographic evidence of hip arthritis while 12–15% of people over the age of 60 have clinical manifestations of this arthritis [39, 40]. In people older than 85, the lifetime risk is quoted as high as 25% with a 10% lifetime risk of total hip replacement [41]. With increasing comorbidities with age, the risk of hip surgery can often outweigh the potential benefits and both surgeons and patients may desire alternate treatment options. The contraindications of hip injection are the same as for other large joints, as outlined in the knee section above.

Evidence

Steroids

The joint-specific nature of research outcomes is highlighted with hip steroid injections. In contrast to knee steroid injections, a 2020 meta-analysis by Zhong et al. demonstrated that intra-articular steroid injections were efficacious in both immediate as well as delayed pain relief. This effect persisted for to 12 weeks [42]. In regard to concern for perioperative infection if a patient had received a steroid injection, a small, 175 patient, retrospective study showed no difference in postoperative infection between patients who did and did not have steroid injections 1 year prior to total hip arthroplasty [43]. No specific data exists on the interaction between steroids and chondrocytes of the hip, unlike the knee and shoulder.

Hyaluronic Acid

Intra-articular injection of hyaluronic acid is commonly used to treat osteoarthritis in multiple other joints, as outlined above. For the hip, meta-analysis indicates that the use of HA for osteoarthritis leads to improved pain control and improved functional capabilities. Unfortunately, this effect was also seen with the saline control group and there was no significant difference seen between HA and saline. There were also no differences in risk between these groups [44].

Platelet-Rich Plasma (PRP)

PRP injection for hip osteoarthritis does appear to provide improved patient outcomes at 6 and 12 months, according to a 2021 meta-analysis by Berney et al. Interestingly, this improvement is similar, with no significant difference, to hyaluronic acid [45]. However, in a 2020 RCT comparing PRP to hyaluronic acid, Villanova–Lopez et al. demonstrated improved hip function, reduced pain, and decreased use of analgesics in the PRP group. Researchers were able to delineate responder and nonresponder groups in the PRP arm and this differentiation correlated with injectate platelet concentration. Responders had an average platelet count of 565 platelets/μL compared to the nonresponders who had an average injectate platelet count of 449/μL. This study also found that patients with early-stage OA had a higher response rate compared to those with late-stage disease [22].

Local Anesthetics

There are no RCT studies evaluating the role of local anesthetics in intra-articular hip injections. When considering the evidence for cartilaginous damage with local anesthetic infusions in shoulders, caution should be taken with medication and concentration choice.

Radiofrequency Ablation

Radiofrequency ablation of the articulating branches of the femoral and obturator nerves is another evolving treatment for various pain-generating pathologies of the hip. Unfortunately, few randomized controlled trials have been conducted on this treatment technique. Most publications on this topic describe a technique or are retrospective analyses of patients, though these studies demonstrate favorable VAS scale improvements at variable follow-up durations (3 months–3 years) [46]. Similar to knee radiofrequency ablation.

(RFA) publications, industry sponsorship confounds the current evidence available on outcomes and independent RCTs are needed to improve the quality of data.

Shoulder

Indications

Glenohumeral joint injections are common for a variety of conditions including osteoarthritis, adhesive capsulitis, labral tears, and rotator cuff tendinopathies. The annual incidence of shoulder pathology has been reported as high as 14.7 per 1000 patients per year with a lifetime prevalence as high as 70% [47]. Though specific technique will not be detailed here, it is important to acknowledge that when choosing a procedural approach, ultrasound and fluoroscopic guidance has demonstrated better outcomes than the blind approach [48, 49].

Evidence

Steroids

Of the various pathologies affecting the shoulder joint, adhesive capsulitis is a commonly studied indication for intra-articular steroid injections. In this population, the outcomes data is mixed with some studies showing no difference between steroid injection and alternate treatment groups while other studies have demonstrated short-term, small improvements in pain and function in favor of steroids [50]. Oh et al. demonstrated improved functional outcomes for patients with adhesive capsulitis at 1 month after receiving steroid injection or steroid plus HA injection compared to saline. Unfortunately, there was no difference at 3 or 6 months outcomes [51].

In patients receiving preoperative steroid injections for partial-thickness rotator cuff injuries, those who received an intra-articular steroid injection 0–3 months prior to their surgery had improved functional outcomes compared to those who did not receive an injection. In the setting of optimizing perioperative outcomes, presurgical ultrasound-guided or fluoroscopic steroid injection should be considered given this promising data.

Hyaluronic Acid

The evidence for hyaluronic acid injection for shoulder pathology remains mixed. In one meta-analysis of frozen shoulder patients, the conclusion was made that patients who received HA injection showed improved function and range of motion (ROM), but no difference in pain control compared to conservative therapy [52]. In contrast, Oh et al., whose paper was included in the meta-analysis above, showed no difference in functional outcomes between saline, HA, steroid, or combination steroid/HA beyond 1 month. At 1 month, steroid or combination steroid/HA outperformed saline and HA alone, however [53].

In osteoarthritis patients, HA injection did not outperform control for VAS pain score at 3 and 6 months [54]. The role of HA in shoulder pathology remains unclear, with conflicting results when comparing meta-analysis versus individual studies as well as comparing diagnoses.

Platelet-Rich Plasma

PRP injection for shoulder pain has also yielded conflicting results. In a meta-analysis of rotator cuff tendinopathy, when compared to sham injection, no intervention, or PT alone, there was no difference in groups out to 12 weeks. After 24 weeks, however, pain improved in the PRP group compared to control. Functional improvement of the shoulder was not statistically different at any point in time, however [55]. One meta-analysis by Chen et al. did conclude that PRP may reduce short- and long-term pain with rotator cuff tendinopathies, though there was a high level of heterogeneity of studies and injectate characteristics [56].

Local Anesthetic

The greatest amount of literature regarding the negative effects of local anesthetic on chondrolysis is published in glenohumeral arthroscopic surgery. Most of these cases (19/23) utilized intra-articular pumps but all 23 had received a single intra-articular injection of 0.25% bupivacaine with 1:200k epinephrine postoperatively [57]. Another meta-analysis pooling data from four studies demonstrated a chondrolysis rate of 40.6% when an intra-articular local anesthetic pain pump was utilized for postoperative pain control [58]. Though this clearly demonstrates the deleterious effects of this medication on joint health perioperatively, it also should inform practitioners to reduce the joint's total exposure to local anesthetic, perhaps even avoided.

Medium Sized Joints

Sacroiliac Joint

Indication

Sacroiliac joint pain is estimated to account for 10–27% of mechanical low back pain. In addition to primary osteoarthritis, there are many causes of SI joint dysfunction. These include advanced age, pregnancy and childbirth, leg length discrepancy, biomechanical changes after spinal surgery, and trauma which can all lead to joint dysfunction [59]. Procedural intervention along with physical therapy and lifestyle modifications are considered the cornerstones of treatment.

Steroids

Similar to the treatment of osteoarthritis in other joints of the body, intra-articular steroid injection has been a gold standard for the treatment of sacroiliitis. Despite this, a review of the available literature in 2012 by Hansen et al. demonstrated limited evidence for intra- or periarticular steroid injections [60]. A 2015 retrospective analysis of 54 patients demonstrated effect in the short term (2 weeks) [61]; however, current high-quality evidence for long-term pain relief is limited at this time.

Hyaluronic Acid

There is little evidence for the use of hyaluronic acid in the treatment of sacroiliac pain. A 2022 RCT trial by Hosny et al. demonstrated improved pain control in patients receiving steroids compared to hyaluronic acid up to 4 weeks. Both groups did have statistically significant pain relief compared to baseline, however [62]. Given the potential side effects of steroids, this may provide a suitable short-term treatment option for patients in which steroid is contraindicated.

Platelet-Rich Plasma

Platelet-rich plasma for sacroiliac pain has some promising initial studies, though randomized controlled studies are lacking. In one study by Ko et al., patients who received an ultrasound-guided PRP intra-articular injection demonstrated statistically significant pain control at 12 and 48 months postinjection [63]. In addition, a prospective open-blinded study by Singla et al. in 2017 demonstrated improved pain control at 6 and 12 weeks compared to steroid therapy [64].

Radiofrequency Ablation

In a 2020 meta-analysis by Shih et al., radiofrequency ablation was evaluated through cooled, traditional as well as pulsed RFA for improvement in SI joint pain. Patients demonstrated significant improvements for all three radiofrequency ablation techniques at 3 months. At 6 months, only cooled and thermal ablation had data to be analyzed which demonstrated continued pain improvement with similar efficacy between the techniques. This was again demonstrated at 12 months follow-up [65]. In a 2018 randomized controlled trial, Dutta et al. looked at pulsed RFA versus steroid injection and demonstrated pulsed RFA had a significantly higher global perceived effect and significantly improved Oswestry Disability Index at 3 and 6 months post-procedure [66].

Facet

Indication

Though there are varying epidemiologic studies on low back pain, it is estimated that the incidence of low back pain is 5–10% with a lifetime prevalence of up to 60–90%. Lumbar facet osteoarthritic disease is a leading cause of this pain and the primary indication for intra-articular or periarticular injection. In fact, facet-related pain is estimated to comprise 15–45% of all chronic low back pain complaints [67]. Patients with chronic cervical pain have an even higher prevalence of facet disease with up to 55% of those patients carrying this diagnosis [68].

Steroids

For lumbar facet disease, intra-articular steroid facet injections have received significant attention. A large placebo-controlled trial by Carette et al. in 1991 demonstrated no benefit in intra-articular steroid injection compared to saline [69]. A later study by Fuchs et al. in 1994 showed improvement in pain relief, function, and quality of life but this was conducted without a control group, rather than comparing it to hyaluronic acid which showed equivalent outcomes [70]. In 2018 and 2019, two papers by Kennedy et al. demonstrated no difference in rates of radiofrequency ablation between groups that received either intra-articular steroid or saline for lumbar facet disease [71, 72]. Additionally, intra-articular and periarticular injections have been shown to be equivalent in short-term (1 week) pain relief in a 2019 study by Kershen et al. [73]

For cervical facet disease, there have been few high-quality studies supporting intra-articular steroid injections. In a 1994 randomized control trial, no difference was seen between local anesthetic and steroid. Additionally, patients reported returning to baseline pain at 3 days post-procedure and no lasting effect at 6 months [74]. Unfortunately, there have been few studies looking at this treatment since then.

Hyaluronic Acid

In 2005, a randomized controlled study compared HA to intra-articular steroid injection for lumbar non-radicular pain. In this study, hyaluronic acid was demonstrated to be non-inferior to triamcinolone [70]. Since intra-articular steroids have low-level support, there have been few studies into this injectate since then.

Platelet-Rich Plasma

There are limited studies looking at platelet-rich plasma as an injectate for lumbar facet disease. A 2017 randomized controlled comparison of steroid and PRP demonstrated higher patient satisfaction with PRP injection compared to steroid injection at 6 months. At 1 and 3 months steroid demonstrated higher satisfaction, however [75]. In a randomized control trial in 2023, Singh et al. demonstrated a similar effect on ODI when comparing intra-articular steroid plus RFA to intra-articular PRP plus RFA, with PRP showing improved ODI at 6 months [76].

Radiofrequency Ablation

Radiofrequency ablation of the medial branch nerves in the lumbar spine has been a keystone for treating facetogenic pain for many years [77]. In a 2020 meta-analysis by Shih et al., three methods of radiofrequency (cooled, traditional, and pulsed) were compared for the treatment of lumbar facet disease. Of the three ablation techniques, cooled RFA was the most effective in pain relief at 6 months. This was followed by traditional thermal ablation and then pulsed ablation. Each of the ablation techniques demonstrated improvement compared to baseline pain. At 12 months, only thermal and pulsed RFA had evidence to be analyzed which demonstrated continued pain improvement compared to baseline, with both techniques being similar in their efficacy [65].

Clinical outcomes also support the success of patients who receive this therapy. In a 2020 retrospective study of commercially insured patients, Starr et al. demonstrated that 33% of patients who received lumbar RFA repeated this procedure within 3 years. Additionally, 24.9% of patients who took opiates preRFA discontinued opiate prescriptions at 180 days post-procedure. Of those who did not take opiates before the procedure, only 6.7% started taking opiates at 180 days post-procedure [78].

Radiofrequency ablation remains a primary treatment regimen for lumbar facet-related pain. As demonstrated above, its efficacy and low side effect profile make it an attractive therapy option for patients, particularly with limited long-term evidence for intra-articular injections.

Elbow

Indications

Elbow epicondylitis is considered the most common indication for elbow injection therapy. Lateral epicondylitis is estimated to affect 1–3% of the adult population per year [79]. Approximately 2% require surgical intervention, however the remainder can be treated conservatively [80]. There are few studies looking at intra-articular joint injections with the majority of evidence for peritendon injection.

Evidence

Steroids

The use of steroid injections along the lateral epicondyle has remained a standard of procedural-based therapy for lateral epicondylitis. Evidence demonstrates a short, 4–8 week, improvement in disability score with this procedure. This result was not shown to be superior to standard NSAID therapy, however [81]. Many patients are unable to tolerate NSAIDs and this procedure would be an excellent option in this case. There is an important procedural consideration which is tendon rupture, which is a rare complication if steroids are deposited directly into the tendon. These are now often performed under ultrasound guidance for this reason.

Platelet-Rich Plasma

Peritendon injection of PRP shows improved long-term outcomes as compared to steroids. Though steroids demonstrate improved pain control in the short-term, PRP demonstrated superior pain and functional improvement at 24 weeks for elbow epicondylitis in a 2019 systemic review and meta-analysis by Li et al. [82] As outlined earlier, standardization of PRP is lacking; however, these outcomes are encouraging.

Small-Sized Joints

The small-sized joints including the hand, foot, and temporomadibular joint (TMJ) are common targets for intra-articular steroid injections for degenerative or inflammatory diseases. Many of these treatment areas have their own subspecialized area of medicine and great detail is needed to fully describe the various individual joints in the hand and foot. When counseling patients on therapy options, there are trends within small joint therapy that are important to know. A 2022 meta-analysis of steroid injections for hand arthritis demonstrated little effect in short-term (4–6 weeks) or long-term (3–12 months) pain improvement [83]. In a single study of trapeziometacarpal degenerative arthritis, hyaluronic acid was found to be more efficacious in improving some fine hand movements in comparison to corticosteroids. Both groups improved in pain and functional capacity out to 6 months [84]. In a separate but similar study looking at hyaluronic acid injection into the first carpometacarpal joint, HA also showed benefit over corticosteroid injection at 6 months [85]. Similar results were found for the treatment of temporomandibular joint dysfunction. In a 2014 study by Gencer et al., HA outperformed corticosteroids, NSAID, or saline control at 1 and 6 weeks [86].

Soft Tissue Injection

Trigger Point

Trigger point injections can be conducted in any muscle group in the body with various injectates including saline, local anesthetic, steroid, botulinum toxin, or no injectate at all. There is no current evidence to suggest that any injectate is superior to another or even that injection has better long-term outcomes than dry needling [87]. Some local anesthetics have been shown to have different degrees of discomfort with injection with ropivacaine having the least discomfort compared to bupivacaine and lidocaine. Steroid use has not been shown to be superior to other injectates, including saline, despite its widespread use in trigger point injections [87].

Carpal Tunnel

Carpal tunnel syndrome is another common soft tissue injection. Steroids are frequently deposited deep into the transverse carpal ligament to reduce inflammation around the nervous bundle. A 2021 meta-analysis of available data demonstrated that in-plane ultrasound-guided carpal tunnel injections provided improved symptom control and functionality for patients [88]. A 2023 review demonstrated a similar outcome with superiority to placebo and delay in surgery up to 12 months after steroid injection [89].

Conclusion

In the review of the available evidence for the treatment of musculoskeletal pain through nonsurgical procedural intervention, it is clear that the evidence is mixed. Studying a disease process that cannot be directly measured (pain) and has many subjective inputs remains a limiting factor in interpreting outcomes. With so many conflicting studies and differential results between joints, it is clear that more research is needed to determine the optimal injectable therapies for musculoskeletal pain. Unfortunately, these results may continue to be as variable as the patients we treat. Many therapies may provide value to the patient, though it may not be shown through reduced pain scores. Many patients improve function, reduce medications, or are able to tolerate strengthening regimens due to injections even if they report similar pain scores. Separating a patient's overall response to therapy is critical in considering therapeutic success in clinical medicine.

One point that is important is that many therapies show short-term but waning long-term patient improvements. Short-term improvement should not be considered a therapeutic failure. These windows of opportunity give patients the chance to optimize their strength and start making the lifestyle changes necessary for long-term success. Without these periods of pain improvement, many would not be able to initiate physical therapy or exercise without high levels of pain, often preventing meaningful progress.

With so many new therapies over the past 20 years and additional treatments likely to be developed, some traditional injectates have garnered increased skepticism in recent literature. The effects of steroids and local anesthetics on joint health are an area of question and should be factored into clinician decision-making. Regardless of this, steroids will likely play a role in providing a short-term interruption in pain. The dose-dependent nature of these outcomes is something that has not been fully studied but should be considered prior to injection. Discussing this with the patient and setting expectations for what defines a successful treatment may also assist in improving patient satisfaction and overall therapeutic motivation.

Bullet Points

- There remains conflicting evidence for the best treatments in injectable musculoskeletal therapies.
- Evidence for each injectable therapy varies depending on the joint treated.
- Steroid and local anesthetics have been shown to cause potentially deleterious effects in large joint chondrocytes.
- Hyaluronic acid derivatives and platelet-rich plasma are treatment options with greater long-term benefits but fewer short-term improvements.
- Platelet-rich plasma research is limited with lack of standardized protocols and preparation.
- Radiofrequency ablation of sensory nerves is a growing procedural target for practitioners, with favorable outcome data and few known side effects.
- Many therapies provide patients with short-term pain relief allowing improved strength and initiation of lifestyle changes which can lead to long-term pain improvement.
- High-quality randomized controlled trials are needed to further determine the short- and long-term benefits of many of the procedural interventions in pain management.

References

1. Benedek TG. History of the development of corticosteroid therapy. Clin Exp Rheumatol. 2011;29(5 Suppl 68):S-5-12. Epub 2011 Oct 21. PMID: 22018177.
2. Derby R, Lee SH, Date ES, Lee JH, Lee CH. Size and aggregation of corticosteroids used for epidural injections. Pain Med. 2008;9:227–34.
3. Yasir M, Goyal A, Sonthalia S. Corticosteroid adverse effects. [Updated 2022 Jul 4]. In: StatPearls [Internet]. Treasure Island (FL): StatPearls Publishing; 2023. Available from: https://www.ncbi.nlm.nih.gov/books/NBK531462/.
4. Williams GH, Dluhy RG. Disorders of the adrenal cortex. In: Harrison T, Braunwald E, editors. Harrison's principles of internal medicine. 15th ed. New York: McGraw-Hill; 2001. p. 2084–105.
5. Coursin DB, Wood KE. Corticosteroid supplementation for adrenal insufficiency. JAMA. 2002;287:236–40.
6. Bowen R. Mineralocorticoids. Vivo pathophysiology. (n.d.). http://www.vivo.colostate.edu/hbooks/pathphys/endocrine/adrenal/mineralo.html
7. Park CH, Lee SH, Kim BI. Comparison of the effectiveness of lumbar transforaminal epidural injection with particulate and nonparticulate corticosteroids in lumbar radiating pain. Pain Med. 2010;11(11):1654–8.
8. Lee JW, Park KW, Chung SK, Yeom JS, Kim KJ, Kim HJ, Kang HS. Cervical transforaminal epidural steroid injection for the management of cervical radiculopathy: a comparative study of particulate versus non-particulate steroids. Skeletal Radiol. 2009;38(11):1077–82.

9. Mehta P, Syrop I, Singh JR, Kirschner J. Systematic review of the efficacy of particulate versus nonparticulate corticosteroids in epidural injections. PM R. 2017;9(5):502–12. https://doi.org/10.1016/j.pmrj.2016.11.008. Epub 2016 Nov 30
10. Hajialilo M, Ghorbanihaghjo A, Valaee L, Kolahi S, Rashtchizadeh N, Amirkhiz MB, Malekmahdavi I, Khabbazi A. A double-blind randomized comparative study of triamcinolone hexacetonide and dexamethasone intra-articular injection for the treatment of knee joint arthritis in rheumatoid arthritis. Clin Rheumatol. 2016;35(12):2887–91.
11. Lento P, Ihm J, Kennedy D, Visco C. Peripheral joint and soft tissue injection techniques. In: Chan L, et al., editors. Braddom's physical medicine & rehabilitation. 4th ed. Philadelphia: Saunders; 2011. p. 517–40.
12. Shin WY, An MJ, Im NG, Oh KR, Choe Y, Yoon SR, Ryu SR. Changes in blood glucose level after Steroid injection for musculoskeletal pain in patients with diabetes. Ann Rehabil Med. 2020;44(2):117–24.
13. Pace CS, Blanchet NP, Isaacs JE. Soft tissue atrophy related to corticosteroid injection: review of the literature and implications for hand surgeons. J Hand Surg Am. 2018;43(6):558–63, ISSN 0363-5023
14. Brinks A, Koes BW, Volkers AC, et al. Adverse effects of extra-articular corticosteroid injections: a systematic review. BMC Musculoskelet Disord. 2010;11:206.
15. Kim S, Hwang B. Relationship between bone mineral density and the frequent administration of epidural steroid injections in postmenopausal women with low back pain. Pain Res Manag. 2014;19(1):30–4.
16. Nah SY, Lee JH, Lee JH. Effects of epidural Steroid injections on bone mineral density and bone turnover markers in patients taking anti-osteoporotic medications. Pain Physician. 2018;21(4):E435–47.
17. McAlindon TE, LaValley MP, Harvey WF, Price LL, Driban JB, Zhang M, Ward RJ. Effect of intra-articular triamcinolone vs saline on knee cartilage volume and pain in patients with knee osteoarthritis: A randomized clinical trial. JAMA. 2017;317(19):1967–75.
18. Marshall KW. Intra-articular hyaluronan therapy. Curr Opin Rheumatol. 2000;12(5):468–74.
19. Felson DT, Anderson JJ. Hyaluronate sodium injections for osteoarthritis: hope, hype, and hard truths. Arch Intern Med. 2002;162(3):245–7.
20. Walker K, Basehore BM, Goyal A, et al. Hyaluronic acid. [Updated 2023 Mar 7]. In: StatPearls [Internet]. Treasure Island (FL): StatPearls Publishing; 2023. Available from: https://www.ncbi.nlm.nih.gov/books/NBK482440/.
21. Karjalainen TV, Silagy M, O'Bryan E, Johnston RV, Cyril S, Buchbinder R. Autologous blood and platelet-rich plasma injection therapy for lateral elbow pain. Cochrane Database Syst Rev. 2021;9:Art. No.: CD010951.
22. Villanova-López MM, Núñez-Núñez M, Fernández-Prieto D, González-López C, García-Donaire J, Pérez-Pérez A, Sandoval Fernández Del Castillo S, Murillo-Izquierdo M, Camean-Fernández M, Gutiérrez-Pizarraya A, Navas-Iglesias N, Roca-Ruiz LJ, Calleja-Hernández MÁ, Ballester-Alfaro JJ. Randomized, double-blind, controlled trial, phase III, to evaluate the use of platelet-rich plasma versus hyaluronic acid in hip coxarthrosis. Rev Esp Cir Ortop Traumatol (Engl Ed). 2020;64(2):134–42.
23. Kim JH, Park YB, Ha CW, Roh YJ, Park JG. Adverse reactions and clinical outcomes for leukocyte-poor versus leukocyte-rich platelet-rich plasma in knee osteoarthritis: a systematic review and meta-analysis. Orthop J Sports Med. 2021;9(6):23259671211011948.
24. Ruetsch YA, Böni T, Borgeat A. From cocaine to ropivacaine: the history of local anesthetic drugs. Curr Top Med Chem. 2001;1(3):175–82.
25. Chu CR, Izzo NJ, Coyle CH, Papas NE, Logar A. The in vitro effects of bupivacaine on articular chondrocytes. J Bone Jt Surg Br. 2008;90:814–20.
26. Park J, Sutradhar BC, Hong G, Choi SH, Kim G. Comparison of the cytotoxic effects of bupivacaine, lidocaine, and mepivacaine in equine articular chondrocytes. Vet Anaesth Analg. 2011;38:127–33.
27. Gulihar A, Robati S, Twaij H, Salih A, Taylor GJ. Articular cartilage and local anaesthetic: A systematic review of the current literature. J Orthop. 2015;12(Suppl 2):S200–10.

28. Zhang Y, Jordan JM. Epidemiology of osteoarthritis. Clin Geriatr Med. 2010;26(3):355–69. https://doi.org/10.1016/j.cger.2010.03.001. Erratum in: Clin Geriatr Med. 2013;29(2):ix.
29. Maricar N, Callaghan M, Felson D, O'Neill T. Predictors of response to intra-articular steroid injections in knee osteoarthritis—a systematic review. Rheumatology. 2013;52(6):1022–32.
30. Hepper CT, Halvorson JJ, Duncan ST, Gregory M, Andrew J, Dunn WR, Spindler KP. The efficacy and duration of intra-articular corticosteroid injection for knee osteoarthritis: A systematic review of level I studies. J Am Acad Orthop Surg. 2009;17(10):638–46.
31. Utamawatin K, Phruetthiphat OA, Apinyankul R, et al. The efficacy of intra-articular triamcinolone acetonide 10 mg vs. 40 mg in patients with knee osteoarthritis: a non-inferiority, randomized, controlled, double-blind, multicenter study. BMC Musculoskelet Disord. 2023;24:92.
32. Kokubun B, Manista G, Courtney PM, Kearns S, Levine B. Intra-articular knee injections before total knee arthroplasty: outcomes and complication rates. J Arthroplast. 2017;32(6):1798–802, ISSN 0883-5403
33. Jayaram P, Kennedy DJ, Yeh P, Dragoo J. Chondrotoxic effects of local anesthetics on human knee articular cartilage: A systematic review. PM R. 2019;11(4):379–400.
34. Wang CT, Lin J, Chang CJ, Lin YT, Hou SM. Therapeutic effects of hyaluronic acid on osteoarthritis of the knee. A meta-analysis of randomized controlled trials. J Bone Joint Surg Am. 2004;86(3):538–45.
35. He W, Kuang M, Zhao J, Sun L, Lu B, Wang Y, Ma J, Ma X. Efficacy and safety of intraarticular hyaluronic acid and corticosteroid for knee osteoarthritis: a meta-analysis. Int J Surg. 2017;39:95–103. ISSN 1743-9191.
36. Kunze KN, Pakanati JJ, Vadhera AS, Polce EM, Williams BT, Parvaresh KC, Chahla J. The efficacy of platelet-rich plasma for ligament injuries: A systematic review of basic science literature with protocol quality assessment. Orthop J Sports Med. 2022;10(2):23259671211066504.
37. Zhao J, Huang H, Liang G, et al. Effects and safety of the combination of platelet-rich plasma (PRP) and hyaluronic acid (HA) in the treatment of knee osteoarthritis: a systematic review and meta-analysis. BMC Musculoskelet Disord. 2020;21:224.
38. Chen A, Mullen K, Casambre F, Visvabharathy V, Brown G. Thermal nerve radiofrequency ablation for the nonsurgical treatment of knee osteoarthritis: A systematic literature review. J Am Acad Orthop Surg. 2021;29(9):387–96.
39. Jordan JM, Helmick CG, Renner JB, Luta G, Dragomir AD, Woodard J, Fang F, Schwartz TA, Nelson AE, Abbate LM, Callahan LF, Kalsbeek WD, Hochberg MC. Prevalence of hip symptoms and radiographic and symptomatic hip osteoarthritis in African Americans and Caucasians: the Johnston County Osteoarthritis Project. J Rheumatol. 2009;36(4):809–15.
40. Christmas C, Crespo CJ, Franckowiak SC, Bathon JM, Bartlett SJ, Andersen RE. How common is hip pain among older adults? Results from the third National Health and Nutrition Examination Survey. J Fam Pract. 2002;51(4):345–8.
41. Murphy LB, Helmick CG, Schwartz TA, Renner JB, Tudor G, Koch GG, Dragomir AD, Kalsbeek WD, Luta G, Jordan JM. One in four people may develop symptomatic hip osteoarthritis in his or her lifetime. Osteoarthr Cartil. 2010;18(11):1372–9.
42. Zhong HM, Zhao GF, Lin T, Zhang XX, Li XY, Lin JF, Zhao SQ, Pan ZJ. Intra-articular Steroid injection for patients with hip osteoarthritis: a systematic review and meta-analysis. Biomed Res Int. 2020;2020:6320154.
43. Meermans G, Corten K, Simon JP. Is the infection rate in primary THA increased after steroid injection? Clin Orthop Relat Res. 2012;470(11):3213–9. https://doi.org/10.1007/s11999-012-2390-8. Epub 2012 May 19. Erratum in: Clin Orthop Relat Res. 2013;471(11):3724.
44. Wu B, Li YM, Liu YC. Efficacy of intra-articular hyaluronic acid injections in hip osteoarthritis: a meta-analysis of randomized controlled trials. Oncotarget. 2017;8(49):86865–76.
45. Berney M, McCarroll P, Glynn L, Lenehan B. Platelet-rich plasma injections for hip osteoarthritis: a review of the evidence. Ir J Med Sci. 2021;190(3):1021–5. https://doi.org/10.1007/s11845-020-02388-z. Epub 2020 Oct 5
46. Cheney C, Ahmadian A, Brennick C, Zheng P, Mattie R, McCormick Z, Nagpal A. Radiofrequency ablation for chronic hip pain: A comprehensive, narrative review. Pain Med. 2021;22(Supplement_1):S14–9.

47. Tafti D, Schultz D. Shoulder joint injection. [Updated 2022 Sep 7]. In: StatPearls [Internet]. Treasure Island (FL): StatPearls Publishing; 2022. Available from: https://www.ncbi.nlm.nih.gov/books/NBK559318/.
48. Lee HJ, Lim KB, Kim DY, Lee KT. Randomized controlled trial for efficacy of intra-articular injection for adhesive capsulitis: ultrasonography-guided versus blind technique. Arch Phys Med Rehabil. 2009;90(12):1997–2002.
49. Amber KT, Landy DC, Amber I, Knopf D, Guerra J. Comparing the accuracy of ultrasound versus fluoroscopy in glenohumeral injections: a systematic review and meta-analysis. J Clin Ultrasound. 2014;42(7):411–6. https://doi.org/10.1002/jcu.22154. Epub 2014 Mar 25
50. Cushman D, Bruno B, Christiansen J, Schultz A, McCormick Z. Efficacy of injected corticosteroid type, dose, and volume for pain in large joints: a narrative review. PM&R. 2018;10(7):748–57, ISSN 1934-1482.
51. Oh SH, Sung WS, Oh SH, Jo CH. Comparative analysis of intra-articular injection of steroid and/or sodium hyaluronate in adhesive capsulitis: prospective, double-blind, randomized, placebo-controlled study. JSES Int. 2021;5(6):1091–104.
52. Donohue NK, Prisco AR, Grindel SI. Pre-operative corticosteroid injections improve functional outcomes in patients undergoing arthroscopic repair of high-grade partial-thickness rotator cuff tears. Muscles Ligaments Tendons J. 2017;7(1):34–9.
53. Mao B, Peng R, Zhang Z, et al. The effect of intra-articular injection of hyaluronic acid in frozen shoulder: a systematic review and meta-analysis of randomized controlled trials. J Orthop Surg Res. 2022;17:128.
54. Zhang B, Thayaparan A, Horner N, Bedi A, Alolabi B, Khan M. Outcomes of hyaluronic acid injections for glenohumeral osteoarthritis: a systematic review and meta-analysis. J Shoulder Elb Surg. 2019;28(3):596–606.
55. Lin MT, Wei KC, Wu CH. Effectiveness of platelet-rich plasma injection in rotator cuff tendinopathy: a systematic review and meta-analysis of randomized controlled trials. Diagnostics (Basel). 2020;10(4):189.
56. Chen X, Jones IA, Park C, Vangsness CT Jr. The efficacy of platelet-rich plasma on tendon and ligament healing: A systematic review and meta-analysis with bias assessment. Am J Sports Med. 2018;46(8):2020–32.
57. Bailie DS, Ellenbecker TS. Severe chondrolysis after shoulder arthroscopy: a case series. J Shoulder Elb Surg/Am Shoulder Elb Surg [et al]. 2009;18:742–7.
58. Gulihar A, Robati S, Twaij H, Salih A, Taylor GJ. Articular cartilage and local anaesthetic: a systematic review of the current literature. J Orthop. 2015;12(Suppl 2):S200–10.
59. Wu L, Tafti D, Varacallo M. Sacroiliac joint injection. [Updated 2022 Sep 7]. In: StatPearls [Internet]. Treasure Island (FL): StatPearls Publishing; 2022. Available from: https://www.ncbi.nlm.nih.gov/books/NBK513245/.
60. Hansen H, Manchikanti L, Simopoulos T, Christo P, Gupta S, Smith H, Hameed H, Cohen S. A systematic evaluation of the therapeutic effectiveness of sacroiliac joint interventions. Pain Physician. 2012;15:E247–78.
61. Scholten PM, Patel SI, Christos PJ, Singh JR. Short-term efficacy of sacroiliac joint corticosteroid injection based on arthrographic contrast patterns. PM R. 2015 Apr;7(4):385–91.
62. Hosny K, Abdelkareem MI, Moshrif A. AB1231 ultrasound-guided injection of low molecular weight hyaluronic acid versus steroid for inflammatory and degenerative sacroiliitis: a randomized controlled trial. Ann Rheum Dis. 2022;81:1727.
63. Ko GD, Mindra S, Lawson GE, Whitmore S, Arseneau L. Case series of ultrasound-guided platelet-rich plasma injections for sacroiliac joint dysfunction. J Back Musculoskelet Rehabil. 2017;30(2):363–70.
64. Singla V, Batra YK, Bharti N, Goni VG, Marwaha N, Steroid vs. Platelet-rich plasma in ultrasound-guided sacroiliac joint injection for chronic low Back pain. Pain Pract. 2017;17(6):782–91.
65. Shih CL, Shen PC, Lu CC, Liu ZM, Tien YC, Huang PJ, Chou SH. A comparison of efficacy among different radiofrequency ablation techniques for the treatment of lumbar facet

joint and sacroiliac joint pain: A systematic review and meta-analysis. Clin Neurol Neurosurg. 2020;195:105854.
66. Dutta K, Dey S, Bhattacharyya P, Agarwal S, Dev P. Comparison of efficacy of lateral branch pulsed radiofrequency denervation and Intraarticular depot methylprednisolone injection for sacroiliac joint pain. Pain Physician. 2018;21(5):489–96.
67. Alexander CE, Cascio MA, Varacallo M. Lumbosacral facet syndrome. [Updated 2022 Sep 26]. In: StatPearls [Internet]. Treasure Island (FL): StatPearls Publishing; 2023. Available from: https://www.ncbi.nlm.nih.gov/books/NBK441906/.
68. Manchikanti L, Boswell MV, Singh V, Pampati V, Damron KS, Beyer CD. Prevalence of facet joint pain in chronic spinal pain of cervical, thoracic, and lumbar regions. BMC Musculoskelet Disord. 2004;5:15.
69. Carette S, Marcoux S, Truchon R, Grondin C, Gagnon J, Allard Y, et al. A controlled trial of corticosteroid injections into facet joints for chronic low back pain. N Engl J Med. 1991;325:1002–7.
70. Fuchs S, Erbe T, Fischer HL, Tibesku C. Intraarticular hyaluronic acid versus glucocorticoid injections for nonradicular pain in the lumbar spine. J Vasc Interv Radiol. 2005;16(11):1493–8. ISSN 1051-0443.
71. Kennedy DJ, Huynh L, Wong J, Mattie R, Levin J, Smuck M, Schneider BJ. Corticosteroid injections into lumbar facet joints: A prospective, randomized, double-blind placebo-controlled trial. Am J Phys Med Rehabil. 2018;97(10):741–6.
72. Kennedy DJ, Fraiser R, Zheng P, Huynh L, Levin J, Smuck M, Schneider BJ. Intra-articular steroids vs saline for lumbar z-joint pain: a prospective, randomized, double-blind placebo-controlled trial. Pain Med. 2019;20(2):246–51.
73. Kershen LM, Nacey NC, Patrie JT, Fox MG. Fluoroscopically guided facet injections: comparison of intra-articular and Periarticular Steroid and anesthetic injection on immediate and short-term pain relief. Am J Neuroradiol. 2018;39(11):21612165.
74. Barnsley L, Lord SM, Wallis BJ, Bogduk N. Lack of effect of intraarticular corticosteroids for chronic pain in the cervical zygapophyseal joints. N Engl J Med. 1994;330(15):1047–50.
75. Wu J, Zhou J, Liu C, Zhang J, Xiong W, Lv Y, Liu R, Wang R, Du Z, Zhang G, Liu Q. A prospective study comparing platelet-rich plasma and local anesthetic (LA)/corticosteroid in intra-articular injection for the treatment of lumbar facet joint syndrome. Pain Pract. 2017;17(7):914–24.
76. Singh C, Yadav S, Loha S, Prakash S, Paswan AK. Comparison of intra-articular lumbar facet joint injection of platelet-rich plasma and steroid in the treatment of chronic low back pain: a prospective study. J Orthop Trauma Rehabil. 2023;30(2):221049172311618.
77. Cohen SP, Bhaskar A, Bhatia A, et al. Consensus practice guidelines on interventions for lumbar facet joint pain from a multispecialty, international working group. Reg Anesth Pain Med. 2020;45:424–67.
78. Starr JB, Gold LS, McCormick Z, Suri P, Friedly J. Repeat procedures and prescription opioid use after lumbar medial branch nerve radiofrequency ablation in commercially insured patients. Spine J. 2020;20(3):344–51.
79. Calfee RP, Patel A, DaSilva MF, Akelman E. Management of lateral epicondylitis: current concepts. J Am Acad Orthop Surg. 2008;16(1):19–29.
80. Degen RM, Conti MS, Camp CL, Altchek DW, Dines JS, Werner BC. Epidemiology and disease burden of lateral epicondylitis in the USA: analysis of 85,318 patients. HSS J. 2018;14(1):9–14.
81. Gaujoux-Viala C, Dougados M, Gossec L. Efficacy and safety of steroid injections for shoulder and elbow tendonitis: a meta-analysis of randomized controlled trials. Ann Rheum Dis. 2009;68:1843–9.
82. Li A, Wang H, Yu Z, Zhang G, Feng S, Liu L, Gao Y. Platelet-rich plasma vs corticosteroids for elbow epicondylitis: A systematic review and meta-analysis. Medicine. 2019;98(51):e18358.
83. Estee MM, Cicuttini FM, Page MJ, et al. Efficacy of corticosteroids for hand osteoarthritis – a systematic review and meta-analysis of randomized controlled trials. BMC Musculoskelet Disord. 2022;23:665.

84. Stahl S, Karsh-Zafrir I, Ratzon N, Rosenberg N. Comparison of intraarticular injection of depot corticosteroid and hyaluronic acid for treatment of degenerative trapeziometacarpal joints. J Clin Rheumatol. 2005;11(6):299–302.
85. Monfort J, Rotés-Sala D, Segalés N, Montañes FJ, Orellana C, Llorente-Onaindia J, Mojal S, Padró I, Benito P. Comparative efficacy of intra-articular hyaluronic acid and corticoid injections in osteoarthritis of the first carpometacarpal joint: results of a 6-month single-masked randomized study. Joint Bone Spine. 2015;82(2):116–21.
86. Gencer ZK, Özkiriş M, Okur A, Korkmaz M, Saydam L. A comparative study on the impact of intra-articular injections of hyaluronic acid, tenoxicam and betametazon on the relief of temporomandibular joint disorder complaints. J Craniomaxillofac Surg. 2014;42(7):1117–21.
87. Srinivasan M, Lam C, Alm J, Chadwick AL. Trigger point injections. Phys Med Rehabil Clin N Am. 2022;33(2):307–33.
88. Yang FA, Shih YC, Hong JP, et al. Ultrasound-guided corticosteroid injection for patients with carpal tunnel syndrome: a systematic review and meta-analysis of randomized controlled trials. Sci Rep. 2021;11:10417.
89. Ashworth NL, Bland JDP, Chapman KM, Tardif G, Albarqouni L, Nagendran A. Local corticosteroid injection versus placebo for carpal tunnel syndrome. Cochrane Database Syst Rev. 2023;2(2):CD015148.

Perioperative Pain Management and Enhanced Recovery Protocols

22

Lisa Gu, Jasmine Liu, and Anthony T. Machi

Why Use an Enhanced Recovery Protocol?

The primary goals of an enhanced recovery protocol are to achieve the highest quality results and fastest recovery for patients, to lead them to optimal health outcomes. The idea for Enhanced Recovery After Surgery® (ERAS) was developed by a group of academic surgeons in Europe in 2001 who aimed to shift the focus of recovery from a singular goal of speed popularized by "fast-track surgery" in the 1990s to quality of recovery [1]. The enhanced recovery concepts leveraged multi-disciplinary teamwork, evidence-based guidelines, and continuous cycles of audit and refinement that they had partially implemented in pilot studies [2–4]. From the outset, the group aimed to modify the endocrine and metabolic response by addressing nutrition, inflammation, and protein metabolism, while also revealing to the surgical community how a complete perioperative care, rather than surgical technique alone, determined postsurgical outcomes [5]. The group formed the ERAS Society in 2010, and they published the first protocols addressing colorectal surgery and pancreaticoduodenectomy in 2012. Their ideas spread to other types of surgery and eventually led to the creation of protocols for orthopedic and spine surgery by both society members and other professionals [6–10]. As the groups developed comprehensive protocols to achieve these goals, analgesia became a critical component.

While published protocols such as those developed by the ERAS Society are a good starting point, forming a pathway involves many components [11, 12]. The first step is forming a multidisciplinary team that includes surgeons, anesthesiologists, nurses, and may include other stakeholders, such as physical therapists, occupational therapists, and care coordinators. This team will then set goals and priorities, review existing evidence-based guidelines and literature, identify concerns for

L. Gu · J. Liu · A. T. Machi (✉)
Anesthesiology, Perioperative and Pain Medicine, Stanford Medicine, Stanford, CA, USA
e-mail: lisa.gu@utsouthwestern.edu; amachi@stanford.edu

C. E. Noe (ed.), *Musculoskeletal Pain*,
https://doi.org/10.1007/978-3-031-86057-7_22

design and implementation, and identify existing resources. The next step is creating a pathway that is service and institution specific that meets the core tenets of enhanced recovery protocols: preoperative medical optimization, nutrition screening and support, patient education, prophylaxis against venous thromboembolism, infection and postoperative nausea and vomiting, comprehensive analgesia, maintenance of homeostasis, early mobilization, restoration of postoperative alimentation, and early discharge from the hospital. Following this, support must be garnered from leadership and additional stakeholders, and users must be educated. The protocol and corresponding pathway may then be implemented for patient care and systems created to collect data, audit, and analyze protocol elements and patient outcomes. Data collection and cyclical review and revision are crucial to the success of enhanced recovery programs.

How Does Perioperative Pain Management Fit into an Enhanced Recovery Protocol?

The analgesic process begins with a preoperative evaluation for the pain experience screening through a strategic assessment that considers the following questions:

1. How much pain is anticipated from the surgery, for how long, and where is the pain?
2. What are the specific postoperative functional goals to facilitate?
3. Will the patient be ambulatory or hospitalized following surgery?
4. Can regional anesthesia be utilized?
5. Does the patient have specific baseline pain modifying considerations, such as:
    (a) Advanced age
    (b) Mental health disorder: anxiety, depression, substance use, post-traumatic stress disorder (PTSD)
    (c) History of pain: chronic, neuropathic, nociplastic
    (d) Opioid tolerance, or central sensitization
    (e) Pain catastrophizing
6. Are there any contraindications to any of the treatments or techniques? [13, 14]

Analgesic elements begin presurgery with multimodal analgesia via oral medication and regional analgesia, continue intraoperatively with intravenous medications and the application of local anesthetics via local infiltration, peripheral blockade, or neuraxial blockade, and continue in the postoperative period with multimodal analgesia by all suitable means to provide the most comfort while incurring the least side effects and permitting the patient to engage in rehabilitation as soon as possible. Newer modalities, such as cryoneurolysis or percutaneous peripheral nerve stimulation (pPNS), may play important roles for longer duration perioperative pain management in the near future. The cornerstones of the approach are the rational selection of pain mechanism specific medications and the strategic use of peripheral and central neural blockade. Because perioperative pain results from a variety of mechanisms: nociception, inflammation, and nerve injury with subsequent neurohumoral physiological consequences: peripheral and central sensitization, transcriptional and post-transcriptional dysregulation, augmented facilitation, structural organization, and disinhibition, multimodal analgesia provides an approach capable of addressing the distinct analgesic requirements of the perioperative patient [15, 16]. Specific medications that are recommended and will be described in detail include acetaminophen, nonsteroidal anti-inflammatory medications, steroids, local anesthetics, opioids, and ketamine. Additional medications that may be considered include gabapentinoids, muscle relaxants, and alpha-2-agonists. Finally, recommended techniques that will be covered include perineural blockade, neuraxial blockade, cryoanalgesia, peripheral neuromodulation, transcutaneous electrical nerve stimulation, acupuncture, and nonpharmacologic nonphysical interventions, such as pain management education and counseling, meditation, and music therapy.

Foundation

The International Association for the Study of Pain (IASP) has been describing pain since the 1970s. The most recent 2018 update defines pain as "an unpleasant sensory and emotional experience associated with or resembling that associated with actual or potential tissue damage" [17]. While a focus on blunting nociceptive and augmenting antinociceptive pathways is most important within the context of perioperative pain management, it is necessary to maintain the value of the "emotional experience" that should be addressed with both pharmacologic and nonpharmacologic methods as well. A full discussion of the emotional experience is beyond the scope of this chapter. Instead, the next sections will discuss multimodal analgesia as a strategy to diminish nociception and augment antinociception. Multimodal analgesia is an effective way to target perioperative pain by using various classes of medications via various routes of administration, to target different receptors while maximizing benefits and minimizing risks. By using a thoughtful combination of multimodal analgesia, we aim to decrease pain, minimize side effects, improve the patient's recovery trajectory, and reduce the uniquely harmful side effects associated with perioperative opioid therapy. Once implemented, the multimodal analgesia approach is refined on an individual basis through reassessment of pain using validated tools that distinguish the severity of pain, its impact on functional recovery, and assessment of any side effects that may arise. Treatments are then adjusted to address patients' evolving needs [13].

Acetaminophen

Acetaminophen is a medication that has been in use since the late 1800s [18]. It crosses the blood-brain barrier and has analgesic and antipyretic properties. When given in appropriate doses, it is efficacious, safe, well-tolerated, widely available, and inexpensive. A single preoperative dose of intravenous acetaminophen 1000 mg is associated with an approximate decrease of 10 mg IV morphine equivalents and is associated with a reduction in postoperative nausea and vomiting with a number needed to treat (NNT) of 3.3 [19]. Intraoperative and postoperative administration of acetaminophen similarly decrease postoperative pain at 4–6 h after surgery with an NNT of 3.6 to achieve a 50% pain reduction and elimination of treatment of breakthrough pain [20–22]. While acetaminophen's definite mechanism is yet to be elucidated, many likely target receptors have been identified.

Though acetaminophen has been used clinically for over 50 years, its mechanism of action is unknown. It may exert its clinical effect at several different receptors in different pain pathways, and numerous potential receptor targets have been identified. Acetaminophen weakly inhibits central COX-1 and COX-2. However, unlike nonsteroidal ant-inflammatory medications (NSAIDs), its anti-inflammatory effects are weak at best and do not cause any of the systemic side effects associated with NSAIDs because the COX inhibition is central, rather than peripheral [23]. Acetaminophen upregulates endogenous cannabinoids both centrally and peripherally, and its metabolite N-acylphenolamine is an agonist for the vanilloid receptor TRPV1 [24, 25]. Acetaminophen may also upregulate serotonin to reinforce the descending serotonergic pain inhibition pathways.

The most effective dose for acetaminophen is 15 mg/kg up to 1000 mg every 8 h [19, 20, 23]. This typically translates to a plasma concentration of 10–20 mcg/mL. Acetaminophen (paracetamol; N-acetyl-p-aminophenol) is well-absorbed from oral administration with oral bioavailability estimated between 63% and 89% in adults [23]. It is metabolized by the liver, via glucuronidation and sulphation to form nontoxic metabolites which are then excreted in the urine. A small amount is oxidized by cytochrome P450 enzymes to N-acetyl-p-benzoquinone imine (NAPQI), which reacts with and can deplete hepatic glutathione. Excessive amounts of acetaminophen can lead to acute hepatic failure by this mechanism. N-acetyl-cysteine reverses acetaminophen toxicity. Hepatotoxicity is thought to occur at plasma concentrations of 150–200 mcg/mL, which is approximately ten times the therapeutic dose [23, 26]. This is usually reflective of at least 10–12 mg of oral acetaminophen. By limiting the total 24 h dose to 3 gm in adults, patients should be well within the safety window. Caution should be taken in calculating total daily acetaminophen dose when combination medications are utilized in addition to acetaminophen by itself (e.g., oxycodone with acetaminophen). Acetaminophen metabolism is reduced in patients who are malnourished, elderly, and with liver cirrhosis, so additional caution should be exercised in these patient populations [27]. While a tight dose response relationship has not been clearly shown for acetaminophen, improved analgesia seems to occur up to a dose of 1000 mg or 15 mg/kg, and not beyond it [19, 20]. Doses as low as 5 mg/kg may be utilized if given intravenously [28]. Scheduled acetaminophen (e.g., 1 g every 8 h) can be a helpful addition to perioperative multimodal analgesia, both to decrease opioid requirement and to decrease pain scores.

Acetaminophen is available both as oral and IV formulations. IV formulation provides faster peak serum and cerebrospinal fluid (CSF) concentration and is more bioavailable since it bypasses first-pass hepatic metabolization [29]. Oral acetaminophen is rapidly absorbed by the duodenum, achieving peak plasma concentrations within 1–2 h [23, 30]. Clinically, oral administration provides equianalgesic effects compared to IV administrations and is usually much less expensive [31, 32]. IV formulation is an excellent alternative for patients unable to take oral medications. Acetaminophen is also available as rectal suppositories, which has less predictable absorption; higher doses around 35–40 mg/kg may be needed for adequate serum concentration [23, 33].

In the perioperative patient population, most patients would benefit from and can tolerate oral acetaminophen 15 mg/kg up to 1 gm immediately before surgery followed by postoperative scheduled acetaminophen 15 mg/kg up to 1 gm every 8 h. For moderate to severe pain, scheduled acetaminophen will not be adequate as a sole analgesic agent but remains a cornerstone component of multimodal postoperative analgesia upon which additional medications and modalities may be added.

Nonsteroidal Ant-inflammatory Medications

NSAIDS are a class of widely used, structurally heterogeneous medications that reversibly inhibit cyclooxygenase enzymes, which in turn prevents the synthesis of prostaglandins and prostacyclin from arachidonic acid. This results in analgesic, anti-inflammatory, and antipyretic effects [34–38]. Additionally, they can reduce perioperative opioid consumption and opioid-related side effects. Most NSAIDs block both COX-1 and COX-2. COX-1 is thought to, in part, provide protective prostaglandins in the gastric mucosa, and inhibition is thought to increase gastrointestinal complications. Although celecoxib is a widely available selective COX-2 inhibitor, other selective COX-2 inhibitors were removed from the market in the United States in the mid-2000s because of association with a potential increased risk of myocardial infarction (MI) and stroke [39].

NSAIDs exert their clinical effect by impacting prostanoid synthesis [40]. This begins with the release of arachidonic acid from the phospholipid membrane of cells in response to inflammatory mediators and active acyl hydrolases. Arachidonic acid is a polyunsaturated fatty acid present in cell membranes throughout the body. Following its release, arachidonic acid is converted to prostaglandin G2 and then prostaglandin H2 by the sequential cyclooxygenase and hydroperoxidase actions of the two isoforms of the cyclooxygenase enzymes, COX-1 and COX-2. PGH2 then takes different pathways leading to the production of thromboxane A2 and other prostaglandins, such as PGE2, PGI2, and PGD2. The prostanoids are then released outside the cell after intracellular biosynthesis and act locally in an autocrine or paracrine fashion. These prostaglandins then sensitize local pain receptors to mechanical and chemical stimulation by lowering the threshold of polymodal nociceptors of C fibers. While COX-1 has roles in regulating normal cell processes, COX-2 is normally expressed at low levels unless triggered by inflammatory mediators. NSAIDs exert their effect on COX enzymes by competitively inhibiting the active sites of the enzymes, which ultimately leads to their analgesic effects.

NSAIDs are clinically shown to decrease pain and opioid requirements after surgery [41–43]. Analgesia from NSAIDs is dose dependent, and the lowest effective dose is recommended for initiation of use. While there are many different NSAIDs to choose from, commonly available medications for oral and IV administration in the perioperative period with NNT between 1.6 and 3 for at least 50% acute pain relief over 4–6 h include: ibuprofen 400–600 mg PO every 6–8 h, celecoxib 200–400 mg PO every 12 h, diclofenac 50–100 mg PO every 8–12 h, meloxicam 7.5–15 mg PO daily, and ketorolac 15–30 mg IV every 6 h [43, 44]. When used with acetaminophen, they provide more pain relief and decreased opioid requirements than each alone [41]. These low NNTs indicate that NSAIDs are some of the most effective treatments for acute perioperative pain. Strong evidence of analgesic efficacy for one NSAID over another is lacking. Rather, medication selection may be driven by the selectivity of inhibition of COX-1 versus COX-2, the resultant side effect profile, and the desired route of administration. Whichever NSAID is chosen should be scheduled around the clock to optimize efficacy.

Despite their utility, the administration of NSAIDs may be limited by several clinically relevant adverse effects in certain patient populations that depend on the degree of alteration of various aspects of the COX pathway: inhibition of platelet aggregation, impairment of renal function, effects on bone healing, gastric mucosa injury, gastrointestinal anastomotic wound healing, and cardiovascular events. These effects can be significant enough to cause nephrotoxicity and gastric and small bowel mucosal injuries. To reduce risk of injury, the lowest effective dose should be selected, and the duration should be limited to the time of greatest utility. For example, gastrointestinal (GI) bleeding was found to be trivially increased with perioperative IV ketorolac unless therapy was extended beyond 5 days [45]. Nonselective NSAIDs mildly inhibit platelet aggregation, which may limit their use in surgical patient populations with open vascular beds or associated with large blood loss [46].

Surgical bleeding associated with perioperative NSAID administration is a controversial topic and concerns for bleeding may hinder the routine use of NSAIDs in perioperative multimodal analgesic regimens. Nonselective NSAIDs reversibly block COX-1, which is responsible for the synthesis of thromboxane A1 from arachidonic acid. Thromboxane A1 mediates platelet activation [47]. However, in most patients without coexisting coagulation deficiencies, NSAID-induced platelet dysfunction does not result in any clinically significant bleeding [45]. Overall, there is little evidence to suggest a significant association between perioperative NSAID use and increased postoperative bleeding in patients [48]. However, it is prudent to evaluate NSAID administration in high bleeding risk surgeries on a case-by-case basis.

In the kidney, prostaglandins promote vasodilation and subsequent renal perfusion, acting as a counterbalance to the renin-angiotensin-aldosterone system [49]. NSAIDs, by reducing prostaglandin synthesis, can reduce renal perfusion, leading to acute renal injury [50]. Additionally, NSAIDs use can result in acute interstitial nephritis, the etiology of which is still unclear but may have a hypersensitivity component [49]. Furthermore, prostaglandins are involved in the renal regulation of sodium reabsorption and potassium secretion, with the role more pronounced in patients with limited renal perfusion [51]. In these patients, NSAIDs can lead to sodium reabsorption, fluid retention, and potentially hyperkalemia. Meta-analyses suggest that in patients with normal renal function, a clinically unimportant, transient decrease in renal function may be seen, but NSAIDs are overall safe in this patient population [52]. However, in patients who are predisposed to renal injury—those with preexisting renal disease, advanced age, hepatic disease, and renal medication use including diuretics, Angiotensin-Converting Enzyme (ACE) inhibitors, and angiotensin receptor blockers—caution should be applied with NSAID use.

NSAIDs have been shown to delay bone healing in animal models, potentially by inhibiting the inflammation that initiate fracture healing, decreasing osteoblast proliferation, and reducing collagen expression [53, 54]. If these animal studies findings were reflective of clinical NSAID use in humans, then NSAID use would be of concern in many orthopedic and spine surgeries. However, clinical studies overwhelmingly do not suggest problems with bone healing, particularly with short-term NSAID therapy in the acute postoperative period [55–57].

Although NSAIDs are associated with small increases in cardiovascular risk with chronic use, such as an increased incidence of ischemic and thrombotic events and heart failure due to COX-2 inhibition of vasodilatory prostaglandins, leading to thrombosis, these risks have not been seen for acute perioperative use [58–60].

In patients without a contraindication to NSAID use, preoperative celecoxib 400 mg, followed by postoperative scheduled celecoxib 200 mg every 12 h, is a recommended regimen. Meloxicam 15 mg is a good alternative to celecoxib for patients with sulfa allergy (subsequent doses of 7.5 mg scheduled daily). Alternatively, IV ketorolac 15–30 mg at the end of the surgery after hemostasis is achieved, followed by scheduled postoperative ibuprofen 400 mg or IV ketorolac 15–30 mg every 6–8 h are other recommended options.

Local Anesthetics

The local anesthetic properties of the coca leaf have been used for centuries by indigenous South American people to numb painful parts of the body. Cocaine was first isolated from the coca leaf in 1860, and in the decades to follow, desire to synthesize new local anesthetics with better safety profiles and less addictive properties led to the discovery of procaine in 1904, lidocaine in 1943, and mepivacaine and bupivacaine in 1957 [61]. Now, local anesthetics are widely available, inexpensive, well-tolerated medications that have a wide array of delivery methods to provide perioperative analgesia. Typical delivery methods include surgical field infiltration, topical (e.g., EMLA cream, benzocaine topical spray), transdermal (e.g., lidocaine patch), parenteral (e.g., IV lidocaine), and via regional anesthesia methods (perineural, interfascial, epidural, and intrathecal). Additional discussions of regional anesthesia will be in subsequent sections.

Local anesthetics block sodium channels within an axon, thereby producing a reversible neural conduction block, interrupting impulse propagation. The local anesthetic molecule consists of a hydrophobic aromatic ring and a hydrophilic tertiary amine. The bond between the two structures contains either amide or ester bonds, which define the two local anesthetic categories: amides and esters [40, 62]. Clinically in the USA, amides are more commonly used than esters. Commonly used amides include lidocaine, mepivacaine, bupivacaine, and ropivacaine. Commonly used esters include chloroprocaine, tetracaine, cocaine, and benzocaine. Esters are broken down by plasma esterases, and amides are metabolized by the liver.

Many of the important properties of local anesthetics are defined by their lipid solubility, protein binding, and pKa. Highly lipophilic molecules can diffuse into nerves more readily, resulting in denser block, thus, greater potency. Local anesthetics with more protein binding properties result in longer duration. Local anesthetics are weak bases. The ionized local anesthetic molecules bind to sodium channels. Therefore, the lower the pKa of the local anesthetic (i.e., closer to physiologic pH), the faster the onset. The increased difference between the local anesthetic pKa mixture and physiologic pH accounts for the decreased efficacy of local anesthetic in acidic, infected tissue. In a similar vein, the addition of sodium bicarbonate can hasten local anesthetic onset.

Epinephrine is often added to local anesthetics as a vasoconstrictor. This decreases vascular absorption of the local anesthetic, increasing the duration of action and decreasing risk of local anesthetic systemic toxicity (LAST). A secondary but important mechanism of action for perioperative pain is that local anesthetics appear to have anti-inflammatory properties by modulating the response of some inflammatory cells, such as polymorphonuclear granulocytes and macrophages [63].

Local anesthetics at high enough doses can exert toxic effects on the CNS and cardiac conduction. Mild LAST symptoms can manifest as altered mental status, perioral numbness, tinnitus, and agitation, whereas severe symptoms include seizures, cardiac dysrhythmias, and cardiac arrest. Treatment involves immediate cessation of local anesthetic administration, IV 20% lipid emulsion, airway support, effective resuscitation, benzodiazepines to control seizures, and modified Advanced Cardiac Life Support (ACLS) if cardiac arrest or hemodynamically significant cardiac dysrhythmia have occurred [64]. LAST should always be on the differential if a patient has unexpected neurologic or hemodynamic changes after the administration of local anesthetic [65].

Local anesthetics can also cause dose- and time-dependent myotoxicity and neurotoxicity [66]. Local anesthetic exposure to myocytes leads to disruption of calcium release and influx, which appears to result in mitochondrial uncoupling and cell death [67]. Myotoxicity has been well described in patients receiving ophthalmic blocks for eye surgery, but has also been documented in patients receiving interscalene blocks, adductor canal blocks, and trigger point injections. The mechanism for local anesthetic associated neurotoxicity is less clear with multiple proposed subcellular pathways [66]. While permanent injury from solely local anesthetic associated myotoxicity and neurotoxicity are rare, care should be taken to avoid injecting high-dose local anesthetics into muscle, and caution exercised with continuous infusions prolonging time-exposure. Overall, using lower concentration local anesthetics may mitigate the risk of myotoxicity and neurotoxicity.

Liposomal Local Anesthetic

Currently there is only one widely used FDA-approved liposomal local anesthetic, that is, liposomal bupivacaine (Exparel; Pacira Pharmaceuticals). Liposomal bupivacaine uses multivesicular liposomes to encapsulate bupivacaine and slowly release its contents over multiple days as the lipid membranes break down. It is used for single injection only. It is currently FDA approved for local surgical site infiltration (including field and plane blocks) and specific nerve blocks including interscalene brachial plexus block, adductor canal block and sciatic nerve block in the popliteal fossa. Current published studies on the postoperative pain scores and opioid consumption comparing liposomal bupivacaine versus unencapsulated bupivacaine with or without adjuncts result in heterogeneous conclusions. Meta-analyses of these studies overall do not find clinically relevant benefits of liposomal bupivacaine over plain bupivacaine [68–70]. Therefore, there is no current recommendation of using liposomal bupivacaine over unencapsulated bupivacaine with or without adjuncts.

When using liposomal bupivacaine, care must be taken to avoid the early release of the encapsulated bupivacaine which could precipitate LAST. This involves limiting the mixture of liposomal bupivacaine to only plain bupivacaine in a 2:1 ratio, avoiding additional concomitant local anesthetic administration, waiting for antiseptics like chlorhexidine to dry before administering liposomal bupivacaine, and counseling patients on avoiding additional local anesthetics in the upcoming days.

Surgical Field Infiltration

Infiltrating the surgical site is one of the easiest, safest, and quickest techniques to administer local anesthetics for postoperative analgesia [71]. However, the analgesic effect of infiltration with plain ropivacaine or bupivacaine only lasts approximately half a day and is limited by infiltration technique. Many adjuncts have been evaluated to prolong or augment the analgesic effect of local anesthetic infiltration, and alpha-2 agonists and dexamethasone probably are the most efficacious with low side effect profiles [72]. Periarticular local anesthetic infiltration is popular among many orthopedic joint surgeons either to complement or to replace regional anesthesia, and many "cocktails" have been described, often including epinephrine, morphine, and ketorolac in addition to long-acting local anesthetic [73]. Some surgeons choose to place wound catheters with continuous local anesthetic infusions, which has been shown to decrease pain and opioid consumption in certain surgeries involving laparotomies and sternotomies, but are contraindicated for articular infusion due to the risk of chondrolysis [74–76]. Additionally, others choose to use liposomal bupivacaine, although there is a lack of evidence of its analgesic benefit over plain bupivacaine [69, 77, 78]. Surgical infiltration with a reduced dose of local anesthetic should be considered if the patient has recently received local anesthetics via any other method of administration as local anesthetics from all sources contribute to the maximum total systemic local anesthetic dose.

IV Lidocaine

Lidocaine was synthesized in 1943 as a quick onset local anesthetic with relatively low toxicity compared to the existing options [79]. Intravenous lidocaine was used starting in the 1980s to treat neuropathic pain. IV lidocaine infusions are often used intraoperatively and sometimes postoperatively as part of multimodal analgesia. However, how IV lidocaine infusions provide clinically significant analgesia in the early postoperative period is less clear, although potential mechanisms have been identified [80, 81].

Like all local anesthetics, lidocaine blocks voltage-gated sodium channels, including those throughout the nervous system. Systemic lidocaine, however, also appears to have N-methyl-D-aspartate (NMDA) inhibitory effects and anti-inflammatory properties [82]. IV lidocaine infusions were shown to decrease inflammatory cytokine levels in patients undergoing laparoscopic cholecystectomies [81]. Lidocaine likely affects gene transcription to inhibit pro-inflammatory molecules while upregulating anti-inflammatory mediators [83].

The best evidence for lidocaine's impact on perioperative analgesia is with laparoscopic and open abdominal surgery, genitourinary surgery, major spine surgery, and thoracic surgery [84, 85]. IV lidocaine is typically given as a loading dose of up to 1.5 mg/kg and infused at 1.5 mg/kg/h of ideal body weight (unless underweight, then actual body weight should be used with avoidance in patients <40 kg) [86]. The therapeutic index is low, and vigilance must be maintained to watch for signs of local anesthetic systemic toxicity. For use outside the operating room, telemetry in a monitored area is recommended and resuscitation equipment and trained staff should be available. Caution should be used in patients with hepatic impairment, acidemia, hypoxemia, and hypoalbuminemia since these patients may be at increased risk for toxicity at lower doses. Additionally, after 12 h of infusion, plasma levels may continue to increase disproportionately to the infusion amount, so caution should be taken for long-term infusions. Some experts suggest decreasing half or even discontinue the infusion, after 24 h to mitigate this risk [86]. IV lidocaine infusions should not be routinely administered to most postoperative patients, but for those with severe pain and unable to have local anesthetic application by infiltration or regional blockade, it can be a useful addition to a robust multimodal regimen.

Topical and Transdermal Local Anesthetic

Using topical or transdermal local anesthetics avoids the discomfort and potentially anatomical distortion of local anesthetic injections. Mucosa generally allows for easy absorption of local anesthetics, but keratinized skin, particularly the stratum corneum, resists penetration. Topical and transdermal local anesthetics depend on their ability to penetrate the skin or mucosa and target the localized nerve endings. Ability to penetrate the mucosa or skin barrier depends on local anesthetic lipophilicity, concentration, time of exposure, and carriers [87]. For example, EMLA cream is an emulsion of 2.5% lidocaine and 2.5% prilocaine in a low melting point oil mixture (eutectic mixture). The cream is applied on intact skin and sealed with an occlusive dressing for 1–3 h to achieve desired level of analgesia [88].

Most single applications of topical local anesthetics do not provide prolonged analgesia and are usually used as procedural analgesia (e.g., prior to intravenous cannulation). However, transdermal lidocaine patches have been successfully used to decrease postoperative pain scores up to 48 h after surgery in certain settings, although their effect on early postoperative opioid consumption is not significant [89]. Lidocaine patches seem to provide better analgesia when applied directly to the incision site. Postoperative patients who are not receiving local anesthetic by other means may benefit from lidocaine patches next to or on the incision site if those do not interfere with surgical healing.

Perineural Blockade

Peripheral nerve blocks allow for selective analgesia of certain areas of the body. They typically involve injection of local anesthetic perineurally, within interfascial planes, or in certain spaces where nerves reside like the paravertebral space. Peripheral nerve blocks are typically performed as single injections or delivered via continuous catheter infusions. When performed for postoperative analgesia, long-acting local anesthetics like ropivacaine or bupivacaine are usually selected. Plain ropivacaine or bupivacaine blocks typically last 12–20 h. Adjuvants like dexamethasone or dexmedetomidine can extend the duration of analgesia, dexamethasone for an additional 4–6 h and dexmedetomidine for 4–5 h [90]. With the addition of liposomal bupivacaine (only FDA-approved for local surgical site infiltration, including field and plane blocks, and specific nerve blocks at this time), there is potential increase of analgesia to 24 h and beyond. Continuous catheter infusions can provide prolonged analgesia for multiple days. With vigilant attention and care to avoid infection, peripheral catheters can be run for up to 7 days (or even beyond in select circumstances) [91, 92]. These are particularly helpful in surgeries where prolonged duration of pain is expected (e.g., amputation) or those where staged surgeries over multiple days are expected. Additionally, continuous peripheral nerve blocks can utilize sophisticated pumps that allow for patient-controlled boluses with lockout on top of a clinician-adjustable basal rate. Some studies have also looked at using programmed intermittent boluses (PIB) instead of continuous infusions, and, while results are heterogeneous, analgesic or local anesthetic-reducing benefits have sometimes been found [93, 94]. More research is needed to determine which perineural or fascial plane targets benefit the most and whether managing the potentially more complicated pumps is worth the benefit [93, 95]. Peripheral nerve catheters are often more resource- and labor-intensive than single injection blocks and can be more technically challenging with additional complications including secondary block failure, catheter migration, and pump malfunction [90].

Commonly performed peripheral blocks include:

Upper extremity: brachial plexus, terminal nerves of the brachial plexus, and intercostobrachial nerve

Lower extremity: femoral nerve (or branches thereof such as adductor canal), sciatic nerve (or branches thereof), obturator nerve, lateral femoral cutaneous nerve, fascia iliaca, lumbar plexus, and pericapsular nerve group (PENG)

Truncal: serratus anterior plane, PECS I/II, erector spinae, transversus abdominis plane, rectus sheath, quadratus lumborum, and thoracic paravertebral

Peripheral blocks are typically well-tolerated and do not cause hemodynamic perturbations. Depending on the complexity and depth of the block, patients with coagulopathies and anticoagulation can potentially receive blocks with caution. Regional anesthesia should be considered in most extremity or truncal surgeries with expected moderate to severe pain including many orthopedic and spine surgeries. Reasons to avoid regional anesthesia include patient refusal or if the regional anesthesia technique will interfere with the surgery or surgical recovery (e.g., local anesthetic distortion of surgical field, nerve block masking surgical nerve injury, and nerve block delaying detection of pain associated with acute compartment syndrome). Complications such as infection, nerve injury, serious catheter related issues, and local anesthetic systemic toxicity are rare [92].

Neuraxial Blockade

Neuraxial blockade involves either medication delivery into the intrathecal space or the epidural space. Typical medications include local anesthetics and opioids. Epidurals for perioperative analgesia typically involve an infusion of longer acting local anesthetic, such as bupivacaine, with or without low dose opioids—typically a lipophilic opioid like fentanyl or sufentanil. The infusion is delivered via an automated pump. Depending on the circumstances and resources, patient-controlled epidural analgesia may be a good option, allowing patients to self-deliver an additional bolus on top of basal infusion with a lockout. In the laboring obstetric population, epidurals with scheduled programmed intermittent boluses (PIB) instead of continuous infusions have shown to provide better analgesia [96]. However, the benefit of epidurals with PIB over continuous epidurals with patient-controlled epidural analgesia (PCEA) for the non-obstetric postoperative patient is not clear [97].

Examples of epidural infusions include 0.0625–0.125% bupivacaine with fentanyl 2 mcg/ml running at 6 mL/h basal rate with 2 mL PCEA as needed every 20 min and 0.2% ropivacaine with fentanyl 2 mcg/ml running at 8 mL/h basal rate with 4 mL PCEA as needed every hour.

Neuraxial local anesthetics provide not only sensory blockade but also motor and sympathetic blockade. Depending on the density and location of the blockade these effects may be undesirable as patients may experience lower extremity weakness, urinary retention, or hypotension (particularly in hypovolemic patients). By using more dilute local anesthetics, the density of motor and sympathetic blockade can be reduced; however, this also reduces the sensory blockade, so patients may have more breakthrough pain. Opioids are synergistic with neuraxial local anesthetic allowing for lower doses of local anesthetic to provide the same level of analgesia. This can allow a reduction in local anesthetic concentration, reducing the undesired effects of profound sympathetic and motor blockade.

Overall, neuraxial techniques for postoperative analgesia have somewhat waned in popularity due to a variety of factors. With the increasing predominance of minimally invasive surgical techniques, such as laparoscopy and robotic assisted techniques, over open surgeries, the discovery of various fascial plane blocks and motor sparing peripheral nerve blocks, and the growing enthusiasm of surgeons infiltrating their surgical site with long-acting local anesthetics, resource- and time-intensive epidurals and their side effects have become less popular. In surgical populations for which epidurals were previously considered gold standard, like those undergoing open colorectal surgeries, or even quite useful, such as total hip arthroplasty, newer studies suggest that other modalities, including other regional anesthesia techniques, can provide clinically equivalent analgesia and postoperative outcomes [98–100]. Previously noted benefits of epidurals for decreasing postoperative respiratory complications and postoperative ileus have become less clear with improvements in surgical technique, better postoperative physical therapy, and pulmonary rehab, and updates in perioperative medication regimen [101]. However, in certain surgical patient populations, like those undergoing open liver resections, open esophagectomies, open thoracotomy, open pancreatectomies, cytoreductive surgery with hyperthermic intraoperative chemotherapy, and large multilevel spine fusions, such as T10-pelvis fusion, epidural analgesia ranges from beneficial to highly recommended [102–109].

Steroids

Corticosteroids provide analgesia in the perioperative setting by modulating the inflammation and neuroendocrine stress response to tissue injury that contribute to postoperative pain. Steroids modulate this response via various pathways including the inhibition of transcription of proinflammatory mediators, inhibition of the cyclooxygenase pathway, and inhibition of the synthesis of cytokines and inflammatory mediators at the site of tissue injury [110, 111]. These inflammatory agents activate peripheral nociceptive receptors on peripheral primary afferent sensory nerves [112]. Reducing their production decreases the signals transmitted to the neurons of the dorsal column of the spinal cord. Thus, decreased signals are projected along central ascending pathways to many other sensory processing areas including the thalamus, hypothalamus, and somatosensory cortex. At higher central nervous system locations, such as the hypothalamus and pituitary, glucocorticoids again inhibit nociception via reduced levels of cytokines and inflammatory mediators [113]. In addition to their analgesic effect, they more generally attenuate early organ dysfunction mediated by the neuroendocrine, inflammatory, and immunological surgical stress response that manifests in a multitude of adverse effects, including postoperative nausea and vomiting, swelling, fatigue, delirium, and weakness [114]. Consequently, they play an important role in many ERAS protocols.

Dexamethasone, a long-acting, nonparticulate glucocorticoid, is frequently studied as the prototypical perioperative corticosteroid. Dexamethasone has a high-level of glucocorticoid and hence anti-inflammatory activity without mineralocorticoid activity, in contrast to other steroids. Additionally, it is nonparticulate, cheap, and widely available. The optimal intravenous single dose for perioperative analgesia is unknown, but studies indicate that it is likely at least 0.1 mg/kg but less than 0.2 mg/kg [115, 116]. Dexamethasone may also be administered as an adjuvant to local anesthetic to prolong duration of perineural blockade [117]. In the orthopedic population, patients undergoing total shoulder, total knee and total hip arthroplasty had better pain control and less opioid requirements with perioperative steroids than without [118, 119]. Increased analgesic benefit after total knee arthroplasty, particularly with quadriceps flexion, was associated with higher dose dexamethasone (16 mg compared to 8 mg) [120]. In the total knee arthroplasty population, two doses of dexamethasone 24 h apart extended the analgesic benefit to 48 h [121]. Because steroids exert a significant portion of their effect by crossing the cell membrane and affecting gene transcription, they can take an hour or two to take effect and cause a longer duration of action [40, 122]. Administering dexamethasone at the beginning of surgery allows time for the inflammatory-modulating effect. Thus, many anesthesiologists prefer to administer dexamethasone immediately after induction of anesthesia.

Concerns regarding perioperative steroid use include steroid-induced hyperglycemia, poor wound healing, and risk of infection. While steroid-induced hyperglycemia is transient and typically not clinically relevant in most patients receiving perioperative steroids (causing hyperglycemia in patients with and without diabetes when given perioperatively—by 13 and 32 mg/dl, respectively), those with poorly controlled or brittle diabetes mellitus may be better served with reduced steroid doses with careful postoperative glucose monitoring and treatment [123]. Perioperative steroids do not increase the risk of delayed wound healing or postoperative infections, although high-risk patients may have been excluded from some studies [116, 123, 124]. In addition, a very large multicenter prospective randomized controlled trial (RCT) found no association of intraoperative dexamethasone IV 8 mg with surgical site infection [125]. Additional steroid side effects that can be problematic with chronic administration, but that do not appear to be problematic in the perioperative short-term setting include: Cushing's syndrome, osteoporosis, myopathy, cataract formation, glaucoma, gastrointestinal effects such as stomach ulcer formation, cardiovascular effects such as hypertension, leukocytosis, psychologic effects such as psychosis and skin changes [126].

Most patients should receive at least 0.1 mg/kg or 8 mg of IV dexamethasone at induction of general anesthesia. Patients with brittle or poorly controlled diabetes may be better served with a reduced dose. For patients undergoing total joint replacements, an additional 8 mg of dexamethasone on postoperative day 1 may be beneficial.

Opioids

Humans have been treating pain with opioids for millennia. Opium, derived from the poppy, *Papaver somniferum*, was isolated by the Sumerians almost 5000 years ago and was used to provide surgical analgesia before the advent of general anesthetics in the mid-1800s. The first clear, documented use of opium as an ingredient in laudanum to treat postoperative pain was recorded in the late 1700s [127]. Morphine was isolated from opium in the early 1800s, initially as an oral formulation, and became popularized with subcutaneous and intravenous delivery. Subsequent opioid discoveries included heroin in 1898, meperidine in 1939, methadone in 1946, and fentanyl in 1959 [128]. Opiates are an even larger group of compounds comprising opioids as well as semisynthetic and synthetic compounds that act as ligands at opioid receptors [40]. Opioids are commonly used for the treatment of moderate to severe surgical pain and are a standard medication for perioperative analgesia due to their profound analgesic effects [129–131]. They range in analgesic potency from relatively weak to very potent. While opioids do not have a ceiling effect for analgesia, they are associated with numerous severe and non-severe side effects that limit their clinical efficacy and utility including respiratory depression and sedation. Moreover, they are associated with the relatively rapid development of tolerance and hyperalgesia [132, 133]. In addition, they cause euphoria and tranquility, which may lead to reward-seeking behavior in some individuals, and have led to a crisis in the United States of opioid addiction, opioid misuse, opioid abuse, and opioid-related overdose deaths [134, 135]. The addictive properties of opioids have been known for centuries if not millennia. Many of the opioid discoveries were at least in part fueled by the desire to find effective analgesics with less addictive properties. In the United States, the Harrison Narcotics Act of 1914 was the first federal attempt at regulating opium, morphine, heroin, and cocaine as part of a worldwide effort to regulate the opium trade [136]. In the 1980s–1990s, there was concern about the under-treatment of pain. In response, the American Pain Society's "pain as a fifth vital sign" initiative in 1995 and subsequent to the Joint Commission's increased emphasis on pain assessments in 2000, in conjunction with the development of oxycodone in 1996, and its subsequent heavy marketing led to liberalization of prescription opioid use. Unfortunately, this aggressive pendulum swing led to increased opioid-related adverse events and is widely thought to have heralded the current epidemic of opioid addiction, misuse, and overdose. Specifically, in the surgical population, of concern is the development of persistent postoperative opioid use (of which the definition widely varies but is often defined as prescription opioid use between 90 and 180 days after surgery). Meta-analyses have found that this ranges from 0.01% to 26% for opioid-naïve patients, and up to 77% for patients exposed to opioids preoperatively [137, 138]. Since the mid-2010s, attempts to correct the errors of the recent past have most clinicians reducing the amount of opioids used in the perioperative setting and restricting the amount patients are prescribed after discharge for postoperative pain. While the most serious opioid-related adverse events include respiratory depression and oversedation, opioids can cause other undesired side effects, like bowel dysfunction, constipation, nausea and vomiting, pruritus, opioid-induced hyperalgesia, and euphoria.

Nevertheless, opioids remain a vital component of perioperative analgesia. Opioids may be administered by many routes: oral, sublingual, intravenous, intramuscular, subcutaneous, neuraxial, and transdermal [139]. Perioperative administration tends to be oral, intravenous, and neuraxial, owing to favorable bioavailability and pharmacodynamic relationships. The intravenous route may also be used in the postoperative period for patient-controlled analgesia (PCA), which permits rapid administration, compensates for interpatient variability in analgesic needs, and relies on a negative feedback loop to provide safety from respiratory depression and sedation [140]. PCAs are particularly useful when hospitalized patients are unable to take analgesics by other routes, though the negative feedback loop may be violated and appropriate monitoring is required [13]. Morphine, hydromorphone, and fentanyl are the most common intravenous opioids for intraoperative analgesia and in the post-anesthesia care unit, while sufentanil, alfentanil, and remifentanil are three rapid, short acting opioids that can be useful for intraoperative analgesia. In the postoperative period, a transition is often made to oral opioids with a longer duration of action including tramadol, hydrocodone, and oxycodone. Common intraoperative doses are morphine 0.025–0.15 mg/kg, hydromorphone 0.01–0.02 mg/kg, and fentanyl 1–2 mcg/kg IV [141]. Patient factors, such as age and comorbidities, should influence empiric dosing decreases [142]. Common PCA doses are hydromorphone 0.2 mg IV demand dose with an 8–10 min lockout interval with or without a loading dose and without a basal infusion, and morphine 1–2 mg IV demand dose with an 8–10 min lockout interval with or without a loading dose and without a basal infusion. One hour and 4-h limits may be used to provide additional safety [143]. Finally, common postoperative oral opioid dose regimens include tramadol 50 mg every 6 h as needed, hydrocodone 5 mg every 4–6 h as needed, and oxycodone 5 mg every 4–6 h as needed [40, 141]. While there is some growing enthusiasm for eliminating opioids from the perioperative setting, universal opioid-free approaches are very difficult to apply universally given our current armamentarium, and the benefits are unclear [144, 145]. There is, however, a clear movement away from the liberal opioid use of the 2000s to early 2010s to a more "opioid-sparing" approach which utilizes careful titration of opioids as part of a larger, multimodal analgesic plan.

Unlike some of the other pain medications, pure opioids do not exhibit a ceiling analgesic effect, allowing for more flexible titration. Opioid receptors are found throughout the body and are divided into four subtypes: mu, delta, kappa, and nociceptin receptor (also called ORL1). Opioid receptor agonist binding leads to analgesia by reduction of neurotransmission in the following manner. The agonist binds to a G-protein-coupled-opioid receptor on the transmembrane portion. This causes the α-subunit of the G-protein to exchange its guanosine diphosphate (GDP) molecule with intracellular guanosine triphosphate (GTP), which then dissociates from the βγ complex resulting in the inhibition of adenyl cyclase, which in turn reduces levels of cyclic adenosine monophosphate (cAMP). This leads to increased potassium conductance (hyperpolarization), calcium channel inactivation, and reduced neurotransmitter release. Opioid receptors are located throughout the central nervous system including the periaqueductal grey, locus coeruleus, rostral ventral medulla, and substantia gelatinosa of the dorsal horn. They are additionally located on peripheral afferent nociceptive nerves and nonnervous system tissue such as the heart, liver, lung, gut, lymphocytes, and mononuclear phagocytes [146–148]. Mu, delta, and kappa receptors are implicated in supraspinal and spinal level analgesia, while each has varying roles in other opioid mediated effects, such as: respiratory depression—μ and decreased gastrointestinal motility—μ and κ- [149, 150]. Because the mu receptor is thought to mediate addiction, there have been many attempts to develop targeted delta and kappa receptor agonists with limited therapeutic success and no current commercial availability [151].

Methadone is an older synthetic opioid that has since found renewed popularity for the treatment of severe chronic pain and opioid use disorder. Unlike other pure opioid agonists, it also has NMDA blocking properties. Methadone's long half-life makes it a perioperative option for patients undergoing long surgeries with expected severe postoperative pain [152]. Caution is warranted with methadone for methadone-naïve patients given the risk of respiratory depression and sedation. Buprenorphine is a partial opioid agonist that is sometimes used for chronic pain and often for opioid use disorder. It has a ceiling effect for respiratory depression, improving its safety profile [153]. There does not seem to be an analgesic ceiling effect, however [154]. Because buprenorphine binds tightly to opioid receptors, patients who continue it perioperatively will require larger doses of opioids to produce adequate analgesic effects. Current consensus by a multidisciplinary expert panel recommends continuing buprenorphine in the perioperative period for patients with opioid use disorder [155]. When used to manage opioid use disorder, buprenorphine is frequently combined with naloxone as an abuse deterrent since naloxone is inactivated by first pass metabolism in the liver when delivered orally, sublingually, or buccally, but not if injected intravenously.

Opioid-only intrathecal or epidural administration is also an option. As a single epidural dose, 2.5–4 mg of morphine can be helpful, particularly if a patient cannot tolerate the sympathetic blockade of epidural local anesthetic. Continuous opioid-only epidural infusions are not commonly used in the acute postoperative setting as evidence for the use is equivocal to systemic opioid administration. If only a single injection of neuraxial morphine is planned, many clinicians would elect for a single dose of 0.075–0.3 mg intrathecal morphine injected in the lower lumbar region [156]. Hydrophilic opioids can reach higher spinal bioavailability than lipophilic ones. Intrathecal injection allows for higher spinal bioavailability and decreases systemic absorption. Neuraxial morphine provides analgesia for typically 20–24 h. The risk of respiratory depression increases significantly with doses of morphine greater than 0.3 mg intrathecal and 4 mg epidural. Lipid solubility determines many pharmacologic effects of neuraxial opioids. Morphine, a hydrophilic opioid, has slower onset and longer duration, whereas lipophilic fentanyl has more rapid onset and shorter duration because of more rapid distribution and clearance from the spinal cord. Additionally, the slow rostral migration of hydrophilic morphine in the CSF to eventually bind to the opioid receptors in the ventral medulla can cause delayed respiratory depression 6–12 h after administration. Neuraxial opioids can cause systemic side effects including respiratory depression, pruritus, nausea and vomiting, and urinary retention but generally do so to a lesser extent than equipotent dosing of systemic opioids, except for pruritus, nausea, and vomiting.

Opioid tolerance can develop quickly with opioid use. Patients chronically taking opioids usually require higher doses of opioids in the perioperative setting to provide adequate analgesia. These patients in particular benefit from a carefully thought-out multimodal analgesic plan with systemic medications that target a multitude of receptors, and other targeted modalities like neuraxial and regional anesthesia. In sum, perioperative opioids are potent analgesics that can be very helpful to treat moderate-severe postsurgical pain but are limited to varying degrees by their many serious adverse effects.

Ketamine

Ketamine is a derivative of phencyclidine and is primarily a noncompetitive N-methyl-D-aspartate (NMDA) receptor antagonist, which affects the nociceptive pathway in the brain and spinal cord [157, 158]. It has also been found to act on several other receptors including μ-opioid receptors, muscarinic receptors, and γ-aminobutyric acid receptors [159]. As an NMDA receptor antagonist, it has been shown to decrease central sensitization, have antihyperalgesical effects, and can reduce or reverse opioid tolerance [160]. Ketamine also acts on a variety of other receptors that may explain additional analgesic effects: decreasing central sensitization, enhancing descending inhibition, neural modulation, and anti-inflammation. These receptors include nicotinic receptors, sodium channels, mu, kappa, and delta opioid receptors, monoaminergic and voltage-gated calcium channels, serotonergic receptors, cholinergic receptors, and cannabinoid receptors [161, 162].

Ketamine produces analgesia at plasma concentrations of 100–200 ng/mL and produces general anesthesia at plasma concentrations of 9000–25,000 ng/mL. It can be administered via multiple routes including intravenous, intranasal, intramuscular, oral, subcutaneous, rectal, and even intrathecal [159]. Intrathecal administration, however, has been associated with neurotoxicity and safety data is lacking. Per consensus guidelines for perioperative analgesia, intravenous bolus initiation of ketamine should be 0.35 mg/kg with or without an infusion of 0.06–0.2 mg/kg/h up to a max dose of 1 mg/kg/h. Lower dose infusions of 0.1–0.5 mg/kg/h IV for the perioperative period may be preferred to achieve analgesia but avoid adverse side effects. A few studies continued ketamine doses for 24–48 h postoperatively but showed moderate to low quality of improving pain [163]. The most common adverse effects of ketamine include hallucinations, agitation, anxiety, dysphoria, euphoria, dizziness, nausea, sedation, and tachycardia. Adverse effects are dose dependent. A lower total dose is recommended to mitigate or avoid such effects. Because ketamine inhibits monoamine transport, it increases the prevalence of psychotomimetic adverse effects as dose increases (hallucinations, agitation, anxiety, dysphoria, and euphoria) [163].

Ketamine undergoes hepatic metabolism by the cytochromes CYP3A4, CYP2B6, and CYP2C9 to the weakly active metabolite norketamine via *N*-demethylation, which is then broken down into 6-hydroxynorketamine, and to the lesser metabolites 4-hydroxyketamine and 6-hydroxyketamine [164]. They are excreted in the urine and bile. The half-life of intravenous ketamine is about 7 min. Contraindications for administering ketamine include severe hepatic dysfunction, poorly controlled cardiovascular disease, active psychosis, pregnancy, elevated intraocular pressure, and elevated intracranial pressure.

Ketamine has been shown to benefit patients undergoing surgery who are opioid tolerant or dependent and those who are experiencing an acute exacerbation of a chronic pain condition. It can result in an absolute reduction in perioperative Visual Analog Scale (VAS) pain score of about one point on a scale of 1–10, 20% approximate relative reduction in opioid requirement, a mild reduction in opioid-related adverse effects and double the time to first postoperative analgesic request [163, 165, 166]. Patients who benefit most are those undergoing surgery associated with severe pain and those who have chronic pain, are opioid tolerant, and have hyperalgesia [159]. Ketamine can be helpful in patients at risk for respiratory depression from opioids since it helps decrease opioid consumption postoperatively [159]. Twenty-four hours postoperative opioid consumption has been shown to be ~7.6 MME less in a collection of opioid-tolerant and opioid-naïve patients who receive ketamine than those who do not, and still continued to require less even 48 h postoperatively [163]. Pain intensity on a visual analogue scale was also modestly reduced in patients who received ketamine. Ketamine has been shown to help with mobilization following total knee arthroplasty, and also decreases pain scores and morphine equivalent consumptions in THAs and TKAs up to 48 h postoperatively, though it is unclear how it affects long-term outcomes [167, 168]. Recent trials have shown that ketamine also has an opioid-sparing effect in patients undergoing complex spinal surgeries, lowering the cumulative morphine consumption in the first 24 h postoperatively by 4 MME and decreasing consumption when combined with another intervention such as administering magnesium or an epidural [169, 170]. Ketamine also decreases opioid consumption when added to an opioid PCA [171]. However, it is unclear if it improves long-term outcomes after spine surgeries; one RCT was unable to show an effect on neuropathic pain prevalence at 6 and 12 months postoperatively [172].

Gabapentinoids

Gabapentin and pregabalin are medications originally intended as antiepileptic agents that were subsequently found to be useful in the treatment of chronic neuropathic pain. Gabapentin was approved by the Food and Drug Administration in 1993, and pregabalin in 2004. Currently, gabapentin and pregabalin are FDA approved for seizures and to treat post-therapeutic neuralgia, while pregabalin is also approved for diabetic neuropathic pain, fibromyalgia, and neuropathic pain associated with spinal cord injury [173, 174]. While gabapentin and pregabalin are gamma-aminobutyric acid analogues, they do not work on GABA receptors. Gabapentinoids bind to the $\alpha_2\delta$ subunit of the voltage-gated calcium channel found in the central nervous system. This is thought to decrease central release of pro-nociceptive neurotransmitters [175]. There also may be additional activation of central noradrenergic pain inhibition pathways and activation of noradrenergic pain-inhibiting pathways [176]. In recent years, gabapentinoids have fallen out of favor as medications to treat acute postoperative pain. While gabapentin and pregabalin were previously commonly used as part of perioperative multimodal analgesia, studies now suggest that they provide modest reductions in perioperative pain that may not be clinically significant [177]. Additionally, they are associated with significant side effects including sedation, visual disturbance, and dizziness [175]. Gabapentinoids may potentiate the respiratory and cognitive depressive effects of opioids [178, 179]. A large retrospective study of patients undergoing colorectal surgery found an association between gabapentinoid use on day of surgery with increased postoperative noninvasive ventilation support and naloxone use [180].

The current recommendation is to avoid gabapentinoids as part of most enhanced recovery after surgery protocols and avoid for routine use for perioperative pain. It is possible that select patients with large neuropathic or hyperalgesic components of their pain may still benefit from gabapentinoids; these should be determined on a case by case basis and weighed against the risks. Due to the relatively common occurrence of neuropathic pain in patients with spine pathologies, that is a subset that may benefit from perioperative gabapentinoids. Perioperative dosing of gabapentin may range from 300 to 600 mg PO three times a day (TID) and of pregabalin may range from 75 to 150 mg PO either twice a day (BID) or TID. Common preoperative single dose regimens are gabapentin 300–600 mg PO and pregabalin 75–150 mg PO with dose reduction recommended in the elderly and those at risk for side effects. Higher single dose perioperative regimens have been utilized—gabapentin 1200 mg and pregabalin 300 mg—but are also associated with a higher incidence of side effects [176]. Typical multi-dose regimens trend toward the low end of the dosing ranges due to the significant incidence of serious adverse effects. There is insufficient evidence to recommend either gabapentin over pregabalin or vice versa in the perioperative setting.

Muscle Relaxants

Muscle relaxants refer to a broad category of medications with various mechanisms of actions, most of which are still not fully understood. They are more commonly used to treat conditions such as back pain and fibromyalgia. Muscle relaxants can be divided into antispasmodic, which help treat muscle spasms, and antispasticity, which helps treat muscles that are stiff and are difficult to move, thereby affecting function [181]. Common side effects of muscle relaxants include sedation, dizziness, bradycardia, and hypotension. Despite these concerns, and the fact that there is limited literature examining the utility of muscle relaxants in any type of surgery, muscle relaxants have been added to many perioperative protocols in attempt to decrease opioid consumption when muscle spasm or muscular discomfort plays a significant role in the perioperative experience (e.g., spine surgery or anterior hip replacement).

Methocarbamol is a muscle relaxant that is used to treat muscle spasm. It is low cost and has both intravenous and oral formulations. The exact mechanism of action is unknown, though it is thought to affect the central nervous system and not skeletal muscle directly. While there are multiple retrospective studies suggesting the benefit of perioperative methocarbamol, prospective studies are lacking, and the evidence for its use is limited and weak. The optimal dose and regimen are not known for perioperative use. Studies have been limited to orthopedic surgery and breast augmentation [182, 183]. Perioperative doses range from 500 mg to 1000 mg IV or oral every 6–8 h [184, 185]. Methocarbamol is metabolized by the liver and excreted by the kidneys. Common adverse effects include sedation and dizziness, while uncommon but serious adverse effects include seizure, leukopenia, and cholestatic jaundice.

Tizanidine is an $\alpha 2$-adrenergic receptor agonist that acts on the central nervous system and is an antispasmodic. The half-life is 2.5 h, with its peak effect at 1–2 h. Adverse effects include dose-dependent sedation, drowsiness, dizziness, ataxia, and lethargy [181]. Clearance is significantly reduced when administered with ciprofloxacin. Significant hypotension, bradycardia, and sedation can occur when given with CYP1A2 inhibitors. There is a single randomized controlled trial that found decreased opioid consumption and improved pain scores when tizanidine was given at a dose of 4 mg for analgesia for laparoscopic cholecystectomy. There have been no studies in orthopedic or spine surgery patients. No recommendation can be made for its perioperative use.

Like tizanidine, baclofen is an antispasmodic. It has a GABA-like structure and may work on GABA type B receptors. Its exact mechanism is not well-understood. Baclofen is renally excreted and can cause increased central nervous system and respiratory depression when used with opiates and benzodiazepines. There are no known studies of baclofen for perioperative use. While patients who are already on baclofen should continue to take it in the perioperative period, initiation of baclofen is not recommended for perioperative indications. Abrupt discontinuation of baclofen can cause a serious, potentially life-threatening withdrawal syndrome [181].

Cyclobenzaprine is an oral 5-HT2 receptor antagonist that has anticholinergic activity and can potentiate the effect of norepinephrine. Because of its anticholinergic activity, it can cause adverse effects including hallucinations, confusion, drowsiness, constipation, urinary retention, and dry mouth. There is also a lack of research regarding the usefulness of cyclobenzaprine in the perioperative period to treat acute pain [181, 186]. Perioperative initiation of cyclobenzaprine is also not recommended.

In general, there is a dearth of research on muscle relaxants and their effects on analgesia and recovery in the perioperative period. Few studies suggest limited benefits of using methocarbamol or tizanidine to help decrease opioid consumption in select patient populations, such as spine surgery. Caution is advised with their use given the risk for serious adverse effects.

Alpha-2-agonists

Clonidine and dexmedetomidine are alpha-agonists with preferential alpha-2 activity at central and peripheral alpha-2 receptors. Clonidine has an alpha-2:alpha-1 activity ratio of 220:1, while dexmedetomidine is much more highly alpha-2 specific with an alpha-2:alpha-1 ratio of 1620:1. Clonidine is available as oral tablets, transdermal patch, and injection, whereas dexmedetomidine is only available as an injection. Clonidine is often prescribed as an antihypertensive or as an antianxiety medication. Its alpha-agonist action in the brainstem decreases CNS mediated norepinephrine release, decreasing peripheral vascular tone [187]. Dexmedetomidine is only available for administration by a clinician at this time, currently only FDA-approved for ICU and procedural sedation but has additional off-label uses. Analgesia may be from peripheral inhibition of C-fibers and Aα fibers and central inhibition of nociceptive transmission via the dorsal horn in the spinal cord. Both medications have a modest analgesic effect, with an approximate 1.5-point reduction on a 10-point scale at 12 h and an approximate 0.7-point reduction on a 10-point VAS scale at 24 h in one meta-analysis across a wide variety of surgeries, while another meta-analysis focusing on abdominal surgery found no significant impact on analgesia [188, 189]. Dexmedetomidine primarily causes anxiolysis and sedation while also causing sympatholytic effects including bradycardia and hypotension. Thus, it is most useful for ICU sedation, procedural sedation, and reducing emergence agitation and delirium in pediatric populations rather than as an analgesic [190, 191]. The α_2-agonists may also be useful in modulating the surgical stress response [192].

The sedating and hemodynamic effects of clonidine and dexmedetomidine somewhat limit the utility of systemic alpha-2-agonists for analgesia. However, they have been shown to decrease intraoperative anesthetic requirements and provide a modest decrease in postoperative opioid use when given as part of a balanced anesthetic. One meta-analysis looking at perioperative clonidine or dexmedetomidine use across a wide array of surgeries found that perioperative clonidine decreased morphine consumption by 0 mg at 2 h after surgery, 9 mg at 12 h, and 4 mg at 24 h. Dexmedetomidine provided more opioid-sparing effect by decreasing morphine consumption by 6 mg at 2 h, 6 mg at 12 h, and 14.5 mg at 24 h [188]. This same meta-analysis found that clonidine resulted in more hypotension, whereas patients receiving dexmedetomidine experienced more bradycardia.

Clonidine and dexmedetomidine are also both common adjuvants in regional anesthesia for both peripheral and neuraxial blocks. In a meta-analysis examining dexmedetomidine as a neuraxial adjunct with bupivacaine or ropivacaine, dexmedetomidine was found to reduce pain scores and prolong analgesia [193]. In this meta-analysis, neuraxial dexmedetomidine was found to result in an increased risk of bradycardia but not of hypotension or sedation. Dexmedetomidine as an epidural adjuvant to bupivacaine seems to provide faster onset of block and prolonged analgesia than clonidine [194].

An optimal dosing regimen for clonidine or dexmedetomidine for perioperative analgesia is unknown. Perioperative clonidine is most commonly administered via oral, intravenous, transdermal, or perineural routes in doses for adults ranging from 150–300 mcg as an oral preoperative dose to 2–5 mcg/kg IV as a one-time intraoperative dose to a transdermal 0.2 mg/24 h application to 100–150 mcg added to local anesthetic for perineural blockade [188, 195]. Perioperative dexmedetomidine administration is typically intravenous, intranasal, or perineural. An infusion as low as 0.2 mcg/kg/h has been shown to produce analgesia [196]. The maximum approved dose for sedation is 0.7 mcg/kg/h and initiation is recommended with a 1 mcg/kg bolus over 10 min. Studies investigating dexmedetomidine for perioperative analgesia all used less than 0.7 mcg/kg/h [197]. Unless the patient is monitored in the ICU, dexmedetomidine is not commonly administered in the postoperative phase due to sedation and hemodynamic effects. When given intranasally, dexmedetomidine produces reliable sedation at 45 min with a peak effect of 90–150 min but the resulting analgesia is uncertain [198]. Dexmedetomidine 30–100 mcg or 0.75–1.0 mcg/kg when added to local anesthetic for peripheral neural blockade prolongs sensory and motor blockade [199].

Clonidine has an elimination half-life of 9–12 h [200]. Approximately half is metabolized by the liver to inactive metabolites, while the remainder is excreted unchanged by the kidneys. Dexmedetomidine has an elimination half-life of 2 h and is highly bound to plasma proteins [201], while the context-sensitive half-life ranges from 4 min after a 10-min infusion to 250 min after an 8-h infusion [202]. It is metabolized by the liver via glucuronidation and cytochrome P450 2A6 oxidation and excreted primarily by the kidneys.

Because clonidine and dexmedetomidine have modest analgesic benefits and are associated with potentially significant adverse effects, they are not recommended as routine analgesic medications for most postoperative patients or as a common analgesic in an enhanced recovery protocol. They may be considered when alternatives have been exhausted or when their other effects, such as anxiolysis or sedation, are primarily desired.

Magnesium

Magnesium is a noncompetitive antagonist of NMDA receptors, which are involved in the transduction of pain [203]. Magnesium can alter the perception and duration of pain by regulating the influx of calcium into the cells, attenuating central sensitization, and impeding cytokine release [204]. Three meta-analyses have shown that there is no one superior way of administering IV magnesium to see the most analgesic benefit (bolus vs. infusion vs. bolus and infusion) [204–206]. Additionally, there is a lack of consensus on the optimal dosing, though studies typically use 30–50 mg/kg for blousing and 10–15 mg/kg/h. Magnesium has been found to cause a modest decrease in cumulative opioid consumption and pain scores, as well as a longer time to first analgesic in the first 24 h postoperatively. The quality of the studies and how magnesium was administered amongst the studies varied widely [204, 205, 207]. Adverse effects of magnesium include dizziness, headache, bradycardia, hypotension, and weakness. While it may be beneficial to add magnesium as an adjunct to a robust multimodal analgesic regimen when trying to avoid other agents (e.g. ketamine or muscle relaxants), its utility is limited [208].

Beta-Blockers

Beta-adrenergic blockade blunts the autonomic nervous system's adrenergic response to intense perioperative stimuli such as endotracheal intubation, surgical incision, organ manipulation, and emergence from anesthesia [209]. While the hemodynamic effects are well-understood, less clear is how beta-blockade leads to analgesia. Nonetheless, there is strong clinical evidence for beta-blockers to have an intraoperative and postoperative opiate-sparing effect with associated decrease in opiate side effects, such as nausea and vomiting [210, 211]. In patients undergoing general anesthesia, the beta-blocker esmolol is also associated with a decreased induction dose requirement of propofol and a reduction in end-tidal volatile anesthetic requirement [210]. In addition, esmolol can hasten time to discharge from PACU [212].

While most medications that block β-adrenergic receptors have some activity at β_1- and β_2-adrenoceptors and sometimes other types of receptors, esmolol is highly selective for the β_1-adrenoceptor where it has a 34-fold higher affinity than at the β_2-adrenoceptor [213]. The β1 receptor is found almost exclusively in the heart, while the β2 receptor is found on organs throughout the body [214]. Thus, esmolol has rapid onset and resolution and highly selective cardiac activity, making it the preferred beta-blocker for perioperative use where these effects are most desirable.

Esmolol has a rapid onset within 2–3 min and a short duration of action with a half-life of approximately 9 min. Esmolol is rapidly metabolized via hydrolysis by erythrocyte esterases [215]. It is unclear if and how esmolol has an analgesic effect. It is also unclear how long the analgesic effect persists, and studies have questioned whether it is truly analgesia or if by treating hemodynamic response to stimulation with esmolol instead of an opioid, the observed analgesia is actually a reflection of decreased opioid consumption and subsequent decrease in acute opioid-induced hyperalgesia and acute opioid tolerance [211, 216, 217]. One proposed mechanism includes that beta-blockers regulate voltage-gated calcium channels that may control the release of neurotransmitters involved in the nociceptive pathway [211, 218]. Another is by blocking hippocampal activation, as it becomes active during times of stress and nociception, so beta-blockade may attenuate the response to noxious stimuli [215, 218]. Nonetheless, studies show that esmolol decreases intraoperative anesthetic requirements, decreases the incidence of postoperative nausea and vomiting, and decreases opioid consumption in multiple types of surgeries [210, 211, 218–220]. Studies examining esmolol and its utility for perioperative pain commonly used bolus doses of 0.5–1 mg/kg at induction of general anesthesia, but infusion rates varied widely from 5 to 50 mcg/kg/min.

Beta-blockade is generally well-tolerated in the perioperative setting, and more specifically, esmolol is not known to have effects beyond the impact of β_1-adrenoceptor antagonism in specific patient contexts [210, 211, 221]. However, there are potential risks to this type of physiologic manipulation. In a meta-analysis of 67 controlled clinical trials with 3766 patients undergoing noncardiac surgery, investigators found that esmolol was associated with an increased incidence of unplanned hypotension when it was administered as a bolus [222]. Overall, esmolol may be considered as an adjunct to an analgesic plan for opioid reduction, if appropriate hemodynamic parameters are maintained. It otherwise plays a limited role in enhanced recovery protocols and perioperative analgesia.

Cryoanalgesia

Cryoanalgesia refers to the technique of cryoneurolysis where a very low temperature is applied to a nerve to cause reversible nerve damage and provide analgesia [223]. A probe creates a small ice ball that is between −20 °C and − 100 °C, which then causes a lesion. Wallerian degeneration occurs distal to the injury, but the endometrium, perineurium, and the epineurium remain intact. The axon then regenerates slowly, 1–2 mm/day. Analgesia can last weeks to months after a single treatment. Because of this, it is indicated for sensory nerves and relatively contraindicated for motor nerves and mixed sensory-motor nerves [224]. Additional relative contraindications also include bleeding disorders, cryoglobulinemia, and Raynaud's syndrome. Risks include frostbite, alopecia, depigmentation or hyperpigmentation of the skin [223].

Cryoneurolysis has been used to treat post-thoracotomy pain since the 1970s and has gained more perioperative applications with the assistance of ultrasound.

Current indications include analgesia for rib fractures, postmastectomy pain, total knee arthroplasty, burns, and limb amputations [224]. Cryoneurolysis reduces pain, decreases opioid consumption, and resolves in 2–16 weeks [225, 226]. However, in one study, two patients subsequently went on to have worse post-thoracotomy pain after cryoneurolysis resolved [227]. The most significant limitation for its use is the amount of time it takes to apply cryoneurolysis—5–10 min per nerve—which can pose a logistical challenge if performing preoperatively, especially when multiple nerves need to be treated [224]. Cryoneurolysis may be considered for patients who have preoperative chronic pain and who would be anticipated to have severe or moderately severe pain lasting many days to weeks in the anatomic distribution of isolated sensory nerves. As an emerging analgesic modality, it may have expanded indications in the future within enhanced recovery protocols and perioperative analgesia.

Percutaneous Peripheral Nerve Neuromodulation

Percutaneous peripheral nerve stimulation (pPNS) or neuromodulation is an analgesic method that has been introduced recently into clinical practice to address perioperative pain [228]. It entails using ultrasound to place a fine wire lead through a needle percutaneously and implanting it adjacent to peripheral nerves in the distribution of a pain generator, such as a joint that has been replaced. The optimal location of a lead may vary slightly depending on the neural target but is in general 1.0–1.5 cm [223]. This distance allows the device to achieve selective stimulation of larger-diameter myelinated sensory neurons that interrupts the transmission of pain signals to the central nervous system thereby providing analgesia [229–231]. The lead is connected to an external pulse generator that delivers the electric current to the nerve. This technology has been used for the treatment of chronic pain for decades via spinal cord stimulation and was limited in the perioperative setting due to the design of the systems, invasiveness, cost, feasibility, and concerns around placement. The invention of smaller leads and commercially available pPNS systems for cheaper, rapid, and easier placement, have increased the perioperative utility of pPNS [232–235].

Utilizing pPNS is an appealing alternative to continuous nerve blocks with perineural catheters with local anesthetic because local anesthetics may cause denser sensory and motor blockade than desired to still achieve adequate analgesia, and perineural catheters are more limited in duration, typically up to a week. In contrast, pPNS causes little motor stimulation and no motor blockade and can be left in the body for up to 60 days [223]. One limitation is that it can take a significant amount of time to place a pPNS system due to the need to trial and finalize lead locations [236]. Multiple pilot studies and case series have shown effectiveness in treating pain in patients after total knee arthroplasty, hallux valgus repair, rotator cuff repair, and ACL repair [232–235]. Overall pPNS seems very promising as a uniquely effective means of providing analgesia throughout the entire postoperative course of healing. Larger studies supporting their use and devices that can be implanted at a low enough cost may take this technology from novel and emerging to having a significant role in perioperative analgesia and enhanced recovery protocols [237].

Acupuncture

Acupuncture has been performed for three millennia, beginning in China. It has grown in popularity in the last half century in North America, mostly in the outpatient settings as an alternative medicine treatment for pain and other ailments [238]. Acupuncture involves inserting very thin, short needles at designated points along the body. The points selected are based on the treatment goal.

Traditional descriptions of how acupuncture works involve the insertion of needles along meridians (channels) where qi (vital life force) flow [239]. These descriptions, of course, are not rooted in modern Western scientific vocabulary. Recent research has sought to describe the mechanisms of this ancient practice via the lens of modern biology and physiology. There is good clinical evidence that acupuncture decreases pain. Proposed mechanisms of action include the release of endogenous opioids and endorphins and involvement in the serotonin, bradykinin, and cannabinoid pathways. Traditional acupuncture involves points on the entire body. Additionally, some acupuncturists will stimulate the needles with electric current during the treatments. As an alternative to whole-body acupuncture, some microsystem acupuncture (e.g., auricular, scalp, hand acupuncture) may be easier to perform in the perioperative period [240]. There is some promising clinical evidence that patients who receive acupuncture during a variety of surgeries ranging from tonsillectomy to craniotomies to knee replacements have decreased postoperative pain [241, 242].

Compared to other nonpharmacologic methods, acupuncture involves slightly more risk since needles are inserted into the skin. However, the needles are fine and filiform. So long as sterile needles and appropriate aseptic technique are used, risk of infection, bleeding, or damage to other tissues are extremely low [243]. Some adverse effects of acupuncture can include insertion pain, fatigue, and dizziness [244].

Acupuncture requires an experienced practitioner to perform and is a regulated practice in most states. Not many healthcare systems have acupuncture trained personnel on staff for perioperative procedures. More research is needed to quantify how much pain relief acupuncture provides in the postoperative setting and which surgical patient populations gain the most benefit from the practice. It is currently unclear if acupuncture should be more widely offered to patients in the perioperative setting. Consequently, acupuncture is not currently featured in enhanced recovery protocols. However, initial evidence shows promise, and further research is needed to determine if it is worth investing resources to provide perioperative acupuncture more widely.

Nonpharmacologic Nonphysical Interventions: Pain Management Education, Counseling, Mind-Body Interventions, Music Therapy, and Virtual Reality:

Education and Counseling

Patient counseling, education, and expectation setting about expected surgical pain and recovery trajectory should begin in the surgery clinic as the patient mentally and physically prepares for their procedure [13]. Patients should understand before they arrive for their procedure that most surgeries involve some postoperative pain and certain types may involve moderate or even severe postoperative pain. They should also be told that no pain is not a realistic goal. Instead, the treatment of pain in both the immediate postoperative period and after they are discharged will aim to make the pain tolerable so that the patient may function in activities of daily living, participate in therapies (e.g., avoiding oversedation), avoid side effects of pain medications (e.g., minimizing opioid-induced nausea and bowel dysfunction), and optimally recover. They should be instructed to have any planned over-the-counter medications like acetaminophen or NSAIDs already available at home prior to arriving for surgery and be counseled on which medications should be scheduled and which medications should be taken only as needed.

Mind-Body Interventions

Mind-body interventions include meditation, cognitive behavioral therapy (CBT), and mindfulness among others. They are all noninvasive techniques with almost no risk involved. Certain versions can be free or extremely inexpensive. The underlying concept of these techniques is to help the individual become more attuned with their own biofeedback and self-modulate responses including sympathetic surge, pain response, and reward system. Of course, these techniques require that the patient can understand and follow instructions.

Mind-body interventions have been used in patients with chronic pain. There is evidence that these interventions can help decrease pain response and opioid consumption in patients with chronic pain [245]. There is a growing movement to implement these techniques in the perioperative patient population.

Mind-body interventions can help augment a patient's parasympathetic system as shown by increases in heart rate variability [246]. Additionally, it can help reorient dysregulated reward pathway feedback associated with opioid use [247]. In-person guidance via a counselor, psychologist, or integrative medicine provider could provide the most personalized intervention; however, many clinical environments do not have these resources. In these settings, patients may choose among the many free or inexpensive phone apps available to guide meditation, mindfulness, and even CBT. They can download and start using them even before surgery takes place. It is also possible to prerecord audio only or audiovisual mind-body intervention guidance tailored to postoperative pain in a specific patient population and have the patient listen to and follow along at their own pace.

Meditation, CBT, and mindfulness are unlikely to dramatically decrease pain intensity; however, there may be a reduction in the perception of pain unpleasantness and in the ability to cope with the pain [246]. Additionally, a recent meta-analysis found that techniques conducted by an in-person provider lasting more than 5 min seem to show more promise over shorter sessions or audio-only versions [248]. Since many mind-body interventions are easily accessible, cheap, and with negligible risks, they are worth adding on as a non-pharmacologic modality to complement pharmacologic treatment of pain.

Music Therapy

There is good evidence that music therapy decreases postoperative pain and anxiety [249, 250]. Like with mind-body interventions, there may be some influence on autonomic nervous system modulation. Music therapy can involve minimal cost (often free if the patient brings his or her own music-capable phone and headphones) and poses negligible risk. The type of music genre in and of itself does not necessarily matter, but patient-selected music seems to provide more benefit [250]. Music therapy appears to provide a small decrease in postoperative pain scores and postoperative pain medication requirement [251]. Music therapy may provide slightly more benefit when begun preoperatively. There may be some small benefit to music therapy for patients under general anesthesia, but conscious patients derive more benefit.

Since music therapy is easily accessible with almost no risk, it should be offered to most patients as an adjunct to their multimodal pain regimen. Patients should be allowed to select their music of choice, and music therapy could be started in preop holding if it does not interfere with any part of the preoperative process. If not feasible to begin in preop, it should be started when the patient is awake after surgery.

Virtual Reality

Virtual reality is a technology that is beginning to be adopted throughout healthcare. It leverages immersive distraction from unpleasant physical sensation towards positive emotional and cognitive processing to help users change their thoughts and perception of pain and cope better [252, 253]. Initial clinical investigations into virtual reality for analgesia addressed burn dressing change pain, dental procedure pain, hospitalized in-patients with acute pain, and total joint arthroplasty [254–258]. More investigations specific to perioperative pain management are ongoing. Limitations to widespread perioperative adoption include FDA approval, device delivery, and financial considerations. Virtual reality seems potentially promising as a future perioperative analgesic adjunct.

Bullet points for main points end of chapter:

- Perioperative pain management attempts to mitigate postsurgical pain and help patients supersede the challenges and stressors of surgery.

- Enhanced recovery protocols aim to decrease physiologic stress, restore homeostasis, and lead patients to faster recovery and optimal quality outcomes.
- Non-opioid pain medications of different classes with relevant regional anesthesia or local anesthetic infiltration provide a foundation of analgesia upon which judicious use of opioids can be added as needed to provide postsurgical pain control while decreasing opioid-related adverse events.
- Interventional acute pain management techniques are effective modalities for patients undergoing surgeries associated with severe and moderately-severe pain.

Example Enhanced Recovery After Surgery Pain Management Protocols

Archetype

- Preop:
  - Acetaminophen
  - NSAID vs COX-2 inhibitor
  - Regional analgesia vs neuraxial analgesia
  - Patient counseling and education
- Intraop:
  - Steroid
  - Ketamine (if opioid tolerant/chronic pain)
  - Short acting opioid IV as necessary
- Postop:
  - Acetaminophen
  - NSAID vs COX-2 inhibitor
  - Muscle relaxant PRN (if spasm may occur)
  - Opioid short acting oral prn
  - Music therapy
  - Meditation
- Consider Emerging Techniques:
  - Cryoanalgesia
  - Percutaneous peripheral neuromodulation
  - Acupuncture

Total Hip or Knee Arthroplasty

- Preop:
  - Acetaminophen scheduled 15 m/kg up to 1000 mg PO
  - Celebrex 400 mg PO
  - Regional analgesia: adductor canal block (TKA) or pericapsular nerve group block (THA)
  - Patient counseling and education

- Intraop:
  - Dexamethasone 0.1–0.15 mg/kg IV at induction of anesthesia
  - Ketamine 0.5 mg/kg IV bolus at induction + 0.1 mg/kg/hr IV bolus (if opioid tolerant/chronic pain)
  - Short acting opioid IV as necessary (fentanyl 1–2 mcg/kg/case)
- Postop:
  - Acetaminophen scheduled 15 m/kg up to 1000 mg PO TID
  - Celebrex 200 mg PO BID
  - Muscle relaxant PRN: such as methocarbamol 500–1000 mg Q8hrs PRN
  - Oxycodone 5–10 mg PO Q6hrs PRN and hydromorphone 0.5 mg IV Q3hrs PRN for breakthrough pain
  - Music therapy
  - Meditation
- Consider Emerging Techniques:
  - Percutaneous peripheral neuromodulation
  - Cryoneurolysis

Total Shoulder Arthroplasty

- Preop:
  - Acetaminophen scheduled 15 m/kg up to 1000 mg PO
  - Celebrex 400 mg PO
  - Regional analgesia: interscalene brachial plexus blockade single injection, bupivacaine 0.5% 6–10 mL with liposomal bupivacaine 10mL
  - Patient counseling and education
- Intraop:
  - Dexamethasone 0.1–0.15 mg/kg IV at induction of anesthesia
  - Ketamine 0.5 mg/kg IV bolus at induction + 0.1 mg/kg/hr IV bolus (if opioid tolerant/chronic pain)
  - Short acting opioid IV as necessary (fentanyl 1-2mcg/kg/case)
- Postop:
  - Acetaminophen scheduled 15 m/kg up to 1000 mg PO TID
  - Celebrex 200 mg PO BID
  - Muscle relaxant PRN: such as methocarbamol 500–1000 mg Q8hrs PRN
  - Oxycodone 5–10 mg PO Q6hrs PRN and hydromorphone 0.5 mg IV Q3hrs PRN for breakthrough pain
  - Music therapy
  - Meditation
- Consider Emerging Techniques:
  - Percutaneous peripheral neuromodulation
  - Cryoneurolysis

Multilevel Spine Fusion

- Preop:
  - Acetaminophen scheduled 15 m/kg up to 1000 mg PO
  - Celebrex 400 mg PO
  - Gabapentin 600 mg PO
  - Patient counseling and education
- Intraop:
  - Dexamethasone 0.15 mg/kg IV at induction of anesthesia
  - Preincisional wound infiltration with long acting local anesthetic OR regional analgesic interfascial plane block, such as erector spinae plane block or thoraco-lumbar interfascial plane block OR continuous epidural placed at end of surgery prior to closure
  - Ketamine 0.35 mg/kg IV bolus + 0.1–0.2 mg/kg/hr IV infusion
  - Methocarbamol 500–1000mg IV at end of surgery
  - Short acting opioid IV as necessary (fentanyl or hydromorphone). Caution as patient may be opioid tolerant and have higher baseline requirements.
  - (consider) Dexmedetomidine 1 mcg/kg IV bolus, 0.5 mcg/kg/hr infusion
- Postop:
  - Acetaminophen scheduled 15 m/kg up to 1000 mg PO TID
  - Celebrex 200 mg PO BID
  - Gabapentin 300–600 mg PO TID
  - Muscle relaxant PRN: such as methocarbamol 500–1000 mg Q8hrs PRN
  - Oxycodone 5–10 mg PO Q6hrs PRN and hydromorphone 0.5 mg IV Q3hrs PRN for breakthrough pain
  - +/– Thoraco-lumbar epidural analgesia (for bigger cases, such as T10-pelvis)
  - (consider) Ketamine 0.1–0.2 mg/kg/h IV infusion
  - (consider)+/– Lidocaine IV infusion 2 mg/kg/h (if no local infiltration or regional/neuraxial technique prior)
  - Music therapy
  - Meditation

In-hospital patients with severe postoperative pain not controlled by standard ERAS multimodal regimen:

- Consider consulting acute pain service or anesthesiology service for evaluation for appropriate additional neuraxial or regional anesthetic technique or the addition of less common analgesic modalities (e.g., alpha-2-agonist or cryoneurolysis).
- Be aware that worsening postsurgical pain can be indicative of underlying pathology (e.g., acute compartment syndrome or infection).

Chart summary of evidence for treatments

Treatment	Evidence base	Endorsed by guideline	Standard or accepted care
Acetaminophen	+++	+++	+++
NSAIDs	+++	+++	+++
Local anesthetics	+++	+++	+++
Corticosteroids	+++	+++	+++
Opioids	+++	+++	+++
Ketamine	++	++	++
Muscle relaxants	+	+	++
Gabapentinoids	++	++	+
Alpha-2-agonists	+	+	+
Magnesium	+	+	+
Beta-blocker	+	+	+
Cryoneurolysis	+	+	+
Peripheral neuromodulation	+	+	+
Acupuncture	+	+	+
Education and counseling on analgesics	+	+++	+++
Mind-body intervention	++	+	+
Music therapy	+	++	++
Virtual reality	+	+	+

Chart summary of evidence for assessment

Assessment	Evidence base	Endorsed by guideline	Standard or accepted care
Preoperative evaluation of medical and psychiatric history	+	+++	+++
Frequent reassessment of perioperative pain	+	+++	+++
Use validated tools to assess pain severity and impact	+	+++	+++
Screen for catastrophizing	+	+++	+++

References

1. Ljungqvist O, Scott M, Fearon KC. Enhanced recovery after surgery: a review enhanced recovery after surgery enhanced recovery after surgery. JAMA Surg. 2017;152(3):292–8.
2. Bardram L, Funch-Jensen P, Jensen P, Crawford ME, Kehlet H. Recovery after laparoscopic colonic surgery with epidural analgesia, and early oral nutrition and mobilisation. Lancet (London, England). 1995;345(8952):763–4.

3. Kehlet H, Mogensen T. Hospital stay of 2 days after open sigmoidectomy with a multimodal rehabilitation programme. Br J Surg. 1999;86(2):227–30.
4. Lassen K, Soop M, Nygren J, Cox PBW, Hendry PO, Spies C, et al. Consensus review of optimal perioperative care in colorectal surgery: enhanced recovery after surgery (ERAS) group recommendations. Arch Surg. 2009;144(10):961–9.
5. Nygren J, Hausel J, Kehlet H, Revhaug A, Lassen K, Dejong C, et al. A comparison in five European Centres of case mix, clinical management and outcomes following either conventional or fast-track perioperative care in colorectal surgery. Clin Nutr. 2005;24(3):455–61.
6. Wainwright T, Middleton R. An orthopaedic enhanced recovery pathway. Curr Anaesth Crit Care. 2010;21(3):114–20.
7. Wainwright TW, Immins T, Middleton RG. Enhanced recovery after surgery (ERAS) and its applicability for major spine surgery. Best Pract Res Clin Anaesthesiol. 2016;30(1):91–102.
8. Wainwright TW, Gill M, McDonald DA, Middleton RG, Reed M, Sahota O, et al. Consensus statement for perioperative care in total hip replacement and total knee replacement surgery: Enhanced Recovery After Surgery (ERAS(®)) Society recommendations. Acta Orthop. 2020;91(1):3–19.
9. Soffin EM, YaDeau JT. Enhanced recovery after surgery for primary hip and knee arthroplasty: a review of the evidence. Br J Anaesth. 2016;117(suppl 3):iii62–72.
10. Kopp SL, Børglum J, Buvanendran A, Horlocker TT, Ilfeld BM, Memtsoudis SG, et al. Anesthesia and analgesia practice pathway options for Total knee arthroplasty: An evidence-based review by the American and European Societies of Regional Anesthesia and Pain Medicine. Reg Anesth Pain Med. 2017;42(6):683–97.
11. Brindle M, Nelson G, Lobo DN, Ljungqvist O, Gustafsson UO. Recommendations from the ERAS® Society for standards for the development of enhanced recovery after surgery guidelines. BJS Open. 2020;4(1):157–63.
12. Lam JY, Howlett A, McLuckie D, Stephen LM, Else SDN, Jones A, et al. Developing implementation strategies to adopt Enhanced Recovery After Surgery (ERAS®) guidelines. BJS Open. 2021;5(2):zraa011.
13. Chou R, Gordon DB, de Leon-Casasola OA, Rosenberg JM, Bickler S, Brennan T, et al. Management of postoperative pain: A Clinical Practice Guideline From the American Pain Society, the American Society of Regional Anesthesia and Pain Medicine, and the American Society of Anesthesiologists' Committee on Regional Anesthesia, Executive Committee, and Administrative Council. J Pain. 2016;17(2):131–57.
14. Shah S, Schwenk ES, Sondekoppam RV, Clarke H, Zakowski M, Rzasa-Lynn RS, et al. ASRA Pain Medicine consensus guidelines on the management of the perioperative patient on cannabis and cannabinoids. Reg Anesth Pain Med. 2023;48(3):97–117.
15. Woolf CJ. Pain: moving from symptom control toward mechanism-specific pharmacologic management. Ann Intern Med. 2004;140(6):441–51.
16. Memtsoudis SG, Poeran J, Zubizarreta N, Cozowicz C, Morwald EE, Mariano ER, et al. Association of Multimodal Pain Management Strategies with perioperative outcomes and resource utilization: a population-based study. Anesthesiology. 2018;128(5):891–902.
17. Raja SN, Carr DB, Cohen M, Finnerup NB, Flor H, Gibson S, et al. The revised International Association for the Study of Pain definition of pain: concepts, challenges, and compromises. Pain. 2020;161(9):1976–82.
18. Ghanem CI, Pérez MJ, Manautou JE, Mottino AD. Acetaminophen from liver to brain: new insights into drug pharmacological action and toxicity. Pharmacol Res. 2016;109:119–31.
19. De Oliveira GS Jr, Castro-Alves LJ, McCarthy RJ. Single-dose systemic acetaminophen to prevent postoperative pain: a meta-analysis of randomized controlled trials. Clin J Pain. 2015;31(1):86–93.
20. Toms L, McQuay HJ, Derry S, Moore RA. Single dose oral paracetamol (acetaminophen) for postoperative pain in adults. Cochrane Database Syst Rev. 2008;2019(4):CD004602.
21. McNicol ED, Ferguson MC, Haroutounian S, Carr DB, Schumann R. Single dose intravenous paracetamol or intravenous propacetamol for postoperative pain. Cochrane Database Syst Rev. 2016;2019(5):Cd007126.

22. McNicol ED, Tzortzopoulou A, Cepeda MS, Francia MB, Farhat T, Schumann R. Single-dose intravenous paracetamol or propacetamol for prevention or treatment of postoperative pain: a systematic review and meta-analysis. Br J Anaesth. 2011;106(6):764–75.
23. Oscier CD, Milner QJ. Peri-operative use of paracetamol. Anaesthesia. 2009;64(1):65–72.
24. Klinger-Gratz PP, Ralvenius WT, Neumann E, Kato A, Nyilas R, Lele Z, et al. Acetaminophen relieves inflammatory pain through CB(1) cannabinoid receptors in the rostral ventromedial medulla. J Neurosci. 2018;38(2):322–34.
25. Ohashi N, Kohno T. Analgesic effect of acetaminophen: a review of known and novel mechanisms of action. Front Pharmacol. 2020;11:580289.
26. Chiew AL, Gluud C, Brok J, Buckley NA. Interventions for paracetamol (acetaminophen) overdose. Cochrane Database Syst Rev. 2018;2(2):Cd003328.
27. Yoon E, Babar A, Choudhary M, Kutner M, Pyrsopoulos N. Acetaminophen-induced hepatotoxicity: a comprehensive update. J Clin Transl Hepatol. 2016;4(2):131–42.
28. Hahn TW, Mogensen T, Lund C, Jacobsen LS, Hjortsoe NC, Rasmussen SN, et al. Analgesic effect of i.v. paracetamol: possible ceiling effect of paracetamol in postoperative pain. Acta Anaesthesiol Scand. 2003;47(2):138–45.
29. Singla NK, Parulan C, Samson R, Hutchinson J, Bushnell R, Beja EG, et al. Plasma and cerebrospinal fluid pharmacokinetic parameters after single-dose administration of intravenous, oral, or rectal acetaminophen. Pain Pract. 2012;12(7):523–32.
30. Forrest JA, Clements JA, Prescott LF. Clinical pharmacokinetics of paracetamol. Clin Pharmacokinet. 1982;7(2):93–107.
31. Patel A, Pai BHP, Diskina D, Reardon B, Lai YH. Comparison of clinical outcomes of acetaminophen IV vs PO in the peri-operative setting for laparoscopic inguinal hernia repair surgeries: a triple-blinded, randomized controlled trial. J Clin Anesth. 2020;61:109628.
32. Hickman SR, Mathieson KM, Bradford LM, Garman CD, Gregg RW, Lukens DW. Randomized trial of oral versus intravenous acetaminophen for postoperative pain control. Am J Health Syst Pharm. 2018;75(6):367–75.
33. Stocker ME, Montgomery JE. Serum paracetamol concentrations in adult volunteers following rectal administration. Br J Anaesth. 2001;87(4):638–40.
34. Ong CK, Lirk P, Tan CH, Seymour RA. An evidence-based update on nonsteroidal anti-inflammatory drugs. Clin Med Res. 2007;5(1):19–34.
35. De Oliveira GS Jr, Agarwal D, Benzon HT. Perioperative single dose ketorolac to prevent postoperative pain: a meta-analysis of randomized trials. Anesth Analg. 2012;114(2):424–33.
36. Ekman EF, Wahba M, Ancona F. Analgesic efficacy of perioperative celecoxib in ambulatory arthroscopic knee surgery: a double-blind, placebo-controlled study. Arthroscopy. 2006;22(6):635–42.
37. Huang YM, Wang CM, Wang CT, Lin WP, Horng LC, Jiang CC. Perioperative celecoxib administration for pain management after total knee arthroplasty – a randomized, controlled study. BMC Musculoskelet Disord. 2008;9:77.
38. Kinsella J, Moffat AC, Patrick JA, Prentice JW, McArdle CS, Kenny GN. Ketorolac trometamol for postoperative analgesia after orthopaedic surgery. Br J Anaesth. 1992;69(1):19–22.
39. El-Malah AA, Gineinah MM, Deb PK, Khayyat AN, Bansal M, Venugopala KN, et al. Selective COX-2 inhibitors: road from success to controversy and the quest for repurposing. Pharmaceuticals (Basel). 2022;15(7):827.
40. Brunton LL, Goodman LS, Gilman AG, Parker KL. Goodman and Gilman's manual of pharmacology and therapeutics. New York: McGraw-Hill; 2008.
41. Thybo KH, Hägi-Pedersen D, Dahl JB, Wetterslev J, Nersesjan M, Jakobsen JC, et al. Effect of combination of paracetamol (acetaminophen) and ibuprofen vs either alone on patient-controlled morphine consumption in the first 24 hours after Total hip arthroplasty: the PANSAID randomized clinical trial. JAMA. 2019;321(6):562–71.
42. Pogatzki-Zahn E, Chandrasena C, Schug SA. Nonopioid analgesics for postoperative pain management. Curr Opin Anaesthesiol. 2014;27(5):513–9.

43. Moore RA, Derry S, Aldington D, Wiffen PJ. Single dose oral analgesics for acute postoperative pain in adults – an overview of Cochrane reviews. Cochrane Database Syst Rev. 2015;2015(9):Cd008659.
44. Recart A, Issioui T, White PF, Klein K, Watcha MF, Stool L, et al. The efficacy of celecoxib premedication on postoperative pain and recovery times after ambulatory surgery: a dose-ranging study. Anesth Analg. 2003;96(6):1631–5. table of contents
45. Strom BL, Berlin JA, Kinman JL, Spitz PW, Hennessy S, Feldman H, et al. Parenteral ketorolac and risk of gastrointestinal and operative site bleeding. A postmarketing surveillance study. JAMA. 1996;275(5):376–82.
46. Rusy LM, Houck CS, Sullivan LJ, Ohlms LA, Jones DT, McGill TJ, et al. A double-blind evaluation of ketorolac tromethamine versus acetaminophen in pediatric tonsillectomy: analgesia and bleeding. Anesth Analg. 1995;80(2):226–9.
47. Schafer AI. Effects of nonsteroidal anti-inflammatory therapy on platelets. Am J Med. 1999;106(5b):25s–36s.
48. Bongiovanni T, Lancaster E, Ledesma Y, Whitaker E, Steinman MA, Allen IE, et al. Systematic review and meta-analysis of the association between non-steroidal anti-inflammatory drugs and operative bleeding in the perioperative period. J Am Coll Surg. 2021;232(5):765–90.e1.
49. Lucas GNC, Leitão ACC, Alencar RL, Xavier RMF, Daher EF, Silva Junior GBD. Pathophysiological aspects of nephropathy caused by non-steroidal anti-inflammatory drugs. J Bras Nefrol. 2019;41(1):124–30.
50. Bell S, Rennie T, Marwick CA, Davey P. Effects of peri-operative nonsteroidal anti-inflammatory drugs on post-operative kidney function for adults with normal kidney function. Cochrane Database Syst Rev. 2018;11:CD011274.
51. Harris RC Jr. Cyclooxygenase-2 inhibition and renal physiology. Am J Cardiol. 2002;89(6a):10d–7d.
52. Lee A, Cooper MG, Craig JC, Knight JF, Keneally JP. Effects of nonsteroidal anti-inflammatory drugs on postoperative renal function in adults with normal renal function. Cochrane Database Syst Rev. 2007;2018(2):Cd002765.
53. Endo K, Sairyo K, Komatsubara S, Sasa T, Egawa H, Ogawa T, et al. Cyclooxygenase-2 inhibitor delays fracture healing in rats. Acta Orthop. 2005;76(4):470–4.
54. Krischak GD, Augat P, Blakytny R, Claes L, Kinzl L, Beck A. The non-steroidal anti-inflammatory drug diclofenac reduces appearance of osteoblasts in bone defect healing in rats. Arch Orthop Trauma Surg. 2007;127(6):453–8.
55. Hassan MK, Karlock LG. The effect of post-operative NSAID administration on bone healing after elective foot and ankle surgery. Foot Ankle Surg. 2020;26(4):457–63.
56. Abdul-Hadi O, Parvizi J, Austin MS, Viscusi E, Einhorn T. Nonsteroidal anti-inflammatory drugs in orthopaedics. J Bone Joint Surg Am. 2009;91(8):2020–7.
57. Aliuskevicius M, Østgaard SE, Hauge EM, Vestergaard P, Rasmussen S. Influence of ibuprofen on bone healing after Colles' fracture: a randomized controlled clinical trial. J Orthop Res. 2020;38(3):545–54.
58. Marsico F, Paolillo S, Filardi PP. NSAIDs and cardiovascular risk. J Cardiovasc Med (Hagerstown). 2017;18(Suppl 1: Special Issue on The State of the Art for the Practicing Cardiologist: The 2016 Conoscere E Curare Il Cuore (CCC) Proceedings from the CLI Foundation):e40-e3.
59. Joshi GP, Gertler R, Fricker R. Cardiovascular thromboembolic adverse effects associated with cyclooxygenase-2 selective inhibitors and nonselective antiinflammatory drugs. Anesth Analg. 2007;105(6):1793–804. table of contents
60. Liu SS, Bae JJ, Bieltz M, Ma Y, Memtsoudis S. Association of perioperative use of nonsteroidal anti-inflammatory drugs with postoperative myocardial infarction after total joint replacement. Reg Anesth Pain Med. 2012;37(1):45–50.
61. Calatayud J, González A. History of the development and evolution of local anesthesia since the coca leaf. Anesthesiology. 2003;98(6):1503–8.
62. Tetzlaff JE. The pharmacology of local anesthetics. Anesthesiol Clin North Am. 2000;18(2):217–33. v

63. Hollmann MW, Durieux ME. Local anesthetics and the inflammatory response: a new therapeutic indication? Anesthesiology. 2000;93(3):858–75.
64. Macfarlane AJR, Gitman M, Bornstein KJ, El-Boghdadly K, Weinberg G. Updates in our understanding of local anaesthetic systemic toxicity: a narrative review. Anaesthesia. 2021;76(Suppl 1):27–39.
65. Neal JM, Barrington MJ, Fettiplace MR, Gitman M, Memtsoudis SG, Morwald EE, et al. The third American Society of Regional Anesthesia and Pain Medicine practice advisory on local anesthetic systemic toxicity: executive summary 2017. Reg Anesth Pain Med. 2018;43(2):113–23.
66. Verlinde M, Hollmann MW, Stevens MF, Hermanns H, Werdehausen R, Lirk P. Local anesthetic-induced neurotoxicity. Int J Mol Sci. 2016;17(3):339.
67. Hussain N, McCartney CJL, Neal JM, Chippor J, Banfield L, Abdallah FW. Local anaesthetic-induced myotoxicity in regional anaesthesia: a systematic review and empirical analysis. Br J Anaesth. 2018;121(4):822–41.
68. Ilfeld BM, Eisenach JC, Gabriel RA. Clinical effectiveness of liposomal bupivacaine administered by infiltration or peripheral nerve block to treat postoperative pain. Anesthesiology. 2021;134(2):283–344.
69. Dinges HC, Wiesmann T, Otremba B, Wulf H, Eberhart LH, Schubert AK. The analgesic efficacy of liposomal bupivacaine compared with bupivacaine hydrochloride for the prevention of postoperative pain: a systematic review and meta-analysis with trial sequential analysis. Reg Anesth Pain Med. 2021;46(6):490–8.
70. Hussain N, Brull R, Sheehy B, Essandoh MK, Stahl DL, Weaver TE, et al. Perineural liposomal bupivacaine is not superior to nonliposomal bupivacaine for peripheral nerve block analgesia. Anesthesiology. 2021;134(2):147–64.
71. Joshi GP, Machi A. Surgical site infiltration: a neuroanatomical approach. Best Pract Res Clin Anaesthesiol. 2019;33(3):317–24.
72. Bai JW, An D, Perlas A, Chan V. Adjuncts to local anesthetic wound infiltration for postoperative analgesia: a systematic review. Reg Anesth Pain Med. 2020;45(8):645–55.
73. Klag EA, Okoroha KR, Kuhlmann NA, Sheena G, Chen C, Muh SJ. Does the use of periarticular anesthetic cocktail provide adequate pain control following shoulder arthroplasty? Shoulder Elbow. 2021;13(5):502–8.
74. Huang XZ, Zhao JH, Gao P, Chen XW, Song YX, Xu Y, et al. Continuous wound infiltration with local anesthetic is an effective and safe postoperative analgesic strategy: a meta-analysis. Pain Ther. 2021;10(1):525–38.
75. Matsen FA 3rd, Papadonikolakis A. Published evidence demonstrating the causation of glenohumeral chondrolysis by postoperative infusion of local anesthetic via a pain pump. J Bone Joint Surg Am. 2013;95(12):1126–34.
76. Rao AJ, Johnston TR, Harris AH, Smith RL, Costouros JG. Inhibition of chondrocyte and synovial cell death after exposure to commonly used anesthetics: chondrocyte apoptosis after anesthetics. Am J Sports Med. 2014;42(1):50–8.
77. Hussain N, Brull R, Sheehy BT, Kushelev M, Essandoh MK, Abdallah FW. The mornings after-periarticular liposomal bupivacaine infiltration does not improve analgesic outcomes beyond 24 hours following total knee arthroplasty: a systematic review and meta-analysis. Reg Anesth Pain Med. 2021;46(1):61–72.
78. Jiang H, Ma Q, Dong J, Ye X. The effect of liposomal bupivacaine for surgical wound infiltration: a meta-analysis of randomised controlled trials. Int Wound J. 2022;20:1591.
79. Gordh T. Lidocaine: the origin of a modern local anesthetic. 1949. Anesthesiology. 2010;113(6):1433–7.
80. Weibel S, Jelting Y, Pace NL, Helf A, Eberhart LH, Hahnenkamp K, et al. Continuous intravenous perioperative lidocaine infusion for postoperative pain and recovery in adults. Cochrane Database Syst Rev. 2018;6:Cd009642.

81. Ortiz MP, Godoy MC, Schlosser RS, Ortiz RP, Godoy JP, Santiago ES, et al. Effect of endovenous lidocaine on analgesia and serum cytokines: double-blinded and randomized trial. J Clin Anesth. 2016;35:70–7.
82. Yang X, Wei X, Mu Y, Li Q, Liu J. A review of the mechanism of the central analgesic effect of lidocaine. Medicine. 2020;99(17):e19898.
83. Lahav M, Levite M, Bassani L, Lang A, Fidder H, Tal R, et al. Lidocaine inhibits secretion of IL-8 and IL-1beta and stimulates secretion of IL-1 receptor antagonist by epithelial cells. Clin Exp Immunol. 2002;127(2):226–33.
84. Kranke P, Jokinen J, Pace NL, Schnabel A, Hollmann MW, Hahnenkamp K, et al. Continuous intravenous perioperative lidocaine infusion for postoperative pain and recovery. Cochrane Database Syst Rev. 2015;(7):Cd009642. https://doi.org/10.1002/14651858.CD009642.pub2.
85. Dunn LK, Durieux ME. Perioperative use of intravenous lidocaine. Anesthesiology. 2017;126(4):729–37.
86. Foo I, Macfarlane AJR, Srivastava D, Bhaskar A, Barker H, Knaggs R, et al. The use of intravenous lidocaine for postoperative pain and recovery: international consensus statement on efficacy and safety. Anaesthesia. 2021;76(2):238–50.
87. Kumar M, Chawla R, Goyal M. Topical anesthesia. J Anaesthesiol Clin Pharmacol. 2015;31(4):450–6.
88. EMLA Cream Prescription Information US Food and Drug Administration. 2023. https://www.accessdata.fda.gov/drugsatfda_docs/label/2017/020235s064_020882s047_021129s046lbl.pdf.
89. Koo CH, Kim J, Na HS, Ryu JH, Shin HJ. The effect of lidocaine patch for postoperative pain: a meta-analysis of randomized controlled trials. J Clin Anesth. 2022;81:110918.
90. Ranganath Y, Seering M, Marian A. Curb your enthusiasm: local anesthetic adjuvants for peripheral nerve blocks. ASRA Pain Med News. 2020;45 https://doi.org/10.52211/asra110120.071.
91. Machi AT, Ilfeld BM. Continuous peripheral nerve blocks in the ambulatory setting: an update of the published evidence. Curr Opin Anaesthesiol. 2015;28(6):648–55.
92. Ilfeld BM. Continuous peripheral nerve blocks: An update of the published evidence and comparison with novel. Alternative Analg. 2017;124(1):308–35.
93. Law WZW, Sara RA, Cameron AJD, Lightfoot NJ. Local anaesthetic delivery regimens for peripheral nerve catheters: a systematic review and network meta-analysis. Anaesthesia. 2020;75(3):395–405.
94. Behrend Christiansen C, Herold Madsen M, Rothe C, Bretlau C, Lundstrøm LH, Lange KHW. Programmed, intermittent boluses versus continuous infusion to the sciatic nerve – a non-inferiority randomized, controlled trial. Acta Anaesthesiol Scand. 2022;66(1):114–24.
95. Aoyama Y, Sakura S, Wittayapairoj A, Abe S, Tadenuma S, Saito Y. Continuous basal infusion versus programmed intermittent bolus for quadratus lumborum block after laparoscopic colorectal surgery: a randomized-controlled, double-blind study. J Anesth. 2020;34(5):642–9.
96. Wang XX, Zhang XL, Zhang ZX, Xin ZQ, Guo HJ, Liu HY, et al. Programmed intermittent epidural bolus in parturients: a meta-analysis of randomized controlled trials. Medicine. 2022;101(5):e28742.
97. Wiesmann T, Hoff L, Prien L, Torossian A, Eberhart L, Wulf H, et al. Programmed intermittent epidural bolus versus continuous epidural infusion for postoperative analgesia after major abdominal and gynecological cancer surgery: a randomized, triple-blinded clinical trial. BMC Anesthesiol. 2018;18(1):154.
98. Cummings KC III, Zimmerman NM, Maheshwari K, Cooper GS, Cummings LC. Epidural compared with non-epidural analgesia and cardiopulmonary complications after colectomy: a retrospective cohort study of 20,880 patients using a national quality database. J Clin Anesth. 2018;47:12–8.
99. Yeung JH, Gates S, Naidu BV, Wilson MJ, Gao SF. Paravertebral block versus thoracic epidural for patients undergoing thoracotomy. Cochrane Database Syst Rev. 2016;2(2):Cd009121.

100. Anger M, Valovska T, Beloeil H, Lirk P, Joshi GP, Van de Velde M, et al. PROSPECT guideline for total hip arthroplasty: a systematic review and procedure-specific postoperative pain management recommendations. Anaesthesia. 2021;76(8):1082–97.
101. Rawal N. Current issues in postoperative pain management. Eur J Anaesthesiol. 2016;33(3):160–71.
102. Dieu A, Huynen P, Lavand'homme P, Beloeil H, Freys SM, Pogatzki-Zahn EM, et al. Pain management after open liver resection: procedure-specific postoperative pain management (PROSPECT) recommendations. Reg Anesth Pain Med. 2021;46(5):433–45.
103. Durkin C, Schisler T, Lohser J. Current trends in anesthesia for esophagectomy. Curr Opin Anaesthesiol. 2017;30(1):30–5.
104. Aloia TA, Kim BJ, Segraves-Chun YS, Cata JP, Truty MJ, Shi Q, et al. A randomized controlled trial of postoperative thoracic epidural analgesia versus intravenous patient-controlled analgesia after major hepatopancreatobiliary surgery. Ann Surg. 2017;266(3):545–54.
105. Bialka S, Copik M, Daszkiewicz A, Rivas E, Ruetzler K, Szarpak L, et al. Comparison of different methods of postoperative analgesia after thoracotomy-a randomized controlled trial. J Thorac Dis. 2018;10(8):4874–82.
106. Lee GC, Fong ZV, Ferrone CR, Thayer SP, Warshaw AL, Lillemoe KD, et al. High performing whipple patients: factors associated with short length of stay after open pancreaticoduodenectomy. J Gastrointest Surg. 2014;18(10):1760–9.
107. Sanford DE, Hawkins WG, Fields RC. Improved peri-operative outcomes with epidural analgesia in patients undergoing a pancreatectomy: a nationwide analysis. HPB (Oxford). 2015;17(6):551–8.
108. Raspé C, Flöther L, Schneider R, Bucher M, Piso P. Best practice for perioperative management of patients with cytoreductive surgery and HIPEC. Eur J Surg Oncol. 2017;43(6):1013–27.
109. Machi A, Kandil E. Epidural catheter infusion for post-operative analgesia for major spine surgery. In: Noe CE, editor. Multidisciplinary spine care. Cham: Springer International Publishing; 2022. p. 723–30.
110. Rhen T, Cidlowski JA. Antiinflammatory action of glucocorticoids–new mechanisms for old drugs. N Engl J Med. 2005;353(16):1711–23.
111. Turan A, Sessler DI. Steroids to ameliorate postoperative pain. Anesthesiology. 2011;115(3):457–9.
112. Li H, Xie W, Strong JA, Zhang JM. Systemic antiinflammatory corticosteroid reduces mechanical pain behavior, sympathetic sprouting, and elevation of proinflammatory cytokines in a rat model of neuropathic pain. Anesthesiology. 2007;107(3):469–77.
113. Westlund K. Pain pathways: peripheral, spinal, ascending, descending pathways. In: Practical management of pain. Elsevier; 2014. p. 87–112.
114. Kehlet H. Glucocorticoids for peri-operative analgesia: how far are we from general recommendations? Acta Anaesthesiol Scand. 2007;51(9):1133–5.
115. De Oliveira GS Jr, Almeida MD, Benzon HT, McCarthy RJ. Perioperative single dose systemic dexamethasone for postoperative pain: a meta-analysis of randomized controlled trials. Anesthesiology. 2011;115(3):575–88.
116. Waldron NH, Jones CA, Gan TJ, Allen TK, Habib AS. Impact of perioperative dexamethasone on postoperative analgesia and side-effects: systematic review and meta-analysis. Br J Anaesth. 2013;110(2):191–200.
117. Chong MA, Berbenetz NM, Lin C, Singh S. Perineural versus intravenous dexamethasone as an adjuvant for peripheral nerve blocks: a systematic review and meta-analysis. Reg Anesth Pain Med. 2017;42(3):319–26.
118. Klag EA, Kuhlmann NA, Tramer JS, Franovic S, Muh SJ. Dexamethasone decreases postoperative opioid and antiemetic use in shoulder arthroplasty patients: a prospective, randomized controlled trial. J Shoulder Elb Surg. 2021;30(7):1544–52.

119. Yue C, Wei R, Liu Y. Perioperative systemic steroid for rapid recovery in total knee and hip arthroplasty: a systematic review and meta-analysis of randomized trials. J Orthop Surg Res. 2017;12(1):100.
120. Chan TCW, Cheung CW, Wong SSC, Chung AYF, Irwin MG, Chan PK, et al. Preoperative dexamethasone for pain relief after total knee arthroplasty: a randomised controlled trial. Eur J Anaesthesiol. 2020;37(12):1157–67.
121. Gasbjerg KS, Hägi-Pedersen D, Lunn TH, Laursen CC, Holmqvist M, Vinstrup L, et al. Effect of dexamethasone as an analgesic adjuvant to multimodal pain treatment after total knee arthroplasty: randomised clinical trial. BMJ (Clinical research ed). 2022;376:e067325.
122. Tsuei SE, Moore RG, Ashley JJ, McBride WG. Disposition of synethetic glucocorticoids. I. Pharmacokinetics of dexamethasone in healthy adults. J Pharmacokinet Biopharm. 1979;7(3):249–64.
123. Polderman JA, Farhang-Razi V, Van Dieren S, Kranke P, DeVries JH, Hollmann MW, et al. Adverse side effects of dexamethasone in surgical patients. Cochrane Database Syst Rev. 2018;11:Cd011940.
124. Corcoran T, Kasza J, Short TG, O'Loughlin E, Chan MT, Leslie K, et al. Intraoperative dexamethasone does not increase the risk of postoperative wound infection: a propensity score-matched post hoc analysis of the ENIGMA-II trial (EnDEX). Br J Anaesth. 2017;118(2):190–9.
125. Corcoran TB, Myles PS, Forbes AB, Cheng AC, Bach LA, O'Loughlin E, et al. Dexamethasone and surgical-site infection. N Engl J Med. 2021;384(18):1731–41.
126. Anitescu M. Pharmacology for the interventional pain physician. In: Practical management of pain. Elsevier; 2014. p. 596–603.
127. Hamilton GR, Baskett TF. In the arms of Morpheus the development of morphine for postoperative pain relief. Can J Anaesth. 2000;47(4):367–74.
128. Brownstein MJ. A brief history of opiates, opioid peptides, and opioid receptors. Proc Natl Acad Sci USA. 1993;90(12):5391–3.
129. Kharasch ED, Brunt LM. Perioperative opioids and public health. Anesthesiology. 2016;124(4):960–5.
130. Quigley C, Wiffen P. A systematic review of hydromorphone in acute and chronic pain. J Pain Symptom Manag. 2003;25(2):169–78.
131. Opioids FK. Miller's anesthesia. Philadelphia: Elsevier; 2010. p. 769–824.
132. Hayhurst CJ, Durieux ME. Differential opioid tolerance and opioid-induced hyperalgesia: a clinical reality. Anesthesiology. 2016;124(2):483–8.
133. Fletcher D, Martinez V. Opioid-induced hyperalgesia in patients after surgery: a systematic review and a meta-analysis. Br J Anaesth. 2014;112(6):991–1004.
134. Kaiko RF, Wallenstein SL, Rogers AG, Grabinski PY, Houde RW. Analgesic and mood effects of heroin and morphine in cancer patients with postoperative pain. N Engl J Med. 1981;304(25):1501–5.
135. Yaster M, Benzon HT, Anderson TA. "Houston, we have a problem!": the role of the anesthesiologist in the current opioid epidemic. Anesth Analg. 2017;125(5):1429–31.
136. Jones MR, Viswanath O, Peck J, Kaye AD, Gill JS, Simopoulos TT. A brief history of the opioid epidemic and strategies for pain medicine. Pain Ther. 2018;7(1):13–21.
137. Jivraj NK, Raghavji F, Bethell J, Wijeysundera DN, Ladha KS, Bateman BT, et al. Persistent postoperative Opioid use: a systematic literature search of definitions and population-based cohort study. Anesthesiology. 2020;132(6):1528–39.
138. Kent ML, Hurley RW, Oderda GM, Gordon DB, Sun E, Mythen M, et al. American Society for Enhanced Recovery and Perioperative Quality Initiative-4 Joint Consensus Statement on Persistent Postoperative Opioid Use: Definition, Incidence, Risk Factors, and Health Care System Initiatives. Anesth Analg. 2019;129(2):543–52.
139. Hanna M. Systemic analgesics: opioids. In: Benzon H, Rathmell JP, Wu C, Turk D, Argoff C, Hurley R, editors. Practicial management of pain. Philadelphia: Elsevier; 2014.
140. Momeni M, Crucitti M, De Kock M. Patient-controlled analgesia in the management of postoperative pain. Drugs. 2006;66(18):2321–37.

141. Stoelting RK. Acute postoperative pain management. In: Basics of anesthesia. Philadelphia: Elsevier; 2007.
142. Macintyre PE, Jarvis DA. Age is the best predictor of postoperative morphine requirements. Pain. 1996;64(2):357–64.
143. VanDercar DH, Martinez AP, De Lisser EA. Sleep apnea syndromes: a potential contraindication for patient-controlled analgesia. Anesthesiology. 1991;74(3):623–4.
144. Shanthanna H, Ladha KS, Kehlet H, Joshi GP. Perioperative opioid administration: a critical review of opioid-free versus opioid-sparing approaches. Anesthesiology. 2021;134(4):645–59.
145. Forget P. Opioid-free anaesthesia. Why and how? A contextual analysis. Anaesth Crit Care Pain Med. 2019;38(2):169–72.
146. Villemagne PS, Dannals RF, Ravert HT, Frost JJ. PET imaging of human cardiac opioid receptors. Eur J Nucl Med Mol Imaging. 2002;29(10):1385–8.
147. Feng Y, He X, Yang Y, Chao D, Lazarus LH, Xia Y. Current research on opioid receptor function. Curr Drug Targets. 2012;13(2):230–46.
148. Vallejo R, de Leon-Casasola O, Benyamin R. Opioid therapy and immunosuppression: a review. Am J Ther. 2004;11(5):354–65.
149. Romberg R, Sarton E, Teppema L, Matthes HW, Kieffer BL, Dahan A. Comparison of morphine-6-glucuronide and morphine on respiratory depressant and antinociceptive responses in wild type and mu-opioid receptor deficient mice. Br J Anaesth. 2003;91(6):862–70.
150. Kojima Y, Takahashi T, Fujina M, Owyang C. Inhibition of cholinergic transmission by opiates in ileal myenteric plexus is mediated by kappa receptor. Involvement of regulatory inhibitory G protein and calcium N-channels. J Pharmacol Exp Ther. 1994;268(2):965–70.
151. Nagase H, Saitoh A. Research and development of κ opioid receptor agonists and δ opioid receptor agonists. Pharmacol Ther. 2020;205:107427.
152. Murphy GS, Szokol JW, Avram MJ, Greenberg SB, Shear TD, Deshur MA, et al. Clinical effectiveness and safety of intraoperative methadone in patients undergoing posterior spinal fusion surgery: a randomized, double-blinded, controlled trial. Anesthesiology. 2017;126(5):822–33.
153. Dahan A, Yassen A, Romberg R, Sarton E, Teppema L, Olofsen E, et al. Buprenorphine induces ceiling in respiratory depression but not in analgesia. Br J Anaesth. 2006;96(5):627–32.
154. Raffa RB, Haidery M, Huang H-M, Kalladeen K, Lockstein DE, Ono H, et al. The clinical analgesic efficacy of buprenorphine. J Clin Pharm Ther. 2014;39(6):577–83.
155. Kohan L, Potru S, Barreveld AM, Sprintz M, Lane O, Aryal A, et al. Buprenorphine management in the perioperative period: educational review and recommendations from a multisociety expert panel. Reg Anesth Pain Med. 2021;46(10):840–59.
156. Sultan P, Gutierrez MC, Carvalho B. Neuraxial morphine and respiratory depression. Drugs. 2011;71(14):1807–19.
157. Domino EF, Chodoff P, Corssen G. Pharmacologic effects of CI-581, a new dissociative anesthetic, in man. Clin Pharmacol Ther. 1965;6:279–91.
158. Urban MK, Ya Deau JT, Wukovits B, Lipnitsky JY. Ketamine as an adjunct to postoperative pain management in opioid tolerant patients after spinal fusions: a prospective randomized trial. HSS J. 2008;4(1):62–5.
159. Schwenk ES, Viscusi ER, Buvanendran A, Hurley RW, Wasan AD, Narouze S, et al. Consensus Guidelines on the Use of Intravenous Ketamine Infusions for Acute Pain Management From the American Society of Regional Anesthesia and Pain Medicine, the American Academy of Pain Medicine, and the American Society of Anesthesiologists. Reg Anesth Pain Med. 2018;43(5):456–66.
160. Bell RF, Kalso EA. Ketamine for pain management. Pain Rep. 2018;3(5):e674.
161. Schmid RL, Sandler AN, Katz J. Use and efficacy of low-dose ketamine in the management of acute postoperative pain: a review of current techniques and outcomes. Pain. 1999;82(2):111–25.

162. Ferreira RCM, Castor MGM, Piscitelli F, Di Marzo V, Duarte IDG, Romero TRL. The involvement of the endocannabinoid system in the peripheral antinociceptive action of ketamine. J Pain. 2018;19(5):487–95.
163. Brinck EC, Tiippana E, Heesen M, Bell RF, Straube S, Moore RA, et al. Perioperative intravenous ketamine for acute postoperative pain in adults. Cochrane Database Syst Rev. 2018;12:Cd012033.
164. Niesters M, Martini C, Dahan A. Ketamine for chronic pain: risks and benefits. Br J Clin Pharmacol. 2014;77(2):357–67.
165. Bell RF, Dahl JB, Moore RA, Kalso E. Peri-operative ketamine for acute post-operative pain: a quantitative and qualitative systematic review (Cochrane review). Acta Anaesthesiol Scand. 2005;49(10):1405–28.
166. Elia N, Tramer MR. Ketamine and postoperative pain–a quantitative systematic review of randomised trials. Pain. 2005;113(1–2):61–70.
167. Aveline C, Gautier JF, Vautier P, Cognet F, Hetet HL, Attali JY, et al. Postoperative analgesia and early rehabilitation after total knee replacement: a comparison of continuous low-dose intravenous ketamine versus nefopam. Eur J Pain (London, England). 2009;13(6):613–9.
168. Wang P, Yang Z, Shan S, Cao Z, Wang Z. Analgesic effect of perioperative ketamine for total hip arthroplasties and total knee arthroplasties: a PRISMA-compliant meta-analysis. Medicine. 2020;99(42):e22809.
169. Waelkens P, Alsabbagh E, Sauter A, Joshi GP, Beloeil H. Pain management after complex spine surgery: a systematic review and procedure-specific postoperative pain management recommendations. Eur J Anaesthesiol. 2021;38(9):985–94.
170. Geisler A, Zachodnik J, Køppen K, Chakari R, Bech-Azeddine R. Postoperative pain treatment after spinal fusion surgery: a systematic review with meta-analyses and trial sequential analyses. Pain Rep. 2022;7(3):e1005.
171. Brinck ECV, Virtanen T, Mäkelä S, Soini V, Hynninen VV, Mulo J, et al. S-ketamine in patient-controlled analgesia reduces opioid consumption in a dose-dependent manner after major lumbar fusion surgery: a randomized, double-blind, placebo-controlled clinical trial. PLoS One. 2021;16(6):e0252626.
172. Czarnetzki C, Desmeules J, Tessitore E, Faundez A, Chabert J, Daali Y, et al. Perioperative intravenous low-dose ketamine for neuropathic pain after major lower back surgery: a randomized, placebo-controlled study. Eur J Pain (London, England). 2020;24(3):555–67.
173. Neurontin (gabapentin). 2017. https://www.accessdata.fda.gov/drugsatfda_docs/label/2017/020235s064_020882s047_021129s046lbl.pdf.
174. Lyrica (pregabalin). 2018. https://www.accessdata.fda.gov/drugsatfda_docs/label/2017/020235s064_020882s047_021129s046lbl.pdf.
175. Eipe N, Penning J, Yazdi F, Mallick R, Turner L, Ahmadzai N, et al. Perioperative use of pregabalin for acute pain-a systematic review and meta-analysis. Pain. 2015;156(7):1284–300.
176. Schmidt PC, Ruchelli G, Mackey SC, Carroll IR. Perioperative gabapentinoids: choice of agent, dose, timing, and effects on chronic postsurgical pain. Anesthesiology. 2013;119(5):1215–21.
177. Verret M, Lauzier F, Zarychanski R, Perron C, Savard X, Pinard AM, et al. Perioperative use of gabapentinoids for the management of postoperative acute pain: a systematic review and meta-analysis. Anesthesiology. 2020;133(2):265–79.
178. Myhre M, Diep LM, Stubhaug A. Pregabalin has analgesic, ventilatory, and cognitive effects in combination with remifentanil. Anesthesiology. 2016;124(1):141–9.
179. Deljou A, Hedrick SJ, Portner ER, Schroeder DR, Hooten WM, Sprung J, et al. Pattern of perioperative gabapentinoid use and risk for postoperative naloxone administration. Br J Anaesth. 2018;120(4):798–806.
180. Ohnuma T, Krishnamoorthy V, Ellis AR, Yan R, Ray ND, Hsia HL, et al. Association between gabapentinoids on the day of colorectal surgery and adverse postoperative respiratory outcomes. Ann Surg. 2019;270(6):e65–e7.
181. O'Rourke MJ, Keshock MC, Boxhorn CE, Correll DJ, O'Glasser AY, Gazelka HM, et al. preoperative management of opioid and nonopioid analgesics: Society for Perioperative

Assessment and Quality Improvement (SPAQI) consensus statement. Mayo Clin Proc. 2021;96(5):1325–41.
182. Looke TD, Kluth CT. Effect of preoperative intravenous methocarbamol and intravenous acetaminophen on opioid use after primary total hip and knee replacement. Orthopedics. 2013;36(2 Suppl):25–32.
183. Hidalgo DA, Pusic AL. The role of methocarbamol and intercostal nerve blocks for pain management in breast augmentation. Aesthet Surg J. 2005;25(6):571–5.
184. Aljuhani O, Kopp BJ, Patanwala AE. Effect of methocarbamol on acute pain after traumatic injury. Am J Ther. 2017;24(2):e202–e6.
185. Forsyth HF. Methocarbamol (robaxin) in orthopedic conditions; preliminary report of one hundred cases. JAMA J Am Med Assoc. 1958;167(2):163–8.
186. de Santana Santos T, Calazans AC, Martins-Filho PR, Silva LC, de Oliveira ESED, Gomes AC. Evaluation of the muscle relaxant cyclobenzaprine after third-molar extraction. J Am Dent Assoc (1939). 2011, 142(10):1154–62.
187. Sullivan PA, De Quattro V, Foti A, Curzon G. Effects of clonidine on central and peripheral nerve tone in primary hypertension. Hypertension. 1986;8(7):611–7.
188. Blaudszun G, Lysakowski C, Elia N, Tramer MR. Effect of perioperative systemic alpha2 agonists on postoperative morphine consumption and pain intensity: systematic review and meta-analysis of randomized controlled trials. Anesthesiology. 2012;116(6):1312–22.
189. Jessen Lundorf L, Korvenius Nedergaard H, Moller AM. Perioperative dexmedetomidine for acute pain after abdominal surgery in adults. Cochrane Database Syst Rev. 2016;2:Cd010358.
190. Chen K, Lu Z, Xin YC, Cai Y, Chen Y, Pan SM. Alpha-2 agonists for long-term sedation during mechanical ventilation in critically ill patients. Cochrane Database Syst Rev. 2015;1:Cd010269.
191. Shukry M, Clyde MC, Kalarickal PL, Ramadhyani U. Does dexmedetomidine prevent emergence delirium in children after sevoflurane-based general anesthesia? Paediatr Anaesth. 2005;15(12):1098–104.
192. Li Y, Wang B, Zhang LL, He SF, Hu XW, Wong GT, et al. Dexmedetomidine combined with general anesthesia provides similar intraoperative stress response reduction when compared with a combined general and epidural anesthetic technique. Anesth Analg. 2016;122(4):1202–10.
193. Wu HH, Wang HT, Jin JJ, Cui GB, Zhou KC, Chen Y, et al. Does dexmedetomidine as a neuraxial adjuvant facilitate better anesthesia and analgesia? A systematic review and meta-analysis. PLoS One. 2014;9(3):e93114.
194. Shaikh SI, Mahesh SB. The efficacy and safety of epidural dexmedetomidine and clonidine with bupivacaine in patients undergoing lower limb orthopedic surgeries. J Anaesthesiol Clin Pharmacol. 2016;32(2):203–9.
195. Brummett CM, Williams BA. Additives to local anesthetics for peripheral nerve blockade. Int Anesthesiol Clin. 2011;49(4):104–16.
196. Hall JE, Uhrich TD, Barney JA, Arain SR, Ebert TJ. Sedative, amnestic, and analgesic properties of small-dose dexmedetomidine infusions. Anesth Analg. 2000;90(3):699–705.
197. Peng K, Liu HY, Wu SR, Cheng H, Ji FH. Effects of combining dexmedetomidine and opioids for postoperative intravenous patient-controlled analgesia: a systematic review and meta-analysis. Clin J Pain. 2015;31(12):1097–104.
198. Yuen VM, Irwin MG, Hui TW, Yuen MK, Lee LH. A double-blind, crossover assessment of the sedative and analgesic effects of intranasal dexmedetomidine. Anesth Analg. 2007;105(2):374–80.
199. Abdallah FW, Brull R. Facilitatory effects of perineural dexmedetomidine on neuraxial and peripheral nerve block: a systematic review and meta-analysis. Br J Anaesth. 2013;110(6):915–25.
200. Maze M, Tranquilli W. Alpha-2 adrenoceptor agonists: defining the role in clinical anesthesia. Anesthesiology. 1991;74(3):581–605.

201. Nguyen V, Tiemann D, Park E, Salehi A. Alpha-2 agonists. Anesthesiol Clin. 2017;35(2):233–45.
202. Venn RM, Karol MD, Grounds RM. Pharmacokinetics of dexmedetomidine infusions for sedation of postoperative patients requiring intensive caret. Br J Anaesth. 2002;88(5):669–75.
203. Urits I, Jung JW, Amgalan A, Fortier L, Anya A, Wesp B, et al. Utilization of magnesium for the treatment of chronic pain. Anesth Pain Med. 2021;11(1):e112348.
204. De Oliveira GS Jr, Castro-Alves LJ, Khan JH, McCarthy RJ. Perioperative systemic magnesium to minimize postoperative pain: a meta-analysis of randomized controlled trials. Anesthesiology. 2013;119(1):178–90.
205. Albrecht E, Kirkham KR, Liu SS, Brull R. Peri-operative intravenous administration of magnesium sulphate and postoperative pain: a meta-analysis. Anaesthesia. 2013;68(1):79–90.
206. Lysakowski C, Dumont L, Czarnetzki C, Tramer MR. Magnesium as an adjuvant to postoperative analgesia: a systematic review of randomized trials. Anesth Analg. 2007;104(6):1532–9. table of contents
207. Tsaousi G, Nikopoulou A, Pezikoglou I, Birba V, Grosomanidis V. Implementation of magnesium sulphate as an adjunct to multimodal analgesic approach for perioperative pain control in lumbar laminectomy surgery: a randomized placebo-controlled clinical trial. Clin Neurol Neurosurg. 2020;197:106091.
208. Naidu R, Flood P. Magnesium: is there a signal in the noise? Anesthesiology. 2013;119(1):13–5.
209. Figueredo E, Garcia-Fuentes EM. Assessment of the efficacy of esmolol on the haemodynamic changes induced by laryngoscopy and tracheal intubation: a meta-analysis. Acta Anaesthesiol Scand. 2001;45(8):1011–22.
210. Watts R, Thiruvenkatarajan V, Calvert M, Newcombe G, van Wijk RM. The effect of perioperative esmolol on early postoperative pain: a systematic review and meta-analysis. J Anaesthesiol Clin Pharmacol. 2017;33(1):28–39.
211. Harkanen L, Halonen J, Selander T, Kokki H. Beta-adrenergic antagonists during general anesthesia reduced postoperative pain: a systematic review and a meta-analysis of randomized controlled trials. J Anesth. 2015;29(6):934–43.
212. Collard V, Mistraletti G, Taqi A, Asenjo JF, Feldman LS, Fried GM, et al. Intraoperative esmolol infusion in the absence of opioids spares postoperative fentanyl in patients undergoing ambulatory laparoscopic cholecystectomy. Anesth Analg. 2007;105(5):1255–62. table of contents
213. Volz-Zang C, Eckrich B, Jahn P, Schneidrowski B, Schulte B, Palm D. Esmolol, an ultrashort-acting, selective beta 1-adrenoceptor antagonist: pharmacodynamic and pharmacokinetic properties. Eur J Clin Pharmacol. 1994;46(5):399–404.
214. Berne R. The autonomic nervous system and its central control. In: Physiology: Mosby; 2004. p. 206–20.
215. Bahr MP, Williams BA. Esmolol, antinociception, and its potential opioid-sparing role in routine anesthesia care. Reg Anesth Pain Med. 2018;43(8):815–8.
216. Ander F, Magnuson A, de Leon A, Ahlstrand R. Does the beta-receptor antagonist esmolol have analgesic effects?: A randomised placebo-controlled cross-over study on healthy volunteers undergoing the cold pressor test. Eur J Anaesthesiol. 2018;35(3):165–72.
217. Booze RM, Crisostomo EA, Davis JN. Beta-adrenergic receptors in the hippocampal and retrohippocampal regions of rats and Guinea pigs: autoradiographic and immunohistochemical studies. Synapse (New York, NY). 1993;13(3):206–14.
218. Gelineau AM, King MR, Ladha KS, Burns SM, Houle T, Anderson TA. Intraoperative esmolol as an adjunct for perioperative opioid and postoperative pain reduction: a systematic review, meta-analysis, and meta-regression. Anesth Analg. 2018;126(3):1035–49.
219. Mendonça FT, Tramontini AJ, Miake HI, Seixas LF, de Carvalho LSF, Sposito AC. Intraoperative esmolol and pain following mastectomy: a randomised clinical trial. Eur J Anaesthesiol. 2021;38(7):735–43.
220. Lee SJ, Lee JN. The effect of perioperative esmolol infusion on the postoperative nausea, vomiting and pain after laparoscopic appendectomy. Korean J Anesthesiol. 2010;59(3):179–84.

221. Byrd RC, Sung RJ, Marks J, Parmley WW. Safety and efficacy of esmolol (ASL-8052: an ultrashort-acting beta-adrenergic blocking agent) for control of ventricular rate in supraventricular tachycardias. J Am Coll Cardiol. 1984;3(2 Pt 1):394–9.
222. Yu SK, Tait G, Karkouti K, Wijeysundera D, McCluskey S, Beattie WS. The safety of perioperative esmolol: a systematic review and meta-analysis of randomized controlled trials. Anesth Analg. 2011;112(2):267–81.
223. Ilfeld BM, Finneran JJ IV. Cryoneurolysis and percutaneous peripheral nerve stimulation to treat acute pain: a narrative review. Anesthesiology. 2020;133:1127.
224. Finneran Iv JJ, Ilfeld BM. Percutaneous cryoneurolysis for acute pain management: current status and future prospects. Expert Rev Med Devices. 2021;18(6):533–43.
225. Mihalko WM, Kerkhof AL, Ford MC, Crockarell JR Jr, Harkess JW, Guyton JL. Cryoneurolysis before Total knee arthroplasty in patients with severe osteoarthritis for reduction of postoperative pain and Opioid use in a single-center randomized controlled trial. J Arthroplast. 2021;36(5):1590–8.
226. Urban JA, Dolesh K, Martin E. A multimodal pain management protocol including preoperative cryoneurolysis for Total knee arthroplasty to reduce pain, Opioid consumption, and length of stay. Arthroplast Today. 2021;10:87–92.
227. Ilfeld BM, Gabriel RA, Trescot AM. Ultrasound-guided percutaneous cryoneurolysis for treatment of acute pain: could cryoanalgesia replace continuous peripheral nerve blocks? Br J Anaesth. 2017;119(4):703–6.
228. Ilfeld BM, Grant SA, Gilmore CA, Chae J, Wilson RD, Wongsarnpigoon A, et al. Neurostimulation for postsurgical analgesia: a novel system enabling ultrasound-guided percutaneous peripheral nerve stimulation. Pain Pract. 2017;17(7):892–901.
229. Melzack R, Wall PD. Pain mechanisms: a new theory. Science. 1965;150(3699):971–9.
230. Strand NH, D'Souza R, Wie C, Covington S, Maita M, Freeman J, et al. Mechanism of action of peripheral nerve stimulation. Curr Pain Headache Rep. 2021;25(7):47.
231. Campbell JN, Taub A. Local analgesia from percutaneous electrical stimulation. A peripheral mechanism. Arch Neurol. 1973;28(5):347–50.
232. Ilfeld BM, Gilmore CA, Grant SA, Bolognesi MP, Del Gaizo DJ, Wongsarnpigoon A, et al. Ultrasound-guided percutaneous peripheral nerve stimulation for analgesia following total knee arthroplasty: a prospective feasibility study. J Orthop Surg Res. 2017;12(1):4.
233. Ilfeld BM, Finneran JJT, Gabriel RA, Said ET, Nguyen PL, Abramson WB, et al. Ultrasound-guided percutaneous peripheral nerve stimulation: neuromodulation of the suprascapular nerve and brachial plexus for postoperative analgesia following ambulatory rotator cuff repair. A proof-of-concept study. Reg Anesth Pain Med. 2019;44:310.
234. Ilfeld BM, Gabriel RA, Said ET, Monahan AM, Sztain JF, Abramson WB, et al. Ultrasound-guided percutaneous peripheral nerve stimulation: neuromodulation of the sciatic nerve for postoperative analgesia following ambulatory foot surgery, a proof-of-concept study. Reg Anesth Pain Med. 2018;43(6):580–9.
235. Ilfeld BM, Plunkett A, Vijjeswarapu AM, Hackworth R, Dhanjal S, Turan A, et al. Percutaneous peripheral nerve stimulation (Neuromodulation) for postoperative pain: a randomized, sham-controlled pilot study. Anesthesiology. 2021;135(1):95–110.
236. Gabriel RA, Ilfeld BM. Acute postoperative pain management with percutaneous peripheral nerve stimulation: the SPRINT neuromodulation system. Expert Rev Med Devices. 2021;18(2):145–50.
237. Ilfeld BM, Finneran Iv JJ, Dalstrom D, Wallace AM, Abdullah B, Said ET. Percutaneous auricular nerve stimulation (neuromodulation) for the treatment of pain following outpatient surgery: a proof-of-concept case series. Reg Anesth Pain Med. 2022;47(9):581–5.
238. Hao JJ, Mittelman M. Acupuncture: past, present, and future. Glob Adv Health Med. 2014;3(4):6–8.
239. Acar HV. Acupuncture and related techniques during perioperative period: a literature review. Complement Ther Med. 2016;29:48–55.

240. Shah S, Godhardt L, Spofford C. Acupuncture and postoperative pain reduction. Curr Pain Headache Rep. 2022;26(6):453–8.
241. Ko HF, Chen CH, Dong KR, Wu HC. Effects of acupuncture on postoperative pain after total knee replacement: systematic literature review and meta-analysis. Pain Med (Malden, Mass). 2021;22(9):2117–27.
242. Cheng SI, Kelleher DC, DeMeo D, Zhong H, Birch G, Ast MP. Intraoperative acupuncture as part of a multimodal analgesic regimen to reduce Opioid usage after Total knee arthroplasty: a prospective cohort trial. Med Acupunct. 2022;34(1):49–57.
243. Mallory MJ, Do A, Bublitz SE, Veleber SJ, Bauer BA, Bhagra A. Puncturing the myths of acupuncture. J Integr Med. 2016;14(5):311–4.
244. Patil S, Sen S, Bral M, Reddy S, Bradley KK, Cornett EM, et al. The role of acupuncture in pain management. Curr Pain Headache Rep. 2016;20(4):22.
245. Zgierska AE, Burzinski CA, Cox J, Kloke J, Stegner A, Cook DB, et al. Mindfulness meditation and cognitive behavioral therapy intervention reduces pain severity and sensitivity in opioid-treated chronic low back pain: pilot findings from a randomized controlled trial. Pain Med (Malden, Mass). 2016;17(10):1865–81.
246. Adler-Neal AL, Waugh CE, Garland EL, Shaltout HA, Diz DI, Zeidan F. The role of heart rate variability in mindfulness-based pain relief. J Pain. 2020;21(3–4):306–23.
247. Garland EL, Froeliger B, Howard MO. Effects of mindfulness-oriented recovery enhancement on reward responsiveness and opioid cue-reactivity. Psychopharmacology. 2014;231(16):3229–38.
248. McClintock AS, McCarrick SM, Garland EL, Zeidan F, Zgierska AE. Brief mindfulness-based interventions for acute and chronic pain: a systematic review. J Altern Complement Med. 2019;25(3):265–78.
249. Koch ME, Kain ZN, Ayoub C, Rosenbaum SH. The sedative and analgesic sparing effect of music. Anesthesiology. 1998;89(2):300–6.
250. Lin CL, Hwang SL, Jiang P, Hsiung NH. Effect of music therapy on pain after orthopedic surgery-a systematic review and meta-analysis. Pain Pract. 2020;20(4):422–36.
251. Hole J, Hirsch M, Ball E, Meads C. Music as an aid for postoperative recovery in adults: a systematic review and meta-analysis. Lancet (London, England). 2015;386(10004):1659–71.
252. Gold JI, Belmont KA, Thomas DA. The neurobiology of virtual reality pain attenuation. Cycberpsychol Behav. 2007;10(4):536–44.
253. Hoffman HG, Richards TL, Van Oostrom T, Coda BA, Jensen MP, Blough DK, et al. The analgesic effects of opioids and immersive virtual reality distraction: evidence from subjective and functional brain imaging assessments. Anesth Analg. 2007;105(6):1776–83. table of contents
254. Carrougher GJ, Hoffman HG, Nakamura D, Lezotte D, Soltani M, Leahy L, et al. The effect of virtual reality on pain and range of motion in adults with burn injuries. J Burn Care Res. 2009;30(5):785–91.
255. Furman E, Jasinevicius TR, Bissada NF, Victoroff KZ, Skillicorn R, Buchner M. Virtual reality distraction for pain control during periodontal scaling and root planing procedures. J Am Dent Assoc (1939). 2009;140(12):1508–16.
256. Tashjian VC, Mosadeghi S, Howard AR, Lopez M, Dupuy T, Reid M, et al. Virtual reality for Management of Pain in hospitalized patients: results of a controlled trial. JMIR Mental Health. 2017;4(1):e9.
257. Barry KS, Nimma SR, Spaulding AC, Wilke BK, Torp KD, Ledford CK. Perioperative outcomes of immersive virtual reality as adjunct anesthesia in primary total hip and knee arthroplasty. Arthroplast Today. 2022;18:84–8.
258. Peuchot H, Khakha R, Riera V, Ollivier M, Argenson JN. Intraoperative virtual reality distraction in TKA under spinal anesthesia: a preliminary study. Arch Orthop Trauma Surg. 2021;141(12):2323–8.

Postoperative Rehabilitation

23

Jake Stephen, Ryan Flowers, Alison Ho, Cathy Nakashima, and Donald Kasitinon

Introduction

Appropriate, well-executed postoperative (post-op) rehabilitation plays a significant role in desired outcomes following surgery. The overall goals of post-op rehabilitation include re-establishing joint mobility, muscle control around the joint, and eventually joint function in a safe manner. There remains variability in post-op rehabilitation protocols, but effort has been placed to find evidence in terms of

Author "Jake Stephen" and "Ryan Flowers" was previously at this institution when majority of work on this chapter was completed.

J. Stephen
Department of Anesthesiology Back and Pain Center, University of Michigan Health, Ann Arbor, MI, USA

Department of Physical Medicine and Rehabilitation, University of Texas Southwestern Medical Center, Dallas, TX, USA

R. Flowers
Department of Physical Medicine and Rehabilitation, University of Texas Southwestern Medical Center, Dallas, TX, USA

Mountain View Physical Medicine and Rehabilitation, Denver, CO, USA

A. Ho
Department of Physical Medicine and Rehabilitation, Baylor University Medical Center, Dallas, TX, USA

C. Nakashima
Health Sciences Digital Library and Learning Center, University of Texas Southwestern Medical Center, Dallas, TX, USA
e-mail: cathy.nakashima@utsouthwestern.edu

D. Kasitinon (✉)
Department of Physical Medicine and Rehabilitation, University of Texas Southwestern Medical Center, Dallas, TX, USA
e-mail: donald.kasitinon@utsouthwestern.edu

C. E. Noe (ed.), *Musculoskeletal Pain*,
https://doi.org/10.1007/978-3-031-86057-7_23

standardization of these protocols. In this chapter, established post-op protocols following some of the most common surgeries are discussed. We also discuss common complications specific to each surgery that providers should be aware of as well as new technologies or more accelerated post-op rehabilitation protocols that may further improve outcomes for certain surgeries.

Spine

Posterior Transpedicular Dynamic Stabilization

Posterior transpedicular dynamic stabilization involves the surgical repair of lumbar degenerative disk disease. Post-op rehabilitation involves three phases. Phase 1 or the Active Rest Phase (0–6 weeks) involves mobilization on post-op day 1. An emphasis is placed on no curving of the lumbar region, no rotation of the lumbar region, no intense abdominal exercises, avoidance of lifting, twisting, and hyperextending, as well as trying to keep the back straight. Phase 2 or the minimum movement phase (6–12 weeks) focuses on pelvic-tilt exercises, walking, and swimming. Phase 3 or the dynamic phase (12 weeks–6 months) focuses on dynamic lumbar stabilization exercises, kinetic chain strengthening exercises, swimming, and jogging. The return-to-sport phase is after 6 months, with an initial focus on low-resistance, and high repetition activities. Contact sports are allowed. Common complications include surgical wound infection and loose/malpositioned screw(s) [1].

Lumbar Decompression Through Minimally Invasive Laminotomy

Lumbar decompression through minimally invasive laminotomy is a surgical procedure performed for individuals with lumbar spinal stenosis. Post-op course involves four phases. Phase 1 (start around 1 week) involves extremity and core muscle conditioning. Initially, exercises are performed in the supine position and then are advanced to the standing stationary position. Phase 2 (start around 1 month) involves balance and stance training to accommodate the upright position, with the goal of increasing the duration of standing with minimal assistance. Phase 3 (start around 2 months) involves cardiovascular conditioning and gait training. Phase 4 (start around 3 months) involves sit-to-stand training. Common complications include surgical wound infection [2].

Lumbar Discectomy

Lumbar discectomy is a surgical procedure to treat lumbar disk herniation. The post-op course involves several phases. 1–3 days post-op, the focus is on limb active movement training, lower extremity passive joint mobility training, and active joint mobility training. From day 4 to 2 weeks, the focus is on active training for the lower extremities in bed, as well as straight-leg raise training and isometric contraction training for lumbar extensors. Weeks 2–3 focus on appropriately increasing lumbar range of motion (ROM), as well as increasing walking distance. Weeks 4–6 focus on gradually strengthening the lower back muscles and abdominal muscles, gradually transitioning to daily activities, gradually resuming walking in the community, participating in daily life activities and non-physical work, and increasing walking distance. The goal is to continue to avoid weightbearing on the waist and straight-leg bending activities, as well as learn to sit correctly and maintain lordosis. Weeks 6–12 focus on completing daily activities independently and gradually performing strength training for the core muscle groups of the spine. Weeks 12–24 focus on performing strength training for the core muscles of the spine with continued avoidance of strenuous exercise and high-intensity weightbearing [3]. Intense and dynamic active exercises are usually the first line, as opposed to isometric exercises or isolated stretching, which appear less effective [4]. Repetitive flexion exercises are not recommended before 6 weeks. Avoiding rotational movements and axial load over 5 kg (~10 lbs) is recommended before 6 weeks [5]. Common complications include surgical wound infection and deep vein thrombosis (DVT) [3].

Lumbar Fusion

Lumbar fusion is a surgical procedure to treat lumbar disease degeneration. For the first days post-op, goal is to perform light walking training and leg muscle stretching, as well as light trunk muscle contraction exercises to relearn a good posture of the upper body [6]. Maintaining prolonged positions for long periods and movements and postures with the trunk in extreme positions are not recommended before 6 weeks [4]. Avoid continuous sitting for more than 30 minutes at a time during the first 4 weeks. Common complications include surgical wound infection [6].

Sacroiliac (SI) Joint Fusion

SI joint fusion is a surgical procedure to treat SI joint degeneration and pain. Post-op course involves several phases. Phase 1 (0–5 weeks) focuses on no bending, lifting >10 lbs, wearing a pelvic belt correctly, and no twisting at the waist. Phase 2 (6–11 weeks) involves tissue mobilization around the surgical site to promote appropriate collagen alignment, evaluating and treating muscle tightness throughout the hip's ROM with stretching of muscles surrounding the SI joint without engaging past end ROM, starting deep abdominal muscle and pelvic floor muscle retraining, as well as starting gait training to decrease step length. Phase 3 (12–19 weeks) involves the addition of resistance exercises, progressing the patient's stabilization exercises, and initiation of single-leg exercises. Phase 4 (>20 weeks) involves incorporating high-impact exercises into the home exercise program

(HEP). Common complications include surgical wound infection and nerve root irritation [7].

Anterior Cervical Discectomy and Fusion (ACDF)

ACDF is a surgical procedure to treat cervical radiculopathy often due to disk herniation or degenerative disk disease [8]. Post-op, a cervical collar is recommended for 2 weeks. Once asymptomatic with radiographic evidence of stability, the patient is allowed to walk and use a recumbent bike and hands-free elliptical [9]. Therapy typically starts 4–6 weeks post-op [8, 9]. Emphasis is placed on endurance exercises, isometric strengthening, stretching, and aerobic activity while placing a lower emphasis on passive modalities [8]. Recommendations start with trunk stabilization exercises, with the goal to build strength and endurance in the lumbar spine-stabilizing muscles, with subsequent progression to chest-out posture and scapular stabilization exercises. The cervical spine rehabilitation program focuses on building strength and endurance of postural spine-stabilizing muscles rather than direct force on the cervical spine musculature. Return-to-sport for professional athletes is typically in the post-op 6–12 month period [9]. Common complications include dysphagia, worsening of preexisting myelopathy, unilateral recurrent laryngeal nerve palsy, and dural perforation [10].

Shoulder

Rotator Cuff Repair

Rotator cuff tears affect individuals across a wide demographic, from young athletes to aging adults [11, 12], and arthroscopic repair has become the mainstay of surgical approaches [13]. The primary goal of rehabilitation after surgery is to promote and support tissue healing, reduce pain, and restore ROM and function while minimizing stiffness and reducing the risk of recurrent tears. Despite the prevalence of rotator cuff tears and subsequent surgical repairs, there remains an absence of definitive guidelines for post-op rehabilitation, with significant heterogeneity in therapeutic timing and progression [11, 12, 14–19]. Furthermore, there is a wide range in the estimated rate of recurrent tears reported in the literature, from 13% to 94% noted by Sgrol and Cilenti, to a re-tear or partially healed rate of 20–90% reported by Tirefort et al. [16, 20] Multiple variables influence the risk of re-tears following repair, including patient factors, type of surgery, characteristics of the tear, tension on the repair, medial retraction, and early mobilization [11].

Consensus in the literature supports a three- to four-phase model structured around the principles of wound/tissue healing and criteria-based progression [19, 20]. These guidelines allow for protocol customization according to patient, injury, and surgical characteristics. While there are no precise criteria for advancement through phases, the International Classification of Function, Disability, and Health outlined a basis for identifying targets [19]. Underlying all the phases of rehabilitation should be early and consistent patient education. Patients should be educated on the guiding principles of the therapeutic stages of recovery to maximize compliance, reduce risk for impaired healing, set realistic goals, and improve participation in therapy.

See Table 23.1 for a proposed post-op rehabilitation protocol following rotator cuff repair. The debate over early versus delayed mobilization remains controversial. Multiple studies have attempted to clarify the benefits and limitations of early versus delayed mobilization following rotator cuff repair [12–15, 17, 19, 21]. While some studies have shown reduced stiffness, improved ROM, and improved quality of life on short-term follow-up at 3 and 6 months following early mobilization, only four studies recorded data 2 years post-op, showing no difference in functional outcomes along with comparable efficacy among accelerated and conservative rehabilitation protocols [12, 14]. Contrasting these findings, additional studies found a statistically significant association between early mobilization and an increased rate of recurrent tears and poor healing, particularly in medium- to large-sized lesions [11–14, 17, 20]. In small- to medium-sized tears, delayed mobilization demonstrated improved tendon healing, but did not provide a significant advantage in shoulder function [14]. Chen et al. demonstrated patients undergoing delayed mobilization had significantly better American Shoulder and Elbow Surgeons (ASES) scores [13]. The consensus statement from the American Society of Shoulder and Elbow Therapists (ASSET) recommends an initial two-week period of strict immobilization [12], whereas the American Academy of Orthopaedic Surgeons (AAOS) does not offer a definitive guideline on timing or progression of ROM or exercises [19]. One should consider the risk of re-tear unique to each patient, relative to initial tear size, and the consequence of managing stiffness versus the potential for a recurrent tear and subsequent prolongation of immobility and rehabilitation. More studies are needed to examine the relationship between tear size and early versus delayed mobilization protocols.

Phase I (0–6 Weeks): Immobilization, Pain Control, and PROM

The goals of phase I are aimed at supporting initial tissue healing, protecting the surgical repair, minimizing adhesions, and reducing pain [19, 20]. This is accomplished with a variable combination of pain control, immobilization, bracing, and passive ROM (PROM).

From post-op day 0, pain control is a priority for short- and long-term success. In addition to medical therapies, cryotherapy has proven effective at reducing pain, reducing narcotic usage, improving sleep, and providing generalized comfort for at least the first 10 days following surgery [11]. Cryotherapy should be initiated immediately following surgery, up to 4–6 times daily [19]. There is some evidence to support the use of transcutaneous electrical nerve stimulation (TENS) for the reduction of pain and opioid use within the first week following rotator cuff repair [17].

Initial mobility in the first phase is restricted to PROM starting between 2 and 4 weeks after surgery [19]. Leading up to this during weeks 0 through 2, the patient can be instructed on open chain active ROM (AROM) at the hand and wrist [20]. To

Table 23.1 Postoperative rehabilitation course for rotator cuff repair [12, 19, 20]

Phase	Goals	Range of motion/precautions	StrengtheningcConditioning/intervention
Phase I (Weeks 0–6)	Immobilization, pain control, PROM, and prevent stiffness	Week 0–2: Strict immobilization (removal from sling only for showers, while eating, and physiotherapy), distal hand/wrist activity (squeezing and AROM) Week 2–4: Continued immobilization, hand/wrist exercises, PROM self-initiated in scapular plane (limit to 90 forward flexion and 30 degrees external rotation), elbow activation with arm at side, and scapular protraction/depression Weeks 4–6: *Discontinuation of sling*, PROM/AROM with therapist (flexion and external rotation), supine shoulder elevation PROM	Week 0–4: Pendulum exercises Week 4–6: Active-assisted exercises in pain-free range, within ROM limitations *Criteria to Advance:* Pain-free PROM, PROM forward flexion 90–120 degrees or beyond, PROM external rotation 30–45 degrees or beyond, and PROM abduction to 90 degrees
Phase II (Weeks 6–12)	Restoration of full ROM, and improve basic functional strength with emphasis on rotator cuff co-activation	Forward flexion and external rotation to tolerance Limit internal rotation to beltline with no aggressive stretching	Week 7–12: Progress from active-assisted ROM to AROM, supine to incline to standing cane forward flexion in scapular plane, towel slide scaption, submaximal and pain-free isometric exercises (starting with internal rotation, followed by external rotation), T-band rows with scapular retraction Week 8–12: Standing shoulder extension exercises *Criteria to Advance:* Full pain-free PROM, full and symmetric AROM without compensation (no shoulder "shrug" sign), pain-free isometric exercises Some patients will not progress beyond this phase

(continued)

Phase III (Weeks 12+)	Maintain FROM, improve strength in multiple planes of motion, and improve scapular and glenohumeral mechanics	Unrestricted forward flexion, external rotation, and internal rotation Focus on scapular kinematics and glenohumeral joint centration with increasing loads. Reduce risk of subacromial impingement	Initiate rotator cuff strengthening in all planes of motion with isometric, isotonic, and light closed-chain exercises, T-band external/internal rotation with towel, standing row, supine punch, side-lying external rotation, proprioceptive neuromuscular facilitation diagonals, prone mid and ascending trapezius Scapular kinematic strengthening, to include trapezius, serratus anterior, rhomboids, and deltoid Timed progressions as appropriate to healing
Phase IV (Weeks ~24+)	Advance functional abilities to sport, daily life, and/or work, integration of trunk posture	Expect full PROM/AROM	Continue prior strengthening protocols with addition of sport/life/work-specific motions Further emphasis on trunk posture and core, integration Duration of phase will vary depending on goals Full return-to-sport varies from 6 to 12 months

minimize active strain on the repaired tissue, PROM should be limited to arm elevation to 90 degrees in the scapular plane, external rotation from 0 to 60 degrees, and pendulum exercises, avoiding internal rotation altogether [11, 20]. When performed properly, EMG studies have demonstrated activity in the supraspinatus to be similar to the resting state during these therapy assisted motions. If there is concern about the ability to properly perform pendulum exercises, these should be avoided in the early course of therapy. Patients with subscapularis injury should avoid external rotation, and forward flexion with inferior tears, during the early post-op period [20]. Adjunct use of continuous passive motion (CPM) therapy with a motorized CPM machine has been shown to reduce visual analog scale (VAS) scores and improve ROM at 2.5 and 6 months without compromising repair integrity, but no difference was observed in outcomes at 12 months [17].

A central focus during phase I should be placed on scapular kinematics, identifying and treating potential dyskinesia [11, 20]. Glenohumeral function is reliant on appropriate scapular positioning and mechanics, which has been shown to be deficient in 68% to 100% of patients with shoulder injuries, even giving rise to glenohumeral dysfunction. Patients can be safely placed in the side-lying position with the shoulder unweighted to perform scapular neuromuscular re-education during the early immobilization period of post-op rehabilitation, preparing a sound foundation for future glenohumeral motions to follow [20].

Phase II (6–12 Weeks): AAROM → AROM

At 6 weeks, the estimated strength of the repair is 19–30% [11]. Premature advancement to this phase, which involves assisted active ROM (AAROM) and AROM, could be deleterious. Progression to Phase II should only occur after minimal-to-no reported pain with PROM, PROM approaching 120 degrees of elevation in the scapular plane, and exercise tolerance without compensation [20].

The goals of Phase II include restoration of full ROM, improving basic and functional strength with emphasis on rotator cuff co-activation versus isolation to reduce risk of reinjury at this stage. Patients are guided through submaximal and subpainful isometric exercises, starting with internal rotation, followed by external rotation [11, 20]. Safe exercises shown to maintain low activation levels in the supraspinatus include standing-resisted shoulder extension and prone extension, as well as seated and prone row. Particular attention should be paid to the shoulder "shrug" sign, indicating possible insufficient activation of the rotator cuff and altered mechanics within the glenohumeral joint [20]. Therapists should be mindful that the time to transition to AROM was positively correlated with the size of the rotator cuff tear, with smaller tears allowing for earlier transition [12].

Phase III (12+ Weeks): Strengthening

Rotator cuff repair strength at approximately 12 weeks post-op is estimated between 29% and 50%. The decision to progress to this phase of strengthening is variable in both timing and appropriateness. Patients with continued pain and stiffness with PROM in forward elevation and external rotation should not progress until these improve [11]. For some, progression past phase II may not occur.

During phase III, strengthening exercises are initiated targeting the rotator cuff in multiple planes of motion with isometric, isotonic, and light closed-chain exercises [11, 20]. External rotation at 0 degrees abduction was reported to produce supraspinatus activation up to 41% of maximal voluntary isometric contraction (MVIC), versus its highest activation with the arm in 90 degrees of abduction. Therefore, progression through varying positions should be timed appropriately as tissue and tendon-to-bone union strengthen and mature. Continued attention should remain on scapular kinematics to ensure positive reinforcement of glenohumeral mechanics with increasing loads. Important at reducing the risk of subacromial impingement, special attention should be directed toward balanced function between the descending, middle, and ascending trapezius, as well as the serratus anterior and deltoid muscles [20].

Phase IV (~24+ Weeks): Return-to-Sport/High Functioning

Phase IV continues to focus on strengthening with an emphasis on regaining functional abilities in sport, daily life, and/or work. Further integration of trunk posture and control may be integrated into this stage of recovery. Depending on patient factors and goals, the duration of this phase may vary widely. Return to sport typically does not occur until the end of this phase when mobility and strength are symmetric side-to-side [19]. There is no official consensus on the time to return-to-sport, with recommendations ranging from 3 months to 12 months, but 6–12 months is most common [12].

Common complications include pain, re-rupture/re-tear, stiffness, nerve injury, complex regional pain syndrome (CRPS), adhesive capsulitis, biceps tendon rupture, infection, DVT, and hardware failure [11–21]. Blood flow restriction training (BFRT) involves the application of a pneumonic tourniquet to occlude blood flow to the targeted muscles during the performance of low-load exercise with the intent of eliciting adaptations in strength and hypertrophy. A single randomized controlled trial (RCT) by Brumitt et al. demonstrated equivalent gains in strength and tendon thickness between the BFRT experimental group versus traditional rotator cuff resistance training over an 8-week period [15]. More research is needed to determine efficacy and safety.

Proximal Humerus Fracture Open Reduction Internal Fixation (ORIF)

Proximal humerus fractures are among the most common in the upper extremity, accounting for approximately 4% to 5% of all fractures in adults; however, when surgery is indicated, multiple factors may influence outcomes [22]. Factors associated with post-op functional outcomes include the type of fracture, age of the patient, osteoporosis, status of the rotator cuff, motivation in therapy, and stability of the greater and lesser tuberosities [23]. In addition to these variables, post-op rehabilitation plays an important role in the return of function and quality of life after a proximal humerus fracture, but authors have not been able to adequately compare approaches to make evidence-based recommendations [22].

While no definitive rehabilitation protocol was found in the literature, there is consensus for general phase progression and timeline [22–24]. Initial post-op precautions center around control of pain and edema, protecting the fracture repair site, minimizing deconditioning, maintaining ROM at distal joints, and preventing glenohumeral joint stiffness [24]. ROM is limited the first 3 weeks during the use of a sling, which can be removed multiple times daily to allow for appropriate exercises and daily activities including eating, bathing, and dressing [22, 24]. Non-weightbearing (NWB) remains under debate, with 67% of surgeons in agreement with 6–12 weeks duration for ORIF, but greater variation in opinion for hemiarthroplasty, ranging from <6 weeks to 6–12 weeks [22]. See Table 23.2 for a recommended rehabilitation course [22–24].

Pain and stiffness are the most commonly reported complications following shoulder surgery, motivating interest in early mobilization [23]. The use of nonsteroidal anti-inflammatories (NSAIDs) and glucocorticoids is generally avoided following fractures due to the known inhibitory effects on bone healing; however, a study by Kim, Lee, and Lee examined the use of an ultrasound-guided glenohumeral glucocorticoid injection 8-weeks post-op in patients treated with ORIF and rehabilitation versus patients only undergoing rehabilitation. They found a single injection of triamcinolone improved ROM, in external rotation and forward flexion, and reduced pain on the VAS at 3 and 6 months in patients following a three-part proximal humerus fracture (PHF), but these differences were no longer evident by 12 months post-op. There were no complications in either group, including screw cut-out, malunion, avascular necrosis, or nonunion, and average time to union was equivalent between groups, at 14.6 weeks in the experimental group and 15.4 weeks in the control ($P > 0.05$) [25]. While the long-term benefit is not evident, given the apparent relative safety of administering glenohumeral joint steroid injections 8 weeks post-op, there may be limited benefit for patients struggling with excessive pain and stiffness. More research is needed to further assess the safety and benefit of steroid injections following ORIF and other surgical techniques for addressing pain and ROM after proximal humerus fractures. Additional complications include loosening of the greater or lesser tubercles, neurovascular/brachial plexus injury, infection, avascular necrosis, malunion/nonunion, rotator cuff dysfunction, CRPS, ectopic bone formation, and glenoid erosion [22, 23, 25–27].

While relatively rare, the incident rate for nonunion in humeral fractures ranges from 2.3% to 11.6% in surgically treated patients and carries a significant burden on patients, families, and the healthcare system. High-energy extracorporeal shock-wave therapy (ESWT) has been shown to be an effective alternative to revision surgery in delayed healing fractures or non-unions at various anatomic sites. Dahm et al. investigated its application specifically for humerus fractures and found healing rates from 52.5% to 66.7%, depending on the anatomic region of the humerus affected, limited by the size of the gap, and additional patient factors. This rate is well below that of surgical revisions with plating and bone grafts between 75% and 98.1%, but ESWT may still be an appropriate alternative in cases where surgical revision is not preferred or viable [28]. More research is needed to elucidate its efficacy and parameters of use.

Table 23.2 Postoperative rehabilitation course for proximal humerus fracture ORIF [22, 24]

Phase	Goals	Range of motion/precautions	Strengthening/conditioning/intervention
Phase I (Weeks 0–4)	Optimize healing, control pain, and inflammation, introduce PROM to reduce stiffness, and maintain elbow, wrist, and hand function	Weeks 0–4: Wear sling with removal at least four times daily for exercises, ROM, and ADLs No abduction past 90 degrees, no driving until adequate ROM, and avoid pain with ROM Shoulder external rotation 0–40 degrees Weeks >2: Consider introducing PROM, depending on fracture type	Weeks 0–4: Pain management (e.g., cryotherapy), ROM/mobility (Codman, PROM), scapular retraction/mobility, and no lifting >1 lb *Criteria to Advance:* Wean from sling at 4 weeks, pain control, full elbow AROM, PROM in shoulder flexion to 140 degrees, external rotation to 40 degrees, and abduction to 90 degrees
Phase II (Weeks 4–8)	Full PROM, initiate AAROM/AROM, initiate elbow and shoulder strengthening, and return to ADLs with precautions	Weeks 4–6: PROM at shoulder Week 6: Initiate AAROM/AROM at shoulder without force at end range	Weeks 4–6: No lifting >1 lb Weeks 6–8: No lifting >2 lbs Weeks 4–8: AAROM (table slides, lawn chair progression, rail slides, wall slides, pulleys), AROM (supine shoulder flexion, side-lying shoulder external rotation, abduction and flexion to 90 degrees low punch), strengthening (biceps curls, triceps extension, prone rows, shoulder isometric flexion/extension/internal and external rotation) Shoulder isotonic prohibited at this phase *Criteria to Advance:* Full shoulder PROM, full elbow AROM, pain control, tolerance to elbow isometrics, and strengthening
Phase III (Weeks 8–12)	Full shoulder AROM, initiate shoulder strengthening, progress elbow/wrist strength, control pain	Stretching in all ranges without pain or force	No lifting >10 lbs Initiate isotonic shoulder strengthening and rotator cuff strengthening for adequate humeral head mechanics Emphasis on scapulothoracic/scapulohumeral strength and rhythm *Criteria to Progress:* Full shoulder AROM with appropriate mechanics and no pain or compensatory strategies
Phase IV (Weeks 12+)	Progress strength, return to normal functional activities or sport, and improve ROM as needed	Continue stretching for full ROM without force or pain	General strength progression, plyometrics, and sport/work-specific strength training *Criteria to Advance:* Return of 80% or greater strength, no pain, and low level to no disability score (e.g., QuickDASH)

Shoulder Instability: Anterior/Posterior Stabilization

The glenohumeral joint of the shoulder provides significant mobility with a wide ROM. This functional advantage stems from a shallow glenoid cavity, which also predisposes the glenohumeral joint to subluxation and dislocation, making it the most dislocated diarthrodial joint in the body [29, 30]. Shoulder instability may present anteriorly (most common), posteriorly, or multi-directionally, necessitating rehabilitation strategies tailored to the pathology, surgery performed, and patient characteristics and goals. For anterior instability, both open and arthroscopic surgical techniques are efficacious in reducing recurrent dislocations and providing positive patient-reported outcomes; however, during open Bankart repairs the subscapularis is either incised or reflected and repaired, necessitating special considerations during post-op rehabilitation [31]. With posterior instability, if there is glenoid bone loss or dysplasia, open posterior bone block augmentation or rotational osteotomy may be indicated [32]. Arthroscopic labral repair and/or reconstruction is typical, with or without capsular repair [29]. Additional procedures may be required for concurrent pathologies, including but not limited to superior labral anterior to posterior (SLAP) tears, rotator cuff tears, and Hill-Sachs lesions [32]. Rehabilitation following potentially complex or multifaceted surgical repairs requires close communication between the surgeon and the therapy team.

Consensus guidelines from ASSET provide a set of principles to consider when formulating a rehabilitation protocol, as there is a paucity of level I or II evidence for a specific protocol following surgery for shoulder instability. These principles are as follows [33]:

1. Understanding the surgical procedure.
2. Understanding of the anatomic structures to be protected, how they are stressed, and the rate at which they heal.
3. Identification and skilled application of techniques to impart appropriate levels of stress on healing tissues.
4. Managing the initial immobilization period and the rate of ROM progression.

The ASSET Consensus Rehabilitation Guideline promotes a three-phase approach centered around tissue-healing timelines and milestone-based progression, as depicted below. Within this framework, adjustments are made according to the principles outlined above. Popchak et al. proposed a treatment-based classification process with three approaches closely aligned with the ASSET phases: symptom modulation, motor control, and functional optimization [33].

- Phase I (weeks 0–6): Symptomatic modulation.
  - Reduce severity of symptoms.
  - Protect healing structures; limit ROM to 20–30 degrees.
  - Improve patient presentation.
- Phase II (weeks 7–12): Motor control.
  - Enhancement of joint proprioception.

  - Improve quality of movement (PROM, AAROM/AROM, scapulohumeral rhythm, basic strength for ADLs).
- Phase III (13–24): Functional optimization.
  - Work toward higher level of activity and optimize performance for work/sport.
  - Pain low to absent.
- Phase IV (optional): Gradual return-to-sport [34].
  - Restoration of proprioceptive feedback.
  - Address kinesiophobia.
  - Incorporation of functional rehabilitation and psychological evaluation leads to better outcomes with lower incidence of recurrent dislocation.

Rehabilitation considerations with different surgical interventions:

- Arthroscopic Bankart Repair [33]
  - Most common in recurrent dislocations and repeated instability.
  - Additional lesions may include rotator cuff tears, Hill-Sachs lesions, and osteochondral lesions.
  - Arthroscopic (most frequent) versus open procedures.
  - Rehabilitation considerations:

    Understanding which static/dynamic structures are stressed throughout ROM.
    - At zero degrees, subscapularis stabilizes glenohumeral joint against external rotation.
    - Both arthroscopic and open procedures require either a subscapularis split or detachment followed by repair.
    - At 45–90 degrees of shoulder abduction, portions of the middle/inferior glenohumeral ligament (often injured in Bankart lesion) provide stability to external rotation forces.
      - During the early rehabilitation phase, prevent excessive force in external/internal rotation which may injure tissues.
- Arthroscopic Bankart with Remplissage of Hill-Sachs Lesion [33]
  - Arthroscopic approach may provide faster recovery, less post-op pain, decreased operative time, improved cosmetic appearance, accurate identification of pathology while minimizing complications.
  - Rehabilitation considerations:

    Concern for potential loss of external ROM due to nonanatomic tethering of infraspinatus tendon.

    Potential loss of external rotation strength, long-term (no evidence of such to date).

    Caution during early phase recruitment of infraspinatus and emphasis on restoration of full external rotation ROM during mid-phase.
    - Gradual progressive infraspinatus loading after initiation of submaximal isometrics.
    - More aggressive measures for restoring ROM if not achieved within 12 weeks.

- Open Bankart [33]
  - Suturing of the avulsed capsulolabral structure back to anterior glenoid rim.

    Minimal risk of neurovascular injury, arthritis, and nonunion.

    Preserves surgical treatment options in the setting of revision surgery.

    Risk for internal rotation weakness due to takedown and repair of subscapularis tendon.

    - Weakness minimized by 3 months post-op, typically resolved by 1 year.
    - Subscapularis weakness associated with less satisfaction with open Bankart repair—most critical factor in determining patient's perception of surgical success.
    - Avoid early aggressive loading of subscapularis that could disrupt healing.
    - Delayed loading of subscapularis can also impair appropriate strengthening and recovery.
    - Proposed protection of subscapularis with PROM only, not to exceed 45 degrees of external rotation and 0–20 shoulder abduction for 6 weeks post-op.
    - AAROM can begin at beginning of sling-weaning process in gravity-eliminated positions.
    - AROM begins at end of sling-weaning process.
    - Initiate submaximal isometric contraction of subscapularis once discharged from sling and AROM fully initiated.
    - Begin progressive resistive exercises once protected period cleared and no signs or symptoms of subscapularis dysfunction.
- Latarjet Coracoid Transfer Procedure [33]
  - Low rate of recurrent instability—0–8% and superior biomechanical resistance to anterior dislocation.

    Gold standard—superior results with respect to recurrent instability.

    However, more often associated with complications.

    - Nonunion of bone block, neurovascular injury, infection, prolonged discomfort due to screw placement, loosening or breakage, and/or dysfunction of subscapularis.

    Rehabilitation considerations:

    - May lead to decreased external rotation in ROM, stiffness (subscapularis), possible rotator cuff tendinopathy, and scapular dyskinesia (detachment of pectoralis minor and relocation of biceps/coracobrachialis).
    - Balance between allowing bone graft union, tendon transfer, and preventing stiffness/loss of ROM.
    - Gradual progression of ROM.
    - Incorporation of proprioceptive activities (joint repositioning and rhythmic stabilization) with strengthening of upper/lower portions of subscapularis.
    - Attention to scapular mechanics.

Common complications include rotator cuff tendinitis, subscapularis detachment, limitation in external rotation, unresolved numbness/tingling from axillary nerve injury, pain, weak internal rotation, coracoid nonunion, and infection [32, 33]. BFRT has been used with success by some authors to introduce low-load resistance training as early as phase II without compromising capsuloligamentous integrity. This technology works by restricting blood flow to target muscle groups during exercise resulting in increased strength and muscle girth under hypoperfusion states [30]. This allows for gains in strength earlier in the rehabilitation process. More randomized controlled trials (RCTs) are needed to demonstrate long-term benefits.

Anatomic Total Shoulder Arthroplasty and Reverse Total Shoulder Arthroplasty

For patients with an intact rotator cuff and adequate glenoid bone, anatomic total shoulder arthroplasty (TSA) remains the gold standard replacement procedure. TSA carries a low incidence of complications, proven longevity, and consistent patient satisfaction. In those requiring higher physical demands or insufficient glenoid bone integrity, alternative procedures may be considered, including humeral head replacement with preservation of the native glenoid (hemiarthroplasty) or a hemiarthroplasty with glenoid reaming, also known as the ream and run procedure. Reverse total shoulder arthroplasty (RTSA) may be considered for those with rotator cuff deficiency and glenohumeral osteoarthritis. With the evolution of surgical techniques comes the necessity to adapt former rehabilitation guidelines. Despite recommendations from leading experts, there are numerous disparities in the literature regarding sling use, ROM, and strength progression [35].

There are several key points that warrant clarification and emphasis prior to starting any rehabilitation protocol. The addition of a “pre-habilitation” session prior to TSA or RTSA is recommended based on the association found between preoperative expectations and post-op outcomes and patient satisfaction following hip, knee, and shoulder arthroplasty alike. Educating patients on the limitations, progression of therapy, influence on ADLs, and pain helps maintain realistic expectations. Furthermore, providing patients with a basic understanding and rationale for early limitations in ROM and activity may help reduce the temptation to accelerate the rehabilitation process and risk repair failures. There remains insufficient evidence to declare the optimum timing and setting of rehabilitation. An RCT comparing immediate versus delayed therapy following TSA found no difference in outcomes at 1 year. A retrospective study comparing a home program versus formal physical therapy revealed better outcomes for flexion and abduction ROM, as well as 36-item Short Form Health Survey physical component scores in the home therapy cohort; however, there were significant differences between the protocols in each group. The formal therapy implemented isometric internal rotation early in the progression (at 4 weeks), whereas the home therapy group performed pendulum exercises alone during the first 8 weeks, likely contributing to the observed outcomes [35]. There is also limited consensus on rehabilitation protocols for RTSA, but there is overwhelming agreement that post-op rehabilitation is imperative [35–38]. There is some evidence that an accelerated rehabilitation protocol without immobilization and with an immediate graduated return-to-activity is noninferior to more conservative regimens implementing 6-week immobilization periods. This accelerated approach produced a quicker return to function and significantly fewer post-op complications related to falls, demonstrating potential benefit over early immobilization-based protocols [39]. See Tables 23.3 and 23.4 for examples of post-op rehabilitation protocols for TSA and RTSA, respectively.

Phase I: Immediately Post-op 0–6 Weeks

Immobilization during the immediate post-op period is important for preserving the integrity of the subscapularis. The majority of members from a survey among the ASES recommends shoulder sling or immobilizer use for at least 4–6 weeks postoperatively throughout the day and night. One study found the use of a neutral rotation sling with an abduction pillow wedge resulted in improved external rotation and adduction at the 1-year follow-up and reduced pain at 2 weeks post-op compared to a traditional internal rotation sling. Sling removal should be reserved for the most basic ADLs with strict adherence to external rotation parameters at the side only, with consensus ranging from 20 to 30 degrees ROM, and avoidance of internal rotation and reaching behind the back. These values may be superseded by the surgeon's determination of the operatively defined "safe zone" [35].

PROM at the shoulder and AROM are permissible and cautiously encouraged in phase I. ASES consensus recommends PROM to 120 degrees of elevation without force, overpressure, or scapular blocking. Methods for achieving PROM that does not exceed 15% MVIC include the seated rope and pulley, table slide, or step back, whereas dowel-assisted elevation was found to exceed this ASES recommended value. Codman pendulum exercises with teaching to ensure appropriate forms are also encouraged. AROM at the elbow may include flexion and extension to preserve mobility following biceps tenodesis, but heavy resistance should be avoided for the first 12 weeks. Active mobilization at the wrist and hand is encouraged to promote circulatory effect and scapular retraction for optimizing scapulothoracic positioning and rhythm. Absolute contraindications include external rotation beyond the established safe zone, external rotation at 90 degrees of shoulder abduction, extension, resisted internal rotation, placing the hand behind the back, weightbearing on the effected upper extremity, and lifting weighted objects [35].

Phase II: Post-op 7–12 Weeks

The primary goal in Phase II is the restoration of shoulder mobility. Introduction of passive stretching beyond the precautionary limits of phase I is permissible, gradually progressing to AAROM followed by AROM. Anticipated ROM goals are greatest for those undergoing TSA for osteoarthritis versus those with rheumatoid arthritis, post-traumatic arthritis, or dislocation arthropathy. Mobility can be introduced using the Jackins' active elevation progression, beginning supine and only lifting the weight of the arm. There is consensus that stretching

Table 23.3 Postoperative rehabilitation course for anatomic total shoulder arthroplasty [35]

Phase	Goals	Range of motion/precautions	Strengthening/conditioning/intervention
Phase I (Weeks 0 to 4–6)	Protect subscapularis, joint capsule, and biceps tenodesis, support healing, prevent infection, control edema, and promote distal circulation PROM to 12 degrees elevation and 3 degrees external rotation	PROM: elevation to 120 degrees in scapular plane (e.g., rope and pulley, table slide, supine well arm assisted), external rotation to 30 degrees in scapular plane with arm at side (e.g., well arm or dowel assisted, or table supported and rotate away) Appropriate sling fit (remove for grooming and exercises up to five times daily) No shoulder AROM, no weightbearing on shoulder, and no reaching hand behind back No submersion in water	Pendulum for shoulder exercise Active exercises for elbow, wrist, hand, and scapular retraction Nonimpact aerobic activities (e.g., walking; stationary bike when incision is healed) *Criteria to Advance:* Pain less than 3/10 on VAS with PROM, appropriately healing incision, clearance from physician following radiographic assessment at postoperative visit
Phase II (Weeks 4–6 to 12)	Optimize PROM, develop AROM to match, and promote dynamic shoulder stability with deltoid, periscapular, and remaining rotator cuff strengthening	Week 4–6: Discontinue sling Motion recovery without force Begin external rotation to 60 degree limit at 90 degrees abduction in scapular plane Functional internal rotation with hand behind back gently Weightbearing for use of an assistive device permitted No closed-chain exercises, but may gradually advance use in ADLs	Stretching beyond precautionary limits in phase I without excessive force (elevation and external rotation) Initiate AROM elevation progression once PROM restored (supine with gradual incline to vertical, short to long-lever arm (bent to straight elbow)) AROM internal and external rotation with arm at side, sitting to side lying Scapular AROM against gravity Aerobic activities: walking, elliptical without UE resistance, stationary bicycle, lower body weight training *Criteria to Advance:* AROM in gravity equals PROM, no pain, requires higher-level demand than typical ADL functions (e.g., work and/or sport)

(continued)

Table 23.3 (continued)

Phase	Goals	Range of motion/precautions	Strengthening/conditioning/intervention
Phase III (Weeks 12+)	Achieve higher-level functional demands for work or sport, pain-free with use, increased deltoid and periscapular strength	Gentle end-range stretching, especially in forward elevation as lifelong routine Keep weight training below shoulder height and anterior to frontal plane Closed-chain exercises permitted (e.g., planks and yoga) Avoid impact loading (e.g., sledgehammer, wood chopping, bench pressing)	Shoulder strengthening with light resistance (free weights, elastic bands, or gym machines) keeping below shoulder level and anterior to frontal plane Biceps strengthening with weighted elbow flexion Functional sport- and/or task-specific training, including core and endurance training Gradual return-to-sport: upper extremity types (e.g., golf and tennis) initiated at 4 months, and full return not prior to 6 months

Table 23.4 Postoperative rehabilitation course for reverse total shoulder arthroplasty [36]

Phase	Goals	Range of motion/precautions	Strengthening/conditioning/intervention
Phase I (Weeks 0–2)	Protect prosthesis from dislocation, support healing, prevent infection, control edema, and promote distal circulation	PROM 90–120 degrees elevation in scapular plane and 30 degrees external rotation in scapular plane Keep arm in anterior frontal plane (see elbow at all times), avoid hand behind back and reaching across body Appropriate sling fit (remove for grooming and exercises up to 5 times daily) No shoulder AROM or weightbearing No submersion in water	Pendulum exercise for shoulder Active exercises for elbow, wrist, hand, and scapular retraction *Criteria to Advance:* Pain less than 3/10 on VAS with PROM, appropriately healing incision, and clearance from physician following radiographic assessment at 2 weeks
Phase II (Weeks 3–6)	PROM elevation to 120 degrees, PROM external rotation to 30 degrees, able to fire all heads of deltoid, and pain less than 3/10 on VAS	Sling only in community PROM for elevation (120 degrees) and external rotation (30 degrees) in scapular plane No active reaching from shoulder and no shoulder extension or hand behind back May use operative arm for basic ADLs with elbow at waist—nothing heavier than cup of coffee May submerge in water after 4 weeks	Discontinue elbow, wrist, and hand exercises with transition to use of arm for ADLs Continue pendulum and scapular retraction Initiate deltoid isometrics (avoid extension beyond frontal plane) and reverse pendulum at 90 degrees elevation in supine *Criteria to Advance:* Passive elevation to 120 degrees and external rotation to 30 degrees, pain-free activation of all deltoid heads, able to position and hold arm at 90 degrees in supine (balanced position)

(continued)

Table 23.4 (continued)

Phase	Goals	Range of motion/precautions	Strengthening/conditioning/intervention
Phase III (Weeks 6–12)	Optimize PROM, develop AROM to match, and promote dynamic shoulder stability with deltoid, periscapular, and remaining rotator cuff strengthening	Discontinue sling Develop AROM to match available PROM without force, and begin internal rotation with hand behind back gently No upper body ergometer due to repetitive loading of deltoid on acromion	Active forward elevation progression, supine to inclined to vertical, short to long-lever arm (bent to straight elbow) AROM in external and internal rotation with arm at side, resistive scapular retraction *Criteria to Advance:* AROM when upright equivalent to PROM in supine, no pain, and requires higher-level demand than ADL functions (e.g., work or sport)
Phase IV (Weeks 12+)	Functional demands for work and/or sport, pain-free, increased deltoid and periscapular strength	Promote maintenance of full PROM and AROM, including gentle end-range stretching in all planes for life Avoid heavy pushing, heavy lifting overhead, or overhead sports May lift no greater than 3 lbs. for deltoid and no upper body ergometer	Deltoid strengthening with no more than 3 lbs. and bent arm (bent elbow) for middle deltoid raise Theraband progressions for scapular muscles, serratus anterior punches

into external rotation with the arm at the side and in the scapular plane with abduction should be limited to 60 degrees. Surveys among surgeons reveal variability in the recommendations for internal rotation, with some allowing progression to reach behind the back and others to the sacrum by the end of phase II. Joint mobilization should be limited to address pain management as needed and address refractory stiffness. Closed-chain exercises are not advised during Phase II, yet AROM with the weight of the arm alone is recommended as able for shoulder muscle activation [35].

Phase III: Post-op 12+ Weeks

The aim of phase III will vary according to anticipated patient activity levels and functional goals. Stretching is continued in all planes of movement without ROM precautions. Those with lesser activity levels may continue with stretching and gentle strengthening, whereas those with higher functional goals will progress through additional strengthening and possible return to sports protocols after post-op month 4. Strength training may now involve closed-chain weightbearing exercises, the use of resistive bands and pulleys, and free weights limiting ROM anterior to the frontal plane and below shoulder level. Return-to-activity or sport is restricted until post-op month 6 to allow for adequate tissue healing and maturation, but this may vary by individual sport. Maximum weight limit recommendations varied among survey respondents, ranging from 15 to 25 lbs., but with agreement advising against heavy impact loading with bench press, wood chopping, or sledgehammer use. It is estimated that approximately 89% of patients are engaged in some type of sport by 2.8 years following surgery [35].

Common complications from TSA and RTSA include acromial or scapular spine stress fracture, dislocation, infection, and nerve palsy. There are new prosthetic components being developed for shoulder arthroplasty that may alter the rehabilitation process. A stemless humeral head may change subscapularis fixation methods [35]. The convertible humeral prosthesis used in RTSA has modified proposed rehabilitation protocols [36, 39]. RTSA is being applied to a wider array of pathological conditions with reliably good outcomes, fewer complications, and equally efficacious accelerated rehabilitation outcomes without the need for immobilization and early ROM [39]. More RCTs are needed to compare rehabilitation protocols and surgical approaches.

Manipulation Under Anesthesia for Adhesive Capsulitis

Adhesive capsulitis of the glenohumeral joint is an often-debilitating condition with a multistage protracted time-course and an estimated prevalence of 10% in the population. When conservative measures fail to control pain and impact ROM, intervention can be escalated to procedures including manipulation under anesthesia (MUA), hydrodilatation, or arthroscopic capsular release [40]. MUA has long been used for refractory adhesive capsulitis despite contradictory findings in the literature and a paucity of well-designed RCTs [40, 41]. Despite continued studies examining the efficacy of MUA, there remains a scarcity of literature on post-procedure therapy or standardized rehabilitation recommendations [40–42].

There are no established or consistent guidelines for post-MUA rehabilitation. Current practice relies on tailoring therapy to the individual toward the management of pain, increasing ROM, and performing functional activities [40, 42]. A survey of physiotherapists by Wilmore et al. found that 45.7% of respondents recommended seeing the patient within one week or less of the procedure date and the majority believed frequency should be once every week or two. The modalities most likely to be used were patient education (99%), AROM/AAROM (91%), and stretching (71%) [40]. While the majority of respondents favored one-to-one treatment, another study by Castelhano et al. comparing post-procedure physical therapy to post-procedure advice/education alone found a statistically significant increase in Oxford Shoulder Scores among the therapy group; however, this difference was below the minimal clinically important difference, putting into question the need for an in-house one-to-one treatment setting [43]. Larger RCTs are needed to help formulate and compare rehabilitation regimens to assess both efficacy and degree of necessity. Complications arising from MUA reported in the literature may include recurrent stiffness, brachial plexus injury, rotator cuff tear, dislocation, or fractures [40, 41].

Superior Labrum Anterior to Posterior (SLAP) Repair

Pathology at the superior aspect of the glenoid labrum, better known as a SLAP tear, is common among the athletic population, especially overhead athletes, and can become a major cause of shoulder dysfunction [44, 45]. Due to the often concurrent injuries associated with SLAP tears, a thorough and targeted physical exam is imperative for both diagnosis and post-op management. Understanding the likely mechanism of injury, surgical procedure(s) performed, and the basic science of tissue healing should provide the basis for post-op rehabilitation [45].

The surgical procedure performed will depend on the type of SLAP tear and other potential injuries present. Detailed description of these surgical methods can be found elsewhere, but generally with exceptions, type I and type III SLAP tears are managed with surgical debridement, and types II and IV are repaired [45, 46]. It is important to be aware of the procedures performed, as this will partially determine the rationale for appropriate restrictions, ROM and exercise progression, and overall rehabilitation timing. The overall goal of post-op rehabilitation is to restore ROM and dynamic stability at the glenohumeral joint while providing adequate protection for healing tissues.

The variability in pathological findings with SLAP lesions inherently leads to significant heterogeneity in post-op rehabilitation protocols, with no single standardized approach defined in the literature. Hermanns et al. analyzed variability among 60 protocols for SLAP lesions from 28 academic institutions and 31 private practice settings and reported their findings as summarized below per major component of rehabilitation [44].

- Immobilization:
  - 97% of protocols mentioned the use of a sling post-op for:
    - 2–4 weeks: 15%
    - 4–6 weeks: 61.7%
    - 6+ weeks: 13%
- ROM:
  - A total of 83.7% of protocols specified ROM recommendations at day or week zero post-op, of which:
    - Permitted PROM of shoulder: 60%
    - Permitted AAROM: 15%
    - Recommend no ROM immediately post-op: 8.3%
    - Certain exercises, including pendulum, wrist, and elbow exercises, were counted as allowing PROM or AAROM.
  - 83% of protocols specified a guideline to full ROM at a specified timeframe, of which the following breakdown was observed.
    - Before 8 weeks: 18.3%
    - 8–10 weeks: 20%
    - 10–12 weeks: 18.3%
    - 12–14 weeks: 23%
    - 14–16 weeks: 3%
    - 16+ weeks: 5%
- Exercises:
  - Scapular strengthening included in 65% of protocols.
  - Upper extremity submaximal isometric exercises in 55% of protocols.
  - Pendulum swings in 53% of protocols, most recommended soon after surgery.
  - Hand/grip, resistance bands, upper body ergometer, and prone exercises were included in at least 40% or more of protocols examined.
- Biceps Engagement and Tenodesis:
  - A total of 36.7% of protocols provided guidelines and timeframes for restricting biceps engagement post-op, as shown below:
    - Before 6 weeks: 1.6%
    - 6–8 weeks: 18.3%
    - 8–10 weeks: 5.0%
    - 10–12 weeks: 11.6%
    - Did not specify biceps engagement or strengthening timeframe: 63%
  - Only 6% of protocols (4/60) specified presence of or difference in rehabilitation due to concomitant biceps tenodesis.
    - Two of these protocols were not modified with the addition of biceps tenodesis.
    - Two added precautions, including no resisted elbow flexion for 6–8 weeks, no resisted shoulder flexion for 8 weeks, and no lifting greater than 1 to 2 lbs. for 8 weeks, and avoid 90/90 stretching with previous instability for 6 weeks.
- Return-to-Sport (RTS) and Throwing:
  - Included in 88.3% of protocols.

- Return-to-sport as follows:
  - 12–16 weeks: 25%
  - 16–20 weeks: 15%
  - 20–24 weeks: 11.6%
  - 24+ weeks: 33%
  - Did not specify: 11.6%
  - Required functional testing: 3%
- Of the 68.3% who included recommendations on return to throwing, the majority (at 38%) allowed some type of throwing to begin at 16–20 weeks.

Rehabilitation Protocol for Arthroscopic Debridement of Type I and III SLAP Lesions

A detailed sample protocol for rehabilitation of type I and type III lesions proposed by Wilk et al. can be found in Table 23.5. Barring complications involving concomitant rotator cuff tears or other pathology, this program can be advanced more aggressively due to an absence of anatomic repair and an intact biceps anchor. A sling is worn for the first 3–4 days immediately post-op, as well as immediate initiation of PROM and AAROM advancing to full PROM by days 10–14. Shoulder flexion is advanced as tolerated and external/internal rotation is initiated at 45 degrees abduction and advanced to 90 degrees abduction by post-op day 4 or 5 [45].

Strengthening is initiated with a similar intention. Isometric pain-free exercises in all planes at submaximal effort are started immediately after surgery for 7 days, followed by light isotonic exercises. Elbow flexion and supination should be avoided to minimize debridement irritation at the biceps anchor. At 2 weeks post-op, light biceps resistance can be introduced. Strength progression continues with the goal of creating muscular balance and dynamic stability at the scapulothoracic and glenohumeral joints. By 4–6 weeks, patients can advance to controlled weight training and plyometric exercises, and athletes can begin sport-specific exercises around 7–10 weeks post-op, depending on the nature and severity of the injury. Starting an interval sport program should be criteria-based, initiated when the patient has minimal pain, full ROM, adequate strength, and dynamic stability [45].

Rehabilitation Protocol for SLAP Repair—Type II

Type II SLAP lesions are the most common and frequently occur in overhead throwing athletes. The detachment of the biceps tendon from the glenoid rim necessitates an anatomic repair and more conservative and time-sensitive progression to protect the repair and allow for tissue healing. Wilk et al. emphasize the importance of being familiar with the extent of the lesion and number of suture anchors used during repair to help guide therapy progression. Sling immobilization is used day and night for an extended 4-week timeframe compared to type I and III lesions. ROM is advanced at a more conservative rate with the goal of obtaining full ROM at 8 weeks post-op and progressing to thrower's motion through 12 weeks [45] (Table 23.6).

Isotonic exercises are initiated immediately postoperatively with rhythmic stabilization drills to promote dynamic joint stability. Resisted biceps activity and weightbearing is avoided during the first 8 weeks to protect the anchor repair, as is

Table 23.5 Postoperative rehabilitation course for arthroscopic debridement of Type I and III SLAP tears [45]

Phase	Goals	Range of motion/precautions	Strengthening/conditioning/intervention
Phase I (Days 1–10) (Motion Phase)	Control pain reduce edema, and minimize atrophy	Pendulum, rope and pulley, L-bar exercises (flexion/extension, abduction/adduction, external/internal rotation starting at 0 degrees abduction, progressing to 45 and 90 degrees abduction), and self-stretching (capsular)	Isometrics, except no biceps isometrics for 5–7 days post-op 7–10 days: initiate tubing for external/internal rotation at 0 degrees abduction Pain control: ice, NSAIDs, modalities *Criteria to Advance:* Full PROM, minimal pain, and adequate manual muscle testing of internal/external rotation and flexion
Phase II (Weeks 2–4) (Intermediate Phase)	Improve strength, and normalize arthrokinematics and scapular kinematics	Continue stretching shoulder (external/internal rotation at 90 degrees abduction) Joint mobilization as appropriate	Week 2: Initiate isotonic shoulder exercises with free weights (scapulothoracic, tubing external/internal rotation at 0 degrees abduction, external rotation side-lying and prone rowing, proprioceptive neuromuscular facilitation manual resistance with dynamic stabilization) Initiate neuromuscular control exercises, proprioceptive training, trunk control exercises, and upper extremity endurance exercises Week 3: Thrower's Ten Program (when indicated), rotator cuff and scapular strengthening, and dynamic stabilization drills *Criteria to Advance:* Full nonpainful AROM and PROM, no pain or tenderness, and strength 70% of contralateral side

(continued)

Table 23.5 (continued)

Phase	Goals	Range of motion/precautions	Strengthening/conditioning/intervention
Phase III (Weeks 4–6) (Dynamic or advanced strengthening phase)	Improve strength, and neuromuscular control, and prepare athlete for throwing (when indicated)	Maintain full PROM/AROM Advance tubing exercises in the 90/90 position for external/internal rotation (slow/fast sets)	Continue Thrower's Ten Program, free weights (supraspinatus and deltoid), scapulothoracic musculature, tubing for biceps, endurance, proprioceptive, and neuromuscular exercises Initiate plyometrics, two-hand drills progressing to one-hand drills *Criteria to Advance:* Full PROM, no pain or tenderness, isokinetic test that fulfills criteria to throw, and acceptable clinical exam
Phase IV (Weeks 7+) (Return-to-activity/sport phase)	Progressive increase in activities to achieve full functional status	Maintain PROM/AROM	Continue program from phase III Initiate sport-specific programs and progress interval programs

Table 23.6 Post-operative rehabilitation course for arthroscopic debridement of Type II SLAP tears [45]

Phase	Goals	Range of motion/precautions	Strengthening/conditioning/ intervention
Phase I (Day 1 to week 6) (Protected motion phase)	Protect the repair, control pain and inflammation, prevent negative effects of mobilization, and promote dynamic stability	Weeks 0–2: Sling for 4 weeks, sleep in immobilizer for 4 weeks, elbow/hand PROM, PROM, and active-assisted gentle ROM (flexion at 60 degrees) (week 2 at 75 degrees), elevation in scapular plane to 60 degrees, and ER (10–15 degrees) and IR (45 degrees) in scapular plane No active external rotation, extension, or abduction Weeks 3–4: Discontinue sling, sleep in immobilizer until week 4, and continue gentle PROM/AAROM (flexion to 90, ER) (25–30) and IR (55–60) in scapular plane No active ER, extension, or elevation Weeks 5–6: Improve ROM (flexion to 145, ER at 45 abduction to 40–50, IR at 45 abduction to 55–60), initiate stretching regimen, initiate light ROM at 90 degrees abduction	Weeks 0–2: Hand-grip exercises, submaximal isometrics for shoulder muscles, and cryotherapy/modalities as indicated Weeks 3–4: Initiate rhythmic stabilization drills and proprioceptive training, tubing ER/IR at 0 degrees abduction, and continue isometrics, and cryotherapy as indicated Weeks 5–6: Continue tubing ER/IR (arm at side), proprioceptive neuromuscular facilitation (PNF) manual resistance, initiate shoulder abduction without resistance, "full can" exercise (weight of arm), prone rowing, and horizontal abduction No biceps strengthening
Phase II (Weeks 7–12) (Moderate protection phase)	Preserve surgical repair integrity, restore strength and balance, and gradually restore full ROM (week 10)	Weeks 7–9: Gradually restore ROM (flexion to 180, ER at 90 degrees abduction to 90–95 degrees, IR at 90 abduction to 70–75 degrees), and begin AROM biceps Weeks 10–12: Increase ER ROM at 90 degrees abduction to 110–115 degrees with introduction of Thrower's motion (weeks 10–12), continue stretching, and progress ROM to functional demands	Week 7–9: Continue progression of isotonic and PNF strengthening and initiate Thrower's Ten Program Weeks 10–12: May increase strengthening program, otherwise continue regimen as in phase I *Criteria to Advance:* Full nonpainful AROM, adequate stability, and strength, no pain or tenderness

(continued)

Table 23.6 (continued)

Phase	Goals	Range of motion/precautions	Strengthening/conditioning/intervention
Phase III (Weeks 12–20) (Minimal protection phase)	Establish and maintain full PROM and AROM, improve strength and endurance, and initiate functional activities	Weeks 12–16: Continue stretching, and maintain Thrower's motion Weeks 16–20: Continue stretching	Weeks 12–16: Continue strengthening as in Phase II, initiate resisted biceps and forearm supination exercises, initiate light plyometrics, and restrict sports activities Weeks 16–20: Continue all exercises, Thrower's Ten Program, plyometrics, and initiate interval sports program *Criteria to Advance:* Full nonpainful AROM, adequate stability, strength 75–80% of contralateral side, and no pain or tenderness
Phase IV (Weeks 20–26) (Advanced Strengthening phase)	Improve muscular strength, progress functional activities, and maintain shoulder mobility	Continue flexibility exercises	Continue isotonic strengthening, PNF, plyometrics, and progress interval sports program *Criteria to Advance:* Full functional ROM, muscular performance isokinetics, adequate shoulder stability, no pain or tenderness
Phase V (Months 6–9) (Return-to-activity phase)	Gradual return-to-sport	Continue stretching program	Continue strengthening program Progress sports activities to unrestricted participation

aggressive biceps strengthening until 12 weeks post-op. An interval sports program may be introduced around week 16 using the same criteria as with type I and type III lesions. Return to play typically occurs between 9 and 12 months postoperatively. Given that type II lesion repairs are often accompanied by glenohumeral stabilization procedures and/or Bankart repairs, it is necessary to modify the rehabilitation protocol to incorporate the required constraints and progression parameters relevant to each procedure [45].

Arthroscopic Labral Repair Protocol—Type IV and Complex Tears

Therapy progression for type IV SLAP lesions is similar to that of type II with the marked exception of biceps protection. Type IV lesions may involve biceps repair, biceps resection, or tenodesis, each requiring unique protection and progressions for healing and functional recovery. Biceps resection allows for earlier activation at 6–8 weeks, compared to biceps tear repair or tenodesis, for which activation and resistive training are prohibited for the first 3 months. At 12–16 weeks, light isotonic exercises with elbow flexion are introduced and progress gradually as tolerated. At 16–20 weeks, full resistive exercises are initiated, followed by plyometrics and the introduction of a sport interval program in a similar manner for type II lesions [45].

The most significant risk for SLAP lesions, particularly type II and IV, pertains to disruption of the repaired tendon or labrum [45]. Patient education can help obviate reinjury or incomplete healing by providing the rationale for restrictions imposed and establishing realistic expectations in relation to tissue healing and remodeling. Common to many shoulder surgeries, pain should be addressed immediately post-op, whereas stiffness must be approached cautiously with strict adherence to mobilization guidelines.

Biceps Tenodesis and Tenotomy

Tendinopathy of the long head of the biceps tendon (LHBT) is usually associated with repetitive, chronic traction and friction forces affecting the tendinous tissue as a microtrauma during shoulder articulation and often secondary to a more significant shoulder disorder [47]. Tenotomy renders this portion of the biceps brachii nonfunctional and involves the release of the tendon from the supraglenoid tubercle with or without a portion of the superior labrum. Tenodesis preserves a portion of contractile force transmission through the long head by resecting the tendon from the supraglenoid tubercle and fixing it to one of multiple bone or soft-tissue locations, including the bicipital groove and supra- or subpectoral attachment sites [48].

There is no consensus on a standardized rehabilitation protocol following tenotomy or tenodesis, but most follow a time-based (dependent on tissue healing) and criterion-based progression, although tenodesis requires additional time and considerations due to the preservation of partial function of the biceps long head [47, 49, 50]. The primary considerations following tenotomy include pain control, incisional healing, restoration of PROM and AROM, and shoulder complex strengthening without concern for tendon healing (Table 23.7) [50]. This results in a shorter rehabilitation timeline, with a return to full strenuous work and/or recreational activities as early as 6–8 weeks post-op, compared to as long as 12–16 months before returning to sport for tenodesis [47, 49–51]. Given that tenodesis involves reattachment of the LHBT, tissue healing necessitates a more gradual therapy progression with additional precautions, as outlined in Table 23.8 [47, 49, 51]. Comparatively, tenotomy has demonstrated earlier pain relief but worsened Popeye deformity of the biceps brachii, whereas tenodesis has shown improved elbow flexion and supination strength at 12 months post-op with equivalent long-term pain outcomes [48]. Both approaches result in high patient satisfaction, good functional outcomes, and equivalent long-term pain relief [47, 52].

The most common complications associated with LHBT tenotomy include cosmetic deformity of the arm, strength deficits in elbow flexion and forearm supination, and soreness or cramping in the biceps muscle. Biceps tenodesis may be subject to greater complications due to the nature of the surgery, which may include loss of fixation with cosmetic deformity, stiffness, residual groove pain, pain or soreness in the biceps brachii, infection, hematoma, neurologic injury, vascular injury, proximal humerus fracture (from anchor placement), or CRPS [53].

Table 23.7 Postoperative rehabilitation course for biceps tenotomy [50]

Phase	Goals	Range of motion/precautions	Strengthening/conditioning/intervention
Phase I (Weeks 1–2)— (Passive range of motion phase)	Incisional care, control of pain and inflammation, enhanced scapular function, and gradual restoration of PROM	Sling for discomfort (wean as able) and sleep with sling as needed (place towel under elbow to prevent shoulder hyperextension) PROM elbow flexion/extension and forearm supination/pronation, begin pain-free shoulder PROM in all planes AROM wrist/hand No AROM at elbow, excessive ER ROM/stretching (stop at first end feel), or lifting objects with affected upper extremity	Pendulum exercise Scapular retraction and clock exercises progressed to isometrics Ball squeezes Cryotherapy for pain and inflammation as indicated Patient education on posture, joint protection, positioning, and hygiene *Criteria to Advance:* Appropriate incisional healing, pain control, full PROM of shoulder and elbow, completion of phase I activities without pain
Phase II (Weeks 2–4) (Active range of motion phase)	Pain and inflammation control, discharge sling, gradual restoration of AROM, and light waist-level activities	Progress shoulder PROM to AAROM and AROM in all planes, AROM in elbow flexion/extension, and forearm supination/pronation No lifting with affected upper extremity	Manual therapy (glenohumeral, scapulothoracic, and trunk joint mobilizations as indicated) (Grade I–IV), posterior capsular stretching (cross-body and sleeper stretch) Cryotherapy for pain and inflammation as indicated Patient education on posture, joint protection, positioning, and hygiene *Criteria to Advance:* Full AROM of shoulder and elbow, proper scapular mechanics with ROM and functional activities, and completion of Phase II activities without pain

(continued)

Table 23.7 (continued)

Phase	Goals	Range of motion/precautions	Strengthening/conditioning/intervention
Phase III (Weeks 4–6) (Initial strengthening phase)	Normalize strength, endurance, neuromuscular control, and return to chest-level functional activities	Continue P/AROM of shoulder and elbow as indicated Do not proceed with strengthening and functional activities until full ROM is achieved in a given plane No heavy lifting	Initiate biceps curls with light resistance, resisted supination/pronation, rhythmic stabilization drills, and a balanced strengthening program with progression in demand and intensity Initiate ER strengthening with tubing at 30 degrees abduction, side-lying ER w/ towel roll, manual resistance ER supine in the scapular plane (light), prone rowing at 30/45/90 degrees of abduction to neutral arm position, and subscapularis strengthening (push-up plus progression, cross-body diagonals with tubing, IR resistive band (0/45/90 degrees abduction), and forward punch Open and closed-chain exercises Cryotherapy for pain and inflammation as indicated *Criteria to Advance:* Appropriate rotator cuff and scapular performance at chest level and completion of phase III activities without pain
Phase IV (Weeks 6+) (Advanced strengthening phase)	Continue stretching, maintain pain-free AROM, and return to full strenuous work/recreational activities	Continue and maintain PROM and AROM Avoid excessive anterior capsule stress, military press, and wide-grip bench press	Continue all exercises as in phase III and progress to isotonic if tolerating well with no pain or soreness Initiate strengthening overhead if strength below 90 degrees is adequate Strength training/stretching at least four times weekly Progressive return to upper extremity weightlifting program emphasizing larger, primary muscles (start light with high repetitions (15–25)) May initiate preinjury activities and vigorous sports if appropriate and medically cleared *Criteria to Advance (to overhead work/sports):* Medical clearance, no pain, adequate ROM, strength, and endurance, and compliance with home exercise program

Table 23.8 Postoperative rehabilitation course for biceps tenodesis [49, 51]

Phase	Goals	Range of motion/precautions	Strengthening/conditioning/intervention
Phase I (Weeks 1–4)—(Passive range of motion phase)	Protect repair, control pain, and inflammation, prevent infection, restore PROM of shoulder and elbow, and maintain scapular function	*Sling use as directed by surgeon (wean at 3 weeks)* No AROM of shoulder or elbow, external rotation (ER) beyond 40 degrees, shoulder abduction or extension past neutral, lifting objects, or friction massage to repair site PROM elbow flexion/extension and forearm supination/pronation	Scapular retractions, mobility exercises, and ball squeezes *Criteria to Advance:* Appropriate incisional healing, pain control, and full PROM of shoulder and elbow
Phase II (Weeks 4–6) (Active range of motion phase)	Pain and inflammation control, gradual restoration of AROM at shoulder and elbow, initiate light waist-level functional activities, submaximal shoulder isometrics, and return to light computer/desk work	Shoulder AAROM (lawn chair, shoulder ER, rail slides, wall slides) Shoulder AROM (supine shoulder flexion, standing scaption, ER in neutral, ER at 90 degrees supported on table) Elbow AROM (elbow flexion/extension and forearm supination/pronation) No lifting with affected upper extremity, loading biceps, elbow flexors, or supinators, friction massage at repair site, running, or over-stressing repair tissue with manual therapy/stretching	Shoulder isometrics (flexion/extension, ER/IR, and abduction) Manual therapy (glenohumeral, scapulothoracic, and trunk joint mobilizations as indicated (Grade I-IV), posterior capsular stretching (cross-body and sleeper stretch) Cardiovascular exercise (walking or stationary bike—avoid excessive weightbearing through arm) *Criteria to Advance:* Full AROM of shoulder and elbow, proper scapular mechanics with ROM and functional activities, and pain control

(continued)

Table 23.8 (continued)

Phase	Goals	Range of motion/precautions	Strengthening/conditioning/intervention
Phase III (Weeks 6–8) (Initial strengthening phase)	Normalize strength, endurance, and neuromuscular control, and return to chest-level activities	Continue shoulder and elbow PROM and AROM No strengthening or functional activities until near full ROM achieved Avoid long-lever arm resistance for elbow flexion and supination	Continue shoulder isometrics—progress as tolerated Initiate resisted biceps curls, supination, triceps extension, and wrist extension/flexion Rhythmic stabilization exercises *Criteria to Advance:* Full shoulder and elbow AROM and tolerance to strengthening without increased symptoms
Phase IV (Weeks 8–12) (Advanced strengthening phase)	Maintain pain-free full shoulder and elbow AROM and progress strength (low load, high repetitions—30–50)	Continue and maintain PROM and AROM	Resisted ER/IR (in neutral), ER/IR (in elevation), full can scapular plane arm elevation, side-lying ER, prone rowing (30/45/90 degrees abduction), push-up plus progression (wall, counter, knees on floor, floor), and PNF diagonals Open- and closed-chain exercises Cardiovascular—initiate to running No swimming *Criteria to Advance:* 5/5 shoulder and elbow strength, full shoulder AROM in all planes, tolerance to strengthening without increased symptoms
Phase V (Months 12–16) (Return-to-sport phase)	Progress strength and function, maintain pain-free ROM, return-to-sport/work activities	Maintain full ROM Avoid anterior capsular stress	Initiate plyometrics training (start below shoulder level and progress overhead), multijoint/compound strengthening, and interval return-to-sport training *Criteria to Advance:* No pain, 90% strength of contralateral upper extremity, within normal limits with field testing (if applicable), and low level to no disability with patient-reported outcome measure (e.g., QuickDASH)

Elbow

Ulnar Collateral Ligament (UCL) Repair (Tommy John Surgery)

UCL repair is a surgical procedure for UCL injuries. The UCL serves as the primary restraint to valgus stress in the elbow [54, 55]. The post-op course involves a 4-phase rehabilitation protocol. The immediate post-op phase (0–3 weeks) has the goal of optimizing healing and protecting the graft. The intermediate phase (weeks 4–7) has the goal of achieving full ROM. The advanced strengthening phase (weeks 8–14) has the goal of increasing strength, power, and endurance. The return-to-activity phase (weeks 14–32) focuses on targeted training and throwing programs to gradually return the patient to preinjury levels of activity. Immobilization in a posterior splint for the first week following surgery is recommended, with the elbow in 90 degrees of flexion, followed by a transition to a hinged elbow brace to gradually increase flexion and extension ROM [54]. Mean time to splint discontinuation is 2.0 weeks. Hinged/functional brace use is discontinued in the 5–6 week range [55]. There is an importance placed on incorporating lower extremity exercises and stretches early in the post-op period, and to progress these activities with the progression of upper extremity exercises. The overhead throwing motion is a complex interaction of kinematic parameters with kinetic energy generated from the foot and the lower extremity and core all the way through the upper extremity. So rehabilitation should not only focus on the injured or at-risk joint, but should involve the entire kinetic chain [54]. The Thrower's Ten Program is initiated at a mean start date of 7.2 weeks and the Interval Throwing Program Phases I and II are started at a mean of 16.3 weeks and 22.6 weeks [54, 55]. Return to play has been reported as soon as 9–10 months, with return to the previous level as high as 81% to 90% [54]. Common complications include ulnar neurapraxia and superficial infection [56]. One new technology is the use of dynamic elbow orthoses in allowing more ROM in the early post-op period as opposed to standard plaster splinting. This has shown greater improvements in pain reduction and recovery of muscle trophism and grip strength in the early post-op period, though similar results are seen after 24 weeks [54]. Common complications include ulnar nerve pathology, medial elbow pain, and superficial wound infections [57].

Arthroscopy for Lateral Epicondylitis (Tennis Elbow)

Arthroscopy for lateral epicondylitis is a surgical procedure for the treatment of lateral epicondylitis, involving tendinosis of the common extensor tendon, most commonly the extensor carpi radialis brevis [58, 59]. During post-op days 0–5, the elbow will be protected with a removable static splint, and the patient is encouraged to remove the splint five times daily for a minimum of 15 minutes, to mobilize the elbow. Normal ROM of the elbow is aimed for after 2 weeks. After achieving the normal ROM, muscular isometric strengthening exercises are started for approximately 4 weeks. Exercises with resistance are initiated 6 weeks after surgery and are indicated for 6 weeks. Unrestricted movements of the limb are allowed after 12 weeks of therapy [58]. Full recovery is to be expected at 3–6 months, but the function is usually good before this time [59]. Common complications include superficial wound infections [58].

Arthroscopy for Medial Epicondylitis (Golfer's Elbow)

Arthroscopy for medial epicondylitis is a surgical procedure for the treatment of medial epicondylitis, involving tendinosis of the common flexor tendon. Post-op, a posterior plaster splint is placed and removed at the first post-op visit in 10–14 days. The patient is then transitioned to a hinged elbow brace. Strengthening exercises are started at 6–8 weeks post-op, with no restrictions at 3–4 months [59, 60]. Common complications include superficial wound infections and ulnar nerve pathology [60].

Open Reduction Internal Fixation (ORIF)

ORIF is the primary surgical repair of distal humerus fractures. ROM exercises of the hand and shoulder are started immediately post-op [61, 62]. The cast is removed partially at week 2, during which guided therapy can be initiated [63]. Therapy includes elbow distraction. This involves the patient lying flat, applying a traction belt around the proximal part of the forearm with the elbow flexed to 90 degrees. With the scooping of both hands along with grasping of belt, a gentle traction is applied and sustained for 20 seconds. Therapy also includes elbow mobilization. This involves the patient lying supine, with a mobilization belt placed around the proximal part of the forearm. A gliding force is applied in lateral direction and the patient is instructed to actively flex and extend his/her elbow. AROM and PROM are encouraged [61]. Due to surgical approaches to the elbow requiring exposure of the radial, median, and/or ulnar nerves, nerve gliding exercises should be used for at least 6–8 weeks post-op. Return to prior level of activity is an average of 29 weeks post-op. Common complications include capsular stiffness and heterotopic ossification [62].

Surgical Intervention for Elbow Instability Following Dislocation

Surgical intervention following a simple elbow dislocation is indicated when there is residual instability in more than 45 degrees of flexion, joint incongruence on post-reduction radiographs, or an open dislocation is present. Surgery typically involves repair of the lateral collateral ligament (LCL) and potentially the medial ulnar collateral ligament. The medial collateral ligament may need to be repaired in rare cases where there is gross instability even after LCL repair. Post-op, the elbow is immobilized in a posterior splint for 1 week before beginning active ROM. Based on the ligaments that are repaired, the elbow can be placed in a hinged braced within 1 week to allow for AAROM as tolerated. At 6 weeks, the brace is used intermittently to begin daily activities. The brace can be discontinued at 3 months to begin strengthening exercises. The patient may begin to participate in sporting activities while in the brace and is recommended to be used for sports activities for a total of 3 months to 6 months post-op. Common complications include stiffness, recurrent instability, and/or dysfunction related to violation of the extensor mechanism [64].

Open Arthrolysis for Post-Traumatic Stiff Elbow

Open arthrolysis for post-traumatic stiff elbow is a surgical procedure for the treatment of a stiff elbow [63, 65, 66]. Post-op, from the first day to 6 weeks, patients are instructed to perform active, assisted, and passive cycles of flexion-extension exercises and forearm-rotation exercises. The hinged external fixator is removed at 6 weeks. From 6 weeks to 3 months, in addition to flexion and extension exercises, a systematic forearm-rotation rehabilitation program is initiated. From 3 months to 1 year, continued exercises are prescribed [65, 66]. Weightbearing exercises are encouraged, starting with 1 kg (~2 lbs) [65]. Common complications include ulnar nerve pathology, heterotopic ossification, and infection [66].

Total Elbow Arthroplasty

Total elbow arthroplasty is a surgical procedure with various indications including treatment of rheumatoid arthritis, osteoarthritis, and post-traumatic arthritis [67]. During the first post-op week, the arm is maintained in extension with an anterior plaster cast to avoid soft-tissue complications [68]. If a triceps-off approach is used, active elbow extension and terminal elbow flexion are avoided for 6 weeks post-op to avoid triceps insufficiency. Triceps strengthening is discouraged until 10 weeks post-op [67, 68]. Early ROM is instituted, and a nighttime extension splint may be used for patients lacking terminal extension. Active supination and pronation are encouraged with the elbow at 90 degrees of flexion [67]. All patients are given permanent activity restrictions, which include weight lifting of maximum 5 kg (~10 lbs) for lifetime [68]. Common complications include ulnar nerve pathology, intraoperative fractures of the humeral condyles, instability because of inadequate soft-tissue healing or component malpositioning, triceps failure or extension weakness, hematoma formation, contracture, implant failure or pullout, disassembly of a linked prosthesis, osteolysis or aseptic loosening, polyethylene bearing wear, and wound healing complication [67].

Wrist/Hand

Carpal Tunnel Decompression/Release

Carpal tunnel syndrome (CTS) is the most common compressive neuropathy in the upper extremity. When bracing/splinting and injections fail to adequately control symptoms or stop progression, surgery may be considered for carpal tunnel decompression [69]. There is strong evidence supporting operative treatment as superior to nonoperative management [69]. There are no definitive guidelines or protocols in the literature for rehabilitation following carpal tunnel decompression and a paucity of high-quality RCTs showing significant benefit [70–73]. The literature also reveals a mix of heterogeneous therapeutic interventions and timeframes [70, 72–74]. An online survey of members of the American Society of Surgeons of the Hand revealed that only 12% of respondents routinely referred post-op patients for formal hand therapy after carpal tunnel decompression. Mack et al. demonstrated that a single occupational therapy visit within 10–14 days post-op may be beneficial for a subset of patients who experience complications or slowed progress following surgery [72]. Based on the lack of high-quality evidence demonstrating efficacy, at this time it is advisable to manage potential complications as needed and provide patients with education for home care and exercise [71, 72]. An initial and single post-op follow-up may prove useful for catching complications earlier and initiating targeted therapy sooner in the recovery phase for patients in need.

Duration of therapy is determined by individual patient needs in relation to post-op healing. General improvement of nocturnal palmer pain, hand weakness, and tingling with the return of functional use of the hand tends to occur within 6 weeks following surgery. To achieve this end, hand therapy sessions may occur 1 to 2 times per week for an undefined duration, as indicated by patient necessity and goal attainment. At minimum, the patient can be educated on a home exercise program for basic ergonomics, body mechanics, adaptive equipment as needed, and adaptations for ADLs as well as general wound care, although there was no difference in pain or wound healing between patients wearing a bulky post-op dressing for 24 hours versus 2 weeks [71]. The use of wrist splinting is generally not indicated following carpal tunnel release and has not been shown to decrease scar pain or improve pinch strength, and may in fact delay recovery [69]. Hand and upper extremity strengthening can begin 3–4 weeks post-op when wounds have healed and inflammation is minimal or resolved. A more intensive regimen can be initiated at 4 weeks post-op in anticipation of return to work and more rigorous daily activities [71]. Of note, patients requiring bilateral carpal tunnel decompression may benefit from simultaneous release, as a return to work is shown to be faster at 2.5 weeks compared to 8.5 weeks following sequentially staged surgeries [69]. Below are common considerations that may be addressed with formal hand therapy or a home exercise program created by a trained therapist.

- Scar management: May commence once Steri-strips have fallen off and light scar massage beginning 2–3 days following suture removal, gradually becoming more vigorous. A desensitization program may be added for pain control [71].
- Edema control: Utilization of compression (Tubi-grip, Coban wrap), icing, mobilization of digits, and elevation is especially important during the immediate post-op period to minimize dependent edema [71].
- Ergonomics education: Emphasis on repetitive work tasks and poor posture, as these are associated with both the development of CTS and poor outcomes following carpal tunnel release [71].

- Mobilization: It is recommended to begin mobilizing the thumb, digits, and wrist immediately post-op to encourage adequate gliding of tendons and the median nerve and reduce the occurrence of restrictive fibrosis. Exercises involving the distal extremity in repetitions of 7 to 10, at a frequency of 3 to 5 times daily. PROM should continue for a minimum of 4 weeks post-op to mobilize stiff joints and elongate shortened tendons, with AROM initially performed at the wrist with relaxed digits [71].
- Tendon-gliding exercises: Recent studies have demonstrated the benefit of individualized tendon gliding for the flexor digitorum superficialis and flexor digitorum profundus, as described by Hayes et al. [71, 75]

Management of possible complications may be the primary indication for rehabilitation following carpal tunnel decompression surgery. While the incidence ranges from 1% to 25% of patients, most complications are minor and transient [69]. Common complications include palmer/pillar pain, paresthesias, reduced grip/pinch strength, edema, hypertrophic scarring, infection, decreased AROM, endurance, and functional use of affected distal extremity.

Blanquero et al. trialed the use of a tablet-based ReHand application within 10 days of surgery for 4 weeks. The experimental group demonstrated improved Disabilities of the Arm, Shoulder, and Hand (QuickDASH) scores compared to a control group who were prescribed a conventional home program on paper, but there was no statistically significant difference in grip strength, pain, or dexterity [76].

Thumb Carpometacarpal Arthroplasty

Osteoarthritis of the first carpometacarpal joint (CMC-1) often presents with pain, decreased pinch and grip strength, and functional limitations with ADLs. CMC-1 arthroplasty may be indicated when conservative management fails to control symptoms, usually with a trapeziectomy with or without ligament reconstruction and/or tendon interposition (LRTI). While post-op rehabilitation is emphasized in some studies, there is a significant lack of high-quality comparative studies and wide variation among protocols. A recent systematic review by Wouters et al. came to similar conclusions as prior authors but was able to identify three phases of rehabilitation: The acute phase, the unloaded phase, and the functional phase [77].

- Three Phases:
  - Acute phase: 0–6 weeks post-op

    Composite finger flexion/extension.

    Thumb interphalangeal (IP)-1 flexion/extension, wrist/elbow/shoulder movements emphasized.

    No CMC-1 or metacarpophalangeal (MCP)-1 movement.
  - Unloaded phase: 1–12 weeks post-op

    ROM for MCP-1 and CMC-1 initiated.

Emphasis on MCP-1 flexion (avoiding hyperextension to prevent Z-deformity) and CMC palmar adduction/extension.
Avoid CMC-1 flexion, adduction, and opposition.
Exercises supplemented with scar management and edema control.
- Functional phase: 3 weeks to 6 months post-op
  Progressive ROM of CMC-1 and MCP-1 allowed.
  Strength exercises initiated.

There is also evidence that early active recovery, including short immobilization and early initiation of ROM and strength exercises, leads to positive outcomes related to pain, ADLs, and grip and pinch strength; however, a conclusion could not be drawn due to a paucity of comparative studies [77]. An accelerated protocol was not associated with worse outcomes (MHQ function, VAS pain, complications, return to work, ROM, satisfaction with treatment, grip, and pinch strength) or increased complications, but higher quality comparative studies are still needed to determine efficacy [77, 78]. Additional protocols have been recently published in further support of the 3-phase model with similar progressions [79]. Common complications include pain, infection, scar tenderness, sensory changes, CRPS, tendon adhesion or rupture, impaired healing, and impaired function.

Flexor Tendon Repair

Flexor tendon injuries of the hand can carry significant morbidity and frequently require surgical repair [80]. Post-op rehabilitation is considered imperative for optimal functional recovery and minimization of complications [80, 81]. Due to the complex anatomy and biomechanics of flexor tendons within the hand, wrist, and forearm, a zone-based classification system was created by Kleinert et al. and Verdan to describe the region of injury, ranging from zones I (most distal) through V (most proximal) (Fig. 23.1) [81]. Surgical techniques and post-op rehabilitation protocols vary by zone with some overlapping principles [80].

The goal of flexor tendon post-op rehabilitation entails a sensitive balance of early motion to reduce adhesions and incremental tensile loading to promote repair strength while minimizing the risk of tendon rupture. Earlier recommendations opted for several weeks of immobilization to protect the repair, but advancements in the field have demonstrated improved outcomes with early controlled mobilization, including increased strength of repair, reduced adhesions, and a decreased incidence of tendon re-rupture [80, 82, 83]. This has given rise to a wide variety of early AROM and PROM protocols [80]. Due to multiple systematic reviews with very low evidence from comparison studies, including a Cochrane review by Peters et al., controversy remains over the safest and most effective protocols [80, 82, 84]. Klifto et al. published their review of current concepts in flexor tendon post-op rehabilitation in the Journal of Hand Surgery with protocol recommendations based

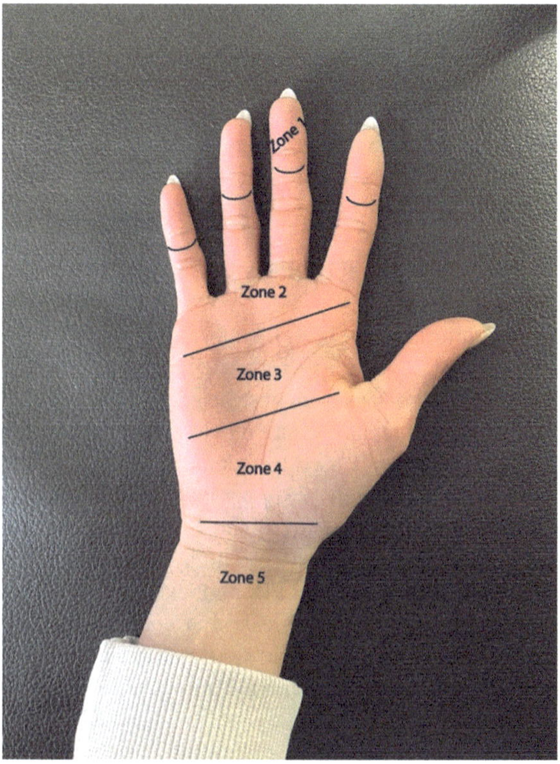

Fig. 23.1 Zone-based classification of flexor tendon injuries

on the zone of injury and supporting evidence [80]. The most frequently studied protocols are as follows, although others are used and cited with apparent success.

- Duran Protocol [81, 85]
  - Low force, low excursion.
  - Early passive-controlled motion for 4–5 weeks post-op
  - Active finger extension with patient-assisted passive finger flexion.
  - Dorsal protective static splint between exercises.
- Kleinert Protocol [81, 85]
  - Low force, low excursion.
  - Active finger extension with dynamic splint-assisted passive finger flexion with rubber bands from fingertips to volar aspects of the wrist.
  - Wrist blocked at 45 degrees of flexion and the MCP joints at 10–20 degrees.
  - Multiple modifications.
- Modified Duran Protocol [86, 87]
- Combined Duran and Kleinert Protocol
  - Controlled passive motion, passive flexion, and active extension.
- Early Active Motion (EAM) [81, 86, 87]
  - Moderate force, potentially high excursion.
  - Dorsal extension-blocking splints.
  - Perform "place and hold" exercises with digits.

Zone 1: Distal to flexor digitorum superficialis (FDS) Insertion

Early mobilization of the distal interphalangeal (DIP) joint (passive followed by active) is important to prevent adhesions at the A4 pulley secondary to post-op edema. This can be achieved with themodified Duran or EAM protocols. Klifto et al. describe two alternate protocols with similar progression through phases of active extension and passive flexion with advancement to active flexion with dorsal splinting in wrist flexion to reduce tensile strain on the flexor digitorum profundus (FDP) tendon [80].

Zone II: Over the A1 Pulley to Flexor Digitorum Superficialis (FDS) Insertion

Zone II injuries have been the most extensively studied and historically referred to as "no-man's land" for their frequent complications. This region is particularly susceptible to adhesions from post-op edema, catching of the repaired tendon under the A2 pulley, and repair rupture due to poor tendon healing. The Duran, Kleinert, and EAM are commonly used for zone II injuries. Active extension with passive flexion is allowed immediately post-operative followed by gentle active flexion at 3–6 weeks (about 3.5 weeks for Duran) and finally resisted flexion around 6–8 weeks. Both protocols are susceptible to proximal interphalangeal joint (PIP) joint contractures, potentially necessitating a PIP joint extension orthosis. The EAM is a more aggressive approach requiring at least four core sutures with cross-locking flexor tendon repair and interlocking horizontal mattress circumferential suturing to ensure adequate strength with early mobilization. AAROM begins as soon as 14 to 21 post-op with the affected finger buddy strapped, and AROM initiated with the strap removed around 28 days. Multiple studies and systemic reviews demonstrated evidence of the superiority of the EAM protocol over early passive mobilization in zone II without an increased risk of rupture. A combined Duran and Kleinert protocol demonstrated improved efficacy and safety, with the lowest risk of repair rupture at 2.3%, whereas Kleinert had the highest at 7.1%. Both the EAM and Duran and Kleinert also demonstrated the greatest recovery in ROM, but additional high-quality RCTs are needed to accurately determine the efficacy of the various protocols [80].

Zone III: Distal from Transverse Carpal Ligament to A1 Pulley

Due to the anatomic location of zone III injuries, patients who sustained proximal injuries receive a concurrent carpal tunnel release and those with distal injuries undergo an A1 pulley release. During the first 4 weeks, patients are placed in a neutral wrist orthosis with the MCP joints at 30 degrees of flexion and the interphalangeal joints at zero degrees. They are permitted to perform full active extension within the orthosis and active flexion within two-thirds of the flexion arc before removing the orthosis at 4 weeks and perform full active extension and flexion. Active flexion with resistance can begin at 6 weeks post-op and contractures are addressed with passive stretching and nightly orthotic use. Evaluation using the Strickland formula demonstrated excellent results among 90% of patients and no reports of rupture [80].

Zone IV: Within the Carpal Tunnel

There is a significant paucity of research on the efficacy of protocols for zone IV protocols. Using the Indiana Hand Protocol, during the first 3 weeks post-op, passive flexion and extension are performed on each finger with a dorsal-blocking orthosis to promote tendon gliding and reduce scar contracture. AROM is initiated at 3 weeks with the wrist positioned in 30 degrees of flexion if nerve injury occurs, gradually decreasing flexion by 10 degrees weekly. If the ulnar nerve is damaged, the 4th and 5th MCP joints should be blocked to prevent hyperextension and clawing distally. Furthermore, in the presence of nerve damage, pressure should be minimized on nerve repairs, and the first web spacer used at night to prevent contracture due to atrophic thenar muscles, blocking all MCP joints if both nerves are injured [80].

Zone V: Proximal to Carpal Tunnel

Concurrent neurovascular injuries are common with zone V injuries, often due to lacerations from glass, knives, or self-inflicted injuries. Active extension and passive flexion for the first 4 weeks demonstrated good to excellent outcomes in one study, with similar results obtained using the modified Duran and Kleinert protocol. The wrist and MCPs are maintained in flexion to reduce strain on the nerves and tendons with extension performed against rubber bands and passive flexion up to four times daily until removal of the brace at 4 weeks and active flexion initiated. Excellent outcomes were obtained in 93% of patients using the Buck-Gramcko evaluation system [80].

FPL: Zones I–IV from Tip of Thumb to Thenar Eminence, Zone V as Above

Surgical repair of flexor pollicis longus (FPL) tendon injuries requires immediate attention to avoid increased retraction and subsequent increased risk for re-rupture after repair. Advances in surgical techniques have lowered the repair rupture rate to as low as 0% from the previously estimated 15% and allowed for early active mobilization. Most case studies use the EAM or Kleinert protocols with relative success, but larger RCTs are lacking for comparison studies [80].

The advancement of surgical techniques has afforded greater opportunity and success with early activation protocols, allowing for the minimization of adhesions while reducing the risk of tendon repair ruptures [80]. Increased risk of rupture is most evident among two-strand core suture repairs compared to four-strand core sutures and greater [82]. Adhesions remain the common complication following flexor tendon repairs, with zone II carrying the greatest risk due to proximity with the pulley systems [80, 84]. In addition to physical therapy, tenolysis can be performed if it is within 4–6 months after tendon repair and there is significant loss of excursion [81, 84]. The rate of repair ruptures varies in the literature, from 4% in systematic reviews to as high as 46% in some early active motion studies [83]. Joint contracture is also a common complication with rates reported as high as 17%. Additional complications may include swan-neck deformity, trigger finger, lumbrical plus finger, and quadrigia [81].

Despite the ubiquitous use of splints in various protocols, there remains insufficient comparative data to provide evidence-based recommendations for or against splints with wrist immobilization [88]. Nonetheless, the premise of limiting wrist extension to relieve tensile strain and protect newly repaired tendons will likely continue to be promoted with the use of orthotic devices.

Distal Radius Fracture

Distal radius fractures (DRFs) are the most common type in the upper extremities, with an increasing incidence across age groups and an estimated fivefold increase in the number of internal fixation procedures from 1996 to 2005 [89]. Surgical treatment is applied to more complex and unstable fracture types and often use an internal fixation approach [90]. It remains unclear in the literature whether post-op rehabilitation improves long-term outcomes. There is some evidence to suggest benefit of at least one educational therapy session with instructions for a home therapy program. Formal hand therapy has shown benefits in short-term outcomes, but many of these studies show no significant difference in long-term outcomes between groups performing home therapy [91]. The AAOS had no clinical guidelines on the type or duration of rehabilitation after surgical fixation of DRFs, mainly offering an optional and weak recommendation for self-directed home therapy [89]. A Cochrane systematic review by Handoll et al. found low-quality evidence in support of post-operative rehabilitation, recommending more robust RCTs with larger sample sizes to establish clear guidelines [91].

The primary focus of rehabilitation is to minimize or prevent complications and optimize functional recovery [92]. The location of DRFs being in proximity to, if not through, the radioulnar and radiocarpal joints warrants some degree of attention to ensure optimal return of function. The principles that guide other intra-articular fractures include precise realignment, stable internal fixation, and early mobilization [93]. These are not often applied to DRFs, yet more studies are showing improved outcomes with early mobilization without the increased risk of displacement [91, 93, 94]. Understanding the type of fracture, location, fixation approach, and potential kinematic changes can safely guide early mobilization strategies. Despite the absence of established guidelines for DRF postoperative rehabilitation, taking the time to understand the injury, the affected structures, and the functional implications will assist in the formulation of a safe treatment plan using evidence-based practices [90].

Most rehabilitation protocols or management plans should revolve around the phases of bone and soft-tissue healing. This leads to a physiologic phase-based approach, as recommended by Naughton and Botsford, and outlined in Table 23.9 [90, 95].

There are multiple potential complications that are important to monitor for following DRFs. A risk associated with many fracture types, malunion, and nonunion can create significant functional impairments and may require revision surgery. Increased compression on the triangular fibrocartilage complex may occur due to a change in load distribution across the wrist from 80/20 (radius/ulnar) to 60/40. Adverse tendon injuries, including tenosynovitis or rupture, were shown to occur following ORIF for DRFs 6.8% of the time in one systematic review. Limitations in ROM can be seen due to the shortening of the joint capsule, decreased tendon gliding, and scar tissue formation. Nerve injury may also occur, including the anterior interosseous nerve, which has also been reported after DRFs. The incidence of CRPS varies widely, from 1% to 37% and DRF is

Table 23.9 Postoperative rehabilitation course for distal radius fracture [90, 95]

Phase	Goals	Interventions/Precautions
Phase I (Days 1–10)	Protect healing with or without orthosis, as indicated	*Weightbearing status:* NWB to involved upper extremity No lifting, pulling, pushing, or forceful gripping
Phase II (Day 11–Week 5)	Begins when immobilization no longer needed, as early as 10 days for ORIF (4–6 weeks for casts, pinning, or external fixation) Increase ROM to wrist and forearm, initiate light functional use of upper extremity wearing splint, wean splint by end of Phase II, improve grip strength (limit to 37.5 lbs or 8 Newtons (N)) (progress with caution, as for every 10 N of grip force, 26 N is transmitted through distal radius metaphysis)	*Weightbearing status:* NWB to involved upper extremity Days 11–14: AROM at wrist and forearm as tolerated with some discomfort expected, edema management, orthotic use except hygiene and exercises, light functional use of hand with orthosis Week 3–6: AAROM/AROM of wrist and forearm, begin weaning splint at 4–5 weeks, except for heavier activities, initiate scar management after sutures removed and incision healed, assess pinch/grip strength and begin strengthening, and introduce functional activities as tolerated *Criteria to Advance:* Improve pain-free ROM
Phase III (Weeks 6–12)	Progressive strengthening, regain functional strength, continue improving ROM as needed, and return to work with full use	*Weightbearing status:* may begin gentle weightbearing (table-top, then to wall, and quadruped) Light grip, isometric, and isotonic wrist and forearm exercises, and advance to close chain and increased load
Phase IV (Weeks 12–20)	Optional phase for more demanding work duties and/or return-to-sport	Hardening/conditioning program

cited as being one of the most commonly associated events preceding onset. Predictors of pain and poor functional outcome include high-energy fracture, a preinjury or prereduction positive ulnar variance, greater injury severity, catastrophic thinking, and the presence of baseline depression Lastly, post-op complications may lead to the development of carpal tunnel syndrome or wrist fusion [90]. Given the increased dexterity required of the hand for functional use, timely and appropriate management of complications is an important component of all post-op rehabilitation regimens.

Given the high incidence rate of DRFs and the subsequent cost to the health care system in combination with an absence of practice guidelines, several authors have investigated alternate post-op rehabilitation strategies. Lara et al. revealed early evidence that a digital media-based home hand therapy program provided for patients following volar plating of DRF produced similar patient-reported and physical outcomes compared to traditional in-person hand therapy, as measured by QuickDASH scores [89]. Further research is needed to assess the efficacy of a home-based model, but this could prove beneficial to health resource management if shown to be equivocal or better than rehabilitation in the traditional setting for select patient populations.

Phalanx Fracture

Phalanx fractures account for an estimated 10% of all fractures, 38% of which involve the 5th digit [96]. In addition to considering the skeletal lesion itself, recognizing the impact of injury and post-op changes on surrounding tissues and neurovascular structures is imperative in devising a comprehensive and effective rehabilitation strategy. There is a rich supply of literature on surgical approaches for the numerous types of phalanx fractures, but a paucity of articles covering the course of rehabilitation [97]. Cannon and Hardy have separately described detailed rehabilitation approaches tailored to each type of phalanx fracture, including the unique splinting and immobilization timeframes recommended for each [97, 98]. We refer to these authors for a more detailed explanation, while offering here a more generalized outline of key principles for successful therapy programs.

There are core principles that underlie all post-op phalanx rehabilitation programs: communication with the surgeon, edema control, early motion as appropriate, and scar desensitization and remodeling [99]. It is crucial to understand the fracture type and location, method of reduction, type of fixation (when applicable), the stability of the fracture, and associated soft-tissue structures [97]. The immediate concern following the fracture is adequate realignment and stabilization of osseous structures, with an immobilization period ranging from 3 to 9 weeks depending on multiple factors related to fracture type and method of reduction [96–98]. After the stabilization of osseous structures, the surrounding soft tissues, pulley systems, and mobile gliding tendons become the central focus in rehabilitation [97, 98]. Particular attention is directed at tendon gliding of FDP, FDS, and extensor digitorum communis. Management of edema and scar tissue deposition and remodeling will impact functional outcomes and if not dealt with appropriately, may lead to complications. Early motion protocols are being utilized more commonly, and are one advantage of external fixation reductions, but motion is nonetheless important for all types to prevent adhesions and promote tendon gliding. The intent to mobilize must be considered in the context of adequate bone healing to prevent nonunion or malunion. This is often initiated with limitations at about 3–4 weeks for bones undergoing secondary healing. For primary healing, bones surgically fixed with compression applied, motion can resume within a few days postoperatively, as the implants provide adequate support. Strengthening programs should be resumed around 6–8 weeks for both primary and secondary healing, as bones healing by closed conservative management and those addressed with open reduction internal fixation achieve the same level of tensile strength at 12 weeks [98].

The most common complication following phalanx fracture is loss of motion. Rehabilitation is important to address decreased ROM following prolonged immobilization, associated joint injury, and extensive surgical dissection. Malunion may lead to malrotation, angulation, or shortening, with surgery indicated if functional impairment is significant. Fracture nonunion is uncommon and most often associated with bone loss or neurovascular compromise leading to resection, bone grafting, plating, ray amputation, or fusion [96]. The risk for phalanx fracture complications is influenced by multiple factors that require individualized attention throughout the post-op period and emphasizes the need for large high-quality RCTs to provide guidelines and standards for safe and effective rehabilitation.

Dupuytren's Contracture

Dupuytren's contracture is a proliferative and progressive fibroplasia of the palmer fascia. Despite the variety of treatment options, success with nonoperative management has been largely limited to short-term effects, often necessitating surgical intervention for appropriate candidates [100]. A limited fasciotomy is now the preferred approach, excising the nodular and/or fibrous bands [101]. While many hand surgeons seem to agree on referral to therapy and the use of an orthosis post-op, there is limited evidence in the literature to support its use or reliably demonstrate the efficacy of different protocols. Nonetheless, the HANDGUIDE study out of Europe aimed to achieve multidisciplinary consensus on treatment guidelines and determined that postoperative care should always consist of education and therapeutic exercise, at minimum [100].

Some authors recommend a single preoperative therapy session to help set expectations and assess baseline function and ROM. Counseling patients can help define realistic expectations, reiterate potential postoperative sequelae, and clarify rehabilitation timelines. The therapist can also measure existing ROM and screen for dynamism, which occurs when a Dupuytren's cord crosses over both the MCP and PIP joints, lessening the extension deficit of one joint due to flexion of another and consequently increasing the extension deficit with extension of the other joint. This can confound measurements post-op if not identified preoperatively. Lastly, preoperative assessment can document sensory function in the hand before surgery and screen for potential concurrent syndromes of finger triggering or symptoms of carpal tunnel syndrome [100].

The goal of post-op rehabilitation is to promote wound healing, prevent infection, control edema, minimize adverse mechanical influences, and support the collagen maturation process. Multiple studies and more recent findings in cellular biology suggest a less aggressive stretching protocol is more appropriate and carries better outcomes in ROM and disease status. Forced and sustained extension, as with stretching and extension-bias splinting is thought to stimulate myofibroblasts in the palmer fascia, impair local circulation to tissues, promote inflammation, and stimulate disease progression. Additionally, there is a lack of consistent evidence in the literature to support the use of a night orthosis; however, some authors have found that the use of a dorsal-blocking orthosis with a no-tension protocol immediately after surgery for the first 2–3 weeks improves outcomes. While there is no established or standardized protocol guiding rehabilitation postoperatively, an example of successful progression is provided in Table 23.10 [100].

Post-op complications are well documented, but rehabilitation protocols to address them are lacking. The most common include infection, flap necrosis, white finger, sympathetic flare, nerve damage, hypertrophic scarring, scar contracture from a poorly designed incision, recurrence, joint stiffness, and disease extension

Table 23.10 Postoperative rehabilitation course for Dupuytren's contracture [100]

Phase	Goals	Interventions/precautions
Phase I (Weeks 1–2)	Wound care and control pain and edema	Dorsal-blocking orthosis—wrist neutral, MCP joints at 35–45 of flexion, and interphalangeal (IP) joints in relaxed extension Thumb in mild abduction if web space released Short-arc digit flexion and extension
Phase II (Weeks 2–3)	Control pain and edema, improve ROM, and scar management	Increase digit ROM in flexion and extension Avoid aggressive active or passive ROM Suture removal at postoperative day 16 or 17, or longer in setting of diabetes or unstable corner flaps, to prevent formation of painful or hypertrophic scarring and wound dehiscence Scar management Continue anti-tension orthosis until week 3
Phase III (Weeks 4–6)	Control edema and improve ROM	Edema control and restore motion May be discharged, or continued 1–2 times weekly as needed Home exercise program—light stretching and strengthening Continue composite digital extension orthoses for 3–6 months

[100]. Patients should be evaluated and treated according to their unique presentation and needs as they arise.

Recent advancements in nonoperative management include collagenase injections (enzymatic fasciotomy) with manipulation and needle fasciotomy. There is limited data on the use of these procedures following surgical intervention, necessitating further studies on safety and efficacy [100].

- Alternate procedures:
  - Needle fasciotomy:
    Limited intervention required.
    Nonaggressive extension orthosis and exercises.
    - Limited evidence to support the use of orthosis.

    Padded gloves for more rigorous activities.
  - Collagenase injection:
    Clostridium collagenase histolyticum injection.
    Nonsurgical treatment.
    Generally positive results.

Proximal Interphalangeal Joint (PIP) Arthroplasty

Arthritis of the PIP joint can be effectively treated with a variety of implant designs, but rehabilitation guidelines are sparse and highly variable based on implant choice, patient characteristics, and institutional experience. See Table 23.11 for an example of one formally proposed post-operative rehabilitation protocol [102]. Common

Table 23.11 Postoperative rehabilitation course for proximal interphalangeal joint arthroplasty [102]

Phase	Goals	Interventions/precautions
Phase I (Days 0–10)	Protect healing with or without orthosis, as indicated, and control pain and edema	Focus primarily on hand Metacarpophalangeal joint maintained at 20–30 degrees flexion, and PIP in full extension AROM of uninvolved fingers, wrist, elbow, and shoulder
Phase II (Day 11–2 Weeks)	Control pain and edema (wraps), improve ROM, and patient education	Custom cylindrical PIP joint orthosis allowing for DIP flexion (used with edema wraps)—orthosis worn day and night with digit sleeve for edema control Scar massage and desensitization therapy Figure-8 orthosis with buddy strap intermittently throughout day during light use of hand Monitor for PIP joint motion extension lag and adjust frequency of active PIP joint flexion to accommodate Patient education is crucial for delicate nature of healing process and importance of graduated therapeutic progression
Phase III (Weeks 2–4)	Protection, improves ROM, and prevents deformities	If no PIP lag, increase light use of hand using figure-8/buddy strap AAROM for PIP joint flexion at least 3× daily, ensuring full extension maintained—progression with flexion dependent on maintenance of near complete extension, goal to achieve 0–45 degrees of PIP joint motion by 4 weeks Avoid lateral stress and protect with night splinting May use Rangor orthosis to allow PIP flexion and block PIP hyperextension and DIP flexion (prevent Swan-neck deformity)
Phase IV (Weeks 4–7)	Control edema, scar management, and 0–60 degrees of PIP joint motion	Motion program continued, along w/ supportive orthosis and edema control Gentle resistance added using light sponge w/ figure-8 orthosis to build tolerance for force and limit rotational and lateral forces Nighttime orthotic use w/ digit in full extension Progression of light functional use
Phase V (Weeks 8–12)	Wean daytime figure-8 orthosis and improve ROM	10–20 extension lag is acceptable Continued daytime orthosis use strongly encouraged for aggressive activities (e.g., yard work and impact sports) up to 4–6 months post-op Nighttime orthosis usually not important after 12 weeks post-op Final hand therapy visit at 12 weeks post-op Final surgeon post-op w/ clinical and radiographic evaluation at 6 months post-op ROM can improve up to 9 months post-op Achieving full extension more important than full flexion, as future surgical correction is far easier to obtain for flexion than extensor lag

complications include implant fracture, lateral instability, silicone synovitis, subsidence, and joint stiffness.

Trigger Finger Release

Unfortunately, there is insufficient evidence, and no definitive post-op rehabilitation guidelines published for trigger finger release. Existing protocols tendon to be practice-specific, and most involve either home rehabilitation or resuming use with limited restrictions unless hand therapy is later required for post-op complications.

Hip

Total Hip Arthroplasty

Total hip arthroplasty (THA) is a common procedure that is indicated for symptomatic end-stage hip osteoarthritis, osteonecrosis, congenital hip disorders (i.e., hip dysplasia, inflammatory arthritis conditions), femur fractures, and hardware failure after previous internal fixation [103]. Post-op, patients are weightbearing as tolerated with the implementation of hip precautions that focus on limiting internal rotation, external rotation, adduction, and flexion of the hip for at least six weeks in order to promote proper healing and prevent hip dislocation during the rehabilitation course [104]. Other complications that are seen post-op include DVT, prosthetic joint infection, joint instability/dislocation, and periprosthetic fractures [105]. The typical rehabilitation course following THA is comprised of five phases over a minimum time frame of 3 months outlined in Table 23.12.

In contrast to the standard rehabilitation protocol stated above, fast-track rehabilitation programs have been recently studied where the rehab process starts three to five hours after surgery with patients being discharged after 3–5 days. The association with early patient mobilization and rapid functional recovery was found to lead to better outcomes and lower risk of complications and readmissions. It was also found to have reduced depression and anxiety in patients with THA and accelerated the post-op recovery period [106]. Overall, mobility on the day of surgery through the first 24 hours has been shown to be crucial in decreasing length of stay, decreasing pain, and improving physical function (balance, muscle strength, etc.) [107].

Hip Arthroscopy

Hip arthroscopy is a minimally invasive surgical procedure that is indicated for symptomatic acetabular labral tears, hip capsular laxity and instability, chondral lesions, osteochondritis dissecans, ligamentum teres injuries, snapping hip

Table 23.12 Postoperative rehabilitation course for THA [103]

Phase	Goals	Interventions
Phase I (Weeks 0–1)	Pain control, increase motor control and strength, increase independence with mobility, hip precaution education	Ankle pumps, quadriceps sets, gluteal sets, and gait training on flat surfaces with appropriate assistive devices
Phase II (Weeks 1–3)	Pain control, increasing ROM while adhering to precautions, increase strength, increase functional independence, and gait training	Passive/Active Assisted/Active ROM (P/AA/AROM) exercises in supine and seated positions: Ankle pumps, heel slides, long arc quads, quadriceps sets in full knee extension, gluteal sets, short-arc quadriceps, hooklying ball/towel squeeze (all within ROM precautions)
Phase III (Weeks 3–6)	Pain control, increase ROM, increase lower extremity and trunk strength, balance, and proprioceptive training to assist with functional activities, and gait training	Stationary bike, level 1 trunk stabilization, three way straight-leg raise, close chain weight shifting activities, balance exercises, lateral step up and step down with eccentric control, front step up and step down, sit-to-stand activities, ascending/descending stairs
Phase IV (Weeks 6–12)	Increase overall strength throughout lower extremities, return to all functional activities, and begin light recreational activities	Progression of phase III exercises by increasing resistance and repetitions, progress trunk stabilization exercises, front lunge and squat activities, progress balance and proprioception activities, initiate overall exercise and endurance training (walking, swimming, progress biking)
Phase V (Weeks 12+)	Return to high-level activities	Continue low-impact activities for aerobic conditioning, and obtain clearance from surgeon for return to impact sports

syndrome, iliopsoas bursitis, intra-articular loose bodies, femoral acetabular impingement, and labral debridement [108, 109]. Post-op, patients are partial weightbearing as tolerated (WBAT) or WBAT to the affected extremity with the immediate goal of preventing post-op joint stiffness and avoiding potential intra-articular adhesions [110]. The literature regarding post-op rehabilitation following hip arthroscopy has not been well-developed, and deficits in strength, endurance, and functional capacity have been seen afterward for up to 2 years, further highlighting the need for additional targeted rehabilitation [111]. Complications seen after hip arthroscopy include lateral femoral cutaneous nerve injury, chondral injury, labral puncture, infection, DVT, pulmonary embolus, hematoma, and heterotopic ossification [109]. The proposed time frame for current rehabilitation varies between 12 and 24 weeks as stated in Table 23.13.

Hip Resurfacing

Hip resurfacing is an alternative surgical approach to THA that is most commonly indicated in end-stage osteoarthritis in a young, active patient [113]. Current literature comparing outcomes and the need for revisions following hip resurfacing and THA for patients with osteoarthritis is still lacking due to lack of consistent post-op definitions and standardized outcome metrics [114]. Complications seen after hip

Table 23.13 Postoperative rehabilitation course for hip arthroscopy [112]

Phase	Goals	Range of motion	Strengthening/conditioning
Phase I (Weeks 1–4)	Reduce joint inflammation, preserve soft-tissue repair, and maintain ROM with pain-free limits	Week 1: Passive internal rotation and external log rolling with pain-free limits Week 2: Prone hip internal rotation with pain-free limits Weeks 2–4: Hip extension in prone lying, prone knee flexion *Limit ER to 20 degrees if capsular closer is performed* *Limit ER and extension if capsulectomy is performed* *Avoid hip hyperextension and passive ER past 20 degrees after labral repair*	Weeks 1–2: Isometric strengthening in all planes except hip flexion Weeks 3–4: Isometric strengthening in all planes except hip flexion, isometric strengthening in hip flexion Core training with advancement to bridging as pain allows, stationary bike (duration increasing from 5 to 30 minutes), hydrotherapy as indicated after adequate wound healing
Phase II (Weeks 4–8)	Advancement through therapy protocol, normalization of gait, functional ROM	Initiation of standard lower extremity stretching program: Standing adductor, iliotibial band, hip flexor, prone quadriceps, seated hamstring, prayer, and V-sit stretches with end-range hold times progressing from 10 to 30 seconds After labral repair, begin bent knee fall outs and stool rotations for external rotation	Standing hip strengthening in all planes utilizing resistance band, clam shell abduction and seated hip ER against resistance band, open chain strengthening of quadriceps, hamstrings, and gastrocnemius muscle groups, standing leg press advancing from two to one-legged press (avoid hip flexion >90 degrees) Weeks 4–6: Continue low-intensity aerobic exercise Weeks 6–8: Nonimpact interval training
Phase III (Weeks 9–12)	Advance strengthening and endurance to restore normal function	End-range stretching in all planes	Step-ups, lateral step off, mini-squats, deadlifts, lunges, core training progression from single plane to multiplane exercises, intro to cross-training (elliptical trainer, stationary bike with resistance, stair stepper with goal of 30 min to continuous exercise at moderate intensity), proprioception exercises
Phase IV and V (Weeks 13–24)	Safe and effective return to sporting or work activities at the preinjury level	End-range stretching in all planes	Multiplanar weightbearing sport-specific exercises, side lunges, split stance cable row, agility training, ladder drills, and plyometric exercise as indicated

resurfacing include femoral or acetabular loosening, femoral neck notching, femoral neck fracture, deep vein thrombosis, stress fracture, nerve palsy, and infection [115]. The post-op rehabilitation course is typically 12 weeks as outlined in Table 23.14 [116].

Femoral Osteoplasty

Femoroacetabular impingement (FAI), more notably FAI due to cam is not an acronym so can be uncapitalized. (CAM) deformity, is the main indication for femoral osteoplasty. It continues to be an important component management of FAI as recent systematic reviews have shown overall improvements in hip function scores and reductions in the severity of symptoms at short-term and midterm follow-ups [117]. In addition, the combination of hip arthroscopy and femoral osteoplasty when compared with hip arthroscopy alone has been shown to demonstrate superior long-term clinical outcomes in some studies [118]. Complications seen after femoral osteoplasty include femoral neck fracture, abdominal compartment syndrome, pulmonary embolism, deep infection of the joint, superficial infection, avascular necrosis of the femoral head, post-operative dislocation, DVT, lateral femoral cutaneous nerve injury, hematoma, and heterotopic ossification [119]. The post-op rehabilitation course is typically at least 10 weeks long as outlined in Table 23.15 with patients being unrestricted at 6 months with a full recovery noted around 1 year [120].

Table 23.14 Postoperative rehabilitation course for hip resurfacing [116]

Phase	Goals	Interventions
Phase I (Weeks 1–4)	Normalize gait, decrease pain, and prevent stiffness	Weeks 1–2: Ankle pumps, quad sets (gluteal squeezes, active heel slides, recumbent bike without resistance as ROM allows, seated "dangle" stretch) Weeks 3–4: SLR hip abduction (progress from standing to side-lying), SLR hip extension, SLR hip flexion, walking as tolerated, stationary bike, fig. 4 stretching, aquatic therapy if wound well healed *Weightbearing status: Partial WBAT with crutches for 2–3 weeks with progression to FWB by weeks 3–4 (may be delayed by 2 weeks if bilateral resurfacing was done)*
Phase II (Weeks 4–12)	Regain hip mobility, gentle stretching, and normal basic activity	Weeks 4–6: initiate hip flexor stretching EOB, add leg presses with lightweight, double leg bridges, clams, resisted ER and IR of hip in standing, single-leg balance and proprioception, stationary biking with resistance Weeks 6–12: Tall kneeling or stool hip flexor stretching, elliptical and stairmaster progression, advanced bridging exercises (single, unsteady surface, resistance), mid-range multidirectional lunges, closed-chain exercise progression *Weightbearing status: FWB without assistive device*
Phase III (Weeks 12+)	Restore normal strength and return to prior level of function	Begin gentle return-to-activity or sport

Table 23.15 Postoperative rehabilitation course for femoral osteoplasty [120]

Phase	Goals	Interventions
Phase I (Weeks 1–3)	Maintaining strength while being restricted weightbearing, regain ROM, decrease pain, decrease inflammation	SLR into extension/abduction/adduction, hip supine AROM IR/ER, prone hip IR/ER isometrics, quad sets/bridging, butterflies, stool hip IR and ER AROM, core stabilization (pelvic tilts, heel walkouts, dead bug), stretching quads/hamstrings/hip flexor, AAROM hip IR/ER, stationary bike with no resistance (<8.2.10 minutes), passive ROM to hip (hip circumduction, flexion to 90 degrees, internal and external rotation prone, internal rotation log roll) *Weightbearing status: Partial weightbearing for at least 3 weeks with use of assistive devices as needed (varies depending on surgeon and extent of surgery)*
Phase II (Weeks 4–6)	Regain ROM to 100% of the uninvolved hip, independent ambulation on all surfaces, and progression of strength as tolerated	Elliptical, leg press, hamstring curls, resisted hip abduction/flexion/extension, mini-squats, resisted hip IR/ER, sidestepping with resistance, advanced bridging, step up and downs, core stabilization (planks, advanced dead bug, crunches, obliques), single-leg stance to restore proprioception *Weightbearing status: FWB as tolerated*
Phase III (Weeks 7–10)	Restore full ROM, restore normal free gait pattern on all surfaces, restoration of 70–80% muscle strength of the uninvolved side, restore muscular strength and cardiovascular endurance, and improve balance reactions	Proprioception drills (cone, side shuffle), continue to progress strengthening of the entire lower extremity, return to social sport when able
Phase IV (Weeks 10+)	Return to play	Exercises are sport dependent and should be geared toward strengthening via more sports-specific exercises

Proximal Hamstring Repair

Hamstring ruptures can either be treated operatively or non-operatively with nonoperative treatments having been shown to be less successful in more severe injuries [121]. Ruptures that include one or two tendons with less than two centimeters (cm) of retraction can often be treated non-operatively while ruptures consisting of two or three tendon avulsions and/or retraction of those tendons greater than two cm are usually recommended to undergo surgical intervention. Post-op complications include hematoma, paresthesias, wound infection, deep venous thrombosis, and re-rupture [122]. General guidelines following hamstring repair surgery include the use of axillary crutches with toe-touching weightbearing for 4–6 weeks with an expected return-to-sport around 6 months with normal gait and running mechanics, greater than 80% hamstring and quad strength versus non-injured extremity with isokinetic testing, and no symptoms with sport-specific dynamic activities (Table 23.16) [123].

Table 23.16 Postoperative rehabilitation course for proximal hamstring repair [124]

Phase	Goals	Precautions/Range of motion	Strengthening/conditioning
Phase I (Weeks 0–2)	Allow healing of repaired tendons, initiate early restricted and protected ROM, prevent muscular atrophy, and decrease pain and inflammation	Precautions: post-op hip brace (limit hip flexion to 45 degrees), brace at all times (aside from exercise and bathing), and avoid hip flexion with knee extension ROM: Active-assisted and passive hip and knee flexion, hip flexion ROM limited to 60 degrees flexion	Nerve gliding (sciatic neural flossing—however, if neural tension exits, do not stretch hamstring), hip flexor stretching in Thomas test position while maintaining neutral pelvis/spine, gastrocnemius and soleus stretching, ankle pumps, quad sets, AAROM and PROM hip flexion (60-degree limit) and knee flexion
Phase II (Weeks 2–6)	Reduce/resolve pain and edema, good motor control, and pain-free functional movements	Precautions: PWB 50% with crutches, continue post-op hip brace (limit hip flexion to 60 degrees), increase brace hip flexion limit at week 4 gradually to 90 degrees by week 6, avoid hip flexion with knee extension, no active hamstring exercises, no active hip extension exercises ROM: Active-assisted and passive hip and knee flexion	Anterior hip glides with and without external rotation at the hip (hip in neutral to slightly extended), posterior/inferior belted hip mobilizations as needed for full flexion (belted quadruped position with active movement into child's pose), hip external rotation in flexion, gluteal sets in prone and supine, low double leg bridge, side-lying hip abduction, standing calf raises
Phase III (Weeks 6–12)	Normalized gait, gradually progresses to full ROM, improves neuromuscular control, increases strength, and enhances proprioception and kinesthesia	Precautions: progressively wean crutches over the next 2 weeks to FWB, discontinue brace at 6–8 weeks per surgeon ROM: progressive active hip and knee flexion, active stretching of all uninvolved muscle groups	Double leg (DL) bridge with band around thighs, DL bridge with ball squeeze, DL bridge with upper back on bench, plank with alternating leg lifts, side plank with leg lift (on left knee until stronger) or oblique twists, SLR, hamstring curls antigravity, hip extension antigravity 10 weeks post-op: SL bridge with back on floor and foot on bench, progress to ankle weight for all leg lifts, wall slides, clam shells, partial squats, step-ups, step-downs Cardiovascular Exercise: stationary bike, progressive slow walking on level surfaces, no running

(continued)

Table 23.16 (continued)

Phase	Goals	Precautions/Range of motion	Strengthening/conditioning
Phase IV (Weeks 13–16)	Full ROM, improve neuromuscular control, improve strength/power/endurance, enhance dynamic stability	Precautions: Thigh compression sleeve as needed, must be pain free during training.	Gentle hamstring stretching, cautious use of weight training machines, single-leg closed-chain exercises, resisted step-ups using sports cord around waist from behind, double leg hamstring ball roll out (eccentric portion only) with progression to DL eccentric and concentric to SL eccentric portion only and then SL eccentric and concentric, DL deadlift (short range) with progression to SL, DL deadlift with wide abducted leg stance (can add resistance band around forefeet), SL with spine rotation deadlift, bridge on ball (eccentric portion only DL with progression to SL) Cardiovascular Exercise: Walk progression on level surface with gradual increase in speed and distance, preparing to run
Phase V (Weeks 16–20)	Emphasis on gradual return to recreational activities	Precautions: Thigh compression sleeve as needed	Progressive strengthening avoiding overload to hamstring, progress speed of resisted steps and add forward lean, SL deadlift with band under stance leg, reverse lunge on slider (progress load bearing and add concentric/eccentric phase), short-range Nordic hamstring to physio ball height, kettlebell swing, retro lunge slide Cardiovascular Exercise: walk-to-jog progression, no sprinting, no speed work
Phase VI (Weeks 20–24)	Progressively increase activities to prepare for unrestricted functional return	Precautions: None	Continued isotonic strengthening, continue ROM exercises, progressive running/speed and agility, and jump training after 22 weeks Cardiovascular exercise: Progress step-ups to resisted jump onto steps, plyometric progression (double leg up/down, double leg forward/back, alternating lateral bounding, single-leg jump, progress plyometrics to resisted plyometrics using sports cord around waist), ladder drills, falling start runs, mini hurdles, sprint progressions

Periacetabular Osteotomy

Acetabular dysplasia has been noted to be a common cause of hip dysfunction in young mature patients that can often lead to osteoarthritis in adulthood. Periacetabular osteotomy (PAO) has been demonstrated to be an effective surgical option for treating acetabular dysplasia in skeletally mature individuals [125]. Complications seen after PAO include nerve lateral femoral cutaneous nerve injury, wound infection, DVT, intraoperative fractures, and conversion to total hip replacement [126]. The post-op rehabilitation course varies between 16 and 20 weeks as outlined in Table 23.17, with most individuals being able to return to an active lifestyle.

Table 23.17 Post-operative rehabilitation course for periacetabular osteotomy [127]

Phase	Goals	Precautions/range of motion	Strengthening/conditioning
Phase I (Weeks 0–6)	Protection of the post-surgical hip through limited weightbearing, reduce pain, normalize gait with assistive device, and restore leg control	Precautions: anterior hip precautions, no active hip flexion with long-lever arm, no open chain isolated muscle activation, avoid prolonged sitting for more than one hour, protected FFWB, no more than 20 lbs of body weight with axillary crutches ROM: continued passive motion machine (8 hours per day) set from 0 degrees extension to 30 degrees flexion, gradual increase after 1 week gradually up to 90 degrees as tolerated	PROM, quat sets, ankle pumps, isometric hip exercises (abduction, adduction, IR, ER, bridge without lifting hips, prone heel squeeze with pillow under hips), short-arc quads, long arc quads, standing hamstring curls
Phase II (Weeks 6–12)	Normalize gait without device (progress to WBAT first with eventual weaning off axillary crutches), core control, pelvic stability, no pain with ADLs	Precautions: assistive device until gait is non-antalgic, avoid post-activity swelling, and avoid active hip flexion if symptomatic	Open chain AROM (standing hip abduction, hip extension to neutral), hip AROM with stable pelvis (bent knee fall out, heel slide, prone windshield wiper), closed-chain exercises (squats, step-ups/downs, static lunge stance, leg press), balance and proprioceptive work, upper extremity resistance training in lunge stance

(continued)

Table 23.17 (continued)

Phase	Goals	Precautions/range of motion	Strengthening/conditioning
Phase III (Weeks 12–16)	Optimize ROM, improve core strength, improve lower extremity strength, pain-free ADLs	Precautions: avoid painful end-range hip flexion, no forced stretching, caution with repetitive hip flexion activities, and no impact activities until at least 3 months out from surgery	Gait and functional movement drills, nonimpact LE and core strength with progression, hip abduction strengthening, hip rotator strengthening, balance, and proprioceptive training, sport/work-specific balance, and proprioceptive drills
Phase IV (Weeks 16–20)	Independence with exercise program, long-distance ambulation		High-level balance and proprioceptive training, maximize ROM, introduction of plyometrics/running/cutting, continue with sport/work-specific balance and proprioceptive drills

Knee

Total Knee Arthroplasty

Total knee arthroplasty (TKA) is a surgical procedure for patients with moderate to severe arthritis who have not responded to medical management. TKA consists of resection of the diseased or degenerative articular surfaces of the knee and replacing the surface with metal and polyethylene prosthetic components. To reduce immediate post-op blood loss and swelling in the first 7 days after surgery, positioning the operated knee in some degree of flexion (30–90 degrees) while resting is optimal. In a previous meta-analysis, long-term ($\geq$24 h) high flexion (>30 degrees) protocol did not only significantly reduce total blood loss, hidden blood loss, and transfusion requirements but did effectively improve ROM one week after the operation [128]. A rapid rehabilitation protocol has come more in favor. This program entails rehabilitation therapies that begin in the post-anesthesia care unit (PACU) on post-op day 0. From this early period, patients perform bed mobility exercises with appropriate assistance, which include rolling to either side, scooting up and down, and moving from the supine position to the sitting position [129]. In the early post-op period, effectiveness of high-intensity resistance training may be limited by muscular inhibition and muscle activation deficits of the quadriceps. Modalities that show post-op benefit include cryotherapy and neuromuscular electrical stimulation (NMES). Cryotherapy shows benefit in early postoperative pain management, while NMES shows improved quadriceps muscle strength, gait performance, performance-based outcomes, and patient-reported outcomes [130]. Common complications include pain, infection, bleeding/thrombosis, and post-op anemia [128]. New technologies being studied include transcranial direct stimulation, electroacupuncture, and Tai chi chuan [131–133]. Transcranial direct stimulation and electroacupuncture showed improvement in VAS pain scores at 3 and 7 days, 3 and 6 weeks after TKA, as well as improved maximum knee flexion at 6 weeks [131, 132]. Tai Chi Chuan showed improvement in physical function and quality of life measures [133].

Anterior Cruciate Ligament Reconstruction (ACLR)

ACLR is the surgical reconstruction of the anterior cruciate ligament, the primary anteriorotary stabilizer of the knee. During ACLR, an autograft (most commonly patellar tendon or hamstring tendon) or allograft is used to replace the damaged ACL. The post-op rehab protocol is most commonly divided into four phases. Phase 1 varies from 2 to 5 weeks and encompasses several components including isometric quadriceps, hamstring, hip abduction, hip adduction, ankle exercises, passive and active ROM exercises, cryotherapy and cold therapy, TENS/NMES, knee brace (locked hinged knee brace), knee and patella mobilization, and gait training. Patients are allowed to weight bear as tolerated, with immediate full weightbearing, provided that no meniscal or cartilage repair was required. Phase 2 varies from 2 to 12 weeks and includes progressive neuromuscular training and proprioception exercises, continued AROM and PROM exercises, promotion of full knee ROM, progressive resistance training, including leg press, calf press, and step-ups, as well as endurance training using a stationary bicycle, stair stepper, or treadmill. Phase 3 varies from 2 to 24 weeks and includes progression of proprioceptive training, balance exercises, introduction of running, as well as performing plyometric exercises and jump training. Phase 4 varies from 2 to 12 weeks and includes progressive resistance training, sport-specific neuromuscular control and proprioception training, sport-specific exercises, agility drills, sprinting, cutting drills, and plyometrics [134]. Return to play ranges from 6 to 12 months [135–137]. Specific metrics used to help with the determination of return to play include the hop test, specific time point after surgery, and the one-legged squat test [135, 137]. Common complications are pain, infection, loss of ROM, and bleeding/thrombosis. New technologies for rehabilitation include vibration training and aquatic rehabilitation [134, 136].

Meniscal Surgery: Partial Meniscectomy, Meniscal Repair, and Meniscus Transplant

Meniscus surgery is a common arthroscopic procedure with several surgical approaches including partial meniscectomy, meniscal repair, and meniscus transplant. Partial meniscectomy is indicated in a patient who has failed conservative treatment with a symptomatic torn meniscus that has a low probability of healing if repaired. Post-op rehabilitation is about 8–12 weeks. Week 1 entails weaning off crutches as tolerated while performing a series of effusion-control and ROM exercises. Week 2 entails performing gait training, balance, stationary bicycle, and strengthening exercises. In weeks 2–4, patients undergo gait normalization and progress through more advanced strengthening and range of motion exercises. In weeks 4–6, along with progressive strength, balance, and ROM exercises, the patient can begin running and cutting drills. If patients have full and painless ROM after week 6, patients can perform sports-specific exercises and gradually return-to-sport. For meniscal repair/transplantation, the rehabilitation protocol is tailored to the tear type, repair technique, and level of activity. An accelerated protocol is recommended for vertical tears, and a weight restriction protocol (WRP) is recommended for radial tears. Finally, a dual restriction protocol (DRP) is recommended for root/

horizontal tears. For the accelerated protocol, TTWB is recommended until week 2 then WBAT afterward, while WRP and DRP are NWB for the first 2–3 weeks. In weeks 0–3 for accelerated, 0–4 for WRP, and 0–6 for DRP, goals are to manage pain and effusion, achieve full passive extension, and improve quadriceps activation. In weeks 3–5 for accelerated, 4–8 for WRP, and 5–10 for DRP, goals are to increase knee AROM, improve strength, normalize gait, and improve balance. In weeks 5–8 for accelerated, 8–12 for WRP, and 10–14 for DRP, goals are preparing for return-to-sport, normalizing jogging and plyometric exercises, achieving full knee AROM, improving jumping and landing mechanics, increasing strength, and improving agility and functional movement. In weeks 8–12 for accelerated, 12–16 for WRP, and 14–20 for DRP, goals are increasing running, sprinting, jumping, and landing exercises. Current return to play recommendations are 3 months for low-impact sports and 6 months for high-impact sports with a mean time of 9 months [138]. Common complications include pain, infection, and bleeding/thrombosis [139]. New technologies include synovial mesenchymal stem cell transplantation, which showed improved Lysholm knee score, and Knee Injury and Osteoarthritis Outcome Scale scores for "pain," "daily living," and "sports activities" after 2 years [140].

Medial Collateral Ligament (MCL) Reconstruction

MCL reconstruction is usually not recommended in isolated MCL injuries. The MCL is the primary medial knee stabilizer. However, in the context of multiple ligament knee injuries, reconstruction of the MCL is advocated. Post-op, early motion is important to ensure that no intra-articular adhesions develop. To avoid elongation of the reconstruction, post-op bracing is recommended [141]. There are differences in recommendations concerning allowed movements in the brace and timing of restricted weightbearing. Most commonly, the brace is placed in full extension versus some degree of flexion 0–90 degrees, with NWB for 2–6 weeks [141, 142]. It is recommended to exercise straight-leg raising in braces until able to do so without knee extension lag. Goal is to gradually wean off the brace at 3 months post-op. Strengthening exercises can be initiated once gait is normalized, commonly after 4–5 months [142]. A common complication is arthrofibrosis [141, 142].

Combined ACL/MCL Reconstruction

Combined ACL/MCL reconstruction is performed for combined ACL/MCL injuries that result from a contact mechanism that involves a valgus stress with external tibial rotation. Post-op rehab protocol is split into five phases. Phase 1 (0–6 weeks) involves active-assisted ROM, quad sets, straight-leg raise exercises in all planes (with brace locked in full extension until quad is strong enough to prevent extension lag), patellar mobilization, prone knee flexion, and hamstring stretching. Phase 2 (6–8 weeks) involves discontinuation of brace and crutches, wall slides from 0 to 45 degrees, use of stationary bike with high seat, closed-chain terminal knee extension, balance exercises, aquatic therapy with emphasis on gait normalization, as well as continued hamstring stretching. Phase 3 (2–6 months) involves stair stepper and/or elliptical use, advanced closed kinetic chain activities (leg press, one-leg mini-squats, and step-ups), progressing proprioceptive activities, and progressing aquatic program to include pool running and swimming. Phase 4 (6–9 months) involves progressing strength, power, and proprioception to prepare for sports-specific retraining. Phase 5 (9+ months) involves sports-specific retraining, including jumping, cutting, and endurance. Common complications include arthrofibrosis, saphenous nerve injury, and postoperative laxity [143].

Medial Patellofemoral Ligament (MPFL) Reconstruction

MPFL reconstruction is the surgical repair of the MPFL, the primary restraint to lateral patellar translation, which plays an important role in centralization and tracking of the patella in the initial 20–30 degrees of knee flexion [144]. Post-op, a knee immobilizer for 2–6 weeks or until able to obtain full extension without lag is recommended. Partial weightbearing using crutches is then initiated for 4–6 weeks. ROM exercises can be performed immediately and without restriction [144, 145]. Active flexion and extension and gluteal activation are emphasized in the third and fourth weeks [146]. Full weightbearing, full knee ROM, progressive strength, and proprioceptive training are recommended after 6 weeks. Return to jogging was initiated based on return of quadriceps function. Progression to sport-specific rehabilitation is around 6 months and one is cleared for return to sports when clinically stable with satisfactory functional and/or isokinetic testing [144]. Common complications include arthrofibrosis [145].

Posterior Cruciate Ligament (PCL) Reconstruction

PCL reconstruction is the surgical repair of the PCL, the primary posterior stabilizer of the knee joint. Post-op, bracing provides posterior stability during the early healing phase. A static posterior stabilizing brace is recommended for the initial 2 weeks post-op, followed by the early implementation of a dynamic PCL brace [141]. Phase 1 (0–6 weeks) focuses on protecting the integrity of the graft while gradually initiating ROM and muscle firing. Within weeks 2–6, an emphasis is placed on early quadriceps muscle activation with prone knee flexion from 0 to 90 degrees of flexion. Phase 2 (4 weeks to 3 months) focuses on return to full ROM, recovery of a normal gait pattern, full weightbearing, and initiating a return to activities of daily living. Around week 6, weightbearing exercises are started alongside low-resistance exercises on the stationary bike. Around week 12, low-impact exercises are begun. Phase 3 (3–6 months) focuses on strengthening and straight-line running. Dynamic bracing is maintained until the sixth month following surgery. Around 6 months, jogging is initiated, along with side-to-side work and proprioceptive exercises. Phase 4 (6–12 months) focuses on higher-level activities including initiation of jumping, agility, and lateral movements. Phase 5 (9–24 months) focuses on sport-specific objective goals and return to play [141, 147]. Isolated hamstring exercises are not allowed for the first 4–6 months, as the posterior shear forces at the tibiofemoral joint can cause increased stress on the PCL graft [141, 147, 148]. Common complications include popliteal artery or tibial nerve injury, osteonecrosis, fractures, persistent laxity, compartment syndrome, heterotopic ossification, and anterior knee pain [149].

Posterior Lateral Corner (PLC) Reconstruction

PLC reconstruction is the surgical repair of the knee ligament complex which encompasses three major static stabilizers including the lateral collateral ligament, the popliteus tendon, and the popliteofibular ligament. Injury to the PLC rarely occurs alone, often with concurrent damage to the ACL and/or PCL. Post-op, as a systematic review showed no significant difference in outcome scores when comparing delayed weightbearing (until post-op week 4) versus progressive weightbearing (partial to full weightbearing by post-op week 6) versus immediate weightbearing (full weightbearing immediately after surgery). Patients in the delayed and immediate weightbearing groups did experience a higher overall complication rate. Progressive weightbearing involves concentrating on the restoration of passive mobility of tibio- and patellofemoral joint motion, reducing post-op pain and swelling, and minimizing quadriceps atrophy. During weeks 0–6, goals are to unload passive ROM efforts immediately after surgery, with the goal of 90 degrees of knee flexion by post-op week 2. Once the milestone of 90 degrees of knee flexion is reached, it is recommended to increase ROM as tolerated and progress gradually to full knee ROM by 6 weeks. During this 6 week period, stretching the knee into hyperextension is avoided. During weeks 6–8, patient progressed to full weightbearing and progressed to closed-chain exercises. After week 8, focus is on single-leg closed-chain exercises to enhance the neuromuscular re-education of the operative limb. During weeks 16–24, sport-specific training is started, including advanced plyometric exercises and multiplane exercises. Estimated return-to-sport is minimum of 6 months, averaging 9–12 months. Common complication includes arthrofibrosis [150].

Multiple Ligament Knee Reconstruction

Multiple ligament knee reconstruction involves the surgical repair of two or more of the four primary knee stabilizers: ACL, PCL, MCL, and LCL. Post-op, a hinged knee brace with a varus mold and locked full extension bracing is recommended for the initial 8 weeks to allow the PCL to begin healing without being stretched [141]. Protected partial weightbearing with the assistance of crutches starts around 3 weeks [141, 151]. Early aim is to prevent stiffness and achieve a target of 90 degrees of knee flexion by 4 weeks following surgery. Maintaining quadriceps activity with protected isometric exercises including in-brace straight-leg raises is also important

[141]. Full active free ROM exercise can start at week 8, with the transition to a dynamic PCL brace with mild varus moment and allow weightbearing as tolerated. Progression to closed kinetic chain exercises as well as avoidance of open kinetic chain flexion is recommended for at least 6 months [151]. Return to full activity ranges between 9 and 12 months after surgery [141]. Common complications include arthrofibrosis [141, 151].

Articular Cartilage Procedures

Articular cartilage procedures involve the surgical restoration/repair of articular cartilage injuries, which can result from significant acute and chronic joint stress associated with impact sports. There are several techniques including restorative techniques (osteochondral autograft transfer system/osteochondral allograft transplantation) and reparative techniques (microfracture/autologous chondrocyte transplantation) [152, 153]. Progression of weightbearing is usually faster with restorative techniques as these techniques rely on bony healing as opposed to cartilage growth. For restorative techniques, recommendations include touch-down loading for 2 weeks, then progression to full weightbearing by 4–6 weeks. For reparative techniques, recommendations include touch-down loading for 2 weeks, then progress by 25% body weight per week. One rehab protocol designed to incorporate all cartilage repair techniques is based on three biological healing phases. This is a criteria-based approach rather than one with fixed timelines. Phase 1 involves protection and joint activation with goals of full passive ROM equal to the non-operated knee, recovery of muscular activation, and recovery of normal gait cycle. Phase 2 involves progressive loading and functional joint restoration with goals of full and painless ROM, maximum peak torque difference of less than 20% between limbs on isokinetic test, hop performance difference of less than 10% between limbs, progression from concentric to eccentric loading, static to dynamic loading, stable to unstable surfaces, uniplanar to multiplanar, and double- to single-limb tasks. Phase 3 involves activity restoration with goals of restoration of symmetry, strength, and flexibility in lower limbs, introducing a loading program with progression to full resistance, functional sport-specific agility training, and increasing intensity and duration of exercise [152]. Common complications include motion restrictions, scar tissue formation, pain, inflammation, and effusion [152, 153].

Foot/Ankle

Achilles Tendon Repair

Achilles tendon ruptures is the most common tendon rupture in the lower extremity, most commonly occurring in adults in their third to fifth decade of life [154]. There is currently no clear consensus in regard to conservative or operative management of acute ruptures. Complications seen after Achilles tendon repair include sural nerve injury, infection, re-rupture, DVT, and hypertrophic scars [155]. Regardless of conservative or operative treatment, functional rehabilitation combined with protected weightbearing and early controlled motion can effectively reduce re-rupture rates with satisfactory outcomes [156]. Support for immediate full weightbearing and early ankle mobilization post-op has been increasing as it has been found to demonstrate significantly increased calf muscle strength, reduced atrophy, and tendon elongation without associated increased re-rupture rate [157]. General rehabilitation goals include preventing re-rupture for the first 2 months after injury and improving calf muscle strength over the next month (between 2 months and 3 months after injury) with the following 3 months (between 3 and 6 months after injury) focused on return-to-sport through vigorous strengthening and proprioceptive exercises [155]. See Table 23.18.

Lisfranc Open Reduction Internal Fixation (ORIF)

Lisfranc injuries include a spectrum of midfoot and tarsometatarsal joint trauma that can range from purely ligamentous injuries-to-bone fracture dislocations depending on the severity of the trauma [160]. ORIF is a common method for treatment for displaced Lisfranc injuries [161]. Postoperative complications after ORIF include post-traumatic osteoarthritis, arthrodesis, hardware failure, infection, compartment syndrome, and DVT [162]. The post-op rehabilitation course is generally 6 months as outlined in Table 23.19.

Jones Fracture ORIF

Fifth metatarsal fractures (Jones Fractures) are classified into zone 1, zone 2, and zone 3 fractures. Zone 1 fractures are usually treated conservatively while zones 2 and 3 can be treated either conservatively or operatively with ORIF depending on the fracture location and patient. Post-op complications include re-fracture, hardware failure, sural nerve injury, malunion, nonunion, and iatrogenic fractures [164]. The post-op course is generally 10 weeks with new literature supporting less rigid immobilization and shorter periods of NWB as they have been associated with better early functional outcomes [165]. See Table 23.20.

Bimalleolar/Trimalleolar Fracture

Bimalleolar and trimalleolar ankle fractures are usually unstable and are treated operatively, most commonly via ORIF. For stable fractures that are treated conservatively, they can gradually WBAT with return to baseline activity as early as six to eight weights after the initial injury [167]. For those treated operatively, common complications include residual pain, infection, post-traumatic ankle osteoarthritis, hardware failure, malunion, arthrofibrosis, and CRPS [168]. The post-op rehabilitation course is generally at least 20 weeks long as outlined in Table 23.21.

Table 23.18 Post-operative rehabilitation course for Achilles tendon repair [158, 159]

Phase	Goals	Interventions
Phase I (Weeks 0–2)	Protect repair, manage swelling, and maintain strength of hip/knee/core	Quad sets, SLR, abdominal bracing, hip abduction, side-lying hip external rotation/clamshell, prone hip extension, prone hamstring curls *Weightbearing status: NWB on crutches in splint and/or walking boot for a minimum of 3 weeks*
Phase II (Weeks 2–6)	Avoid overelongation of Achilles, reduce pain, minimize swelling, restore ankle plantar flexion/inversion/eversion, dorsiflexion to neutral, and normalize gait as much as possible while in the boot by utilizing a shoe leveler for the uninvolved side	Passive plantarflexion, AROM and PROM dorsiflexion to neutral, AROM inversion and eversion with ankle in plantarflexed position to 30 degrees, knee and hip exercises without ankle involvement, start light seated soleus stretching and NWB gastrocnemius stretching, NuStep while following weightbearing restrictions *Weightbearing status:* *Weeks 3–4: begin partial progressive weightbearing (25%) on crutches in boot with three heel wedges (1" in height each)* *Weeks 4–5: 50% PWB (remove 1 wedge)* *Weeks 5–6: 75% PWB (remove 1 wedge)*
Phase III (Weeks 7–9)	Avoid overelongation of Achilles (no overt stretching of Achilles), normalize gait in Achilles boot without wedges, restore full ROM (including DF), safely progress strengthening, promote proper movement patterns, avoid post-exercise pain/swelling, FWB in boot without wedges and crutches with good tolerance and normalized gait pattern by week 8	Full PROM in all planes, full AROM except into dorsiflexion, seated heel slides for DF ROM (gentle progression), toe stretching as needed, stationary bike with boot and heel pedaling, isometric ankle exercises for DF/inversion/eversion, progress active PF to seated heel raises *Weightbearing status:* *Week 6–7: 100% WBAT with walking boot and removal of last heel wedge* *Weeks 8–10: FWB with walking boot with progression to normal shoe as tolerated*

(continued)

Table 23.18 (continued)

Phase	Goals	Interventions
Phase IV (Weeks 10–14 weeks)	Maintain full ROM, normalize gait in supportive sneakers without heel-lift, avoid overelongation of Achilles, safely progress strengthening, promote proper movement patterns, avoid extreme DF combined with active PF	May begin weightbearing gastrocnemius and soleus stretching as needed, lower limb muscle strength work with specifics to plantar flexors with progression of seated heel raise to bilateral standing heel raise and single heel raise, ankle stability exercises, double limb standing balance utilizing uneven surface (wobble board)
Phase V (Weeks 14 +)	Safely progresses strengthening, promotor proper movement patterns, good tolerance with progression to plyometrics and agility training	Jogging on flat surfaces at 5 months post-op if strength is 70% of uninvolved leg, start eccentric lowering exercises, single-leg hopping and higher level plyometrics can be initiated at 24 weeks post-op if strength and stability goals are achieved, sports-specific rehab exercises

Table 23.19 Postoperative rehabilitation course for Lisfranc ORIF [163]

Phase	Goals	Precautions/Interventions
Phase I (Weeks 0–6)	Reduce inflammation and pain, protect surgical repair, and maintain strength and ROM of nonoperative joints	Open chain hip strengthening, gait training *Weightbearing status* *Weeks 0–2: post-operative splint, NWB at all times with crutches* *Weeks 2–6: transition to CAM boot, NWB with crutches, no ROM at operative ankle and foot*
Phase II (Weeks 6–12)	Reduce inflammation and pain, protect surgical repair, weightbearing progression, initiate ROM at foot/ankle, initiate strengthening at foot/ankle	Normalize gait pattern, stationary bike or NuStep, bilateral and unilateral closed kinetic chain strengthening program consistent with weightbearing status, isometric ankle/foot strengthening once FWB, intrinsic foot strengthening *Precautions: gradual progression of weightbearing while in CAM boot* *Weightbearing progression:* *Week 6: 25% weightbearing* *Week 7: 50% weightbearing* *Week 8: WBAT with progression to FWB*
Phase III (Weeks 12–18)	Weightbearing progression, normalize gait pattern, progression of single-limb strength, full ROM	Progression of closed-chain strengthening, initiate balance/proprioceptive drills, stationary bike, elliptical *Weightbearing progression:* *Weeks 12–13: transition out of CAM boot for household ambulation and PT only* *Week 14: transition out of CAM boot at all times*
Phase IV (Weeks 18+)	Full ROM, symmetrical strength, and power	Basic ladder series, linear jogging progression, gym strengthening progression, initiate plyometrics progressing from double to single limb Functional test performed at 18 weeks, return-to-sport functional test between 24 and 26 weeks Potential hardware removal at 20 weeks if indicated per surgeon

Table 23.20 Post-operative rehabilitation course for Jones fracture ORIF [166]

Phase	Goals	Precautions/Interventions
Phase I (Weeks 0–2)	Reduce inflammation and pain, protect surgical repair, and maintain strength and ROM of nonoperative joints	Open chain hip strengthening, gait training *Weightbearing status:* *Weeks 0–2: post-operative posterior splint, NWB at all times with crutches*
Phase II (Weeks 2–6)	Reduce inflammation and pain, protect surgical repair, progress ROM at ankle and foot, progress strength in limb	Gait training, initiate closed-chain exercises in double limb progressing to single limb in CAM boot, at 4 weeks can progress to Alter-G treadmill with full-length carbon fiber insert in shoe or pool running *Precautions: transition to CAM boot* *Weightbearing status: progress from NWB to WBAT*

(continued)

Table 23.20 (continued)

Phase	Goals	Precautions/Interventions
Phase III (Weeks 6–8)	Protect surgical repair, normalize gait pattern, initiate strength and proprioceptive/balance drills, and progress to full ROM	Normalization of gait pattern, introduce bike and elliptical, proprioceptive and balance drills, unilateral closed kinetic chain strengthening program *Weightbearing status: progress to FWB* *Week 6: transition to running shoe with full-length carbon fiber insert*
Phase IV (Weeks 8–10)	Full ROM, symmetrical strength and power, initiation of plyometrics with progression from double to single limb	Basic ladder series, linear jogging progression, basic plyometric box progression, gym strengthening progression Preliminary functional test at 8 weeks, return-to-sport functional test at 10 weeks Potential hardware removal at 20 weeks if indicated per surgeon

Posterior Tibialis Tendon Repair

Posterior tibialis tendon dysfunction is the most common cause of adult acquired flatfoot deformity [171]. Surgical management is usually indicated in more severe cases, for those that have failed conservative methods, and for cases that are associated with inflammatory arthropathies [172]. Complications seen post-operatively include thromboembolic events, infection, wound dehiscence, neurologic injury, hardware failure, and/or painful hardware [171]. The post-op rehabilitation course usually begins with the patient NWB in a cast or splint for 6–8 weeks with varying specific progressive courses as outlined in Table 23.22.

Tarsal Tunnel Release

Tarsal tunnel syndrome is an entrapment neuropathy that is associated with compression of the structures within the tarsal tunnel. It can be treated conservatively or operatively with surgical management indicated when conservative management fails or if a definitive cause of entrapment is identified [174]. Post-op complications include impaired surgical wound healing, infection, and scar formation [175]. The post-op rehabilitation course begins with the patient being NWB in a short leg splint for the first two weeks with return to full activity ranging from 6 to 18 months [176]. See Table 23.23.

Bunionectomy

Hallux valgus (also known as bunions) can be surgically corrected if conservative measures fail to relieve pain or if there is severe misalignment, associated osteoarthritis, or if it is affecting daily activities/sports [178]. Post-op complications include recurrent hallux valgus, hallux varus, infection, malunion, nonunion, and avascular

Table 23.21 Post operative rehabilitation course for ankle fracture ORIF [169, 170]

Phase	Goals	Precautions/Interventions
Phase I (Weeks 0–6)	Manage swelling, minimize the loss of strength in core/hips/knees/upper extremities, performing ADLs in a modified independent or minimum assist manner, and safe ambulation with weightbearing precautions	Gait training on level surfaces and stairs within weightbearing precautions, initiate ankle PROM/AAROM/AROM (ankle pumps, inversion, eversion, circles, seated heel slides for ankle DF ROM), joint position retraining, proximal/core strengthening (quad sets, SLR, abdominal bracing, hip abduction, prone hip extensions, prone hamstring curls), upper body strengthening with weights with modifications for precautions *Precautions: No joint mobilization near fracture site or mobilization that requires stabilization over fracture site* *Weightbearing status:* *Weeks 0–3: NWB, boot/cast per surgeon* *Weeks 3–6: WBAT progression and boot/case per surgeon*
Phase II (Weeks 7–12)	Full ROM of foot/ankle, safely progress strengthening, normalized gait pattern on all surfaces (wean from boot/brace), gradually return to regular activities as able	Continue ankle AROM/PROM exercises and toe stretching as needed, progress to standing ankle dorsiflexion stretch on step, gentle stretching of proximal muscle groups as indicated (standing quad stretch, standing hamstrings stretch, Thomas hip flexor stretch, piriformis stretch), standing gastrocnemius and standing soleus stretching (once weakened from boot), gentle ankle mobilizations once fracture is radiographically healed or cleared by surgeon, stationary bike, treadmill walking (once boot is off and gait is normalized), isometrics for ankle planes that are not near full AROM, ankle exercise with resistance bands once near full ankle ROM, once boot is weaned can begin standing calf raise progression, double limb standing balance utilizing uneven surface (wobble board), single-limb balance *Precautions: No joint mobilizations near fracture site or mobilization that requires stabilization over fracture site* *Weightbearing status: progress to FWB and wean boot per surgeon*

(continued)

Table 23.21 (continued)

Phase	Goals	Precautions/Interventions
Phase III (Weeks 13–16)	Good balance and control of the involved leg in all planes, promote proper movement patterns, and avoid post-exercise pain/swelling	Stationary bike, treadmill walking, seated calf machine, wall sit with bilateral calf raises, unilateral heel raises, hip hikes, forward lunges, bilateral squats progressing to single-leg squats, single-limb balance *Precautions/weightbearing status: no precautions if healing is complete*
Phase IV (Weeks 17–20)	Progress to plyometrics and sports-specific movement patterns, progress to low-impact fitness activities, and gradual return to minimal or low-impact sports	Elliptical, stair climber, treadmill walking, initiate beginner-level plyometric progression (bilateral standing heel raises with equal weightbearing, rebounding heel raises bilateral stance, rebounding unilateral heel raises, hopping in place bilateral stance, unilateral hopping in place)
Phase V (Weeks 21 +)	Gradual return to higher impact activities (jogging, running, jumping), gradual return to activities with multiplanar movements on uneven surfaces, safe initiation of sport-specific training programs, symmetrical performance with sport-specific drills, good lower extremity mechanics with plyometrics/agility/running gait	Continue interventions as above, sport-specific training and conditioning with progression to high-impact movements/activities as tolerated

Table 23.22 Postoperative rehabilitation course for posterior tibialis tendon repair [173]

Phase	Goals	Precautions/Interventions
Phase I (Weeks 0–6)	Protect repair, control pain and swelling	Seated open chain intrinsic foot exercises, toe ROM, ankle ROM (avoiding active eversion), ankle isometrics *Precautions: no eversion AROM for 6 weeks* *Weightbearing status: NWB for 6 weeks in cast*
Phase II (Weeks 6–8)	Full ankle ROM in all planes, progression of weightbearing status from cast to CAM boot	Standing gastrocnemius/soleus stretch, standing calf raises, three-way ankle resistance avoiding resistance to eversion for 8 weeks, foot intrinsic strength in weightbearing, bilateral balance and proprioception activities, stationary bike, aquatic walking *Precautions: no resistance to eversion for 8 weeks* *Weightbearing status: progress to WBAT in CAM boot*
Phase III (Weeks 8–12)	Normalize gait pattern, return to functional movement patterns, single-leg strength, and mechanics	Initiate eversion strength with resistance bands, start single-leg balance and proprioception, bilateral eccentric strength of lower extremities, squats, lunges, step up/downs, biking, swimming, walking, and hiking *Precautions/weigh bearing status: discontinue CAM boot when normal gait pattern present, no running for 4–6 months*
Phase IV (Weeks 12–18)	Normal involved lower extremity eccentric control for functional activities, agility, and control with lateral motions and when initiating cutting motions	Single calf raises, single eccentric lower extremity strength and mechanics, agility training, slow return to running (between 4 and 6 months), must pass return to sports test prior to beginning sports-specific exercises.

Table 23.23 Post-operative rehabilitation course for tarsal tunnel release [177]

Weeks	Goals	Precautions/Interventions
Weeks 0–4	Decrease pain and inflammation	Walking boot/cast should remain in place for at least 3 weeks *Precautions: no eversion AROM for 6 weeks* *Weightbearing status: NWB for 2 weeks in walking boot or short leg cast per surgeon*
Weeks 4–8	Decrease inflammation and pain, increase ROM, normalize gait, and improve biomechanics	Increase strength/flexibility/balance throughout lower extremity, resisted dorsiflexion/plantarflexion/eversion with resistance band, initiation of resisted inversion as tolerates, weightbearing gastrocnemius/soleus strengthening (avoid excessive pronation), static balance training, closed-chain strengthening (e.g., squats and weight shift lunges), bicycle for ROM and light endurance training *Precautions: no resistance to eversion for 8 weeks* *Weightbearing status: progress to WBAT in CAM boot*
Weeks 8–10	Independent with ADLs	Dynamic balance training, dynamic lunges, endurance training on bicycle as tolerated
Weeks 8+	Return to unrestricted work and sports-related activities as determined by surgeon	Begin sport-specific training

necrosis [179]. The post-op rehabilitation course generally ranges from 5 to 6 months as outlined in Table 23.24. The implementation of physiotherapy throughout the rehabilitation course has been shown to have beneficial effects with reductions in pain and correction of deformity [180].

Plantar Fasciotomy

Plantar fasciitis is usually treated conservatively with activity modification, nonsteroidal anti-inflammatory drugs, stretching, strengthening exercises, heel padding, shock wave therapy, corticosteroid injections, and/or platelet rich plasma (PRP) injections [182, 183]. Plantar fasciotomy is normally only considered when conservative therapies have been ineffective and significant symptoms persist for over 6–12 months [184]. Post-op complications include persistent pain, paresthesias or numbness, soft-tissue healing problems, and superficial infection [185]. The post-op rehabilitation course normally allows patients to be immediately PWB with CAM boot as outlined in Table 23.25.

Table 23.24 Postoperative rehabilitation course for bunionectomy [181]

Weeks	Goals	Precautions/Interventions
Weeks 0–2	Manage swelling and pain, and adherence to weightbearing restrictions	AROM of hip and knee, edema management, rest, and elevation of involved lower extremity *Weightbearing status: NWB with post-operative splint*
Weeks 2–6	Manage swelling, protect surgical site, increase ROM at 1st MTP and ankle, minimize loss of strength of core/hips/knees	Ankle and 1st MTP joint AROM and PROM while avoiding pressure on surgical sites, strengthening for core/hips/knees, and gait training *Precautions: No joint mobilization of fused joints, depending on surgery can gradually progress to PWB or touch-down weightbearing*
Weeks 6–10	Full ROM of foot/ankle, increase strength of foot and ankle and maintain hip/knee ROM and strength, normalize gait pattern on all surfaces in boot	Ankle and MTP AROM/PROM stretching, foot and ankle strengthening exercises, joint mobilization techniques to restore motion of foot and ankle with proper stabilization, begin stationary bike while avoiding pressure on the forefoot, gait training to wean off assistive devices and normalize gait in boot *Weightbearing status: Depending on surgeon and surgeon can begin progressing to FWB with boot*
Weeks 10–14	FWB in shoe, restore normal gait pattern, normalize motor control of lower extremity	Start weakening out of boot to support shoe, continue with strength/ROM/conditioning as above, begin closed-chain proprioceptive/balance/motor control exercises, stationary bike, aquatics if surgical site healed
Weeks 14–20	Good balance and control on involved leg in all planes, return to all activities (not sports) if strength/gait/ROM goals met	Activity progression as tolerated, continue exercises as above, single-leg activities on varying surfaces, advance functional training to include sports-specific movement patterns
Weeks 20+	Gradual return to minimal or low-impact sports, once low-impact sports are tolerated can start gradual return to high-impact sports	Continue treatments as above, sports-specific training and conditioning beginning with low impact (cycling, rowing, swimming, stairmaster, elliptical) and progressing to high impact (running, jumping)

Table 23.25 Postoperative rehabilitation course for plantar fasciotomy [177]

Weeks	Goals	Precautions/interventions
Weeks 0–2	Protect surgical foot, reduce swelling, manage pain, and slowly initiate ankle ROM	Ice and elevation as tolerated, ankle AROM/AAROM exercises without resistance, isometric ankle strengthening in PF/DF/inversion/eversion/hallux PF, foot intrinsic exercises (toe crunching, toe extensions, toe spreading, arch doming), calf stretching with knee flexion and hallux dorsiflexion (soleus stretch, FHL stretch) *Weightbearing status: PWB in CAM boot with progression toward walking in boot toward the end of week 1*
Week 2	Discontinuation of walking boot, ankle strengthening, full ankle ROM	Manual plantar fascia stretching, initiation of manual (joint and soft tissue) interventions, isotonic ankle strengthening, initiation of heel-raise progression, stationary bike without boot, gentle swimming, and pool exercise when wound is healed *Precautions: Discontinuation of boot with progression to normal shoes and gait normalization*
Weeks 3–5	Advancing lower extremity strengthening, balance/proprioception	Progress strengthening exercises with the addition of resistance, begin eccentric heel-raise progression to neural (progress beyond neutral and with weight as tolerated), begin balance exercises (single-leg stance on stable surfaces with progression to unstable surfaces), elliptical, increase walking pace, PWB plyometric training as tolerated *Weightbearing status: FWB*
Weeks 6–8	Return to impact activities as tolerated	Increase intensity of biking/swimming/elliptical/resistance exercises as pain/symptoms allow, begin return to impact activities (plyometric training in FWB, proximal lower extremity and trunk strength exercises as tolerated), and continue concentric/eccentric loading and heel-raise progression
Weeks 8+	Return-to-sport and high-impact activities	Return to jogging/running progression, progress to directional changes and variable surfaces, sport-specific training, and continue single-leg balance training

Peroneal Tendon Repair

Peroneal tendon disorders typically refer to peroneal tendonitis, peroneal subluxation, and peroneal tendon tears. Peroneal tendon tears are more often seen in active young patients. Peroneal tendon repairs are indicated in severe cases of peroneal subluxations and in cases where there is more than 50% tearing of the peroneal tendon [186]. Complications seen with peroneal tendon repairs include skin paresthesia due to damage of the small branches of the sural nerve, skin healing complications, recurrent tendon tears, degeneration of the remaining tendon, and revision surgery [187]. The post-op rehabilitation course is generally at least 6 months with patients initially being NWB as outlined in Table 23.26.

Table 23.26 Postoperative rehabilitation course for peroneal tendon repair [188]

Weeks	Goals	Precautions/Interventions
Phase I (Weeks 0–2)	Protect surgical repair, maintain strength of hip/knee/core, manage swelling and pain, and gait training with emphasis on adhering to precautions	Passive hamstring stretching, quad sets, straight-leg raise, hip abduction, side-lying hip external rotation (clamshell), prone hip extension, prone hamstring curls *Weightbearing status: NWB on crutches in splint/cast*
Phase II (Weeks 2–4)	Reduce pain, minimize swelling, improve scar mobility once incision is healed, initiate ankle range of motion, progression to PWB	Joint position retraining, seated heel raises, seated toe raises, initiation of great toe DF, and PF stretching *Precautions: if superior peroneal retinaculum (SPR) is not repaired ankle PROM, AAROM, AROM can be started. If SPR is repaired, no inversion/eversion until 6 weeks post-op* *Weightbearing status: partial progressive weightbearing on crutches in boot/cast with crutches once cleared by surgeon*
Phase III (Weeks 4–8)	Restore full ROM of ankle, safely progress strengthening, promote proper movement patterns, and avoid post-exercise pain/swelling	Foot and ankle joint mobilizations, once boot is weaned begin standing gastrocnemius stretch and standing soleus stretch, stationary bicycle, Alter-G walking, inversion with resistance, DF/PF with resistance once AROM full in these planes, lumbopelvic strengthening, if SPR is not repaired continue with foot/ankle mobility exercises from previous phase and begin isometric eversion at post-op week 4, if SPR is repaired may begin inversion/eversion after postoperative week 6 *Weightbearing status: FWB in boot without crutches*
Phase IV (Weeks 9–12)	Normalize gait in supportive shoe, promote proper movement patterns, increase ankle strength and continue to progress ankle ROM if still limited, improve balance and proprioception	Ankle/foot mobilization (talocrural, subtalar, midfoot, MTPs) as indicated, stationary bike, swimming/pool jogging, Alter-G/treadmill walking, bilateral standing heel raises, bilateral squats progressing to single-leg squats, double limb standing balance utilizing uneven surface, single-limb balance with progression to uneven surface
Phase V (Weeks 12–24)	Full strength and ROM of ankle, good tolerance with progression to plyometrics and agility training	Elliptical, stair climber, Alter-G jogging progression, single-leg heel-raise progressing to eccentric heel raises off edge of step, hip hike, forward/lateral lunges, single-leg progression, rebounding heel raises bilateral stance, rebounding unilateral heel raises, hopping in place bilateral stance with progression to unilateral hopping in place, running progression program
Phase VI (Weeks 24+)	Continuation of strengthening and proprioceptive exercises, safe initiation of sport-specific training program, symmetrical performance with sport-specific drills, safe progression to full sport participation	Sport-specific training and conditioning

Summary

- Postoperative rehabilitation can play a key role in the success (or failure) of a surgery.
- Surgeries can vary significantly, and thus so do the post-op rehabilitation protocols.
- The overall goals of post-op rehabilitation include protecting the surgical repair, regaining range of motion, strengthening, and finally return-to-activity/sport in a safe manner.
- Following the appropriate timelines, precautions, and progressions allow for more favorable post-op outcomes.

Evidence-Based Evaluation and Treatment

Each musculoskeletal surgical case is unique, and thus post-operative rehabilitation protocols can also vary. Established guidelines allow for protocol customization according to patient, injury, and surgical characteristics. Underlying all the phases of rehabilitation should be early and consistent patient education. This chapter discusses some established and example post-op rehabilitation protocols as well as common complications to be avoided. Additionally, some new technologies emerging within post-op rehabilitation are also discussed.

References

1. Canbulat N, et al. A rehabilitation protocol for patients with lumbar degenerative disc disease treated with posterior transpedicular dynamic stabilization. Turk Neurosurg. 2017;27:426–35. https://doi.org/10.5137/1019-5149.JTN.16326-15.1.
2. Hoffman H, Bennett SS, Li CH, Haakana P, Lu DC. Minimally invasive decompression and physiotherapy for lumbar spinal stenosis in geriatric patients. Cureus. 2018;10:e2785. https://doi.org/10.7759/cureus.2785.
3. Lyu Z, Bai J, Chen S, Liu J, Yu W. Efficacy of lumbar kinetic chain training for staged rehabilitation after percutaneous endoscopic lumbar discectomy. BMC Musculoskelet Disord. 2021;22:793. https://doi.org/10.1186/s12891-021-04674-y.
4. Dupeyron A, et al. Rehabilitation and lumbar surgery: the French recommendations for clinical practice. Ann Phys Rehabil Med. 2021;64:101548. https://doi.org/10.1016/j.rehab.2021.101548.
5. Bredow J, Eysel P, Oikonomidis S. Postoperative management of weight bearing and rehabilitation after lumbar spinal surgery. Orthopade. 2020;49:201–10. https://doi.org/10.1007/s00132-019-03799-2.
6. Ilves O, et al. Effectiveness of a 12-month home-based exercise program on trunk muscle strength and spine function after lumbar spine fusion surgery: a randomized controlled trial. Disabil Rehabil. 2022;44:549–57. https://doi.org/10.1080/09638288.2020.1772383.
7. Buchanan P, et al. Best practices for postoperative management of posterior sacroiliac joint fusion. J Pain Res. 2022;15:1149–62. https://doi.org/10.2147/JPR.S357123.
8. Swanson B, Robin R. Physical therapy following anterior cervical discectomy and fusion: a study of current clinical practice and therapist beliefs. Int J Physiother. 2015;2:399. https://doi.org/10.15621/ijphy/2015/v2i2/65249.

9. Watkins RGT, Chang D, Watkins RG. Return to Play After Anterior Cervical Discectomy and Fusion in Professional Athletes. Orthop J Sports Med. 2018;6:2325967118779672. https://doi.org/10.1177/2325967118779672.
10. Yadav R, Chavali S, Chaturvedi A, Rath G. Post-operative complications in patients undergoing anterior cervical discectomy and fusion: a retrospective review. J Neuroanaesthesiol Crit Care. 2017;4:170–4. https://doi.org/10.4103/jnacc-jnacc-18.17.
11. Ratte-Larouche M, Szekeres M, Sadi J, Faber KJ. Rotator cuff tendon surgery and postoperative therapy. J Hand Ther. 2017;30:147–57. https://doi.org/10.1016/j.jht.2017.05.008.
12. Coda RG, et al. A review of online rehabilitation protocols designated for rotator cuff repairs. Arthroscop Sports Med Rehabil. 2020;2:e277–88. https://doi.org/10.1016/j.asmr.2020.03.006.
13. Bakti N, Antonios T, Phadke A, Singh B. Early versus delayed mobilization following rotator cuff repair. J Clin Orthop Trauma. 2019;10:257–60. https://doi.org/10.1016/j.jcot.2019.01.016.
14. Longo U, Risi Ambrogioni L, Berton A, et al. Conservative versus accelerated rehabilitation after rotator cuff repair: a systematic review and meta-analysis. BMC Musculoskelet Disord. 2021;22 https://doi.org/10.1186/s12891-021-04397-0.
15. Sheps DM, et al. Early active motion versus sling immobilization after arthroscopic rotator cuff repair: a randomized controlled trial. Arthroscop J Arthroscop Relat Surg. 2019;35:749–760.e742. https://doi.org/10.1016/j.arthro.2018.10.139.
16. Tirefort J, et al. Postoperative mobilization after superior rotator cuff repair: sling versus no sling: a randomized prospective study. J Bone Joint Surg Am. 2019;101:494–503. https://doi.org/10.2106/JBJS.18.00773.
17. Matlak S, Andrews A, Looney A, Tepper KB. Postoperative rehabilitation of rotator cuff repair: a systematic review. Sports Med Arthrosc Rev. 2021;29:119–29. https://doi.org/10.1097/JSA.0000000000000310.
18. Boland K, Smith C, Bond H, Briggs S, Walton J. Current concepts in the rehabilitation of rotator cuff related disorders. J Clin Orthop Trauma. 2021;18:13–9. https://doi.org/10.1016/j.jcot.2021.04.007.
19. Jung C, et al. Rehabilitation following rotator cuff repair: a work of the Commission Rehabilitation of the German Society of Shoulder and Elbow Surgery e.V. (DVSE) in collaboration with the German Association for Physiotherapy (ZVK) e.V., the Association Physical Therapy, Association for Physical Professions (VPT) e.V. and the Section Rehabilitation-Physical Therapy of the German Society for Orthopaedics and Trauma e.V. (DGOU). Obere Extremitat. 2018;13:45–61. https://doi.org/10.1007/s11678-018-0448-2.
20. Sgroi TA, Cilenti M. Rotator cuff repair: post-operative rehabilitation concepts. Curr Rev Musculoskelet Med. 2018;11:86–91. https://doi.org/10.1007/s12178-018-9462-7.
21. Choi S, Seo KB, Shim S, Shin JY, Kang H. Early and delayed postoperative rehabilitation after arthroscopic rotator cuff repair: a comparative study of clinical outcomes. Clin Shoulder Elbow. 2019;22:190–4. https://doi.org/10.5397/cise.2019.22.4.190.
22. Patch DA, et al. Understanding postoperative rehabilitation preferences in operatively managed proximal humerus fractures: do trauma and shoulder surgeons differ? J Shoulder Elb Surg. 2022;31:1106–14. https://doi.org/10.1016/j.jse.2021.12.045.
23. Caforio M, Maniscalco P. The importance of early rehabilitation in proximal humeral fracture: a clinical trial of efficacy and safety of a new endomedullary nail. J Back Musculoskelet Rehabil. 2017;30:195–202. https://doi.org/10.3233/BMR-160732.
24. Rehabilitation protocol for proximal humeral fracture open reduction. https://www.massgeneral.org/assets/mgh/pdf/orthopaedics/sports-medicine/physical-therapy/rehabilitation-protocol-for-proximal-humeral-fracture-with-orif.pdf.
25. Kim YS, Lee KG, Lee HJ. Effect of triamcinolone acetonide on stiffness after surgical treatment of proximal humerus fractures: a randomized controlled study. Arch Orthop Trauma Surg. 2020;140:1731–7. https://doi.org/10.1007/s00402-020-03425-3.
26. Bucci G, et al. Axillary artery injury and brachial plexus palsy as a complication of proximal humerus fractures. J Orthop. 2017;14:340–1. https://doi.org/10.1016/j.jor.2017.06.001.

27. Altintas B, Anderson NL, Boykin R, Millett PJ. Operative treatment of torsional humeral shaft fractures in throwers leads to an earlier return to sport: a survey of expert shoulder and elbow surgeons. Knee Surg Sports Traumatol Arthrosc. 2019;27:4049–54. https://doi.org/10.1007/s00167-019-05733-7.
28. Dahm F, et al. High-energy extracorporeal shockwave therapy in humeral delayed and non-unions. Eur J Trauma Emerg Surg. 2022;48:3043–9. https://doi.org/10.1007/s00068-021-01782-1.
29. Koczan B, Stryder B, Mitchell C. Postoperative rehabilitation of posterior Glenohumeral joint instability surgery: a systematic review. Sports Med Arthrosc Rev. 2021;29:110–8. https://doi.org/10.1097/JSA.0000000000000317.
30. Ma R, Brimmo OA, Li X, Colbert L. Current concepts in rehabilitation for traumatic anterior shoulder instability. Curr Rev Musculoskelet Med. 2017;10:499–506. https://doi.org/10.1007/s12178-017-9449-9.
31. Lloyd G, et al. Postoperative rehabilitation of anterior Glenohumeral joint instability surgery: a systematic review. Sports Med Arthrosc Rev. 2021;29:54–62. https://doi.org/10.1097/JSA.0000000000000305.
32. Goldenberg BT, et al. Rehabilitation following posterior shoulder stabilization. Int J Sports Phys Ther. 2021;16:930–40. https://doi.org/10.26603/001c.22501.
33. Popchak AJ, Christain H, Poploski K. Postoperative rehabilitation and return to play criteria after anterior shoulder stabilization procedures. Oper Tech Orthop. 2021;31:100863. https://doi.org/10.1016/j.oto.2021.100863.
34. Kelley TD, Clegg S, Rodenhouse P, Hinz J, Busconi BD. Functional rehabilitation and return to play after arthroscopic surgical stabilization for anterior shoulder instability. Sports Health. 2021;19417381211062852 https://doi.org/10.1177/19417381211062852.
35. Kennedy JS, et al. The American Society of Shoulder and Elbow Therapists' consensus statement on rehabilitation for anatomic total shoulder arthroplasty. J Shoulder Elb Surg. 2020;29:2149–62. https://doi.org/10.1016/j.jse.2020.05.019.
36. Kennedy JS, et al. Protocol for a multicenter, randomised controlled trial of surgeon-directed home therapy vs. outpatient rehabilitation by physical therapists for reverse total shoulder arthroplasty: the SHORT trial. Arch Physiother. 2021;11:28. https://doi.org/10.1186/s40945-021-00121-2.
37. Edwards PK, Ebert JR, Joss B, Ackland T, Wang A. A randomised trial comparing two rehabilitation approaches following reverse total shoulder arthroplasty. Shoulder Elbow. 2021;13:557–72. https://doi.org/10.1177/1758573220937394.
38. Hagen MS, et al. A randomized single-blinded trial of early rehabilitation versus immobilization after reverse total shoulder arthroplasty. J Shoulder Elb Surg. 2020;29:442–50. https://doi.org/10.1016/j.jse.2019.10.005.
39. Lee J, et al. Accelerated rehabilitation following reverse total shoulder arthroplasty. J Shoulder Elb Surg. 2021;30:e545–57. https://doi.org/10.1016/j.jse.2020.11.017.
40. Willmore E, McRobert C, Foy C, Stratton I, van der Windt D. What is the optimum rehabilitation for patients who have undergone release procedures for frozen shoulder? A UK survey. Musculoskelet Sci Pract. 2021;52:102319. https://doi.org/10.1016/j.msksp.2021.102319.
41. Kim DH, et al. Early clinical outcomes of manipulation under anesthesia for refractory adhesive capsulitis: comparison with arthroscopic capsular release. CiOS Clin Orthop Surg. 2020;12:217–23. https://doi.org/10.4055/cios19027.
42. Hanchard NCA, Goodchild L, Brealey SD, Lamb SE, Rangan A. Physiotherapy for primary frozen shoulder in secondary care: developing and implementing stand-alone and post operative protocols for UK FROST and inferences for wider practice. Physiotherapy. 2020;107:150–60. https://doi.org/10.1016/j.physio.2019.07.004.
43. Castelhano R, et al. Optimising the use of physiotherapy resources after manipulation under anaesthetic for frozen shoulder. Ann R Coll Surg Engl. 2022; https://doi.org/10.1308/rcsann.2022.0016.
44. Hermanns CA, et al. Variability in rehabilitation protocols after superior labrum anterior posterior surgical repair. Kansas J Med. 2021;14:243–8. https://doi.org/10.17161/kjm.vol14.15286.

45. Wilk KE, et al. Current concepts in the recognition and treatment of superior labral (SLAP) lesions. J Orthop Sports Phys Ther. 2005;35:273–91. https://doi.org/10.2519/jospt.2005.35.5.273.
46. Dodson CC, Altchek DW. SLAP lesions: an update on recognition and treatment. J Orthop Sports Phys Ther. 2009;39:71–80. https://doi.org/10.2519/jospt.2009.2850.
47. Zabrzynski J, et al. Biceps Tenodesis versus Tenotomy with fast rehabilitation protocol-a functional perspective in chronic tendinopathy. J Clin Med. 2020;9 https://doi.org/10.3390/jcm9123938.
48. Vajda M, et al. Tenodesis yields better functional results than tenotomy in long head of the biceps tendon operations-a systematic review and meta-analysis. Int Orthop. 2022;46:1037–51. https://doi.org/10.1007/s00264-022-05338-9.
49. Rehabilitation guidelines for biceps tenodesis. https://www.massgeneral.org/assets/mgh/pdf/orthopaedics/sports-medicine/physical-therapy/rehabilitation-protocol-for-biceps-tenodesis.pdf.
50. Biceps tenotomy protocol - Brigham and Women's Hospital., https://www.brighamandwomens.org/assets/bwh/patients-and-families/rehabilitation-services/pdfs/shoulder-biceps-tenotomy.pdf.
51. Domnisch C. https://medicine.osu.edu/-/media/files/medicine/departments/sports-medicine/medical-professionals/shoulder-and-elbow/bicep-tenodesis-2020.pdf?la=en&hash=CB21C9AA08DE6E12271187BDC5047BB1CA3F83F8#:~:text=Indications%20for%20tenodesis%20include%20partial%20tears%20%3E25%25%2C%20tendon,surgical%20team%20the%20most%20limiting%20protocol%20to%20utilize.
52. Pozzetti Daou J, Nagaya DY, Matsunaga FT, Sugawara Tamaoki MJ. Does biceps Tenotomy or Tenodesis have better results after surgery? A systematic review and meta-analysis. Clin Orthop Relat Res. 2021;479:1561–73. https://doi.org/10.1097/CORR.0000000000001672.
53. Plath J. Complications in biceps tendon management: long head of biceps tenotomy and tenodesis. Compl Arthrosc Shoulder Surg. 2019:103–111. https://doi.org/10.1007/978-3-030-24574-0_11.
54. Douoguih WA, et al. Postoperative rehabilitation of ulnar collateral ligament reconstruction: a systematic review. Sports Med Arthrosc Rev. 2021;29:e9–e17. https://doi.org/10.1097/JSA.0000000000000318.
55. Lightsey HM, et al. Rehabilitation variability after elbow ulnar collateral ligament reconstruction. Orthop J Sports Med. 2019;7 https://doi.org/10.1177/2325967119833363.
56. Somerson JS, Petersen JP, Neradilek MB, Cizik AM, Gee AO. Complications and outcomes after medial ulnar collateral ligament reconstruction: a meta-regression and systematic review. JBJS Rev. 2018;6:e4. https://doi.org/10.2106/JBJS.RVW.17.00138.
57. Rothermich MA, et al. Early complications of ulnar collateral ligament repair with collagen-coated suture tape augmentation. Orthop J Sports Med. 2021;9:23259671211038320. https://doi.org/10.1177/23259671211038320.
58. do Nascimento AT, Claudio GK. Arthroscopic surgical treatment of medial epicondylitis. J Shoulder Elb Surg. 2017;26:2232–5. https://doi.org/10.1016/j.jse.2017.08.019.
59. Verstuyft L, Caekebeke P, van Riet R. Postoperative rehabilitation in elbow surgery. J Clin Orthop Trauma. 2021;20:101479. https://doi.org/10.1016/j.jcot.2021.101479.
60. Alrabaa RG, Sonnenfeld J, Trofa D, Ahmad C. Elbow common flexor tendon repair technique. Arthrosc Tech. 2019;8:e1367–71. https://doi.org/10.1016/j.eats.2019.07.016.
61. Ramo L, et al. Effect of surgery vs functional bracing on functional outcome among patients with closed displaced humeral shaft fractures: the FISH randomized clinical trial. JAMA. 2020;323:1792–801. https://doi.org/10.1001/jama.2020.3182.
62. Midtgaard KS, Ruzbarsky JJ, Hackett TR, Viola RW. Elbow fractures. Clin Sports Med. 2020;39:623–36. https://doi.org/10.1016/j.csm.2020.03.002.
63. Akhtar A, Hughes B, Watts AC. The post-traumatic stiff elbow: a review. J Clin Orthop Trauma. 2021;19:125–31. https://doi.org/10.1016/j.jcot.2021.05.006.
64. Rezaie N, Gupta S, Service BC, Osbahr DC. Elbow dislocation. Clin Sports Med. 2020;39:637–55. https://doi.org/10.1016/j.csm.2020.02.009.

65. Sun Z, et al. What range of motion and functional results can be expected after open Arthrolysis with hinged external fixation for severe posttraumatic elbow stiffness? Clin Orthop Relat Res. 2019;477:2319–28. https://doi.org/10.1097/CORR.0000000000000726.
66. Sun Z, Liu W, Li J, Fan C. Open elbow arthrolysis for post-traumatic elbow stiffness: an update. Bone Joint Open. 2020;1:576–84. https://doi.org/10.1302/2633-1462.19.BJO-2020-0098.R1.
67. Marsh J, Graham J. Total elbow arthroplasty. Oper Tech Orthop. 2013;23:253–64. https://doi.org/10.1053/j.oto.2013.09.002.
68. Hackl M, Leschinger T, Uschok S. Rehabilitation of elbow fractures and dislocations. Obere Extremitat. 2017;12:201–7., https://doi-org.foyer.swmed.edu/10.1007/s11678-017-0425-1.
69. Calandruccio JH, Thompson NB. Carpal tunnel syndrome: making evidence-based treatment decisions. Orthop Clin North Am. 2018;49:223–9. https://doi.org/10.1016/j.ocl.2017.11.009.
70. Whitehead L. Rehabilitation following carpal tunnel release: a Cochrane review summary. Int J Nurs Stud. 2018;79:167–8. https://doi.org/10.1016/j.ijnurstu.2017.08.012.
71. Standard of Care: Carpal Tunnel Release - Brigham and Women's Hospital. Brigham and Women's Hospital, 2007. https://www.brighamandwomens.org/assets/BWH/patients-and-families/rehabilitation-services/pdfs/wrist-carpal-tunnel-release-pt.pdf?TRILIBIS_EMULATOR_UA=nsclpfpr%2cnsclpfpr.
72. Mack EM, Callinan NJ, Reams M, Bohn DC, Chmielewski TL. Patient-reported outcomes after open carpal tunnel release using a standard protocol with 1 hand therapy visit. J Hand Ther. 2017;30:58–64. https://doi.org/10.1016/j.jht.2016.03.007.
73. Mahmoodi R, et al. Effect of rehabilitation interventions on sensation, function, and pain of the patients with carpal tunnel release. Iran Rehabil J. 2019;17:263–70.
74. Zaralieva A, Georgiev GP, Karabinov V, Iliev A, Aleksiev A. Physical therapy and rehabilitation approaches in patients with carpal tunnel syndrome. Cureus. 2020;12:e7171. https://doi.org/10.7759/cureus.7171.
75. Hayes E, Carney K, Wolf J, Smith J, Akelman E. Rehabilitation of the hand and upper extremity. Mosby; 2002.
76. Blanquero J, et al. Exercises using a touchscreen tablet application improved functional ability more than an exercise program prescribed on paper in people after surgical carpal tunnel release: a randomised trial. J Physiother. 2019;65:81–7. https://doi.org/10.1016/j.jphys.2019.02.008.
77. Wouters RM, Tsehaie J, Hovius SER, Dilek B, Selles RW. Postoperative rehabilitation following thumb base surgery: a systematic review of the literature. Arch Phys Med Rehabil. 2018;99:1177–1212.e1172. https://doi.org/10.1016/j.apmr.2017.09.114.
78. Tsehaie J, et al. Shorter vs longer immobilization after surgery for thumb carpometacarpal osteoarthritis: a propensity score-matched study. Arch Phys Med Rehabil. 2019;100:2022–2031.e2021. https://doi.org/10.1016/j.apmr.2019.02.016.
79. Valdes K. Rehabilitation of the hand and upper extremity, vol. 2. Elsevier; 2021. p. 1261–77.
80. Klifto CS, Bookman J, Paksima N. Postsurgical rehabilitation of flexor tendon injuries. J Hand Surg Am. 2019;44:680–6. https://doi.org/10.1016/j.jhsa.2019.02.010.
81. Allen L, Bamberger B, Wang J, et al. Flexor tendon injuries. Orthobullets. https://www.orthobullets.com/hand/6031/flexor-tendon-injuries.
82. Xu H, et al. Outcome of surgical repair and rehabilitation of flexor tendon injuries in zone II of the hand: systematic review and meta-analysis. J Hand Surg Am. 2022; https://doi.org/10.1016/j.jhsa.2021.11.013.
83. Jokinen K, Hakkinen A, Luokkala T, Karjalainen T. Clinical outcomes after aggressive active early motion and modified Kleinert regimens: comparison of 2 consecutive cohorts. Hand (New York, NY). 2021:15589447211017222. https://doi.org/10.1177/15589447211017222.
84. Peters SE, Jha B, Ross M. Rehabilitation following surgery for flexor tendon injuries of the hand. Cochrane Database Syst Rev. 2021;1:CD012479. https://doi.org/10.1002/14651858.CD012479.pub2.

85. Cetin A, Dincer F, Kecik A, Cetin M. Rehabilitation of flexor tendon injuries by use of a combined regimen of modified Kleinert and modified Duran techniques. Am J Phys Med Rehabil. 2001;80:721–8. https://doi.org/10.1097/00002060-200110000-00003.
86. Cannon N. Rehabilitation of the hand and upper extremity, vol. 1. Elsevier; 2021. p. 421–31.
87. Hand rehabilitation protocols - UK healthcare, https://ukhealthcare.uky.edu/sites/default/files/m21-0609_ortho_protocols-final.pdf.
88. Woythal L, Holmer P, Brorson S. Splints, with or without wrist immobilization, following surgical repair of flexor tendon lesions of the hand: a systematic review. Hand Surg Rehabil. 2019;38:217–22. https://doi.org/10.1016/j.hansur.2019.05.004.
89. Lara TR, et al. Traditional versus digital media-based hand therapy after distal radius fracture. J Hand Surg. 2022;47(291):e291–291.e298. https://doi.org/10.1016/j.jhsa.2021.06.018.
90. Naughton N. Rehabilitation of the hand and upper extremity, vol. 1. Elsevier; 2021. p. 833–48.
91. Handoll HH, Madhok R, Howe TE. Rehabilitation for distal radial fractures in adults. Cochrane Database Syst Rev. 2002:CD003324. https://doi.org/10.1002/14651858.CD003324.
92. Roh YH, Noh JH, Gong HS, Baek GH. Effect of low appendicular lean mass, grip strength, and gait speed on the functional outcome after surgery for distal radius fractures. Arch Osteoporos. 2017;12:41. https://doi.org/10.1007/s11657-017-0335-2.
93. Quadlbauer S, et al. Early rehabilitation of distal radius fractures stabilized by Volar locking plate: a prospective randomized pilot study. J Wrist Surg. 2017;6:102–12. https://doi.org/10.1055/s-0036-1587317.
94. Kaji Y, et al. Postoperative early and proactive grip strength training program for distal radius fractures promotes earlier recovery of grip strength: a retrospective study. Medicine (United States). 2022;101:E29262. https://doi.org/10.1097/MD.0000000000029262.
95. Department of Rehabilitation Services Hand Therapy Guidelines, https://www.brighamandwomens.org/assets/BWH/patients-and-families/rehabilitation-services/pdfs/distal-radius-fracture-postop-hand-therapy-guideline.pdf.
96. Patel S, Schulte S, Yousif M, Mahmoud S. Phalanx fractures. Orthobullets. https://www.orthobullets.com/hand/6114/phalanx-fractures.
97. Cannon NM. Rehabilitation approaches for distal and middle phalanx fractures of the hand. J Hand Ther. 2003;16:105–16. https://doi.org/10.1016/s0894-1130(03)80006-6.
98. Hardy MA. Principles of metacarpal and phalangeal fracture management: a review of rehabilitation concepts. J Orthop Sports Phys Ther. 2004;34:781–99. https://doi.org/10.2519/jospt.2004.34.12.781.
99. Phalanx fractures of the hand - statpearls - NCBI bookshelf, https://www.ncbi.nlm.nih.gov/books/NBK557625/.
100. Evans R, Skirven T, DeTullio L. Rehabilitation of the hand and upper extremity, vol. 1. Elsevier; 2021. p. 238–49.
101. McCullough C, Sinnerton R. Surgical management of Dupuytren's disease. Curr Orthop. 1996;10:37–42. https://doi.org/10.1016/s0268-0890(96)90068-7.
102. Ramanathan D, Koludrovich J, Evans P. A new controlled motion program for rehabilitation of the proximal interphalangeal joint arthroplasty. J Hand Ther. 2021;34:151–5. https://doi.org/10.1016/j.jht.2019.04.003.
103. Total hip replacement, https://www.physio-pedia.com/Total_Hip_Replacement.
104. Barnsley L, Barnsley L, Page R. Are hip precautions necessary post total hip arthroplasty? A systematic review. Geriatr Orthop Surg Rehabil. 2015;6:230–5. https://doi.org/10.1177/2151458515584640.
105. Chiung-Jui S, Yuan K, Weng S, et al. Can early rehabilitation after total hip arthroplasty reduce its major complications and medical expenses? report from a nationally representative Cohort. Biomed Res Int. 2015; https://doi.org/10.1155/2015/641958.
106. Elmoghazy AD, Lindner N, Tingart M, Salem KH. Conventional versus fast track rehabilitation after total hip replacement: a randomized controlled trial. J Orthop Trauma Rehabil. 2022;29 https://doi.org/10.1177/22104917221076501.

107. Zhong M, et al. Impacts of the perioperative fast track surgery concept on the physical and psychological rehabilitation of total hip arthroplasty: a prospective cohort study of 348 patients. Medicine. 2021;100:e26869. https://doi.org/10.1097/MD.0000000000026869.
108. Kelly B, Williams R, Philippon M. Hip arthroscopy: current indications, treatment options, and management issues. Am J Sports Med. 2003;31:1020–37. https://doi.org/10.1177/03635465030310060701.
109. Larson C, Beaule PE, Kelly BT, Giveans M, Samuelson K. Complications after hip arthroscopy: a prospective, multicenter study using a validated grading classification. Arthroscopy. 2013;29:e204. https://doi.org/10.1016/j.arthro.2013.09.046.
110. Enseki KR, Kohlrieser D. Rehabilitation following hip arthroscopy: an evolving process. Int J Sports Phys Ther. 2014;9:765–73.
111. Heerey J, et al. Impairment-based rehabilitation following HIP arthroscopy: postoperative protocol for the HIP ARThroscopy international randomized controlled trial. J Orthop Sports Phys Ther. 2018;48:336–42. https://doi.org/10.2519/jospt.2018.8002.
112. Spencer-Gardner L, et al. A comprehensive five-phase rehabilitation programme after hip arthroscopy for femoroacetabular impingement. Knee Surg Sports Traumatol Arthrosc. 2014;22:848–59. https://doi.org/10.1007/s00167-013-2664-z.
113. McMinn DJ, Daniel J, Ziaee H, Pradhan C. Indications and results of hip resurfacing. Int Orthop. 2011;35:231–7. https://doi.org/10.1007/s00264-010-1148-8.
114. Marshall DA, et al. Hip resurfacing versus total hip arthroplasty: a systematic review comparing standardized outcomes. Clin Orthop Relat Res. 2014;472:2217–30. https://doi.org/10.1007/s11999-014-3556-3.
115. Kohan L, Field CJ, Kerr DR. Early complications of hip resurfacing. J Arthroplast. 2012;27:997–1002. https://doi.org/10.1016/j.arth.2012.01.030.
116. Frykberg B. JOI Birmingham hip resurfacing protocol, https://www.joionline.net/library/show/birmingham_hip_resurfacing_protocol/.
117. Chow RM, Kuzma SA, Krych AJ, Levy BA. Arthroscopic femoral neck osteoplasty in the treatment of femoroacetabular impingement. Arthrosc Tech. 2014;3:e21–5. https://doi.org/10.1016/j.eats.2013.08.007.
118. Nepple J, Parilla F, Ince D, Freiman S, Clohisy J. Does femoral osteoplasty improve long-term clinical outcomes and survivorship of hip arthroscopy? A 15-year minimum follow-up study. Am J Sports Med. 2022;50:3586–92. https://doi.org/10.1177/03635465221123048.
119. O'Rourke RJ, El Bitar Y. in StatPearls, 2022.
120. O'chiai D, Little M. Femoroacetabular impingement osteoplasty post-operative protocol, https://www.nirschl.com/pdf/femoroacetabular-impingement-osteoplasty-post-operative-protocol.pdf.
121. Arner JW, Freiman H, Mauro CS, Bradley JP. Functional results and outcomes after repair of partial proximal hamstring avulsions at midterm follow-up. Am J Sports Med. 2019;47:3436–43. https://doi.org/10.1177/0363546519879117.
122. Willinger L, et al. Excellent clinical outcome and low complication rate after proximal hamstring tendon repair at mid-term follow up. Knee Surg Sports Traumatol Arthrosc. 2020;28:1230–5. https://doi.org/10.1007/s00167-019-05748-0.
123. Proximal Hamstring re-attachment rehabilitation guideline, https://www.sanfordhealth.org/-/media/org/files/medical-professionals/resources-and-education/proximal-hamstring-reattachment-rehabilitation-guideline.pdf.
124. Rehabilitation for Proximal Hamstring Repair, https://www.massgeneral.org/assets/mgh/pdf/orthopaedics/sports-medicine/physical-therapy/rehabilitation-protocol-for-proximal-hamstring-tendon.pdf.
125. Millis MB, McClincy M. Periacetabular osteotomy to treat residual dysplasia in adolescents and young adults: indications, complications, results. J Child Orthop. 2018;12:349–57. https://doi.org/10.1302/1863-2548.12.180068.
126. Ali M, Malviya A. Complications and outcome after periacetabular osteotomy - influence of surgical approach. Hip Int. 2020;30:4–15. https://doi.org/10.1177/1120700019871195.

127. Rehabilitation Guidelines for Periacetabular Osteotomy (PAO) of the Hip, https://bynder.uwhealth.org/m/f0914c067052f435/original/Rehab-Guideline-Periacetabular-Osteotomy-PAO-of-the-Hip.pdf.
128. Wang HY, Yu GS, Li JH, Zhang SX, Lin YB. An updated meta-analysis evaluating limb management after total knee arthroplasty-what is the optimal method? J Orthop Surg Res. 2019;14:97. https://doi.org/10.1186/s13018-019-1140-y.
129. Davila Castrodad IM, et al. Rehabilitation protocols following total knee arthroplasty: a review of study designs and outcome measures. Ann Transl Med. 2019;7:S255. https://doi.org/10.21037/atm.2019.08.15.
130. Jette DU, et al. Physical therapist management of total knee arthroplasty. Phys Ther. 2020;100:1603–31. https://doi.org/10.1093/ptj/pzaa099.
131. Li X, Yu W, Li H, Wang B, Xu J. Prospective, single-center comparison of transcranial direct current stimulation plus electroacupuncture and standard analgesia in patients after total knee arthroplasty: effect on rehabilitation and functional recovery. Med Sci Monit. 2021;27:e930363. https://doi.org/10.12659/MSM.930363.
132. Zhang T, et al. Effect of early Electroacupuncture combined with enhanced recovery after surgery (ERAS) on pain perception and dysfunction in patients after total knee arthroplasty (TKA). Biomed Res Int. 2022;2022:6560816. https://doi.org/10.1155/2022/6560816.
133. Li L, Cheng S, Wang G, Duan G, Zhang Y. Tai Chi Chuan exercises improve functional outcomes and quality of life in patients with primary total knee arthroplasty due to knee osteoarthritis. Complement Ther Clin Pract. 2019;35:121–5. https://doi.org/10.1016/j.ctcp.2019.02.003.
134. Nelson C, Rajan L, Day J, Hinton R, Bodendorfer BM. Postoperative rehabilitation of anterior cruciate ligament reconstruction: a systematic review. Sports Med Arthrosc Rev. 2021;29:63–80. https://doi.org/10.1097/JSA.0000000000000314.
135. Marshall NE, Keller RA, Dines J, Bush-Joseph C, Limpisvasti O. Current practice: postoperative and return to play trends after ACL reconstruction by fellowship-trained sports surgeons. Musculoskelet Surg. 2019;103:55–61. https://doi.org/10.1007/s12306-018-0574-4.
136. Glattke KE, Tummala SV, Chhabra A. Anterior cruciate ligament reconstruction recovery and rehabilitation: a systematic review. J Bone Joint Surg Am. 2022;104:739–54. https://doi.org/10.2106/JBJS.21.00688.
137. Andrade R, Pereira R, van Cingel R, Staal J, Espregueira-Mendes J. How should clinicians rehabilitate patients after ACL reconstruction? A systematic review of clinical practice guidelines (CPGs) with a focus on quality appraisal (AGREE II). Br J Sports Med. 2020;54:512–9. https://doi.org/10.1136/bjsports-2018-100310.
138. Hanna T, Smith NP, Sebastianelli WJ. Treatment, return to play, and performance following meniscus surgery. Curr Rev Musculoskelet Med. 2022;15:157–69. https://doi.org/10.1007/s12178-022-09754-7.
139. Pan H, Zhang P, Zhang Z, Yang Q. Arthroscopic partial meniscectomy combined with medical exercise therapy versus isolated medical exercise therapy for degenerative meniscal tear: a meta-analysis of randomized controlled trials. Int J Surg. 2020;79:222–32. https://doi.org/10.1016/j.ijsu.2020.05.035.
140. Sekiya I, et al. Additional use of synovial mesenchymal stem cell transplantation following surgical repair of a complex degenerative tear of the medial meniscus of the knee: a case report. Cell Transplant. 2019;28:1445–54. https://doi.org/10.1177/0963689719863793.
141. Strauss MJ, et al. The use of allograft tissue in posterior cruciate, collateral and multi-ligament knee reconstruction. Knee Surg Sports Traumatol Arthrosc. 2019;27:1791–809. https://doi.org/10.1007/s00167-019-05426-1.
142. Vosoughi F, Rezaei Dogahe R, Nuri A, Ayati Firoozabadi M, Mortazavi J. Medial collateral ligament injury of the knee: a review on current concept and management. Arch Bone Jt Surg. 2021;9:255–62. https://doi.org/10.22038/abjs.2021.48458.2401.
143. Dale KM, Bailey JR, Moorman CT 3rd. Surgical management and treatment of the anterior cruciate ligament/medial collateral ligament injured knee. Clin Sports Med. 2017;36:87–103. https://doi.org/10.1016/j.csm.2016.08.005.

144. Krych AJ, et al. Functional testing and return to sport following stabilization surgery for recurrent lateral patellar instability in competitive athletes. Knee Surg Sports Traumatol Arthrosc. 2018;26:711–8. https://doi.org/10.1007/s00167-016-4409-2.
145. Puzzitiello RN, et al. Primary medial patellofemoral ligament repair versus reconstruction: rates and risk factors for instability recurrence in a young, active patient population. Arthroscopy. 2019;35:2909–15. https://doi.org/10.1016/j.arthro.2019.05.007.
146. Yanasse RH, et al. Surgical technique: anatomic medial patellofemoral ligament retensioning repair. Arthrosc Tech. 2018;7:e569–74. https://doi.org/10.1016/j.eats.2018.02.001.
147. Simhal RK, Bovich M, Bahrun EA, Dreese JC. Postoperative rehabilitation of posterior cruciate ligament surgery: a systematic review. Sports Med Arthrosc Rev. 2021;29:81–7. https://doi.org/10.1097/JSA.0000000000000307.
148. Freychet B, et al. All-inside posterior cruciate ligament reconstruction: surgical technique and outcome. Clin Sports Med. 2019;38:285–95. https://doi.org/10.1016/j.csm.2018.11.005.
149. Marom N, Ruzbarsky JJ, Boyle C, Marx RG. Complications in posterior cruciate ligament injuries and related surgery. Sports Med Arthrosc Rev. 2020;28:30–3. https://doi.org/10.1097/JSA.0000000000000247.
150. Morris BL, et al. Weightbearing protocols after posterolateral corner reconstruction: a systematic review. Orthop J Sports Med. 2021;9:2325967120988274. https://doi.org/10.1177/2325967120988274.
151. Duethman NC, Martin RK, Krych AJ, Stuart MJ, Levy BA. Surgical treatment of combined ACL PCL medial side injuries. Sports Med Arthrosc Rev. 2020;28:e18–24. https://doi.org/10.1097/JSA.0000000000000287.
152. Mithoefer K, et al. Current concepts for rehabilitation and return to sport after knee articular cartilage repair in the athlete. J Orthop Sports Phys Ther. 2012;42:254–73. https://doi.org/10.2519/jospt.2012.3665.
153. Wilk KE, Macrina LC, Reinold MM. Rehabilitation following microfracture of the knee. Cartilage. 2010;1:96–107. https://doi.org/10.1177/1947603510366029.
154. Shamrock AG, Varacallo M. in StatPearls, 2022.
155. Park SH, Lee HS, Young KW, Seo SG. Treatment of acute Achilles tendon rupture. Clin Orthop Surg. 2020;12:1–8. https://doi.org/10.4055/cios.2020.12.1.1.
156. Yang X, et al. Management of acute Achilles tendon ruptures: a review. Bone Joint Res. 2018;7:561–9. https://doi.org/10.1302/2046-3758.710.BJR-2018-0004.R2.
157. Brumann M, Baumbach SF, Mutschler W, Polzer H. Accelerated rehabilitation following Achilles tendon repair after acute rupture - development of an evidence-based treatment protocol. Injury. 2014;45:1782–90. https://doi.org/10.1016/j.injury.2014.06.022.
158. Rehabilitation Protocol for Achilles Rupture Repair, https://www.massgeneral.org/assets/mgh/pdf/orthopaedics/sports-medicine/physical-therapy/rehabilitation-protocol-for-achilles-tendon-repair.pdf.
159. Achilles Tendon Repair Rehabilitation Post-Operative Guideline, https://www.sanfordhealth.org/-/media/org/files/medical-professionals/resources-and-education/014000-01098-booklet-pt-guideline-post-operative-achilles-tendon-repair.pdf.
160. Mascio A, Greco T, Maccauro G, Perisano C. Lisfranc complex injuries management and treatment: current knowledge. Int J Physiol Pathophysiol Pharmacol. 2022;14:161–70.
161. Sun C, et al. Lisfranc injuries with dislocation the first tarsometatarsal joint: primary arthrodesis or internal fixation (a randomized controlled trial). Int Orthop. 2022;46:2529–37. https://doi.org/10.1007/s00264-022-05478-y.
162. Moracia-Ochagavia I, Rodriguez-Merchan EC. Lisfranc fracture-dislocations: current management. EFORT Open Rev. 2019;4:430–44. https://doi.org/10.1302/2058-5241.4.180076.
163. Lisfranc ORIF, https://www.kansashealthsystem.com/-/media/Files/PDF/Ortho-Sports-Med/lisfrancorif.pdf.
164. Chloros GD, et al. Fifth metatarsal fractures: an update on management, complications, and outcomes. EFORT Open Rev. 2022;7:13–25. https://doi.org/10.1530/EOR-21-0025.
165. Bowes J, Buckley R. Fifth metatarsal fractures and current treatment. World J Orthop. 2016;7:793–800. https://doi.org/10.5312/wjo.v7.i12.793.

166. Jones Fracture ORIF, https://www.kansashealthsystem.com/-/media/Project/Website/PDFs-for-Download/PT-protocols/jonesfractureorif.pdf.
167. Wire J, Hermena S, Slane VH. in StatPearls, 2022.
168. Macera A, Carulli C, Sirleo L, Innocenti M. Postoperative complications and reoperation rates following open reduction and internal fixation of ankle fracture. Joints. 2018;6:110–5. https://doi.org/10.1055/s-0038-1653949.
169. Rehabilitation Protocol for Ankle Fracture with ORIF, https://www.massgeneral.org/assets/mgh/pdf/orthopaedics/sports-medicine/physical-therapy/rehabilitation-protocol-for-ankle-fracture-with-orif.pdf.
170. Physical Therapy Guidelines for Ankle Fracture with Surgery, https://www.massgeneral.org/assets/mgh/pdf/orthopaedics/foot-ankle/pt-guidelines-ankle-fracture-with-orif-final.pdf.
171. Knapp PW, Constant D. in StatPearls, 2022.
172. Ling SK, Lui TH. Posterior Tibial tendon dysfunction: an overview. Open Orthop J. 2017;11:714–23. https://doi.org/10.2174/1874325001711010714.
173. Knecht S. Rehabilitation guidelines for posterior Tibial Tendon repair, https://www.mammothortho.com/pdf/ankle-posterior-tibial-tendon-repair.pdf.
174. Kiel J, Kaiser K. in StatPearls, 2022.
175. Rodriguez-Merchan EC, Moracia-Ochagavia I. Tarsal tunnel syndrome: current rationale, indications and results. EFORT Open Rev. 2021;6:1140–7. https://doi.org/10.1302/2058-5241.6.210031.
176. Tarsal Tunnel Release Protocol, https://www.sbortho.com/pdfs/therapy-protocols/dr-thomas-b/tb-pt-tarsal-tunnel-release-protocol.pdf.
177. Martin S. Tarsal Tunnel Release/Plantar Fascia release protocol, https://www.orthopedicarizona.com/wp-content/uploads/2013/01/Tarsal-Tunnel-Release-protocol.pdf.
178. InformedHealth.org. Cologne, Germany, 2018.
179. Belczyk R, Stapleton JJ, Grossman JP, Zgonis T. Complications and revisional hallux valgus surgery. Clin Podiatr Med Surg. 2009;26:475–84., Table of Contents. https://doi.org/10.1016/j.cpm.2009.04.002.
180. Mortka K, Lisinski P. Hallux valgus-a case for a physiotherapist or only for a surgeon? Literature review. J Phys Ther Sci. 2015;27:3303–7. https://doi.org/10.1589/jpts.27.3303.
181. Physical therapy guidelines for Hallux Valgus correction (Bunion reconstruction) https://www.massgeneral.org/assets/mgh/pdf/orthopaedics/foot-ankle/pt-guidelines-hallux-valgus-correction-final.pdf.
182. Trojian T, Tucker AK. Plantar Fasciitis. Am Fam Physician. 2019;99:744–50.
183. Hurley ET, et al. Platelet-rich plasma versus corticosteroids for plantar fasciitis: a systematic review of randomized controlled trials. Orthop J Sports Med. 2020;8:2325967120915704. https://doi.org/10.1177/2325967120915704.
184. Wheeler P, Boyd K, Shipton M. Surgery for patients with recalcitrant plantar fasciitis: good results at short-, medium-, and long-term follow-up. Orthop J Sports Med. 2014;2:2325967114527901. https://doi.org/10.1177/2325967114527901.
185. Malahias MA, Cantiller EB, Kadu VV, Muller S. The clinical outcome of endoscopic plantar fascia release: a current concept review. Foot Ankle Surg. 2020;26:19–24. https://doi.org/10.1016/j.fas.2018.12.006.
186. Walt J, Massey P. in StatPearls, 2022.
187. Danna NR, Brodsky JW. Diagnosis and operative treatment of peroneal tendon tears. Foot Ankle Orthop. 2020;5:2473011420910407. https://doi.org/10.1177/2473011420910407.
188. Rehabilitation Protocol for Peroneal Tendon Repair, https://www.massgeneral.org/assets/mgh/pdf/orthopaedics/sports-medicine/physical-therapy/rehabilitation-protocol-for-peroneal-repair.pdf.

Pain Management in Metastatic Bone Disease

24

Mikayla Roof, Shengqing Wang, and Alexandra Callan

Introduction

Metastatic bone disease (MBD) occurs when cancer cells migrate to the skeleton from their primary tumor origin. Although bone is one of the most common sites of metastatic disease, the management of metastatic bone disease is complex and requires multidisciplinary effort. The main goal of managing metastatic bone disease is to alleviate pain and adverse sequelae of pathologic fractures. Accordingly, this reduces medical complications, helps maintain their quality of life, and decreases the morbidity of metastatic cancer. As clinicians, an understanding of the disease process, the available diagnostic and treatment options, as well as the variations of metastatic bone disease due to the primary tumor is crucial to being able to accomplish these goals. *This chapter aims to help physicians manage metastatic bone disease by introducing them to a basic understanding of the mechanism of metastasis, the proper diagnostic work-up, and treatment options for patients suffering from pain or immobility.*

Epidemiology

The epidemiology of metastatic bone disease is important for clinicians to understand. Bone is the third most affected organ of metastatic disease after the liver and lungs [1–3]. Though difficult to accurately quantify, one study estimates about 400,000–600,000 new cases of metastatic bone disease occur each year in the

M. Roof · S. Wang
UT Southwestern Medical School, Dallas, TX, USA
e-mail: Mikayla.Roof@UTSouthwestern.edu; Shengqing.Wang@UTSouthwestern.edu

A. Callan (✉)
Department of Orthopaedic Surgery, UT Southwestern Medical Center, Dallas, TX, USA
e-mail: Alexandra.callan@utsouthwestern.edu

C. E. Noe (ed.), *Musculoskeletal Pain*,
https://doi.org/10.1007/978-3-031-86057-7_24

USA. However, these numbers may underestimate the incidence of metastatic bone disease, as some autopsy studies have suggested that the incidence is up to 70% in patients who die of cancer. The high incidence may be attributed to the skeleton being a common site of metastasis as well as the increased number of patients living with cancer due to improved detection, targeted systemic treatments, and multidisciplinary management of cancers [4].

In adults, bone metastases are much more common than primary bone tumors [5]. Nearly all types of cancers can metastasize to the bones; however, clinicians should be especially watchful for metastatic bone disease in patients with lung, prostate, breast, kidney, and thyroid cancers [6–9]. This is especially significant since breast, prostate, and lung cancers represent the top three most common types of cancers in new cases of cancers diagnosed annually (CDC). In terms of age, it has been shown that in those older than 25, the lung seems to be the most common primary site followed by the prostate and breast. [6] In patients less than 20 years old, endocrine and soft-tissue sarcomas seem to be the primary source of metastasis [6]. Clinicians should use the epidemiology framework to understand which patients are most at risk of developing metastatic bone disease.

Clinical Significance

From a clinical perspective, bone metastasis can have important prognostic significance. Metastatic bone disease is often an ominous marker of primary cancer progression [10]. Furthermore, depending on the type of primary cancer, the presence of bone metastasis can play an important predictive role in determining the median survival of patients from the time of diagnosis [10, 11].

Clinically, the metastatic pattern in bone metastasis usually comprises multiple lesions involving the axial and appendicular skeleton [11]. Since these lesions are preferentially localized in the most vascularized skeletal parts, the most commonly involved bones include the vertebrae, ribs, pelvis, and hips [10]. The type of bone lesion can also range from osteolytic to osteoblastic lesions or a mixed pattern of both [1, 7, 11, 12]. Depending on the size, duration, and location of the lesion, bone metastasis can cause major adverse sequelae such as hypercalcemia pain, impaired mobility, pathological fractures, spinal cord compression, and bone marrow aplasia [2, 3, 11]. Out of these adverse skeletal-related events, skeletal pain is the most common. [4] Prevention and proper management of these adverse skeletal-related events are crucial to the patient's quality of life and mortality [13, 14].

Thus, it is important for all clinicians to understand the pattern of metastasis in the skeleton, the symptoms of adverse skeletally related events (SREs), and the available treatment currently available to manage these symptoms. Clinical suspicion is important when caring for any patient with a remote cancer history or a new cancer diagnosis. Appropriate work up includes taking a careful history, learning symptoms such as pain and impaired mobility, obtaining blood work (lab values such as alkaline phosphatase (ALP) and calcium can be important markers of bone tunrover), and imaging studies such as x-rays, computed tomography (CTs), magnetic resonance imaging (MRIs) and often PET (Positron emission tomography) CT or bone scan (scintigraphy) [10, 11]. Diagnosis is confirmed with a biopsy. Treatment options depend on a variety of factors such as primary cancer, localization of lesion, type of lesions, and patient factors. Available treatments include radiotherapy, radiopharmaceuticals, surgery, and bisphosphonates [3, 7, 10–12]. The following sections will go into more depth about the mechanism, the proper diagnostic work-up, and the most up-to-date management of metastatic bone disease.

Mechanism of Bone Metastasis

To understand the proper management of metastatic bone disease, especially the therapeutic targets of the prescribed pharmacotherapy, it is important to have a general framework of the mechanism of the disease process. Metastasis occurs as a three-step process. In the migration step, cancer cells break away from their primary origin to enter the body's circulating system, such as the lymph or blood [1]. Next, during adhesion, cancer cells establish residence in bone via a series of interactions between adhesion molecules, chemo-attractive factors, and cell surface receptor interactions [1, 12, 15]. The skeletal system is a particularly attractive place for metastasizing cancer cells because the sinusoidal blood vessels in the bone marrow are fenestrated and increase the likelihood of cancer cell extravasation through the vessel wall. [16] Finally, in the settlement step, cancer cells colonize the perivascular and endosteal niche to disrupt the normal modeling of bone formation and resorption patterns [1, 7, 11, 12, 15].

Osteolytic Disease

As mentioned in the introduction, the clinical appearance of metastatic bone disease can range from lytic to sclerotic lesions. Osteolytic lesions are predominantly seen in metastasis from primary cancers such as breast, multiple myeloma, renal, non-small cell lung, malignant melanoma, thyroid, and non-Hodgkin's lymphoma [11, 12, 15]. The important takeaway from this section is that these lesions mainly result from the direct action of stimulated osteoclasts on bone, NOT via direct tumor cell destruction of bone [10, 12, 15]. Thus, bisphosphonates are a common and effective therapeutic strategy in the prevention and treatment of metastatic bone disease as they inhibit osteoclast activity [10, 12]. The main mediators of osteolytic bone metastasis are increased parathyroid hormone-related peptide (PTHrP) in the bone microenvironment due to tumor cells and the ratio of Osteoprotegerin (OPG) to Receptor Activator of Nuclear Factor Kappa-B Ligand (RANKL) [1, 12]. Accordingly, zoledronic acid (bisphosphonate) and denosumab (RANKL inhibitor) can be very effective.

Osteoblastic Disease

Osteoblastic lesions result from increased bone formation and decreased resorption. The most common type of primary cancer to result in an osteoblastic pattern of bone metastasis is prostate cancer, some 15%–20% of breast cancers, small cell lung cancer, Hodgkin's lymphoma, and medulloblastoma commonly produce osteoblastic patterns [12]. Although less common than osteolytic bone metastasis, endothelin-1 is one of the most studied mediators of osteoblastic metastases and is found to be increased in circulation with osteoblastic metastases from prostate cancer, as well as a minority of those with osteoblastic metastases from breast cancer [7, 10, 15].

Mixed Presentation

Although it would be simple to think of osteoblastic and osteolytic metastasis as mutually exclusive presentations, they are rather separate ends of a spectrum. Patients can present with lesions of both lytic and blastic characteristics. For example, metastasis from breast cancer, GI cancers, and squamous cell cancers can all have a presentation of a mixed pattern [11, 15]. With a better understanding of the mechanism and patterns of presentation for metastatic bone disease, the rest of the chapter will discuss how to evaluate and manage the symptoms and complications.

Evaluation of Metastatic Bone Disease

Work-Up

Clinical Evaluation

Metastatic bone disease can often be asymptomatic and incidentally found during the initial work-up of a primary malignancy or subsequent surveillance. However, in symptomatic metastatic bone disease, pain is usually the most common symptom and may lead to the identification of a new bone lesion [17]. Despite the presentation, the work-up following the identification of a new bone lesion should be thorough and tailored to the clinical presentation.

The first step in working up a newly discovered bone lesion is diagnosing the pathological process. Identifying the pathological process begins with a thorough history, including a review of systems and pertinent family history, as well as a physical exam of the affected anatomical site. Patients with MBD will often have pain that tends to be worse at night and is progressive over time. The characteristic of MBD pain varies but can be intermittent, mild to constant, and severe with disease progression or local invasion [18]. Assessing for thyroid, breast, or prostate nodules may help in identifying the potential pathological process. Furthermore, laboratory studies can be conducted to diagnose certain primary tumors that may have led to a bony metastasis or exclude multiple myeloma. Serum calcium and alkaline phosphatase are recommended in the setting of potential MBD [19]. In patients with a known primary malignancy, it is important to still complete a thorough work-up on a newly found bone lesion to ensure that the lesion is not due to a benign process or a new primary malignancy.

Imaging

In addition to a thorough clinical examination, imaging is important in characterizing the bone lesion and determining the diagnosis. The Musculoskeletal Tumor Society recommends plain radiographs of the affected anatomical site as the initial evaluation of all possible bone tumors. Plain radiographs are good for assessing structure and alignment [17]. However, it is important to note that some lesions may not be reliably detectable on plain radiographs until up to 25–50% of bone destruction occurs [20]. If there is no lesion apparent on plain radiographs but clinical suspicion for a bone lesion remains high, CT or MRI are indicated. [21]

Following the identification of bone lesions on plain radiographs, advanced imaging can be used to further aid in diagnosis, local staging, and treatment decisions. Advanced imaging to assess potentially malignant lesions should include the entire bone as well as the proximal and distal joints [19]. For bone lesions that are larger than 5 cm or for painful lesions in which the etiology is unknown, MRI is the preferred advanced imaging [21]. MRI has excellent soft-tissue resolution and can detect intramedullary metastatic disease prior to cortical destruction making it very sensitive to identifying MBD. Contrast-enhanced CT scans also provide excellent skeletal resolution and may be used for patients who have contraindications to MRI. Of important note, for lesions of the ribs, CT is preferred over MRI [22].

To complete the diagnosis and staging of malignant lesions, additional imaging, including a whole body bone scan or FDG-PET/CT, may be obtained to assess for additional osseous or metastatic lesions [17]. However, this additional imaging should be done at the discretion of the oncologic specialist and is outside the scope of this chapter [21].

Biopsy

Indications for biopsy of a newly found bone lesion are dependent on several factors, including the patient's oncologic history, whether clinical evaluation and imaging were sufficient for diagnosis, the need for histological evaluation to confirm metastasis, and the need for surgery [19].

For patients with a known primary malignancy with a new bone lesion, especially multiple lesions, that have a typical appearance on imaging and features consistent with the primary cancer, metastatic disease may be presumed without biopsy. However, over 20% of new bone lesions found in these patients are unrelated to the primary malignancy. Among newly found lesions that are symptomatic, over 81% are due to the primary malignancy; however, in newly found asymptomatic lesions, only 50% are due to the primary malignancy [23]. Biopsy of new lesions for pathological confirmation of initial bone metastasis is recommended in these patients. Fine needle aspiration and core biopsy are acceptable methods to confirm metastatic disease in these patients.

In patients who present with apparent metastatic bone disease, but the primary malignancy is unclear following evaluation, a biopsy of the bone lesion is recommended to provide pathological information on the likely primary malignancy as well as confirm metastatic bone disease.

Biopsy is also required prior to surgical fixation for patients presenting with impending or pathologic fracture through a solitary bone lesion to rule out primary sarcoma (mesenchymal malignancy). The biopsy tract should be planned such that it can be excised during surgical treatment if biopsy confirms a primary sarcoma such as chondrosarcoma or osteosarcoma.

Patient's Overall Medical Condition

Understanding the patient's overall medical condition is important to guiding treatment plans in MBD, and therefore, the work-up should assess the patient's life expectancy, overall comorbidities, pain level, and surgical candidacy. Obtaining laboratory studies, including Complete Blood Count (CBC) with differential, complete metabolic panel (CMP), LFTs, and renal function tests, and validating estimations of survival, are useful in determining the patient's overall condition and candidacy for various medical and surgical therapies.

Common Causes of Metastatic Bone Lesions in Adults

MBD can occur in any bone and can be secondary to nearly any type of cancer, but recognizing the most common sites and causes of MBD is important in the clinical evaluation and diagnosis of new bone lesions.

Over 400,000 malignant bone metastases are diagnosed annually in the US with the spine being the most common site of bone metastasis [24–26]. MBD of the spine is found during autopsy in up to 70% of patients with malignancy [18]. Due to the frequency of spinal metastases, there should be a high index of suspicion for MBD in patients with a known primary malignancy and new-onset back pain or neurologic symptoms. [27] Vertebral MBD will progress to spinal cord compression in approximately 10% of patients, and early detection of spinal metastases can reduce morbidity. In addition to the spine, the pelvis and long bones are frequent sites of MBD, with the femur being the most affected long bone followed by the humerus and tibia. MBD less commonly affects the hands or feet and is seen most often secondary to primary lung malignancy.

Bone metastases are most common secondary to carcinoma, particularly in primary breast, prostate, renal, and lung carcinomas [16, 25]. Multiple myeloma, thyroid cancer, and melanoma also frequently cause metastatic bone lesions. Knowing a patient's primary malignancy is important in understanding their risk of MBD as the relative incidence of bone metastasis varies by type of tumor [28]. Among patients with advanced metastatic disease, the relative incidence of bone metastasis is 65–75% in breast cancer, 65–75% in prostate cancer, 60% in the thyroid, 30–40% in lung cancer, 20–25% in renal cell carcinoma, and 14–45% in melanoma.

MBD can arise at any time following the development of a primary malignancy. As treatment options for cancer continue to improve and patients live longer, MBD may arise years after diagnosis. The average time between the diagnosis of a primary malignancy and the development of MBD varies based on cancer type. One study reports that the diagnostic intervals were 67.8 months for breast cancer and

50.1 months for kidney cancer. The diagnostic intervals were much shorter for lung and liver cancer at 20.6 months and 29.1 months, respectively [23].

Pathologic Fracture

Early detection and treatment of MBD are important in reducing skeletal-related events (SREs). One common skeletal-related event in MBD is pathologic fracture, a fracture through a weakened bone that occurs with much less force than normally required for fracture. Studies report that anywhere from 5–29% of patients with MBD will develop a pathologic fracture. Pathologic fractures increase morbidity and mortality but may be the first sign a patient has MBD [29, 30]. Of those patients who present with pathologic fracture through MBD, 3–4% will have an undiagnosed primary malignancy [31]. Understanding the common causes and location of MBD is important to preventing pathologic fracture as the incidence varies based on the type of MBD. Pathologic fractures are most common in patients with primary multiple myeloma and breast cancer with an incidence of 43% and 35%, respectively. This is followed by prostate and lung cancer with incidences of 19% and 17%, respectively [29]. Approximately half of pathologic fractures occur in the femur, with the femoral neck being the most common, and 15% of pathologic fractures occu in the humerus [32].

Treatment

Treatment of metastatic bone disease is complex and often requires a multidisciplinary approach. Early referral of patients with MBD to a multidisciplinary team can reduce morbidity and mortality and improve patient quality of life [30]. There are many approaches to managing MBD, but the goals of all treatments include minimizing pain and maintaining function and motion to improve patient quality of life [27]. Treatment decisions must consider the patient's oncologic status, comorbidities, and life expectancy, as well as the local biomechanical requirements of the patient's skeletal metastasis [17].

Current treatment options for metastatic bone disease include analgesics, regional nerve blocks, ablation, systemic medical therapies, radiation treatment and radiopharmaceuticals, and surgery. Often, a combination of these treatments is employed for palliation of MBD symptoms, including pain, pathologic fracture, nerve root or spinal cord compression, and reduced mobility, which all impair the quality of life in patients with metastatic cancer [33].

Analgesics

Most patients with MBD will experience significant pain at some point during their disease. Analgesic medications are a common method of pain management that can be initiated at pain onset and tailored to the severity and type of pain [33]. A stepwise approach using non-opioid and opioid medications is recommended to reduce patients suffering from MBD pain.

Acetaminophen and NSAIDs are well-established in managing cancer-related pain and are often initial treatments for patients without contraindications experiencing mild-to-moderate pain [34–36]. There is not sufficient evidence to support the efficacy or safety of one Non-steroidal anti-inflammatory Drug (NSAID) over another [37].

For patients with moderate-to-severe pain or pain refractory to NSAIDs, opioids may be initiated for improved pain relief. Continuing non-opioid medication may reduce the required opioid dose for effective pain relief and minimize opioid-induced side effects. Opioid therapy often begins with weak opioids, including codeine, hydrocodone, and tramadol. If patients experience severe or persistent pain, potent opioids, including oxycodone, morphine, hydromorphone, methadone, and fentanyl, are indicated. [33]

Referral to palliative care physicians or pain specialists can be beneficial for patients with refractory pain or side effects from high-dose systemic analgesics who may benefit from interventional options, including nerve blocks, spinal cord stimulators, epidurals, or implanted pain pumps.

Radiotherapy

External beam radiation therapy (EBRT) is a safe and effective treatment for pain in MBD and is the most common treatment. Radiation therapy reduces pain in up to 80% of patients and results in complete pain relief in approximately 30% of cases [27]. Recent studies suggest that single-fraction treatments have similar efficacy on pain relief as multiple-fraction radiation treatments for previously unirradiated bone metastases [38]. Single-fraction treatments have a higher rate (20%) of need for retreatment compared to multiple-fraction treatments (8%). However, the rates of retreatment in the first three months post-treatment do not differ significantly between single and multiple fractions, making single-fraction radiation therapy an effective treatment for patients with limited life expectancy. Retreatment with radiation therapy for painful bone metastases has a pain response rate of 58% [39]. Recent evidence suggests that postoperative use of radiation therapy for patients with spinal cord compression may improve patient outcomes [18].

Stereotactic body radiation therapy (SBRT) is a more recent evolving treatment that uses advanced image guidance to allow for the precise delivery of high doses of radiation to tumor sites. This technique is particularly useful in spinal metastases as the advanced conformal technique can minimize radiation exposure to the spinal cord and reduce potential neurological deficits while effectively reducing pain. The American Academy of Radiation Oncology recommends reserving SBRT for patients with a life expectancy longer than six months or for persistent or recurrent pain following EBRT.

Radiopharmaceuticals are an additional treatment option for managing diffuse pain that may not be easily targeted with local radiation therapy. Radiopharmaceuticals are administered systemically and localized to sites of bony metastasis to deliver radiation. These compounds are beneficial in osteoblastic metastases and are generally reserved in the US for patients with persistent or recurrent multifocal bone pain following other treatment modalities. Current agents include samarium-153 lexidronam and strontium-89, which reduce pain in 40–95% of patients but may take several weeks to provide pain relief [40].

Systemic Therapy

Systemic therapies for MBD are diverse but are specific to cancer type. Chemotherapy, hormone therapy, and targeted therapies provide pain relief by killing tumor cells, reducing tumor mass, and interfering with tumor-related pain-signaling pathways. Systemic therapies are recommended for patients with malignancies responsive to available agents and those able to tolerate treatment.

Additional systemic therapies in the treatment of MBD include osteoclast inhibitors, particularly bisphosphonates and denosumab. These agents prevent the recruitment and activation of osteoclasts to reduce bone resorption at sites of bony metastases [41]. Some studies suggest osteoclast inhibitors may reduce or delay skeletal related events Skeletal Related Events (SREs) in MBD as well as provide an alternative treatment to multifocal bone pain [27, 41–43]. Denosumab may have an increased analgesic benefit over bisphosphonates but is associated with increased costs [33]. Overall, osteoclast inhibitors have limited analgesic effects and are not first-line agents for pain management in MBD. These agents can result in jaw necrosis or hypocalcemia and initiation of therapy should consider patient-specific factors.

In patients with spinal metastases resulting in spinal cord compression, high-dose glucocorticoid therapy may aid in reducing cord compression, edema, and pain until definitive decompressive surgery can be performed. [44]

Surgical Interventions

The goals of surgical intervention in MBD include skeletal stabilization, promoting early mobilization and weight-bearing, and reducing pain [19]. Surgical intervention is mostly reserved for impending or pathological fractures as well as lesions causing mechanical instability or spinal cord compression. In select cases where a solitary bone lesion is the only site of cancer beyond the primary tumor, surgical resection may be indicated to aid in tumor control, pain relief, and enhancing patient survival. Indications and options for surgery in MBD depend on the tumor location and size as well as patient-specific factors, including life expectancy. Pathological fractures do not have an optimal environment for healing and patients with MBD are often undergoing chemotherapy or radiotherapy during the perioperative period, further impairing healing potential. [19] Therefore, the surgical construct must provide long-term stability.

There are three main types of surgical intervention in MBD. The first is osteosynthesis (plate and screw fixation) with or without cement augmentation. Pathological fractures can be treated via open reduction and internal fixation with plates and screws. Following the curettage of the lesion, bone cement can be injected if necessary for additional stability. The second option includes an intramedullary nail (IMN) for impending or pathological fractures in long bones. IMN is a safe and effective option that can allow for immediate weight bearing and decreases the risk of pathologic fracture. Unfortunately, due to the underlying pathology in the bone that impairs healing potential, discontinuous cortical bone may not heal following surgical stabilization [19]. Application of cement in addition to IMN may be needed to reduce pain. Lastly, endoprosthetic reconstruction allows for surgical excision of the affected bone and tumor with large bone and joint reconstruction using a metal replacement. Usually, after endoprosthetic reconstruction immediate weight-bearing, joint stability, decreased pain, and durable construction makes this an important option in the treatment of MBD. Endoprosthetic reconstruction techniques are most commonly used when there is massive bony destruction and the lesion or pathological fracture involves the hip, knee, or shoulder joints [19]. There are newer techniques for stabilizing pathologic bone including percutaneous cement-screw fixation or use of photodynamic balloons. These options can be appealing due to minimally invasive approach, rapid recovery, and minimal time needed off of systemic treatments. Patients who have an impending fracture but are not surgical candidates should be made non-weight-bearing or protected weight bearing on the affected extremity. Often times, walkers, wheelchairs, braces or slings can be helpful for mobilization.

Vertebral Metastases

Radiation and systemic therapy do not treat spinal instability. Therefore, surgical intervention is recommended for spine metastases causing vertebral column instability or spinal cord compression to reduce pain and prevent the development or progression of neurological compromise. The mechanical stability of the spine in patients with MBD is often assessed using the spine instability neoplastic score (SINS). SINS accounts for imaging and patient characteristics, including vertebral body locations, bone lesion quality, spinal alignment, degrees of vertebral involvement and collapse, posterior element involvement, and mechanical pain. Referral for surgical evaluation is recommended in patients with a SINS score of 7 or greater [18]. Recent studies show that surgical decompression and stabilization are more effective than laminectomy alone [45].

Nonvertebral Metastases

Surgical intervention is often indicated in impending and complete pathologic fractures to minimize morbidity and pain. The Mirel criteria are used to assess the risk of pathologic fracture and are used to determine if prophylactic surgical intervention is indicated. The Mirels score accounts for pain, size, location, and radiographic appearance of pathologic bone lesions. Lesions with a Mirels score of 9 or greater indicated prophylactic intervention, but clinical discretion should be used as patient factors such as mechanical pain may warrant a lower threshold for surgical management. The surgical principles for prophylactic treatment of impending pathologic fractures are the same as those for displaced pathologic fractures. Prophylactic intervention for impending pathological fractures reduces pain, postoperative rehabilitation time, and in-hospital morbidity compared to intervention following pathological fracture. Importantly, the overall cost of treatment is lower for prophylactic treatment without fracture than for pathological fractures [46].

Surgical Treatment Recommendations Vary Based on the Bone Affected

Humerus

Surgical intervention is indicated in most complete or displaced pathological fractures of the humerus. Proximal humerus fractures that involve the articular segment, humeral head, or proximal metaphysis are often treated with endoprosthetic replacement. Goals should include the stability of the glenohumeral joint and pain relief. Humerus fractures involving the meta-diaphysis or shaft are commonly treated with either proximal plate fixation or IMN with or without cement. Extra-articular, distal humerus fractures are commonly treated with plate fixation and cement or prosthetic arthroplasty as IMN usually does not provide adequate stability in this area and often leads to failure. Distal intra-articular humerus fractures are often treated with total elbow arthroplasty.

Femur

There are several surgical options for treating pathological fractures of the hip and proximal femur. The patient's clinical picture, including life expectancy, lesion type, and fracture displacement, must be considered in determining the most appropriate fixation type. Cemented hip hemiarthroplasty is preferred if there is no acetabular pathology [47]. Total hip arthroplasty can be used if there is significant acetabular pathology, but it requires longer surgical time and has higher complication profiles. Arthroplasty allows for immediate mobilization and weight-bearing while rapidly decreasing pain [48]. Importantly, long stems may lead to higher intraoperative and postoperative complications and therefore should be reserved for patients with additional femoral lesions (MSTS CPG 2020) [47]. Pathological fractures in the distal diaphysis or meta-diaphysis are commonly fixed with lesion curettage and cemented plate osteosynthesis. If the pathologic fracture is intra-articular, endoprosthetic reconstruction should be considered.

Tibia/Fibula

Tibial bone metastases are rare, but the treatments are like those of the humerus and femur. Proximal tibial fractures involving the articular surface are commonly fixed with total knee arthroplasty. If the lesion involves a significant portion of the proximal third of the tibia, a cemented endoprosthesis should be used. Proximal tibial fractures that are extra-articular may be fixed with a plate and screw or IMN. Diaphyseal fractures are most commonly fixed with IMN due to the lack of a robust soft-tissue envelope. Curettage with plate osteosynthesis with or without cement augmentation may also be considered in distal tibial lesions.

Foot/Ankle

Metastatic disease of the ankle and foot are often initially treated with nonoperative measures. However, in cases of continued pain or instability, curettage and cementation can be performed. Surgical intervention can be augmented with internal fixation if required.

Surgical intervention for patients with MBD is associated with higher risks of complications. The 30-day postoperative complication rate in patients with MBD may be over 30% and can be associated with reduced survival. Postoperative complication rates are higher in patients with rapidly growing primary tumors, multiple metastatic bone lesions, and surgical intervention for the lower extremities. The most common complications include urinary tract infection (UTI), pneumonia, delirium, pulmonary embolism, and atrial fibrillation [49]. Therefore, careful consideration of patient-specific factors is important in deciding on surgical intervention in patients with MBD.

Key Points for Evaluation

- A thorough history should elucidate the patient's personal and family history of malignancy as well as his/her risk factors for cancer.
- Plain radiographs are an important initial diagnostic modality in the setting of suspected metastatic bone disease.
- Malignant features on plain radiographs include tumors larger than 5 cm, cortical disruption, periosteal reaction, and pathologic fracture.
- The physical exam should identify the precise location of pain.
- Laboratory tests, including serum calcium and ALP, can be useful in diagnosing metastatic bone disease. Hypercalcemia can often be seen in metastatic bone disease or patients with multiple myeloma. Cancer specific labs such as CBC with diff, CMP, PSA, TSH, CA-15, SPEP/UPEP can be useful to identify the potential primary malignancy.

Key Points for Treatment

- Treatment of metastatic bone disease involves a multimodal approach.
- An understanding of the patient's life expectancy is important in guiding the treatment approach.
- Treatment may consist of analgesics, systemic therapy, radiotherapy, and/or surgical intervention.
- Pain is the most common symptom patients experience in MBD and NSAIDs and/or opioids should be used to minimize patient suffering.
- Radiotherapy is the most common treatment for MBD and is a safe and effective method for managing pain and disease in bony metastases.
- Patients at risk for a pathologic fracture who are surgical candidates may benefit from prophylactic fixation to provide pain relief, preserve function, and provide a construct that is long-lasting and allows for early weight-bearing.

Key Takeaways

- Bone is the third most affected organ of metastatic disease and is a major health issue in the US with 400,000–600,00 new cases per year.

- Metastatic bone disease is most commonly due to carcinomas of the breast, prostate, kidney, and lung. Multiple myeloma is a common cause of primary bone tumors in adults.
- Clinical suspicion of metastatic bone disease should be high in patients with known malignancy and new-onset bone pain.
- Metastatic bone disease can occur in any bone but most commonly affects the spine, pelvis, ribs, and long bones, particularly the femur and humerus.
- Clinical management of metastatic bone disease is complex and should involve multidisciplinary care.
- Pain is the most common skeletal-related event in metastatic bone disease and treatments available for pain management include analgesic medication, radiation therapy, systemic therapies, and surgery.
- Pathologic fractures of long bones should be stabilized with surgery to improve pain, increase mobility, and allow patients to continue tolerating systemic treatments.
- A combination of treatment options is often best at minimizing pain in metastatic bone disease and maximizing quality of life.

References

1. Nayir E. Pathogenesis of bone metastasis. J Oncol Sci. 2016;1:13–6. https://doi.org/10.1016/j.jons.2015.11.004.
2. Schulman KL, Kohles J. Economic burden of metastatic bone disease in the U.S. Cancer. 2007;109(11):2334–42. https://doi.org/10.1002/cncr.22678.
3. Coleman RE. Metastatic bone disease (MBD): clinical features, pathophysiology and treatment strategies. Cancer Treat Rev. 2001;27(3):165–76. https://doi.org/10.1053/ctrv.2000.0210.
4. DiCaprio MR, Murtaza H, Palmer B, Evangelist M. Narrative review of the epidemiology, economic burden, and societal impact of metastatic bone disease. Ann Joint. 2021;7. https://aoj.amegroups.com/article/view/6807
5. Bussard KM, Gay CV, Mastro AM. The bone microenvironment in metastasis; what is special about bone? Cancer Metastasis Rev. 2008;27(1):41–55. https://doi.org/10.1007/s10555-007-9109-4.
6. Ryan C, Stoltzfus KC, Horn S, et al. Epidemiology of bone metastases. Bone. 2022;158:115783. https://doi.org/10.1016/j.bone.2020.115783.
7. Mundy GR. Metastasis to bone: causes, consequences and therapeutic opportunities. Nat Rev Cancer. 2002;2(8):584–93. https://doi.org/10.1038/nrc867.
8. McCabe FJ, Jadaan DY, Jadaan MM, McCabe JP. The rise of metastatic bone disease in Ireland. Clin Exp Metastasis. 2020;37(6):693–702. https://doi.org/10.1007/s10585-020-10059-7.
9. Kendal JK, Abbott A, Kooner S, Johal H, Puloski SKT, Monument MJ. A scoping review on the surgical management of metastatic bone disease of the extremities. BMC Musculoskelet Disord. 2018;19(1):279. https://doi.org/10.1186/s12891-018-2210-8.
10. Selvaggi G, Scagliotti GV. Management of bone metastases in cancer: a review. Crit Rev Oncol Hematol. 2005;56(3):365–78. https://doi.org/10.1016/j.critrevonc.2005.03.011.
11. Macedo F, Ladeira K, Pinho F, et al. Bone metastases: an overview. Oncol Rev. 2017;11(1):321. https://doi.org/10.4081/oncol.2017.321.
12. Vicic I, Belev B. The pathogenesis of bone metastasis in solid tumors: a review. Croat Med J. 2021;62(3):270–82. https://doi.org/10.3325/cmj.2021.62.270.

13. Barton KI, Hazenbiller O, Freeman G, et al. Communication in surgical decision-making while managing metastatic bone disease (MBD): matching patient expectations with surgical goals. Support Care Cancer. 2021;29(2):1111–9. https://doi.org/10.1007/s00520-020-05595-7.
14. Liu Z, Xu Y, Liu ZL, Tian YZ, Shen XH. Combined application of diclofenac and celecoxib with an opioid yields superior efficacy in metastatic bone cancer pain: a randomized controlled trial. Int J Clin Oncol. 2017;22(5):980–5. https://doi.org/10.1007/s10147-017-1133-y.
15. Yin JJ, Pollock CB, Kelly K. Mechanisms of cancer metastasis to the bone. Cell Res. 2005;15(1):57–62. https://doi.org/10.1038/sj.cr.7290266.
16. Buenrostro D, Mulcrone PL, Owens P, Sterling JA. The bone microenvironment: a fertile soil for tumor growth. Curr Osteoporos Rep. 2016;14(4):151–8. https://doi.org/10.1007/s11914-016-0315-2.
17. Yu HH, Tsai YY, Hoffe SE. Overview of diagnosis and management of metastatic disease to bone. Cancer Control. 2012;19(2):84–91. https://doi.org/10.1177/107327481201900202.
18. Mossa-Basha M, Gerszten PC, Myrehaug S, et al. Spinal metastasis: diagnosis, management and follow-up. Br J Radiol. 2019;92(1103):20190211. https://doi.org/10.1259/bjr.20190211.
19. Scolaro JA, Lackman RD. Surgical management of metastatic long bone fractures: principles and techniques. J Am Acad Orthop Surg. 2014;22(2):90–100. https://doi.org/10.5435/JAAOS-22-02-90.
20. Rosenthal DI. Radiologic diagnosis of bone metastases. Cancer. 1997;80(8 Suppl):1595–607. https://doi.org/10.1002/(sici)1097-0142(19971015)80:8+<1595::aid-cncr10>3.3.co;2-z.
21. Miller BJ. Use of imaging prior to referral to a musculoskeletal oncologist. J Am Acad Orthop Surg. 2019;27(22):e1001–8. https://doi.org/10.5435/JAAOS-D-19-00109.
22. O'Sullivan GJ, Carty FL, Cronin CG. Imaging of bone metastasis: an update. World J Radiol. 2015;7(8):202–11. https://doi.org/10.4329/wjr.v7.i8.202.
23. Zhang L, Wang Y, Gu Y, Hou Y, Chen Z. The need for bone biopsies in the diagnosis of new bone lesions in patients with a known primary malignancy: a comparative review of 117 biopsy cases. J Bone Oncol. 2019;14:100213. https://doi.org/10.1016/j.jbo.2018.100213.
24. Damron TA, Mann KA. Fracture risk assessment and clinical decision making for patients with metastatic bone disease. J Orthop Res. 2020;38(6):1175–90. https://doi.org/10.1002/jor.24660.
25. Siegel RL, Miller KD, Jemal A. Cancer statistics, 2017. CA Cancer J Clin. 2017;67(1):7–30. https://doi.org/10.3322/caac.21387.
26. Biermann JS, Holt GE, Lewis VO, Schwartz HS, Yaszemski MJ. Metastatic bone disease (MBD): diagnosis, evaluation, and treatment. J Bone Joint Surg Am. 2009;91(6):1518–30. https://www.ncbi.nlm.nih.gov/pubmed/19487533
27. Kapoor R, Saxena AK, Vasudev P, Sundriyal D, Kumar A. Cancer induced bone pain: current management and future perspectives. Med Oncol. 2021;38(11):134. https://doi.org/10.1007/s12032-021-01587-7.
28. Jiang W, Rixiati Y, Zhao B, Li Y, Tang C, Liu J. Incidence, prevalence, and outcomes of systemic malignancy with bone metastases. J Orthop Surg (Hong Kong). 2020;28(2):2309499020915989. https://doi.org/10.1177/2309499020915989.
29. Saad F, Lipton A, Cook R, Chen YM, Smith M, Coleman R. Pathologic fractures correlate with reduced survival in patients with malignant bone disease. Cancer. 2007;110(8):1860–7. https://doi.org/10.1002/cncr.22991.
30. Ardakani AHG, Faimali M, Nystrom L, et al. Metastatic bone disease (MBD): early referral for multidisciplinary care. Cleve Clin J Med. 2022;89(7):393–9. https://doi.org/10.3949/ccjm.89a.21062.
31. Hage WD, Aboulafia AJ, Aboulafia DM. Incidence, location, and diagnostic evaluation of metastatic bone disease. Orthop Clin North Am. 2000;31(4):515–28., vii. https://doi.org/10.1016/s0030-5898(05)70171-1.
32. Jan MY, Campbell TC. The establishment and future of integrated onco-palliative care. Cancer. 2021;127(12):1963–4. https://doi.org/10.1002/cncr.33475.

33. von Moos R, Costa L, Ripamonti CI, Niepel D, Santini D. Improving quality of life in patients with advanced cancer: targeting metastatic bone pain. Eur J Cancer. 2017;71:80–94. https://doi.org/10.1016/j.ejca.2016.10.021.
34. Eisenberg E, Berkey CS, Carr DB, Mosteller F, Chalmers TC. Efficacy and safety of nonsteroidal antiinflammatory drugs for cancer pain: a meta-analysis. J Clin Oncol. 1994;12(12):2756–65. https://doi.org/10.1200/JCO.1994.12.12.2756.
35. Magee DJ, Jhanji S, Poulogiannis G, Farquhar-Smith P, Brown MRD. Nonsteroidal anti-inflammatory drugs and pain in cancer patients: a systematic review and reappraisal of the evidence. Br J Anaesth. 2019;123(2):e412–23. https://doi.org/10.1016/j.bja.2019.02.028.
36. Nabal M, Librada S, Redondo MJ, Pigni A, Brunelli C, Caraceni A. The role of paracetamol and nonsteroidal anti-inflammatory drugs in addition to WHO Step III opioids in the control of pain in advanced cancer. A systematic review of the literature. Palliat Med. 2012;26(4):305–12. https://doi.org/10.1177/0269216311428528.
37. Ahmad I, Ahmed MM, Ahsraf MF, et al. Pain Management in Metastatic bone disease (MBD): a literature review. Cureus. 2018;10(9):e3286. https://doi.org/10.7759/cureus.3286.
38. Chow R, Hoskin P, Hollenberg D, et al. Efficacy of single fraction conventional radiation therapy for painful uncomplicated bone metastases: a systematic review and meta-analysis. Ann Palliat Med. 2017;6(2):125–42. https://doi.org/10.21037/apm.2016.12.04.
39. Lutz S, Balboni T, Jones J, et al. Palliative radiation therapy for bone metastases: update of an ASTRO Evidence-Based Guideline. Pract Radiat Oncol. 2017;7(1):4–12. https://doi.org/10.1016/j.prro.2016.08.001.
40. Goyal J, Antonarakis ES. Bone-targeting radiopharmaceuticals for the treatment of prostate cancer with bone metastases. Cancer Lett. 2012;323(2):135–46. https://doi.org/10.1016/j.canlet.2012.04.001.
41. Gralow J, Tripathy D. Managing metastatic bone pain: the role of bisphosphonates. J Pain Symptom Manag. 2007;33(4):462–72. https://doi.org/10.1016/j.jpainsymman.2007.01.001.
42. Wong R, Wiffen PJ. Bisphosphonates for the relief of pain secondary to bone metastases. Cochrane Database Syst Rev. 2002;2002(2):CD002068 https://doi.org/10.1002/14651858.CD002068.
43. Hoskin P, Sundar S, Reczko K, et al. A multicenter randomized trial of Ibandronate compared with single-dose radiotherapy for localized metastatic bone pain in prostate cancer. J Natl Cancer Inst. 2015;107(10):djv197. https://doi.org/10.1093/jnci/djv197.
44. Leppert W, Buss T. The role of corticosteroids in the treatment of pain in cancer patients. Curr Pain Headache Rep. 2012;16(4):307–13. https://doi.org/10.1007/s11916-012-0273-z.
45. Patchell RA, Tibbs PA, Regine WF, et al. Direct decompressive surgical resection in the treatment of spinal cord compression caused by metastatic cancer: a randomised trial. Lancet. 2005;366(9486):643–8. https://doi.org/10.1016/S0140-6736(05)66954-1.
46. Blank AT, Lerman DM, Patel NM, Rapp TB. Is prophylactic intervention more cost-effective than the treatment of pathologic fractures in metastatic bone disease? Clin Orthop Relat Res. 2016;474(7):1563–70. https://doi.org/10.1007/s11999-016-4739-x.
47. Houdek MT, Wyles CC, Labott JR, Rose PS, Taunton MJ, Sim FH. Durability of Hemiarthroplasty for pathologic proximal femur fractures. J Arthroplast. 2017;32(12):3607–10. https://doi.org/10.1016/j.arth.2017.06.040.
48. Vermesan D, Prejbeanu R, Haragus H, et al. Case series of patients with pathological dyaphiseal fractures from metastatic bone disease. Int Orthop. 2017;41(10):2199–203. https://doi.org/10.1007/s00264-017-3582-3.
49. Bindels BJJ, Thio Q, Raskin KA, Ferrone ML, Lozano Calderon SA, Schwab JH. Thirty-day postoperative complications after surgery for metastatic long bone disease are associated with higher mortality at 1 year. Clin Orthop Relat Res. 2020;478(2):306–18. https://doi.org/10.1097/CORR.0000000000001036.

Pediatric Musculoskeletal Medicine 25

Andrew Dinh and Ardin Berger

Challenges in Treating Pediatric Musculoskeletal Pain in Children

Lack of Evidence and Epidemiology

Despite such a common prevalence, musculoskeletal research in the medical literature for the adult population remains in the minority. This gap in epidemiological studies further inhibits the identification and management of this population. Musculoskeletal conditions and pathologies in the pediatric population are vast ranging, from common injuries to more systemic conditions requiring specialty attention. Prevalence can vary widely (8.5–40%) in terms of chronic and recurrent musculoskeletal pain with knee, neck, and back pain listed as the most commonly affected areas (excluding headaches) [2]. Review of medical literature notes a range of 6.1–25.6% of visits to primary care and urgent or emergency care were related to musculoskeletal complaints, with up to 15% of the adolescent population fitting criteria for chronic musculoskeletal pain [2–4]. Further, many musculoskeletal pain conditions have been considered "typical" as a child goes through developmental milestones as well as growth spurts and hormonal progression—eventually further delaying treatment and making diagnosis more challenging.

Differences from Adult Musculoskeletal Medicine

With the paucity of medical research investigating musculoskeletal pain in children, practitioners have often had to rely on extrapolation of adult literature to help guide treatment. This can be helpful, as there is no binary separation between patients

A. Dinh · A. Berger (✉)
Stanford Children's Health, Pediatric Anesthesiology and Pain Management, Stanford, CA, USA
e-mail: ardinberger@edscomfortclinic.com

C. E. Noe (ed.), *Musculoskeletal Pain*,
https://doi.org/10.1007/978-3-031-86057-7_25

experiencing pain before reaching the age of majority versus those who have continued into adulthood. Further, both adult and pediatric chronic pain follows the biopsychosocial model of treatment—addressing anatomical and physiologic inputs for pain, psychological tangents (beliefs, social constructs, and mood), as well as social factors (relationships, social factors, and culture) [4]. However, childhood and adolescence differ from adulthood as it is a time for physical, mental, and social growth for an individual—substantial physical growth of the musculoskeletal system in a relatively short period of time leads to new neurosensory inputs; the challenges of emotional and cognitive development are clustered during this period, as well as the expected hormonal and mood changes; social relationships and cultural growth that are closely linked to expectations and individual experiences are also important factors that can greatly affect a person's pain experience. These challenges and differences between childhood and adulthood must be considered to tailor an appropriate treatment plan for those suffering from chronic musculoskeletal pain at a young age.

Difficulty with Diagnosis

Musculoskeletal pain in children and adolescents can be difficult to diagnose and treat due to key differences in characterizing symptoms and a common lack of consistent laboratory and imaging abnormalities, which would typically guide caretakers and practitioners of adult pain patients to appropriate treatment [2]. Thus, it is important for the pediatric pain clinician to maintain an eye for nuance and an appreciation for both medically verifiable and less conspicuous causes of musculoskeletal pain in children. By opening oneself up to the consideration of nuance in the presentation of various pediatric pain conditions, many benefits can be found including a limitation of laboratory and imaging work-up to only that which is necessary and useful, an expedition of appropriate and goal-directed treatment including the alleviation of discomfort, and a facilitation of functional rehabilitation as early in the disease process as possible.

Anatomical Differences Between Pediatrics and Adults

Starting from birth, the structure of bone allows it to be more pliable and resilient to external forces as it goes through multiple stages of growth [4]. With less density and increased porosity in the earlier years, there is an increase in resistance to fracture and a different growth and healing pattern to repair fractures that do arise. The absence of a thick periosteum in the bones of children allows for accelerated remodeling and healing of fractures, though it also allows for greater susceptibility to fluid-filled pathologies, including purulence and hematoma [4].

As a child progresses into adulthood, constant turnover and ossification of the bony structures can make radiographic interpretation difficult. Often, the use of contralateral imaging is more advantageous when attempting to establish what might be considered normal for the growing patient. Due to the high degree of variability on plain films, suspected fractures are often treated empirically with a diagnosis being made on plain films in retrospect [1].

The presence of the physes in young bone allows for a significant difference in the pathophysiology of both traumatic and atraumatic musculoskeletal injuries in the pediatric population. Growth plates represent regions of hypertrophy that are vulnerable to shear forces as compared to the mature bones in adults. The vulnerabilities of skeletal structure can often lead to certain pathologies that are common and well-defined in pediatric medicine [5].

Take-Home Points

- *Pain in pediatric patients is commonly less defined, resulting in decreased treatment options relative to those found for adult patients.*
- *Though extrapolating pain management techniques from those used in adults may be commonplace, it is key to remain mindful of the nuanced differences in anatomy and physiology present in each age group.*

Common Pediatric Musculoskeletal Disorders

Slipped Capital Femoral Epiphysis (SCFE)

Synonyms

Slipped upper femoral epiphysis, Epiphyseolysis of femoral head.

ICD-10 Codes

M93.00.

Description

SCFE is a condition in which there is a displacement of the capital femoral epiphysis from the femoral neck and the physeal plate—a shearing or slipping of the femoral growth plate at the junction of the femoral head and neck. As one of the most common hip disorders of adolescence, it is important for clinicians to avoid delays in diagnosis, which have been shown to worsen prognosis [7].

Clinical Presentation

Hip pain and altered gait are the two most common presenting symptoms related to SCFE. Factors that might place patients at increased risk for development of SCFE include conditions that weaken the physeal junction of the femoral head and neck [6, 7]:

- Obesity (additional shear force and stresses under exercise).
- Trauma.
- Endocrine and metabolic disorders.

- Irradiation in pediatric oncology.
- Non-radiating, dull pain in the hip, groin, or thigh that increases with activity should raise suspicion for SCFE. At or around the time of initial diagnosis, SCFE is only found to be bilateral in roughly 1/3 of cases. Of those cases that are initially unilateral, approximately 1/3 will progress to include the contralateral side at some point in the future.

Physical Examination

With pain being the most common initial symptom, abnormal gait and difficulty with weight-bearing are also typical presenting symptoms.

Limited internal rotation of the hip joint has been the most historical physical examination finding leading to the diagnosis of SCFE.

Obligatory external rotation (Drehmann sign) is noted in the involved hip of patients with SCFE when the hip is passively flexed to 90°.

Unstable, severe forms of SCFE present with external rotation and shortening of the ipsilateral limb.

Diagnostic Work-Up

The gold standard for diagnosis of SCFE is x-ray radiography. X-ray views should be ordered based on the clinical suspicion of severity:

- Stable SCFE: Anteroposterior and frog-leg lateral views of both hips.
- Unstable SCFE: Anteroposterior and cross-table lateral views of the involved hip.

On anterior-posterior views, widening, lucency, and irregularity of the physis may be noted. The most reliable sign of an early stage SCFE may be the blurring of the junction between the metaphysis and the growth plate.

Lateral views are recommended to aid in identifying cases of posterior displacement and step-off of the epiphysis on the femoral neck, which are better demonstrated in this plane.

MRI is another modality that can be employed in cases where suspicion is high with normal film studies. Confirmation of diagnosis is important; in up to 25% of cases in which SCFEs are missed, radiographs were misinterpreted, or the diagnosis could not be established with the radiographs that were obtained.

Ultrasound has been identified as an additional modality to aid in diagnosis, but x-ray films remain the gold standard [7–9].

Treatments

The treatment of slipped capital femoral epiphysis is surgical fixation. Prophylactic pinning of the contralateral hip is currently considered controversial, and consideration thereof should be based on the complete clinical context, including other patient factors and comorbidities. Early operative treatment is preferred to prevent known secondary outcomes, including osteonecrosis of the femoral head, chondrolysis, and femoroacetabular impingement [11, 12].

Following a pinning of the femoral epiphysis, it is recommended that patients rely exclusively on crutches for mobility and practice non-weight bearing for 6–8 weeks [12].

Due to the elevated risk of contralateral slipping or re-injury of the ipsilateral hip, close follow-up with this subset of patients is recommended through later stages of bone maturity [10].

Take-Home Points

- *Slipped capital femoral epiphysis is a common condition of childhood defined by a slipping of the femoral growth plate at the junction of the femoral head and neck.*
- *Adolescents with SCFE commonly present with pain or abnormal gait in the presence of elevated body mass index or a history of trauma.*
- *Diagnosis involves x-ray imaging and treatment involves surgical fixation.*

Juvenile Idiopathic Arthritis—Polyarticular Disease Variant

Synonyms

Juvenile Rheumatoid Arthritis, Still's Disease, JRA, JIA.

ICD-10 Codes

M08.00.

Description

Juvenile Idiopathic Arthritis is a chronic inflammatory condition that primarily involves the joints. Epidemiology and pathophysiology are vast and variable due to the autoimmune etiology of the condition [13, 14]. The pathogenesis of JIA further subdivides the disease into subsets of variants with unique extraarticular manifestations that require their own treatment pathways. Overall, as in all treatment of pediatric-focused conditions, treatment pathways should include pacing of activities, reduction of stress on affected joints, and maintenance of function; well-informed, effective management of the pain arising secondary to JIA can be tremendously helpful for the attainment of all these stated goals [15]. For brevity, subtypes of JIA and descriptions of their unique pathogenesis will be deferred to other texts.

Clinical Presentation

Peak incidence of JIA occurs at 1–3 years of age with a majority being identified in assigned-female patients in this age range. Further studies have noted a separate peak in assigned-male patients from 8–10 years of age. Autoimmune conditions as well as physical, infectious, and immunologic stresses have also led to seasonal and populational groups with consistency. Patients with hypermobility spectrum disorders and Ehlers-Danlos syndrome can be considered to be of greater risk, due to both structural disintegrity and the predisposition for autoimmune disease [13, 14].

Arthralgia is a typical chief complaint from patients with JIA, although appreciable arthritic changes may not be present on examination. Further variability in the interval between the onset of arthralgias and the appearance of objective arthritis can prolong treatment and increase the risk for the development of more severe and systemic manifestations of the disease [17].

In children, presenting complaints typically involve pain and discomfort in 1 or 2 joints, but can quickly progress to an oligoarticular process within months. Younger children typically present with pain in the knees, wrist, and/or ankles and often follow asymmetric patterns early in the disease process before becoming more widespread and symmetrical in nature.

Physical Examination

Typical presenting physical examination involves pain in the joints upon movement and mechanical stress on the affected joints. Disease progression to arthritis can present with edematous and warm joints, but the typical lag interval between arthralgia and arthritis has been well-documented [15, 17].

Diagnostic Work-Up

As a clinical diagnosis, JIA requires arthralgias in more than four joints [15]. Blood work is recommended on clinical suspicion of other subsets of JIA and is often ordered on initial work-up to streamline targeted therapy, when warranted. Blood work to identify subsets of JIA include:

- Complete Blood Count (CBC)
- Comprehensive metabolic panel (CMP).
- Inflammatory markers.
  - Erythrocyte sedimentation rate (ESR).
  - C-reactive protein CRP).
  - Antinuclear antibody (ANA).
  - Rheumatoid factor (RF).
  - Antibodies to cyclic citrullinated peptide (CCP).
  - Human leukocyte antigen (HLA) B27.

Management

Management is based on multiple factors, including disease severity and which subsets of the condition are identified. Early treatment is preferred to quickly control the progression of any associated inflammatory process. Disease-modifying antirheumatic drugs (DMARDs) and biologic agents are often started at the time of diagnosis to minimize requisite medication escalation and an associated increases in side effects. Methotrexate is one typical DMARD started by many rheumatologists in this setting; active monitoring of blood counts and concurrent folic acid therapy are recommended to help reduce side effects. Patients with a higher degree of severity (juvenile arthritis disease activity score [cJADAS]of >2.5) have been shown to benefit from oral glucocorticoid therapy alongside DMARDs and biologic therapy [19].

Nonsteroidal anti-inflammatory drugs are typically used in the setting of JIA to help limit inflammation and reduce symptoms on an as-needed basis. Many patients also find benefit from long-term NSAID therapy, although long-term NSAID use places patients at an increased risk of gastritis and renal injury. Therefore, active monitoring is required when NSAIDs are scheduled, and it is recommended to limit their use to an as-needed basis [17, 19].

Interventions

Intraarticular injections of glucocorticoids as targeted therapy for singular joints have shown to help reduce symptoms, disease process, and drug therapy burden in JIA [18]. Intraarticular interventions have shown a place in supporting functional rehabilitation such as PT/OT in the management of the disease [18]. The risks of infection, the need for sedation/anesthesia in the pediatric population, and potential articular trauma should be weighed with each injection, especially in cases where many joints are affected. The risks of chronic steroid exposure must also be considered.

Rehabilitation

Physical and occupational therapy comprise the foundation for disease management. However, strength and range of motion exercises can be limited by active inflammation and should be tailored to a patient's specific functional ability, with greater levels of involvement being reserved for periods of minimal active disease. Strengthening of the muscles surrounding joints can be protective of the joint overall and may lead to a decreased risk for subsequent inflammatory flares, especially in patients who are hypermobile [15, 17].

Take-Home Points

- *Juvenile idiopathic arthritis is a condition with multiple etiologies and treatment strategies.*
- *Presentation is bimodal, with many assigned-females-at-birth (AFABs) presenting in early childhood and assigned-males-at-birth (AMABs) presenting in late childhood.*
- *Interventional treatment is variable and may include NSAIDS, DMARDS, and local steroid injections.*
- *Maintenance of function should be emphasized and encouraged in the setting of supportive care.*

Legg-Calvé-Perthes Disease

Synonyms

Perthes disease, idiopathic avascular necrosis of the hip, juvenile osteonecrosis of head of femur.

ICD-10 Codes

M91. 1.

Description

Legg-Calvé-Perthes (LCP) refers to idiopathic avascular necrosis of the hip. Disruption of the blood supply to the femoral head is the first phase of the disease and eventually leads to limited growth of the subchondral cortical bone. Risk factors known to the disease include [20]:

- Inherited coagulopathies (e.g., Factor V Leiden).
- Thrombophilia (increased coagulation) and hypofibrinolysis (decreased ability to dissolve clots).
- Human immunodeficiency virus (HIV).
- Secondhand smoke exposure.
- Low socioeconomic status.
- Birth weight less than 2.5 kg in assigned-male patients.

Clinical Presentation

Legg-Calvé-Perthes disease often presents with a limp in childhood. Pain is typically mild and can be vague, with referred pain most commonly being experienced in the knee and/or anteromedial thigh [22].

Physical Examination

Weakness with internal rotation and abduction of the affected hip should lead to a high clinical suspicion for LCP. Other signs of antalgic gait and compensation include atrophy of the thighs and buttocks of the affected side and should further add to the suspicion of a pathologic process in the hip [22].

Trendelenburg gait is a sign of compensation and chronic pain in the hip, which is defined by a downward pelvic tilt away from the affected hip during the swing phase of ambulation [22].

Diagnostic Work-Up

Plain films (anteroposterior pelvis and frog-leg lateral "Lauenstein" views) are preferred during the initial diagnostic phase, though these images are commonly "normal" early in the disease process [21].

MRI can aid in diagnosis if uncertainty remains and can provide information on the staging of the disease process.

Findings on MRI in the early stages describe subchondral and epiphyseal transformations ("Crescent Sign") while late-stage findings show fragmentation and decreased perfusion of the femoral head. Marrow changes of the femoral head are also indicative of long-term sequelae of hypoperfusion to the region [21].

Blood work is often taken at the time of suspicion with the goal of excluding other diagnoses (e.g., ESR and CBC).

Management

Nonoperative treatment entails symptomatic management as well as activity pacing to allow for healing of the joint. Activity restriction and joint protection must be balanced with the maintenance of perfusion to the joint and range of motion exercises to prevent compensation and subsequent atrophy. There is little evidence for known benefit from the use of braces, casts, and orthotics during the healing phase of treatment. With early treatment and activity pacing, outcomes remain satisfactory, with return to function being noted in 60%–80%. NSAIDs are typically prescribed for symptom management throughout the rehabilitation process [24, 25].

If conservative management fails—or if indicated based on severity and rapidity of progression—operative management by pediatric orthopedic surgery may be indicated [25].

Take-Home Points

- Legg-Calvé-Perthes Disease involves osteonecrosis of the femoral head, though presenting pain commonly is commonly noted in the ipsilateral, anteriomedial thigh, or knee.
- Treatment may be operative or supportive, depending on the clinical presentation.

Ehlers-Danlos Syndrome

Hypermobility syndrome, Benign joint hypermobility.

ICD-10 Codes

Q79.6.

Description

Ehlers-Danlos syndrome (EDS) is a collection of connective tissue disorders in which collagen, or the structural support thereof, is disadvantageously impacted resulting in a hypermobile connective tissue support structure. To date, 14 subtypes of Ehlers-Danlos syndrome have been identified [26], all of which are genetically verifiable with a single exception: Hypermobile Ehlers-Danlos syndrome (formerly termed "Type III"). The hypermobile subtype is thought to be the most common form of EDS and—though some clinical presentations may appear spontaneous in origin—is currently considered to be autosomal dominant in inheritance with incomplete penetrance and variable expressivity. Therefore, the clinical presentation thereof is widely variable.

The pediatric pain clinician's understanding of Ehlers-Danlos syndrome is critically important, as—contrary to the widespread belief that these conditions affect the musculoskeletal system in isolation—Ehlers-Danlos Syndrome implies multisystem involvement, with the capacity to affect virtually every body system. Resultantly, for the undiagnosed patient, significant time and resources are commonly spent in pursuit of individual diagnoses for each secondary condition and an accurate diagnosis is frequently never attained. Furthering the delay in diagnosis and proper treatment, clinicians commonly reverse the origin and outcome of these pain conditions, placing the onus for musculoskeletal pain complaints on patients' secondary neuropsychological comorbidity rather than the primary connective tissue disease itself. Therefore, a holistic understanding of these conditions by any pediatric pain-focused clinician is of utmost importance. Recognition, understanding, and acknowledgment of this unifying diagnosis are beneficial in the following ways:

- Mitigation of undue worry on behalf of the patient.
- Prevention of furthered medical and social stigmatization.
- Abbreviation of latency to accurate diagnosis of secondary conditions
- Cultivation of an environment for proper symptomatic support.

Clinical Presentation

Though they remain commonly undiagnosed, cases of Ehlers-Danlos Syndrome and hypermobility spectrum disorders (HSD, formerly "joint hypermobility syndromes" or JHS) have been found to be some of the most common primary conditions in patients presenting to the pediatric pain clinic. Patients with Ehlers-Danlos Syndrome have often been provided misdiagnoses—frequently in the form of a diagnosis of exclusion, including somatization, psychogenic pain, or fibromyalgia—prior to their arrival in the pediatric pain clinic. A large number have been told by clinicians that the pain is "in their head" or that proper psychological support and physical activity are the only treatment modalities available for their condition. Beyond simple pain complaints, presenting signs and symptoms are often multisystem and include:

- Diffuse musculoskeletal pain (e.g., myalgias, myofascial pain, and arthralgias).
- Joint subluxations or dislocations in the absence of trauma.
- Recurrent injury.
- Chronic fatigue.
- Headaches.
- Gastrointestinal complaints (e.g., dysmotility, constipation, and avoidant restrictive food intake disorder).
- Symptoms of mast cell activation (e.g., flushing, pruritis, urticaria, abdominal cramps, diarrhea, vomiting, syncope, hypotension, collapse, and respiratory symptoms).
- Signs and symptoms of dysautonomia (e.g., pallor, peripheral mottling, orthostasis, and tachycardia).
- Secondary neuropsychological comorbidity (e.g., attention deficit hyperactivity disorder, anxiety, speech disability, autistic traits, depression, and functional neurological symptom disorders).
- Sensory abnormalities (e.g., textural aversions, hyperosmia, and hyperacusis).

Physical Examination

To the scrupulous eye, physical differences upon examination of the patient with EDS may be clear from afar. However, at minimum, every pediatric pain physician should make it a regular part of their practice to incorporate the Beighton scoring system (often confused with the outdated Brighton criteria) into their physical examination as a screening for generalized joint hypermobility. The Beighton scoring examination assesses the passive range of motion of the bilateral fifth-digit metacarpophalangeal joints, wrists, elbows, knees, and spine. A positive Beighton score is age-dependent, with an expected decrease in scoring with the advancement of age. If screening is positive, the physical examination should be continued to assess for a generalized connective tissue difference. Specific criteria incorporated into the clinical diagnosis of hEDS and commonly found in varying degrees in other Ehlers-Danlos syndrome subtypes include:

- Unusually soft or velvety skin, commonly described as a "doughy" appearance to the subcutaneous regions.
- Skin hyperextensibility.
- Unexplained presence of striae distensae or rubae.
- Piezogenic papules on the heels, wrists, and/or elbows.
- Recurrent or multiple hernia(s).
- Abnormal scarring (hypotrophic in the hypermobile subtype and atrophic or hemosideric in certain genetically-verifiable subtypes).
- Prolapses (pelvic, rectal, or uterine).
- Dental crowding and a high or narrow palate (often s/p corrective orthodontia, including braces and/or palate expanders).
- Arachnodactyly (positive, bilateral Walker-Murdoch, and/or Steinberg signs).
- Arm-span-to-height ratio ≥ 1.05.
- Cardiac structural abnormalities (mitral valve prolapse or aortic root dilation).

Diagnostic Work-Up

Aside from one, all subtypes of Ehlers-Danlos syndrome are genetically verifiable. However, for diagnosis of the hypermobile subtype, the clinician must rely on a thorough history and physical examination using the current, recently revised diagnostic criteria as defined by the International Consortium on Ehlers-Danlos sndrome in 2017 [27]. This clinical work-up includes specific Beighton scoring requirements ($\geq$6 for pre-pubertal, $\geq$5 for pubertal patients to 50 years of age, and $\geq$ 4 for patients over 50 years of age, with some exceptions for patients missing a single point on the scoring system) and assessment of the above physical examination findings, as well as either a positive family history of hypermobile Ehlers-Danlos syndrome or one or more of the following secondary criteria:

- *Musculoskeletal pain in two or more limbs, recurring daily for ≥ 3 months.*
- *Chronic, widespread pain for ≥ 3 months (e.g., myofascial pain syndrome or "fibromyalgia").*
- *Recurrent joint dislocations or frank joint instability in the absence of trauma.*

Finally, the clinician must rule out less-common, higher-risk subtypes of Ehlers-Danlos syndrome (most commonly the classical subtype, with the hypermobile and classical subtypes making up 90% of cases [28]) and alternative diagnoses, which may better explain the patient's presentation (lupus, rheumatoid arthritis, Loeys-Dietz syndrome, Marfan syndrome, osteogenesis imperfecta, etc.) prior to providing the patient with a diagnosis of hypermobile Ehlers-Danlos syndrome.

Treatments

Though terms including "benign" have previously been used in reference to the hypermobile subtype of Ehlers-Danlos syndrome, the clinician must remain aware that—although not all are verifiable by genetic testing—each of these conditions may be accompanied by comorbidities which are far from benign in clinical impact, and must take note of the multisystem effects of each of the subtypes of Ehlers-Danlos syndrome. By their time of presentation to the pain clinic, patients have often survived years of being told that they have manifested their pain and illness from within, often with loose insinuation of a moral origin to a well-established, clinically-verifiable—though widely underdiagnosed—condition.

The treatment of Ehlers-Danlos Syndrome and its associated comorbidity is largely supportive. Specifically regarding the musculoskeletal manifestations of this condition, rehabilitation, and maintenance of function are foundational, though not curative. The patient must be advised to limit their physical activities to those which are low-impact in order to help prevent worsening of the musculoskeletal manifestations of this condition. They should be encouraged to maintain adequate levels of cardiovascular exercise on a daily basis but should be advised to pace the implementation of all activities to avoid escalated discomfort and pervasive fatigue, which commonly present for days to weeks after significant over-exertion. Patients with comorbid dysautonomia should limit their activities to those which do not involve significant orthostatic stress, and the maximum intensity of their activities should also be limited to moderate levels, as greater exertion can flare episodes of dysautonomic symptoms and thereby worsening their physical status.

Exercise plans beginning with minimal amounts of movement (e.g. 3–5 min of light-to-moderate levels of cardiovascular exercise in the heavily deconditioned), which are then gradually increased by prolonging the daily duration of exercise by just a couple of minutes weekly tend to be successful at avoiding these post-exertional flares in pain and discomfort. Pacing is key in successfully establishing a continuous, consistent cardiovascular exercise regimen. The patient should avoid hyperextension of the joints during each activity in which they choose to participate. Due to the hypotonicity of muscle and the increased load placed on the muscles secondary to hypermobility of the joints, the muscles are at high risk for pathology, and patients will often benefit from muscular strengthening routines of equally-moderated introduction. Though conditioning and psychological support for secondary illness is of high importance, the clinician must remember to avoid prescribing only cardiovascular exercise and psychotherapy and should instead assist the patient with a holistic approach to symptom management, connecting with appropriate specialties as necessary in order to properly address secondary comorbidities.

Take-Home Points

- *Ehlers-Danlos Syndrome (EDS) and hypermobility spectrum disorders are current terms for joint hypermobility syndromes.*
- *Most forms of EDS are genetically verifiable; however, the most common form—the hypermobile form—is not.*
- *Diagnosis of hypermobile EDS is determined by clinical diagnostic criteria based on connective tissue abnormalities.*
- *The secondary effects of Ehlers-Danlos syndrome are frequently extensive, and with multisystem involvement; the pediatric pain clinician's knowledge of its effects on each involved body system may have tremendous cost-saving outcomes.*

Resources

Challenges in Treating Pediatric Musculoskeletal Pain in Children

1. Black, Karen JL, et al. Musculoskeletal disorders in children. In: Tintinalli JE, et al., editors. Tintinalli's emergency medicine: a comprehensive study guide. 8th ed. McGraw Hill; 2016. https://accessmedicine.mhmedical.com/content.aspx?bookid=1658&sectionid=109408415.
2. King S, Chambers, Christine TB, Huguet A, MacNevin Rebecca CB, McGrath Patrick JB, Parker L, MacDonald, Amanda JC. The epidemiology of chronic pain in children and adolescents revisited: a systematic review. Pain. 2011;152(12):2729–38. https://doi.org/10.1016/j.pain.2011.07.016.
3. Jaime de I. Musculoskeletal pain in primary pediatric care: analysis of 1000 consecutive general pediatric clinic visits. Pediatrics. 1998;102(6):e63. https://doi.org/10.1542/peds.102.6.e63.
4. Kamper SJ, Henschke N, Hestbaek L, Dunn KM, Williams CM. Musculoskeletal pain in children and adolescents. Braz J Phys Ther. 2016;20(3):275–84. https://doi.org/10.1590/bjpt-rbf.2014.0149. PMID: 27437719; PMCID: PMC4946844.
5. Lefèvre H, Loisel A, Meunier BB, Deslandre C, Lemoine N, Moro MR, Quartier P, Lachal J. Chronic idiopathic musculoskeletal pain in youth: a qualitative study. Pediatr Rheumatol Online J. 2019;17(1):86. https://doi.org/10.1186/s12969-019-0389-3. PMID: 31882011; PMCID: PMC6935211.

Common Pediatric Musculoskeletal Disorders

6. Mathew SE, Larson AN. Natural history of slipped capital femoral epiphysis. J Pediatr Orthop. 2019;39(Issue 6, Supplement 1 Suppl 1):S23–S27.
7. Loder RT, Skopelja EN. The epidemiology and demographics of slipped capital femoral epiphysis. ISRN Orthop. 2011;2011:486512.
8. Cowell HR. The significance of early diagnosis and treatment of slipping of the capital femoral epiphysis. Clin Orthop Relat Res. 1966;48:89–94.
9. Uvodich M, Schwend R, Stevanovic O, Wurster W, Leamon J, Hermanson A. Patterns of pain in adolescents with slipped capital femoral epiphysis. J Pediatr. 2019;206:184–189.e1.
10. Georgiadis AG, Zaltz I. Slipped capital femoral epiphysis: how to evaluate with a review and update of treatment. Pediatr Clin North Am. 2014;61(6):1119–35.
11. Aprato A, Conti A, Bertolo F, Massè A. Slipped capital femoral epiphysis: current management strategies. Orthop Res Rev. 2019;11:47–54.
12. Otani T, Kawaguchi Y, Marumo K. Diagnosis and treatment of slipped capital femoral epiphysis: Recent trends to note. J Orthop Sci. 2018;23(2):220–8.

Juvenile Idiopathic Arthritis—Polyarticular Disease Variant

13. Horton DB, Shenoi S. Review of environmental factors and juvenile idiopathic arthritis. Open Access Rheumatol. 2019;11:253–67.
14. Rigante D, Bosco A, Esposito S. The etiology of juvenile idiopathic arthritis. Clin Rev Allergy Immunol. 2015;49(2):253–61.
15. Giancane G, Alongi A, Ravelli A. Update on the pathogenesis and treatment of juvenile idiopathic arthritis. Curr Opin Rheumatol. 2017;29(5):523–9.
16. Malattia C, Rinaldi M, Martini A. The role of imaging in juvenile idiopathic arthritis. Expert Rev Clin Immunol. 2018;14(8):681–94.
17. Macaubas C, Nguyen K, Milojevic D, et al. Oligoarticular and polyarticular JIA: epidemiology and pathogenesis. Nat Rev Rheumatol. 2009;5:616.
18. Lanni S, Bertamino M, Consolaro A, et al. Outcome and predicting factors of single and multiple intra-articular corticosteroid injections in children with juvenile idiopathic arthritis. Rheumatology (Oxford). 2011;50:1627.
19. Ravelli A, Davì S, Bracciolini G, et al. Intra-articular corticosteroids versus intra-articular corticosteroids plus methotrexate in oligoarticular juvenile idiopathic arthritis: a multicentre, prospective, randomised, open-label trial. Lancet. 2017;389:909.

Legg-Calvé-Perthes Disease

20. Vosmaer A, Pereira RR, Koenderman JS, Rosendaal FR, Cannegieter SC. Coagulation abnormalities in Legg-Calvé-Perthes disease. J Bone Joint Surg Am. 2010;92(1):121–8.
21. Laine JC, Martin BD, Novotny SA, Kelly DM. Role of advanced imaging in the diagnosis and management of active Legg-Calvé-Perthes Disease. J Am Acad Orthop Surg. 2018;26(15):526–36.
22. Loder RT, Skopelja EN. The epidemiology and demographics of legg-calvé-perthes' disease. ISRN Orthop. 2011;2011:504393.
23. Lee WY, Hwang DS, Ha YC, Kim PS, Zheng L. Outcomes in patients with late sequelae (healed stage) of Legg-Calvé-Perthes disease undergoing arthroscopic treatment: retrospective case series. Hip Int. 2018;28(3):302–8.

24. Heesakkers N, van Kempen R, Feith R, Hendriks J, Schreurs W. The long-term prognosis of Legg-Calvé-Perthes disease: a historical prospective study with a median follow-up of forty one years. Int Orthop. 2015;39(5):859–63.
25. Nguyen NA, Klein G, Dogbey G, McCourt JB, Mehlman CT. Operative versus nonoperative treatments for Legg-Calvé-Perthes disease: a meta-analysis. J Pediatr Orthop. 2012;32(7):697–705.

Ehlers-Danlos Syndrome

26. Blackburn PR, Xu Z, et al. Bi-allelic alterations in AEBP1 lead to defective collagen assembly and connective tissue structure resulting in a variant of Ehlers-Danlos syndrome. Am J Hum Genet. 2018;102(4):696–705.
27. Bloom L, Byers P, Francomano C, Tinkle B, Malfait F. Steering committee of the international consortium on the ehlers-danlos syndromes. Am J Med Genet C, Semin Med Genet. 2017;175(1):5–7.
28. Steinmann B, Royce PM, Superti-Furga A. The Ehlers-Danlos syndromes. In: Steinmann B, Royce PM, editors. Connective tissue and its heritable disorders. Wilmington: Wiley-Liss Inc.; 2002. p. 431–523.

Interdisciplinary Pain Treatment 26

William G. Brose, Dokyoung S. You, Corrine Cooley,
Allie Schmeissing, and Fei Cao

History (Including Trauma and Occupation)

A relevant history regarding pain should contain a detailed appraisal of current pain complaints, along with system reviews, past medical and surgery history, and current and past pain medication trials (it is better to document why those medications were stopped alongside any side effects), family history, social history, etc. Based on the updated definition of pain [1], pain involves both sensory and emotional components. It is essential for clinicians to evaluate the patient's behavior and subjective body language, interaction with their families and/or friends, along with the patient's own insight about perception on how their pain influences their functions and relationship with others, the root cause(s) of their chronic pain, ideal management for them, and treatment goal, etc.

For example, "obsessive thought" to specific therapy without the willingness to try alternative treatments, such as opioid only pain management, may reveal underlying substance use issues instead of uncontrolled chronic pain. To optimize the evaluation of a patient with pain, extra attention to certain barriers for accurate and precise communication needs to be overcome. Cross-cultural and cross-linguistic barriers to communication may call for interpretation by bilingual and bicultural interpreters and may be facilitated by the presence of family caregivers for optimal understanding (e.g., for immigrant patients with chronic pain, clinicians should be

W. G. Brose (✉) · D. S. You · A. Schmeissing · F. Cao
Stanford University, Stanford, CA, USA
e-mail: wbrose@brosemd.com

C. Cooley
Stanford Health Care, Palo Alto, CA, USA

C. E. Noe (ed.), *Musculoskeletal Pain*,
https://doi.org/10.1007/978-3-031-86057-7_26

aware that those patients might perceive chronic pain differently in the context of different cultural backgrounds.) [2].

The comprehensive history will not only help to find the correct diagnosis but also dictate the next-step management. Some key questions related to current pain complaints that clinicians should obtain include pain: Location—onset, intensity, and duration, character—pattern of occurrence, initiating, aggravating, and relieving factors, quality (descriptive adjectives)—sharp/dull, electrical, burning, etc., and associated nonpain conditions—nausea, photophobia, sonophobia, etc). An accurate history can prevent repetitive testing with over-interpretation of diagnostic imaging and/or laboratory results, which provide important supplementary information. The primary utility of pain-specific diagnostic testing should be the elimination of sinister threats and a focus on clear communication of that goal being achieved is necessary for each patient throughout the course of their interdisciplinary treatment. If the pain diagnostics cannot reassure the patient that there is not a sinister cause of the pain, each painful moment will provide a recurrent threat of such an unknown sinister threat. A patient who is fearful of the meaning of their pain will not be able to focus on developing an acceptance of that pain. As a result, this critical step in pain diagnosis cannot be skipped without threatening the potential best outcome of their interdisciplinary treatment plan.

While this complex patient history taking is time-consuming the elaborate and detailed history collection allows clinicians to build rapport by pursuing the most efficient information exchange. This will allow recovery of that time invested as treatment ensues. Often traditional allopathic treatment follows a course of monthly to perhaps even less frequent quarterly care. This type of metered care is often promoted to reduce the unintended reinforcement of the patient's dependency on the provider with more frequent visits, but it does not facilitate the evolution of an increasingly independent model of care. With interdisciplinary care, there is a large teaching opportunity that must be pursued by the care team in order to shift the patient from a model of provider-dependent care delivery to more independence in their own care.

Optimal timing of interdisciplinary provider contacts can vary from multiple interactions with the provider team throughout the day as would be seen with an inpatient treatment program, to several daily contacts seen with an intensive outpatient daily treatment program to multiple times per week in a moderate intensity ambulatory treatment program. Even the longitudinal treatment in such an interdisciplinary program will often benefit from a structure of concurrent medical, rehabilitation, and psychological appointments on the same day with a recurrent visit frequency of weekly to monthly. These recurrent visits always have a core educational content that has been developed by the provider delivering the session and is usually complimented by open patient participation with questions about that content. This frequent longitudinal treatment is almost always improved by the patient receiving care in a group format where the treatment experiences of others in the group can provide useful teaching points for all members as the medical, rehab, or psychological staff reinforce the optimal management of issues interjected into the regular curriculum by the group participants.

The frequency of care coordination for the interdisciplinary team members is generally informed by the frequency of the care provided such that coordination of day-long treatment on an inpatient or intensive outpatient treatment plan will need daily conferencing of patients to optimize their care while moderate intensity treatment may need weekly conferencing and monthly group treatments need monthly conferencing.

Physical Examination

The physical examination is the most significant diagnostic tool, surpassed in importance only by the pain history [3].

It helps to narrow down the differential diagnoses and establish a sense of authority and agency of the medical provider with the patient. Usually, the medical pain physical examination starts with a general checking of all systems, with the emphasis on neurologic, musculoskeletal, and psychiatric parts. An in-depth understanding of knowledge of the motor, sensory, and reflex examinations within the examined region is essential to integrate those findings with patients' individualized psychosocial risks, to further reveal underlying pathological mechanisms of patients' chronic pain. Finally, the provocative maneuvers of the affected body region(s), such as straight leg raise testing for lumbar radiculopathy or Cluster of Laslett for sacroiliac joint pain [4], should provide important values for the provisional diagnoses.

Combined the history with examination findings, the clinician evaluates whether the existing data can explain the patient's symptoms, identify potential pain generators, lead to the appropriate conclusion of certain diagnoses, and necessitate further workups (including labs or imagining studies) for further diagnostic clarification, and appraise functional changes or limitations due to chronic pain. This application of the allopathic method to initial pain examination is necessary to assist the patient in feeling listened to and evaluated traditionally such that the examiner's sense of authority and agency can be trusted in developing diagnostic and treatment plans.

Pain Assessment Tools

There are a variety of pain assessment tools available for evaluating the pain characters in both research and clinical settings, among which the three most popular tools for pain intensity (unidimensional pain assessment tools) are verbal rating scales (VRSs), numerical rating scales (NRSs) [5], and visual analog scales (VASs), whereas the common multidimensional pain assessment tools are listed below as well [3].

Those tools have become invaluable when understanding patients' pain from multiple disciplinary perspectives. Meanwhile, they provide relatively objective values to measure patients' responses to pain management and then guide clinicians to adjust their future treatment plans. The primary value of these tools is to provide cross-patient comparisons and interpatient comparisons as patient treatment ensues. Repeated measures may offer an opportunity for reinforcement and education of the patient using their own self-report data, which can in turn reinforce the value of these measurements given the measurement burden associated with the repeated measures.

Common unidimensional pain assessment tools

Pain intensity tool	Route	Comments
Numerical rating scale (NRS)	Verbal or visual	Numerical scale (0–10, 0–100) Most commonly used Less reliable in very young or elderly patients
Visual analog scale (VAS)	Visual	Easy to administer Challenging for patients with cognitive impairment
Verbal rating scale (VRS)	Verbal	Challenging for patients with language barriers or cognitive impairment

Common multidimensional pain assessment tools [6–8]

Tool	Comments
Oswestry low back pain disability question	The "gold standard" of low back pain functional outcome Provides a percentage score reflecting the amount of restriction that pain imposes on the individual
PROMIS pain interference	Measures the extent to which pain hinders an individual's engagement with physical, mental, cognitive, emotional, recreational, and social activities Also includes items related to enjoyment in life and sleep
McGill pain questionnaires (MPQ)	Measure pain quality and location Take 5 to 15 min to complete
Brief pain inventory (BPI)	Measure pain intensity and interference with family and social functions Appropriate for follow-up patients with progressive conditions
Pain catastrophizing scale (PCS)	Evaluate catastrophizing thoughts related to pain Takes less than 5 min Need at least the 6th-grade reading level

Pain Types

Pain can be classified as nociceptive, neuropathic, and nociplastic pain. Nociceptive pain is the most common form of chronic pain, including a variety of arthritis and most forms of spinal pain. It is secondary to actual stimuli or stimuli that might potentially injure tissues.

Neuropathic pain is caused by damage or disease impacting the somatosensory nervous system. Compared with nociceptive pain, neuropathic pain is usually accompanied by sensory abnormalities, encompassing numbness and tingling, more prominent pain paroxysms, and various neurological findings [9].

The most common conditions of neuropathic pain encompass cervical/lumbar radiculopathy, diabetic neuropathy, postherpetic neuralgia, and radiculopathy [10].

Although the correlation between disability and pain intensity is not strong, neuropathic pain might be associated with greater compromise in the quality of life [11].

In contrast to many forms of nociceptive pain and acute nerve injury, chronic neuropathic pain is always maladaptive.

In 2017, International Association for the Study of Pain (IASP) introduced the new concept of "nociplastic pain," as a third mechanistic pain descriptor in addition to nociceptive and neuropathic pain. It is defined as "pain that arises from altered nociception despite no clear evidence of actual or threatened tissue damage causing the activation of peripheral nociceptors or evidence for disease or lesion of the somatosensory system causing the pain" [11].

The underlying pathophysiological mechanisms primarily involve decremental inhibitory pathways and/or augmented sensory processing [12].

These conditions include fibromyalgia, irritable bowel syndrome, and possibly nonspecific back pain. We should keep in mind that nociplastic pain generally responds poorly to procedural interventions when compared with nociceptive (such as various joint injections) or neuropathic (such as various nerve blocks) pain [9].

However, in practice, there is a significant overlap among those three types of pain mechanisms, and as a consequence, many clinicians view chronic pain classification as a continuum instead of separate entities. Numerous clinical guidelines, along with research outcomes, strongly recommend a personalized multimodal, interdisciplinary treatment approach, including pharmacotherapy, psychotherapy, integrative treatments, and invasive procedures [9].

Diagnostic Imaging

The primary value of diagnostic imaging is the opportunity to reinforce the patient's personal understanding of the cause of their pain with this scientific modality. Most patients have at least a rudimentary understanding of "x-rays," which include X-ray, ultrasound, MRI, CT PET, and virtually any diagnostic imaging as taking a current still picture of the painful body part from which one can begin to determine the underlying cause of the pain. In this way, imaging studies provide an essential bridge for patients and providers to the secret information that is contained beneath the skin, which cannot be seen by the eye or felt by the examiner's hand. The essential job of the provider in translating the information from that secret is to educate the patient about what is shown and what it means in terms of prognosis and treatment options.

X-Ray

X-ray is quick, inexpensive, and readily available in almost any medical facility, used for initial screening of skeletal system changes, but with limited values of appraising pathological changes of soft tissues. For sustained pain, an X-ray should be considered as the first step to rule out any potential fractures, especially for patients who have recent trauma or a history of osteoporosis and compression fractures. For lumbar X-rays, sometimes flexion-extension views are required to provide more information for patients with spondylolisthesis or a history of spinal fusion surgery [13, 14].

Due to the access and speed that accompany plain film X-ray imaging, this is a preferred method of diagnostic testing to reassure and inform patients of a current and evolving pain condition. Relying on dated imaging information to educate the patient will introduce a vulnerability to the educational foundation, and therefore, current and accurate diagnostic imaging is always preferred.

Magnetic Resonance Imaging(MRI)

MRI provides tremendous advantages over X-ray to evaluate soft tissues, such as tendons, ligaments, cartilage, spine disks, spinal cord, and nerve roots. It also has a high sensitivity to detect tumors and infections. An MRI without contrast is sufficient for most cases, whereas an MRI with contrast (such as gadolinium) can provide better imaging quality for detecting tumors, infections, or fibrosis. T1-weighted images offer better detail to detect end-plate reactive changes, osteophytic narrowing, lateral disk herniation, postoperative scarring, spondylolisthesis, and infiltrative disease; in contrast, T2-weighted images provide further details in intramedullary disease, infection, and inflammation because of the higher sensitivity to water content in these conditions [13].

These technical aspects remain of little importance to all but the most sophisticated of patients. Their need to learn about the anatomy and the pathology far exceeds their need to understand any nuances of imaging technology.

MRI also has some important limitations. First, MRI generally has higher expense when compared with other imaging methods, longer procedure time, limited access in some localities, and inability to detect calcification and visualize bone cortex architecture directly; second, due to the strong magnetic field, MRI precludes patients with intraocular metallic foreign bodies, pacemakers, ferromagnetic aneurysm clips, and ferromagnetic cochlear implants [14].

Many chronic patients may have a variety of orthopedic implants within their bodies, and MRI might be permissible based on a recent study [15].

If there are risks to MRI for the imaging of a painful condition that risk needs to be explored helping the patient understand the risk benefits of the imaging and the unique advantage associated with that risk is recommended. The patient who better understands the reasons for a test to be performed will be more likely to accept the results of the test as it relates to treatment planning.

Computed Tomography (CT)

CT can provide imaging on both bony structures and soft tissues. Compared with MRI, CT is quicker, less expensive, and provides better bone details. CT can be a surrogate for MRI in patients who are precluded by MRI due to ferromagnetic devices. It can clearly establish the extent of bone fractures, which are detected by X-ray, detect subtle fractures which are unable to be found by X-ray not previously seen, or determine the degree to which the bony spurs affect the spinal canal [13].

In combination with myelography, CT could have great values in certain situations. For example, CT myelography is considered the gold standard for diagnosing and locating CSF leaks [16].

EMG

Electromyography (EMG) often includes both needle studies of muscles and nerve conduction studies (NCS). The three most common diagnoses from EMG/NCS are peripheral neuropathy, carpal tunnel syndrome, and lumbosacral radiculopathy, all of which can cause pain [3].

As EMG is meant to be an extension of the neurologic examination, the question emerges, "What are the neurologic examination findings in patients with chronic pain?" Patients tend to have unremarkable results when pain is their only complaint [17].

Considering the fact that EMG can be time-consuming, costly, and painful, it is important for clinicians to consider before ordering EMG/NGS: (1) whether patients have pain alone or pain along with other neurological symptoms; (2) what diagnostic question an EMG might answer. If EMG/NGS studies will affect the diagnosis or treatment plan, or if a comprehensive neurologic examination is limited due to pain, it is more warranted to obtain those studies [18].

Even so, clinicians should keep in mind that *EMG/NCS are primarily tests of nerve and muscle function, meaning they only provide complementary information* [19].

Avoiding any invalidation that can be introduced by a negative EMG/NCS into the treatment planning of a patient who is being told they have a radiculopathy is advised as these patients may unintentionally become confused by the negative test being interpreted as the patient not really experiencing pain. Care needs to be taken in introducing complementary language that supports the overall treatment plan where EMG NCS findings can be used to encourage and support healthy rehabilitation while explaining barriers that are being experienced. In this way, the positive predictive value of a negative EMG/NCS and a positive test can both be used to the patient's advantage in pain rehabilitation.

Laboratory Studies

Laboratory investigations are usually performed to reveal disorders that could be primary or contributory causes of chronic pain disorder. Unfortunately, so far, few laboratory studies are able to make substantial contributions, among which inflammatory markers are arguably the most important. Erythrocyte sedimentation rate (ESR) and C-reactive protein (CRP) are acute phase reactants that suggest systemic inflammatory responses in a relatively nonspecific manner. For example, both ESR and CRP are used as markers of active rheumatoid arthritis [20].

Besides, elevated levels of ferritin (also known as hyperferritinemia) can suggest inflammation, infections, or malignancies [21]; for elder patients with widespread pain, 1,25$(OH)_2$ vitamin D level should be checked to rule out the responsible etiology due to vitamin deficiency [22].

Interventional Diagnostics

Differential Block—For Reinforcement of Tissue-based Diagnosis and Validation of Patient

The exact origin of the pain is frequently uncertain, which provides a challenge in developing targeted treatments. Diagnostic procedures under either fluoroscopy or ultrasound guidance, such as selective peripheral nerve block with anesthetics, can be used to localize a potential cause at a specific painful site with the goal of making an accurate diagnosis of pain, e.g., lumbar medial branch block for lumbar facet joint pain. Furthermore, those diagnostic procedures can instruct more durable interventional therapy, such as the abovementioned medial branch block for radiofrequency ablation or selective nerve root block for a variety of peripheral nerve stimulation [23].

Patients' response to those diagnostic procedures, such as pain disappearance in the specific block area, which provide significant values to differentiate among a variety of pain generators, reinforcement of findings from physical examinations and diagnoses tests (such as MRI), and validation of patients' complaints and suffering may all be achieved.

The value of interventional diagnostic neural blockade cannot be overstated in certain patients who are very experiential learners. When a pain specialist uses his or her knowledge and skill to alleviate pain, even temporarily, two very important things occur: (1) The patient experiencing pain relief will be reinforced in believing the provider who relieved the pain understands the cause of that pain and (2) the patient experiencing that relief will have the locus of control for their pain taken away from them and assigned to the pain-relieving procedure. These two consequences combine to create an opportunity for interdisciplinary treatment. By having the provider of this interventional treatment optimize the benefits of both the locus of control and prophetic impact to the patient's advantage, the interdisciplinary treatment can be reinforced. (e.g., the interventionalist needs to have used their knowledge of the immediate consequences of the procedure to educate the patient about what they are going to experience and in so doing become a prophet to the patient with regards to the pain experience.) Communicating that the pain relief being pursued, whether achieved or not, provides valuable information to reinforce the treatment plan the intervention can be coordinated into the care. Interdisciplinary care, which includes education, rehabilitation, and psychological skills, reinforces the diagnostic block outcome and can take on a powerful dimension in care. Alternatively, if that provider simply approaches the intervention as a step in an interventional treatment plan, which is only followed with positive responses that same provider introduces a bias into the treatment response, which may unintentionally disadvantage the long-term outcome (e.g., the patient desiring treatment will provide the necessary response to continue to engage the treater even as their locus of control and belief in the treater continue to escalate.) This less well-informed approach to interventional treatment almost always leads to abandonment when the patient has lost all feelings of internal control and the provider describes that they have nothing else to offer.

To take advantage of the longitudinal treatment response possible with interdisciplinary treatment, even these simple diagnostic procedures need to be pursued with knowledge of these consequences. Providers who neither know nor practice the treatment planning integration of the diagnostic procedures will run the risk of poor or low-yield therapeutic effect and risk worsening a patient's condition because of frustration due to unmet expectations, invalidation, abandonment, or, at minimum, delay in effective therapies and unnecessary cost.

Interdisciplinary Rehabilitation Evaluation

The Health & Human Services Interagency Pain Management Best Practices Task Force Report advocates for interdisciplinary, person-centered care with an emphasis on quality of life, improved functioning, and engagement in activities of daily living [24].

The report highlights the efficacy of coordinated and interdisciplinary programs in improving the outcomes above. Interdisciplinary pain treatment with the inclusion of non-pharmacologic treatment options has been found to be more effective at improving physical function, decreasing medication use, and improving quality of life compared to medical treatment alone [25].

In addition to physicians, psychologists, nurses, and social workers, occupational and physical therapists are key members of interdisciplinary teams and facilitate comprehensive, biopsychosocial assessment [26].

Occupational and physical therapists are uniquely poised to facilitate a comprehensive evaluation of baseline functionality and collaborate with patients to create a roadmap toward achieving individual goals. This chapter will discuss common occupational and physical therapy evaluations and assessments, evidence-based interventions, and future directions in both research and clinical care.

Physical Therapy Evaluation

In order to capture the difficulties associated with pain, several assessments exist to evaluate a patient's thoughts, fear, anxiety, and efficacy for their pain, the impact of pain on their function, in addition to their pain intensity, duration, and quality (Table 26.1).

Interdisciplinary Psychological Evaluation

Because chronic musculoskeletal pain is a sensory, psychological, and sociocultural experience, multidisciplinary team assessment is essential to understand the complex needs of people with chronic pain [27].

When Melzack and Wall presented the gate control theory of pain in 1965, they noted that psychological factors could open and close the gate in the spinal cord [28].

Table 26.1 Common pain questionnaires

Pain-related questionnaires	Clinically elevated significant score cutoffs	Measures
Fear-avoidance beliefs questionnaire—FABQ	FABQ-PA >15 FABQ-W >34	Fear regarding back pain, shoulder pain, cervical, and LE pain
Tampa Scale of Kinesiophobia—(TSK 11)	>30/52	Fear of movement and tissue injury
Pain catastrophizing scale (PCS)	>30/52	Thoughts around pain questions include three subscales: rumination, helplessness, and magnification
Chronic pain acceptance questionnaire (CPAQ)	CPAQ Full: 0–120, lower is less acceptance CPAQ-12: 0–48	Two subscales for activity engagement and pain willingness despite having a chronic pain condition
Patient Health Questionnaire—(PHQ-9)	The PHQ-9 consists of nine items with a potential score range of 0 to 27, with higher scores indicating elevated depressive symptoms	Degree of depressive symptoms
Pain Anxiety Symptom Scale (PASS-20)	0 to 100, with higher scores indicating elevated symptoms of pain-related anxiety	Degree of pain-related anxiety symptoms for individuals with pain disorders
Pain Self Efficacy Short Form PSES-2	PSES- 0-12, <5 is low self-efficacy for pain self-management	Degree of self-efficacy beliefs in the context of pain
OSPRO-YF (Yellow Flag) Assessment Tool	136-item bank was used to develop the OSPRO-YF for patients with chronic MSK	17-item questionnaire with mood, fear avoidance, and positive coping/affect domain to demonstrate pain vulnerability or resilience

For example, a positive mood and distraction can close the gate and reduce the pain signal to the brain, whereas depression and worry about pain can open the gate and send more pain signals to the brain. This gate control theory has been investigated and verified in neurophysiological and brain imaging studies. So far, multiple psychosocial and lifestyle factors have been identified to modulate pain signals and affect pain-related disability. Subsequently, the goal of pain psychology evaluation is to identify pain-modulating psychosocial factors and ultimately to help patients (a) develop and use optimal pain management strategy, (b) restore and maintain optimal function, and (c) live quality life. Health psychologists can help a medical team formulate an individualized, comprehensive treatment plan based on the biopsychosocial model of chronic pain.

Biopsychosocial Assessment

Pain psychology evaluation focuses on biopsychosocial factors affecting pain and disability so the evaluation is commonly called biopsychosocial assessment. The biopsychosocial model of pain was first presented in 1977 as the reductionistic biomedical model was limited in treating a disease [29].

Specifically, the biomedical model is limited in that the objective disease grades based on MRI findings have no relationship with pain intensity and disability [30–35].

In addition, a controlled clinical trial has demonstrated no significant differences between the outcomes after placebo and the standard medical procedures (i.e., arthroscopic lavage or arthroscopic debridement) for knee osteoarthritis [36].

Cumulative evidence has indicated that placebo treatment can improve disease symptoms and reduce pain and that opioid and dopaminergic systems are the mechanisms underlying placebo analgesia [37–41].

The biopsychosocial model embraces a systematic approach, which includes biological (e.g., organ systems, tissues, and cells), personal (e.g., experience and behavior), and social factors (e.g., family, coworkers, and culture) to treat a person with a disease [42, 43].

Over time, more clinicians and researchers have accepted this model and further investigated its clinical implications [9, 44–46].

The next section will explain psychosocial factors influencing musculoskeletal pain and pain-related disability and introduce measures assessing the relevant biopsychosocial factors.

Assessment of Psychological Factors

Depression is one of the most common and critical psychological factors that a clinician should assess initially and ongoingly in treating people with musculoskeletal pain. The prevalence rate of major depressive disorder (MDD) is up to 57.1% of people with back pain or fibromyalgia, which is higher than 4.7% of people with any chronic health conditions and up to 10.4% of the general population [47–51].

More severe depression symptoms are associated with greater pain intensity, more disability, more opioid medications, and poorer quality of life [52–63].

Patients who report high levels of depression prior to an intervention report no or little improvement in pain and function after a surgery or a procedure [64–66].

Therefore, assessment of depression should be a standard practice in treating musculoskeletal pain. Patients may develop symptoms of low mood, tearfulness, and feelings of hopelessness within 3 months of the onset of chronic pain. These mild depression symptoms can influence the daily function and adjustment of people with musculoskeletal pain. Lower levels of mood symptoms in adjustment disorders can be improved after surgery and reduce pain symptoms [67].

Furthermore, chronic pain has long been identified as a risk factor for suicide, and untreated depression increases the risk for *suicide* [68–71].

It is estimated that people with chronic pain are three times more likely to have suicidal ideation than people without chronic pain [69].

More important to clinicians, about 5–24% of patients with chronic pain report having suicidal ideation when visiting outpatient pain clinics [69].

The prevalence rates of current and lifetime suicidal attempts in patients with chronic pain are 5% and 15%, respectively [69, 72], and 2% die by suicide [72].

Greater suicidality is associated with higher pain intensity [73, 74] but also with hopelessness and helplessness about chronic pain, pain catastrophizing [70], perceived burdensomeness to caregivers [75], and low sense of belongingness [72, 76, 77].

Other risk factors for suicide include a previous suicide attempt, female gender, and comorbid insomnia [78]. Unrecognized and untreated depression is associated with not only poor treatment outcomes [64–66] and higher medical costs [79] but also with loss of life by suicide [72].

To assess the DSM-5 diagnostic criteria for psychiatric symptoms, the Structured Clinical Interview for DSM-5: Clinical Version (SCID-5) can be used [80].

The SCID-5 MDD module can be administered to determine whether someone has significant depression symptoms that meet the diagnostic criteria. A clinician conducts a clinical interview to go over the lifetime and current depression symptoms. Similar to the SCID-5, the Mini International Neuropsychiatric Interview (MINI) [81] and Composite International Diagnostic Interview (CIDI) [82] can be used to assess comprehensive psychiatric symptoms listed in ICD-10 and DSM-5.

In order to assess depression symptoms, clinicians do not need to administer all modules in the SCID-5, MINI, and CIDI. Only the depression module can be administered.

There are several brief questionnaires to assess depression symptoms: The Patient Health Questionnaire (PHQ) [82–85], Center for Epidemiological Studies-Depression Scale (CES-D), [86–88] Hospital Anxiety and Depression Scale (HADS) [89, 90], Depression Anxiety and Stress Scale (DASS-21) [91], Symptom Checklist-90 (SCL-90) [92, 93], and Beck Depression Inventory (BDI) [94, 95].

Except the BDI, all measures are in the public domain. The PHQ has 9-item and 2-item versions. The 2-item PHQ is commonly used for a brief screening. The CES-D is another widely used measure, and there are 20-item and 10-item versions. The HADS, DASS-21, and SCL-90 assess depression and anxiety symptoms. To assess depression, a clinician can use a depression scale only. Finally, the Patient-Reported Outcomes Measurement Information System (PROMIS)®-Depression is an extensively validated measure to assess depression in various clinical samples. PROMIS-depression is available free of charge. The PROMIS-Depression can be administered in a paper format and there are the 4, 6, and 8-item short forms. Additionally, the PROMIS-Depression item bank can be administered in a computer adaptive testing (CAT) format. CAT administration method has the advantage of calculating a precise symptom score with a minimum number of items, and therefore reduced patient burden [96].

The PROMIS-depression has normalized T-scores. A T-score of 50 (SD = 10) represents the mean score of the US population.

To assess suicide risk, clinicians can use the Beck Scale for Suicide Ideation (BSS) [97, 98], Columbia–Suicide Severity Rating Scale (C-SSRS) [99, 100], and the Suicide Ideation and Behavior Assessment Tool (SIBAT). [101]

The BSS assesses suicidal thoughts, behaviors, and plans during the past week. The C-SSRS assesses the recent and lifetime suicide risk. The SIBAT assesses suicidal ideation and behaviors. Different from the BSS and C-SSRS, the SIBAT is computer-administered and completed by both patients and clinicians [101].

Anxiety is another common psychological symptom in patients with musculoskeletal pain. About 25–35% of people with chronic pain report any anxiety disorders, whereas 17% of the general population report any anxiety disorders [102, 103].

The common anxiety disorders are generalized anxiety disorder (GAD), panic disorder, and post-traumatic stress disorder (PTSD) [102, 104, 105].

Most anxiety disorders (77%) appear to present prior to the onset of chronic pain [102].

However, some musculoskeletal pain condition starts after musculoskeletal injuries or trauma such as a car accident [106], surgery [107], physical assault, and combat [108, 109].

About 11.2% develop any type of anxiety disorder [107], and 26.6% develop PTSD symptoms after musculoskeletal injuries [110].

Anxiety symptoms are associated with worse pain intensity, and the presence of more than one psychiatric disorder is associated with an increased risk of disability in patients with chronic pain [104].

Some anxiety symptoms are specific to pain conditions, such as fear of pain and pain/fear avoidance [111–113].

The pain-fear relationship has received high research and clinical interest for many decades. Fear about pain is thought to originate from fear of experiencing pain or fear of having an injury [114, 115].

Naturally, human beings have negative appraisal of pain and people usually attempt to avoid pain and fear-provoking behaviors. Although fear of pain is expected to a certain degree, high levels of fear may be problematic. For example, if someone has pain after a car accident, they may become hypervigilant about driving, riding a car, or even seeing a car. Subsequently, they may avoid such fear-provoking behaviors. Unfortunately, people experience pain after basic activities like walking, sitting, and eating so fear avoidance behavior can lead to disuse of the body, deconditioning, disability, and depression.

The generalized anxiety disorder (GAD) is a commonly used survey to assess anxiety symptoms and the GAD has the 7-item and 2-item versions [116–118].

Other anxiety measures include the State-Trait Anxiety Inventory, [119] Beck Anxiety Inventory [120], and PROMIS-Anxiety [121, 122]. Additionally, anxiety symptoms can be assessed using the anxiety subscale of HADS [89, 90], DASS-21 [91], and SCL-90 [92, 93].

To assess anxiety symptoms related to pain, the pain anxiety symptoms scale [123, 124] and fear of pain [125, 126] can be used to assess pain-related anxiety symptoms.

The Tampa Scale for Kinesiophobia [127, 128] can be used to assess fear of painful movements.

In addition to depression and anxiety, *Somatic Symptoms and Related Disorders* are common psychological disorders in patients with musculoskeletal pain. Somatic symptom disorder is diagnosed when one or more distressing somatic symptoms significantly disrupt daily life for at least 6 months and excessive thoughts, feelings, or behaviors related to the somatic symptoms or health concerns are present [129].

Specifically, patients may perceive their pain condition as being more serious than their symptom, have high levels of anxiety related to the somatic symptom or health, or spend excessive time and energy on health concerns. The prevalence rate of somatic symptom disorder is unknown in patients with musculoskeletal pain, but one study has compared somatization severity scores in patients with temporomandibular disorder (TMD) sub-diagnoses myalgia, myofascial pain with referral, and fibromyalgia. Among these pain conditions, somatization tendency scores are higher in patients with fibromyalgia than patients with myofascial pain and, then, TMD myalgia [130].

More somatic symptoms are associated with more medical services, greater pain catastrophizing [131], more disability, higher pain ratings, poor quality of life, and reduced likelihood of returning to work [132].

Other related disorders are illness anxiety disorder, conversion disorder, factitious disorder, and malingering. Illness anxiety disorder is characterized by a "preoccupation" with having or acquiring a serious illness. People with an illness anxiety disorder may seek more (care-seeking type) or avoid medical care (care-avoidant type) [129].

Identification of conversion disorder in chronic pain is difficult, and we do not have a reliable diagnostic tool for conversion disorder. Previously, conversion disorder was called functional neurological symptom disorder, and it is diagnosed when one or more symptoms of altered voluntary motor or sensory function and such symptoms are not compatible with known neurological and medical conditions. While its direct relationship with pain conditions is unknown, psychological profiles are found to be similar between patients with complex regional pain syndrome and conversion disorder.

Additionally, some symptoms of conversion disorders like chronic fatigue syndrome and psychogenic nonepileptic seizures can coexist in patients with musculoskeletal pain [133].

The person with conversion disorder is likely to have poor insight into somatic symptoms [134, 135], so clinicians may need to obtain information from family members.

Multidisciplinary team assessment and review of all subjective and objective biopsychosocial data are also needed to diagnose someone with conversion disorder. Different from the abovementioned somatic symptoms, factitious and malingering are the two somatic symptom disorders that are involved in the conscious and effortful process of symptom presentation. The aim of the former condition is to assume the sick role, and the latter is to obtain secondary gain (e.g., sick leave and money) [129].

Somatization tendency and health-related anxiety can be measured with the PHQ-15 somatization module [136], SCL-90-R somatization subscale [137], Pennebaker Inventory of Limbic Languidness [138], Whiteley-7 scale [139], and Health Anxiety Inventory [140, 141].

Currently, no measures are available to assess conversion disorder, factitious disorder, and malingering.

Next, *personality disorders* are relevant psychological factors in people with musculoskeletal pain. Up to 65.5% of patients with musculoskeletal pain [142] have some type of personality disorder [143, 144].

The common personality disorders are borderline, histrionic, obsessive-compulsive, and avoidant or dependent personality disorders, of which prevalence rates are wide-ranging (5–71%) [143, 144, 145].

According to the Diagnostic and Statistical Manual of Mental Disorders Fifth Edition (DSM-5), borderline personality disorder refers to a pattern of *instability in interpersonal relationships, self-image, and affects, and marked impulsivity*. Histrionic personality disorder is described as a pattern of *excessive emotionality and attention seeking*, and obsessive-compulsive personality disorder is described as a pattern of *preoccupation with orderliness, perfectionism, and control*. Avoidant and dependent personality disorders are a pattern of *social inhibition, feelings of inadequacy, and hypersensitivity to negative evaluation*, and a pattern of *submissive and clinging behavior related to an excessive need to be taken care of*, respectively.

Personality disorders affect the patient-physician interactions. The treating physician needs to understand each personality disorder and have effective interpersonal skills to maintain a therapeutic alliance with patients with personality disorders [146, 147].

Especially when a patient with borderline personality disorder repeatedly reports suicide ideation and presents non-life-threatening self-harming behaviors, clinicians may address personality-related issues in parallel with or even prior to the treatments for chronic pain [148].

To date, similar to mood disorders, personality disorders are associated with worse pain at present [149] and after surgery [150].

Evidence has been inconsistent supporting a link between personality disorders and disability [1, 151–153].

The Minnesota Multiphasic Personality Inventory-2 (MMPI-2) [154] and Personality Assessment Inventory (PAI) [155] are the two major instruments used to assess a wide range of personality traits.

The MMPI-2 and PAI are well-validated, reliable, and widely used instruments. However, the former with 567 questions takes 60–90 minutes and the latter with 344 items takes about 60 minutes to complete. Brief instruments are available to assess borderline personality features: the McLean Screening Instrument for Borderline Personality Disorder [156], Borderline Personality Questionnaire [157], Borderline Symptom List [158, 159], and Zanarini Rating Scale for Borderline Personality Disorder [156, 160].

The Pathological Obsessive-Compulsive Personality Scale [161, 162] and the SCL-90 subscale [163] can be used to assess the Obsessive-Compulsive Personality Disorder trait.

Cognitive function should be assessed routinely as cognitive impairment is commonly observed in patients with musculoskeletal pain [164–166].

Cognitive function can be defined as "*brain's acquisition, processing, storage, and retrieval of information*" [167].

Among patients with chronic pain, cognitive impairment has been observed in attention and executive function (working memory, verbal memory, mental flexibility, inhibition, and processing speed) [168–170].

Attention is the ability to selectively process relevant information and working memory is the ability to retain task-relevant information while performing a task [141, 171].

Pain contributes to cognitive impairment [165, 172–174], but other factors (medications [175–177], substances [178–180], and emotional distress) [174, 181, 182] may also contribute to cognitive impairment in patients with pain.

Assessment of cognitive function is critical, especially for elderly patients. Higher pain, more painful sites, and greater pain interference are associated with reduced cognitive function in this elderly population [183–185] and increased risk of dementia [186–188].

It is critical to identify and treat cognitive impairment and dementia as early as possible. Patients' perceived changes in cognitive function are not always consistent with objective cognitive measures [189–191].

A clinician may ask both patients and their partners about symptoms related to cognitive decline [192, 193] or administer a screening tool (e.g., the mini-mental state examination [MINI] [194] and the Montreal cognitive assessment [MoCA]) [195].

If suspecting mild cognitive impairment, a clinician should consider a neurology or neuropsychology consultation for brain imaging, neurological exams, and neuropsychological testing to have an in-depth assessment of neurocognitive functioning. The NIH toolbox is also freely available to researchers and clinicians to assess cognitive function [196, 197].

Pain coping is cognitive and behavioral strategies to manage pain and its impact. Pain coping can be classified into active and passive coping [198].

Active coping is an "approaching" strategy to manage pain and maintain function, whereas passive coping is an "avoiding" strategy to withdraw and give up activities causing pain. The most frequently used coping strategies are medications (72–78%), followed by exercise (33–35%), cognitive strategy (31–37%), religious activities (18–21%), pacing (15%), or hot/cold modalities (13%) [199, 200].

Other coping strategies include activity engagement despite pain, coping statements, distraction/diverting attention, catastrophizing, ignoring pain, and praying [201, 202].

Exercising, engaging in activity, pacing, and coping statements are active coping, whereas medication, hot/cold modalities, catastrophizing, and ignoring pain are passive coping. Passive coping predicts worse pain, function, and disability [203–207].

Especially, pain catastrophizing has been extensively studied for its relationship with adverse pain-related outcomes. Pain catastrophizing is defined as rumination on pain, magnification of pain, and helplessness about pain [208].

Evidence consistently supports that pain catastrophizing predicts worse pain and disability concurrently [201, 209–211] and prospectively [207, 212–214].

In contrast, active coping predicts less pain and disability [215–218].

Pain self-efficacy is another active and adaptive pain coping strategy [219–221].

Pain self-efficacy is perceived as one's ability and confidence to engage in activities despite pain [189, 220].

Coping strategies can also be classified into (a) problem-focused, (b) emotion-focused coping, and (c) seeking social resources [222].

Problem-focused coping aims to control or change pain and emotion-focused coping aims to manage emotional responses to pain [198].

Both coping strategies can be adaptive when they are used appropriately. Generally, problem-solving and active coping strategies are considered adaptive, but putting substantial efforts into using multiple problem-focused strategies to achieve a goal of "pain free" may be maladaptive. Unfortunately, curative treatment options may be limited for some pain conditions, so emotion-focused coping with acceptance [222–224], mindfulness [225–230], and distress tolerance skills may help reduce emotional distress in people living with chronic pain.

Emotion-focused coping is alternatively called an adaptation of goals [222] and accommodative coping [231].

When there is no curative solution, we need to accept and embrace the situation and then, we set up achievable goals in living with chronic pain [231].

When needing additional resources in coping with pain, individuals may seek social resources and support [222].

The pain catastrophizing scale (PCS) is the most widely used measure to assess pain-related thoughts and feelings [208].

Other pain coping measures are the chronic pain acceptance questionnaire [232, 233], chronic pain coping inventory [234, 235], coping strategies questionnaire [236], pain coping questionnaire [237], psychological inflexibility in pain scale [238], survey of pain attitudes [239], and worry about pain questionnaire [240].

The pain resilience scale has also been developed to assess the tendency to use adaptive, active pain coping strategies (e.g., I still work to accomplish my goals) [241].

Pain behaviors have been explained by *operant conditioning, positive or negative reinforcement*. Pain behaviors refer to behavioral, verbal, and facial expressions in responding to pain, such as avoiding activity, guarding, moaning, and grimacing [242].

Pain behaviors are considered adaptive for acute pain but maladaptive and dysfunctional for persistent pain in the absence of tissue damage [242, 243].

In the context of acute pain associated with tissue damage, pain as a threat signal motivates people to protect the injured tissue and avoid activity. Here, pain provides a strong negative reinforcement of activity avoidance [244–246].

When people experience persistent pain after the damaged tissues are healed, activity avoidance and fear of pain lead to deconditioning, disability [247, 248], and pain hypersensitivity [249, 250].

A study on people with chronic low back pain has demonstrated that brain responses to imagined strenuous exercise are not significantly different between pain-free individuals and patients with high fear avoidance, whose brain responses are significantly different from those of patients with low fear avoidance [251].

In other words, only the low fear avoidance group shows less activation of the hippocampus. This result suggests that pain is unconditioned fearful and adverse stimuli and fear avoidance is a natural, default response. People with chronic pain may need to develop and learn strategies to break the default association, which is no longer adaptive for chronic pain. The PROMIS pain behavior measure is available to assess the degree of pain behaviors in patients with chronic pain conditions [252].

Finally, *lifestyle factors* associated with musculoskeletal pain are physical activity, sleep, diet, and substance use [253].

Low physical activity is a well-known risk factor for musculoskeletal pain. A sedentary lifestyle (e.g., prolonged sitting, TV watching, and computer use) is associated with an increased risk of musculoskeletal pain [253–256].

On the other hand, a longitudinal study has found that compared to inactive people (no exercise), active people (i.e., hard physical activity at least 2 hours per week) are 35% less likely to have chronic widespread at baseline and that those who have increased physical activity are 28% less likely to have chronic widespread pain 11 years later [257].

Chronotype is another activity factor associated with musculoskeletal pain. Chronotype is the individual timing of sleep-wake rhythms [258].

A study reports that about 43% of people are highly active in the morning (morning type), and 13% are active in the evening (evening type) [259].

Birth cohort study has found that the evening type is associated with a higher likelihood of having disabling pain in adults [258] and a much-worsened quality of life [259].

People with fibromyalgia who sleep later time report more perceived stress, memory problems, fatigue, and depression symptoms than those who sleep early [260].

Sleep disturbance is also critical for chronic pain and insomnia, and pain has a bidirectional relationship [261–263].

A 3-year prospective study observed that more adults with widespread pain (48.7%) developed insomnia symptoms than pain-free adults (20.3%) [264].

Another prospective study reported insomnia increased the risk of developing fibromyalgia by 3.1 times over an 11-year observation period. Despite this known bidirectional relationship, a few studies noted that the impact of insomnia on pain ($b = 0.24$) was greater than the other way around ($b = 0.09$) [262].

The same pattern was observed in a treatment study for musculoskeletal pain. Greater sleep disturbance 3 months after treatment predicted higher pain at 12 months post-treatment ($b = 0.29$), and the opposition prediction (pain as a predictor for insomnia) was less strong ($b = 0.15$) [263].

Physical activity and sleep can be assessed with objective and self-report measures. Objective measures for physical activity and sleep are wearable devices (e.g., ActiGraph [263, 265]), smartphone applications [266], polysomnography [267], and sleep sensors [268, 269].

Self-report measures to assess physical activities are the PROMIS-Physical Function [270, 271], Baecke Physical Activity Questionnaire [272–274], and International Physical Activity Questionnaire [275].

Diet and substance use can be lifestyle factors, but also pain coping. Certain types of nutrition and diet may affect inflammatory responses and oxidative stress conditions. Vegetables, fruits (e.g., citrus and blueberries), healthy oils (e.g., olive oil and fish oil), plant-based proteins, and fibers can reduce inflammatory and oxidative stress actions, whereas excessive intake of sugar, meat-based protein, and fat can enhance inflammatory action [276, 277].

Diet intervention studies have demonstrated to be effective in lowering pain. One study on people with chronic musculoskeletal pain has shown on average 3.1 point reduction of pain ratings on a 0–10 scale after an 8-week plant-based diet program [278].

Another study has shown that a 1-month low glutamate diet (less meats, less monosodium glutamate) reduces pain intensity and fatigue in Gulf War illness, which is characterized as widespread chronic pain, fatigue, and gastrointestinal problems [279].

To cope with pain and stress, people with musculoskeletal pain may have emotional eating patterns (also known as stress-induced eating). In exposure to a stressor, the two major stress systems (sympathetic-adrenal modulatory and hypothalamic-pituitary-adrenal axes) are activated and then, may alter appetite and eating. Specifically, the release of noradrenaline and corticotropin-releasing hormone suppresses appetite during acute stress and the release of cortisol stimulates appetite during recovery from stress [280].

In general population, about 20.5% endorse emotional eating often or very often and they frequently eat fast food. It is found younger age and impatience are associated with a greater likelihood of having emotional eating habits [281].

People with chronic pain appear to prefer high-calorie foods and have overeating habits [282, 283].

Emotional eating can be assessed with the Dutch Eating Behavior Questionnaire [284], Emotional Appetite Questionnaire [285], Emotional Eating Scale [286], Three-Factor Eating Questionnaire [287, 288], and Yale Emotional Overeating Questionnaire [289].

A referral to a dietician consult and psychotherapy for stress management may be indicated for patients who are interested in learning diet management for pain and adaptive coping skills for pain and stress.

Caffeine, alcohol, marijuana, and nicotine are common substances that US adults use in daily life. Over 74.7% of US adults drink caffeinated coffee daily. About 3.4 million American adults (18.8%) drink three or more caffeinated coffee daily [290].

Caffeine consumption is known to have some health benefits [290] and indeed, caffeine is used as an active ingredient of over-the-counter pain medication.

However, excessive or evening intake of caffeine (e.g., coffee, chocolate, and soda) can result in insomnia, especially in the elderly [291].

Notably, caffeine half-life for healthy individuals is 4–6 hours, with a shorter half-life in smokers and a longer half-life in people with chronic liver disease or pregnant women [292–294].

Therefore, limiting caffeine intake is recommended for sleep.

According to a national survey of US adults in 2020, 54.2% reported drinking alcohol (18.3% had heavy drinking episodes), 50.8% reported marijuana use, and 20.6% reported cigarette use in the past months [295].

The 2020 national survey revealed that about 21.4% reported any illicit drug use in the past year. Marijuana was the most common (17.9%), followed by prescription pain medication (3.3%), hallucinogens (2.6%), sedative misuse (2.2%, Benzodiazepine 1.7%), cocaine (1.9%), prescription stimulant misuse (1.8%), methamphetamine (0.9%), and heroin (0.2%). Several measures are available to screen substance use: the Alcohol, Smoking, and Substance Involvement Screening Test (ASSIST) [296], Drug Abuse Screening Test (DAST), Tobacco, Alcohol, Prescription Medication, and Other Substance Use (TAPS) [297], Screening to Brief Intervention (S2BI) [298, 299], and Alcohol Use Disorders Identification (AUDIT).

For people taking opioid pain medications, clinicians need to assess opioid misuse periodically. Prescription opioid misuse measures include the Current Opioid Misuse Measure (COMM) [300], the Pain Medication Questionnaire (PMQ) [301], and the PROMIS-Misuse of Prescription Pain Mediation [302, 303].

To assess the risk of developing aberrant opioid use behaviors prior to the start of opioid medications, clinicians can use the Screener to Predict Opioid Misuse-Revised (SOAPP-R) [206] and the revised opioid risk tool (ORT) [304].

In addition to surveys, objective measures such as urine drug screen and a prescription drug-monitoring program are currently utilized to ensure the safety of patients taking controlled substance prescriptions.

Assessment of Social Factors

Patients with chronic pain can experience *life stressors*. Life stressors are not limited to traumatic life events causing PTSD and encompass any type of life stressors and minor daily hassles affecting individuals' health and well-being. Stressful life events during childhood [305, 306] and adulthood [307] are risk factors for developing musculoskeletal pain such as fibromyalgia and widespread body pain.

A birth cohort study has revealed that adverse experiences such as maternal separation, institutional care, general family difficulties (parents' divorce or desertion), a family member with alcoholism, and financial difficulties before age 7 are associated with an increased risk of chronic widespread pain in middle-aged adults [306].

Adults' cumulative stressors or certain life events such as separation from partners, serious financial problems, and workplace violence are also associated with an increased risk of musculoskeletal pain [307–310].

Of patients with musculoskeletal pain, more adverse life events and daily hassles are associated with greater emotional distress (depression and anxiety), poor quality of life, more fatigue, and worse pain-related outcomes (pain interference, pain catastrophizing, and low pain self-efficacy) [311–314].

When assessing life stressors, *current* safety-related stressors should be paid extra attention. Safety-related stressors such as intimate partner violence, abuse of children, older adults, and dependent adults, and homicidal ideation may require immediate actions, which include a report to the police, emergency hospitalization, or consultation with a social worker. Assessment of *lifetime* trauma and interpersonal violence is also important because life traumas shape one's view of self, others, and the world. Patients who have conflicted relationships with most people in their life or with a primary caregiver may have difficulty with trusting a clinician. Empirical data show that the patient-physician relationship and trust predict the treatment outcome in patients with fibromyalgia [315] and chronic low back pain [316].

Additionally, clinicians need to assess trauma history to avoid re-traumatization and establish safety within healthcare encounters [317–319].

Individual coping strategies [320, 321], social support [314, 321, 322], and partner's coping strategy [323] can mitigate the impact of life stressors on health.

The following measures can be used to assess life stressors: The Adverse Childhood Experiences [324], Childhood Trauma Questionnaire [325], Elders Life Stress Inventory [326], Perceived Stress Scale [327], Stressful Life Event Questionnaire [328], Daily Stress Inventory [329], Daily Hassles Scale-Revised [330], and Traumatic Life Events Questionnaire [331].

Although these life stress measures are lengthy (10 or more items) and not practical at a busy outpatient clinic, clinicians who are particularly working with vulnerable populations may need to assess and address childhood and ongoing adulthood stressors in treating people with musculoskeletal pain conditions.

Social isolation, stigma, and perceived family burden are important social factors. Among these social factors, *social isolation* and loneliness have long been identified as a critical factor influencing the health and well-being of human beings and specifically patients with musculoskeletal pain. As noted earlier, reaching out to social support is one of the coping strategies for chronic pain [222].

A national cohort study has revealed that people with musculoskeletal pain reach out to their social support and are less likely to experience social isolation, but more likely to experience loneliness compared to people without it [332].

Of people with chronic pain, social isolation predicts greater pain interference [333, 334] and more depression symptoms [334].

Older adults with chronic musculoskeletal pain are particularly vulnerable to social isolation and they report having insufficient social support and feeling more lonely [335]. The PROMIS-Social Isolation [336], Social Isolation Scale [337], Social Provisions Scale [338, 339], Social Connectedness and Social Assurance Scales [340], UCLA Loneliness Scale [341], and Loneliness Questionnaire [342] are available to assess social isolation, loneliness, perceived social connectedness, and social supports.

Stigma is "a mark of shame, disgrace or disapproval that results in an individual being rejected, discriminated against and excluded from participating in a number of different areas of society" [343].

Patients with chronic pain report being dismissed, blamed, or misled by a romantic partner, relatives, friends, and healthcare providers [344].

During healthcare encounters, patients perceive that healthcare providers think their pain is exaggerated or imagined and that colleagues are hostile against them at work [344].

Stigma around sexual differences in pain is a well-known problem. Women's pain is viewed as being just more sensitive to pain, being related to hysteria, and fitting more into medically unexplained conditions [345].

Some evidence indicate that higher levels of perceived stigma and unfairness are associated with poor physical health [346, 347] and mental health in patients with chronic pain [348].

Perceived stigma is a barrier to treatment so clinicians need to pay attention to the levels of perceived stigma and its impact on patients' health and treatment engagement.

Identity threat is a concept related to stigma. Identity threat theory has been introduced to understand whether minority students are adversely impacted in their academic performance by perceived *stereotype threat* in school [349].

This theory explains that *stereotype threat* imposes a limitation on one's performance. In the case of math performance, women are stereotyped to have lower math ability so women perceive a threat when they are put in a situation to demonstrate their math ability. Subsequently, women perform worse than men as being stereotyped [349].

This identity threat theory has been applied to health matters [350–354].

In the context of chronic pain, studies have examined illness-related identity threats at work and gender identity in intimate relationships. Perceived threat at work is predicted by less boundary flexibility, lower levels of job self-efficacy, and more perceived devaluation of their work in people with chronic health conditions, including pain [352].

Greater perceived threat at work is associated with greater job-related strain and reduced work ability. Men and women with chronic pain perceive themselves as being less masculine and feminine so they have less positive sense of self as being men or women [355] and worry about not meeting their partner's needs [356].

The three-stage model of adjustment of chronic pain has been proposed [357].

Stage I focuses on returning to their former lifestyle, followed by a focusing on making changes to adjust their life and identity (Stage II) and establishing the new course of life with adjusted social roles and self-image (Stage III) [357].

This model explains that improving adjustment to and living well with chronic pain conditions may require changes in lifestyle, social role, and identity.

Pain conditions create a burden for the family when a family member with pain is limited in his or her ability to do daily roles (e.g., bringing household income, managing household chores, dropping off and picking up a child at school, and completing self-care activities independently). It is found that more than 70% of patients perceive an increase in burden on their family members [358].

Patients' *perceived burden* on the family is positively associated with their symptom burdens (pain intensity, pain duration, general health, functional limitation, and depression symptom) and caregiver burden [358, 359].

Perceived burden is linked to a safety issue. Those who perceive themselves as being a burden report having suicidal ideation [75, 358–360].

Patients are at *high risk of suicide* when they endorse a perceived burden ("I am a burden") in combination with social isolation ("I don't belong anywhere") and the capability of suicide with lethal methods ("I have a gun") [361].

A protective factor against perceived burden is understandably pain self-efficacy [358].

The patient's perceived burden can be assessed using the Self-Perceived Burden Scale [358, 362].

Several social determinants of musculoskeletal pain conditions need to be assessed in treating patients with musculoskeletal pain. It has been estimated that socioeconomic status (SES) factors account for 40% of the health and recovery of patients with musculoskeletal impairments, followed by behavioral patterns (30%), medical care (20%), and environmental factors (10%) [363, 364].

A systematic review concludes low SES (income, education, job status, and house ownership) is a social risk factor for poor low back pain outcomes [365].

Generally, social determinants of musculoskeletal pain conditions are not easily addressable, but healthcare providers should be aware of them and their impact on health outcomes. People with low SES may not have access to the best available or even minimum pain care [366].

Clinicians may need to help patients with low SES connect with a social worker and additional or alternative resources.

Assessment for Invasive Medical Procedure

Biopsychosocial assessment is recommended to avoid negative consequences of invasive medical procedures (e.g., surgery, spinal cord stimulation [SCS] [367, 368], neural engineering [369, 370], as well as to optimize the outcomes [371]).

Assessment for invasive medical procedures generally focuses on patients' (a) understanding of a planned procedure, risks, and benefits, expected outcomes, aftercare activity (short-term and long-term), (b) readiness to make behavioral and lifestyle modifications if any (e.g., change in occupation), and (c) coping ability for potential negative consequences [372].

Personal, cultural, and religious belief is also an important variable to assess. Some patients with body dysphoria may not be okay with having a foreign SCS material on the body surface. Electric medical devices may not be acceptable in some cultures (e.g., Amish). Additionally, abovementioned psychosocial factors may impact the outcomes [372–374].

Psychosocial factors can be classified into three categories: Contraindication, risk factor, and positive factor. The psychiatric contraindications for SCS are unresolved major psychiatric disorders, active or untreated substance use disorder, and inability to understand and manage the devices [372, 375].

The risk factors for poor outcomes are smoking [376], high BMI ($\geq$36.5) [377], pending litigation [373], and psychological factors (depression, anxiety, somatization, and poor coping) [378].

Contraindications generally make people ineligible for SCS, but some contraindications like active PTSD and suicidality can be treated and SCS can be reconsidered after psychiatric treatments. Risk factors can be addressed prior to and in parallel with the procedure to optimize the treatment outcomes. Positive factors such as younger age, [379, 380], strong social support [373], and effective coping strategy [381, 382] may reduce the impact of risk factors on treatment outcomes [374].

When recommending invasive medical procedures, clinicians also recommend patients engage in interdisciplinary treatment for musculoskeletal pain to optimize patients' pain care, function, and quality of life.

Interdisciplinary Treatment

Medical Pre-IPRP Medical Treatment Planning

The assessment strategies described above are critical for establishing the foundation of an interdisciplinary care plan. That plan will integrate the patient's understanding of the cause of their pain and the reasons for pursuing a rehabilitatively focused treatment. It will include some level of patient acceptance of their pain being inevitable but their suffering is optional and through a rehabilitative care plan, they will be able to pursue a return to the most normal activity possible. The care plan should be careful to avoid specific surgical and interventional treatment, which will risk distracting the patient from developing their own internal locus of control over their pain. Often when patients look to a particular intervention as a part of the treatment plan this intervention will erode their self-efficacy by having them look to the therapeutic response rather than their own learning and behavior as the most important elements in the care plan.

Medication treatment can be continued through the interdisciplinary plan and a focus that allows "optimization of medication" aligned with rehabilitative achievements is appropriate as it does not threaten the internal locus of control so long as the medication is used optimally. Some interdisciplinary care plans actually include the reduction of medication, especially dependence-producing medications like opioids or benzodiazepines as the regular conversation about the risk and benefits of these dependence-producing therapies can be helpful in aligning the patient in health-oriented goals to minimize medications.

Topical

Topical pain medications are local analgesics that are applied to the skin or mucous membranes to achieve pain relief through acting on the underlying soft tissue and peripheral nerve endings. They can reduce or block the induction and transmission of pain signals to the central nervous system (CNS) [383].

The formulations of topical pain medications include solutions, ointments, creams, gels, foams, sprays, patches, or plaster [14].

The three most commonly used topical pain medications are local anesthetics, nonsteroidal anti-inflammatory drugs (NSAIDs), and neurolytic substances (e.g., capsaicin). Lidocaine, as the local anesthetic, blocks sodium-gated channels, which is involved in the initiation and maintenance of a variety of pain. Pain models have demonstrated an upregulation of abnormal sodium channels in damaged peripheral sensory nerves [384].

Diclofenac, as one of the NSAID medications, can block cyclooxygenase, which converts arachidonic acid to prostaglandins, and then decrease the sensitization of peripheral nerve endings to histamine, bradykinin, and other inflammatory factors, and makes those nerve endings less likely to transmit pain [385].

Capsaicin is an active ingredient from chili pepper. It eradicates small peptides (e.g., substance P in C fibers) stored in cutaneous nerves, which are involved in pain transmissions from the peripheral nervous system to the central nervous system. Although it can excite the peripheral nerve endings initially, prolonged exposure brings insensitivity to capsaicin as well as other noxious stimuli [386, 387].

Lidocaine patches are FDA approved for postherpetic neuralgia (PHN) [388]; however, in practice, it is often used to manage a variety of painful conditions, such as peripheral neuropathy, post-thoracotomy pain syndrome, postmastectomy pain syndrome, and scar neuroma pain.

The topical diclofenac is useful for both musculoskeletal pain [389] and osteoarthritis [390].

Capsaicin is FDA approved for the treatment of PHN; it is also useful in osteoarthritis and diabetic neuropathy [391, 392].

Systemics—Antidepressant Versus Anticonvulsant Versus Opioid Optimization

Antidepressant

Antidepressants are one of the important analgesics of managing chronic noncancer pain. It is generally accepted that inhibiting the reuptake of serotonin and norepinephrine for antidepressants is the mainstay for analgesia. However, the exact mechanism of action remains unknown [393].

At present, two classes of antidepressants are FDA approved for chronic pain, including tricyclic antidepressants (TCAs) and serotonin-norepinephrine reuptake inhibitors (SNRIs).

The most commonly used TCAs are amitriptyline, nortriptyline, imipramine, and desipramine. Based on the structure, TCA can also be classified [394] as follows:

1. Tertiary amines, which have two methyl groups at the end of the side chain, are widely used in the US for chronic pain management, including amitriptyline and imipramine, Generally, they are potent in inhibiting reuptake of serotonin when compared with norepinephrine.
2. Secondary amines, which have one methyl group at the end of the side chain, include desipramine and nortriptyline for pain control. Desipramine is the active metabolite of imipramine, while nortriptyline is the active metabolite of amitriptyline. Secondary amines are more potent in inhibiting the reuptake of norepinephrine.

In addition to blocking the presynaptic reuptake of serotonin and norepinephrine, TCAs are also believed to act on other targets, including voltage-gated sodium channels, adrenergic α1 and α2 receptors, histamine H1 receptors, and muscarinic receptors, all which have been involved in with increased pain or neuronal hypersensitivity [393].

Tertiary tricyclics are less favored by clinicians because they are more sedating (due to central antihistamine effects) and have more anticholinergic side effects (such as constipation, urinary retention, and blurred vision) when compared with secondary tricyclics. Regardless, TCAs are often associated with multiple side effects due to their broad pharmacologic profiles, which inspire the interest in using other antidepressants with fewer side effects to treat chronic pain [14].

In the 1990s, serotonin-norepinephrine reuptake inhibitors (SNRIs) came on the market, and duloxetine is the first SNRI in the USA to be approved for chronic pain management, followed by venlafaxine, desvenlafaxine, and milnacipran. Like TCAs, they are able to inhibit presynaptic serotonin and norepinephrine intake with equivalent antidepressant and potential equal analgesics proprieties; in contrast to TCAs, they have significantly less alpha-1, cholinergic, and histamine reactions, and consequently much fewer side effects than TCAs. Although SNRIs are more selectively acting on serotonin and norepinephrine, they are also associated with some other adverse reactions. For example, the typical analgesic dosage of venlafaxine is 150 mg to 225 mg/day. However, for dosages more than 150 mg daily, venlafaxine can increase systolic blood pressure by 10 mm or even more, which is likely due to the onset of NE reuptake inhibition [3].

As for selective serotonin reuptake inhibitors (SSRIs), there is little evidence showing independent analgesic activities of SSRIs, although some chronic pain patients with the comorbidity of depression may respond to an SSRI with diminished pain, which is mainly attributed to improvements of the affective components of their pain [395].

Anticonvulsant

Anticonvulsants, aka antiepileptic drugs (AEDs), were originally introduced for treating epilepsy. However, they have been used to treat a variety of chronic pain conditions for a long time. In 1960s, carbamazepine was first anticonvulsant to treat trigeminal neuralgia [396, 397].

Many AEDs have pharmacological effects which can interfere with neuronal hyperexcitability, through modulation of ion channels (sodium, calcium, and potassium channels), augmentation of inhibitory effects (potentiating the inhibitory neurotransmitter gamma-aminobutyric acid [GABA]), and suppression of abnormal neuronal excitability such as inhibition of glutamate receptors or suppression of neurotransmitter release [14, 398, 399].

Through this, anticonvulsants can bring down peripheral and central sensitization along with ectopic activity, which are likely underlying mechanisms of a variety of chronic pain conditions [399].

However, the exact mechanisms by which AEDs manage chronic pain remain unknown.

Anticonvulsants embrace a broad range of medications. Based on their individual structures and mechanisms of action, they could be further subdivided. For example, both gabapentin and pregabalin are GABA analogs with similar structure and mechanism of action. Instead of acting on GABA receptors, both block the alpha-2 subunit of voltage-dependent calcium channels on the neuronal cells of central nervous systems [398–400].

Carbamazepine can block sodium channels to reduce the neuronal excitability and discharge that has been proposed to cause neuropathic pain. Lamotrigine has its effect on sodium channels and also suppresses the neuronal release of glutamate, an excitatory neurotransmitter (NT). Valproic acid works to elevate the level of GABA (an inhibitory neurotransmitter) in the CNS and therefore treats pain that is related to the pathological overexcitation of the nervous system [398, 399].

Three anticonvulsants, including gabapentin, pregabalin, and carbamazepine, are approved by FDA to treat neuropathic pain, whereas many others are used off labeled, such as lamotrigine and valproic acid [400].

Some of pain conditions, which have good responses to anticonvulsants include diabetic neuropathy, postherpetic neuralgia, and HIV-related neuropathic pain.

The common side effects of anticonvulsants include sedation, tiredness, ataxia, vertigo, and even diplopia. Serious skin reactions [401], including Stevens-Johnson syndrome and toxic epidermal necrolysis, are more likely related to carbamazepine and lamotrigine, especially in Asian populations.

Other rare reactions to these medications include bone marrow suppression (aplastic anemia and agranulocytosis) [402]; therefore, monitoring of blood counts is recommended.

On the other hand, drug interactions are very common among anticoagulants, because they are either inducer or inhibitor for liver enzymes involved in medication metabolism. For example, Carbamazepine, can induce its own metabolism and lead to a serum level decrease within the first 3 to 5 weeks after initiation and may require dosage adjustment [403], it also causes a significant reduction in the anticoagulant effect of warfarin [404].

Gabapentin, when co-administered with antacid, can have a moderate decrease in absorption [405].

Opioid Optimization

The role of opioids in managing chronic noncancer pain has been controversial and recently drawn more attention due to an emerging global opioid crisis, especially in the United States [406, 407].

With the increased awareness about risks and harms related to opioids, such as overdose and death [408], actions have been already initiated by policymakers, regulatory entities, and clinicians to overcome the opioid crisis.

In 2016, the Centers for Disease Control and Prevention published the Guideline for Prescribing Opioids for Chronic Pain, which provides recommendations for primary care clinicians who prescribe opioids for chronic pain outside of active cancer treatment, palliative care, and end-of-life care [409].

This guidance is often utilized by policymakers, such as medical boards in different states, in determining the standard of care and defining specific rules for the prescription of opioids for pain. Unfortunately, these actions have resulted in unintended consequences for people living with pain who were using opioids as part of their overall pain management [410].

This illustrates the importance of maintaining access to appropriate and safe use of opioids for patients with chronic pain while balancing benefits and harms. In 2019, the CDC advised against a misapplication of its guidelines for prescribing opioids for chronic pain. Specifically, CDS is raising awareness about misapplication of guidelines to populations outside of scope; setting hard dose limits or "cutting off" opioids; abrupt tapering or sudden discontinuing opioids; misapplication of guidelines to patients receiving medical assisted treatment for opioid use disorder, etc. [409, 411].

Opioids manage pain through acting on mu-, kappa-, and delta-opioid receptors in the central and peripheral nervous systems, inhibiting the nociceptive input and/or the pain perception. Moreover, opioids are classified as pure agonist (e.g., fentanyl, oxycodone, and hydromorphone), mixed agonist-antagonists (e.g., buprenorphine and butorphanol), and mixed-mechanism drugs (e.g., tramadol and tapendol). Opioids also have immediate-release/short-acting (IR/SA) and extended-release/long-acting (ER/LA) preparations. Usually, ER/LA opioids are not indicated for as-needed pain management and should be reserved for severe continuous pain because the risks of overdose and misuse are greater with EA/LA opioids [409].

As for opioid selection, dosing, and titration, the treatment plan should be individualized based on patient's health status, age, and previous experience with opioids (including responses and side effects).

To date, there is no strong evidence supporting long-term efficacy when compared with placebo or non-opioid medications [412–414].

From our perspective, opioids should *only be considered* when nonopioid management fails to provide sufficient pain control and/or patients are unable to tolerate non-opioid approach. For example, nonsteroidal anti-inflammatory drugs (NSAIDs) are not appropriate for patients who have kidney diseases and high bleeding risks; acetaminophen is contraindicated for patients with liver failure. Before starting opioid therapy, risks of opioid overdose and misuse should be always assessed. For patients who have high risks, either avoiding opioid therapy or consulting an addiction medicine specialist to reappraise patients' conditions is strongly recommended. Furthermore, opioid therapy should be always initiated as the trial, with the understanding between prescribers and patients that opioids will be stopped when opioids are unable to achieve the treatment goal (such as reasonable pain relief along corresponding function improvement), or brings more harms than benefits. After a trial of therapy, opioids should be only maintained when both patients and prescribers reach a consensus that continuous therapy is necessary (such as benefits outweigh harms).

When patients are not responsive to maintenance opioid therapy or develop intolerance side effects, opioid-induced hyperalgesia, opioid misuse, diversion or use disorder, or parents request to go off opioids due to a variety of reasons, opioids should be discontinued along with initiation of alternative pain management if indicated. Unless opioids were used for diversion, it is extremely important for prescribers, prior to discontinuing opioids, to develop an appropriate plan to help patients taper off opioids appropriately. Prescribers should keep in mind that even short-term exposure to an opioid could make a patient dependent, and then sudden reduction or discontinuation of opioids, especially for patients who use opioids for a long time, can provoke withdrawal symptoms, which could make tapering-off process more challenging.

Interventional Treatments During Interdisciplinary Rehabilitation

There are six treatment modalities for chronic pain, such as pharmaceuticals, physical and/or occupational therapies, psychological interventions, interventional procedures, surgeries, and a combination of all of aforementioned (i.e., multidisciplinary team approach) [415].

A multidisciplinary team approach places primary focus on pain management (rather than cure) and function improvement (rather than pain alleviation) [416].

In the past 30 years, research has consistently demonstrated the therapeutic superiority of a multidisciplinary approach compared to less comprehensive therapies or single-modality interventions [417].

As a result, the interdisciplinary program reached its peak development in the late 1990s and/or early 2000s.

Unfortunately, due to a variety of reasons, including alternations of reimbursement systems and health insurance regulations, multidisciplinary team approach for pain management hit the skids and had been gradually supplanted by interventional pain management. Nowadays, interventional pain medicine is a thriving subspecialty of pain management that includes a variety of techniques, from the peripheral nerve block, epidural steroid injection, facet injections and medial branch blocks, sympathetic blocks, to different flourishing neuromodulations (peripheral nerve stimulation [PNS], dorsal root ganglion stimulation [DRG], spinal cord stimulation [SCS], and transcranial magnetic stimulation [TMS]). Although some of these procedures are also offered within multidisciplinary treatment clinics, survey data strongly demonstrate that the majority is performed by pain clinics that either only offer short-term consultations or provide IPM as the main therapeutic modality for managing pain [418, 419].

Unfortunately, there is no sufficient data supporting the efficacy of invasive procedures for chronic pain [420].

Meanwhile, other limitations of interventional pain techniques include ephemeral pain relief, risks of complications (sometimes could be serious), no concurrent function improvements, and work returning with pain intensity reduction.

In sum, from our perspective, we recommend using interventional pain management as one part of interdisciplinary treatments so long as the patient is educated to limit the erosion of the internal locus of control necessary to develop long-term self-management.

Surgical Treatment During Interdisciplinary Rehabilitation

Surgical treatment as a general rule should be optimized before planning any interdisciplinary care plan. The enormous transition of self-efficacy from the patient to the surgical procedure predictable disrupts even the best-intended treatment plan. It always requires careful crafting of the messages to help patients understand the meaning of their pain to prevent fear from overwhelming their rehabilitation efforts. Many patients suffering from sustained pain have spent months or even years to look for an elusive cure to relieve most if not all their pain. When all else fails, they become so desperate and oftentimes resort to surgery to ease their pain. In doing so they take the locus of management outside of themselves and place that locus with the surgeon or the procedure as they look to that cure to relieve suffering. Sometimes people with chronic back pain choose spine surgery because they feel it is the fastest or most effective treatment for their pain. Unfortunately, in many with chronic pain unless there is a clear structural issue that leads to chronic pain the resultant postoperative pain is only worse [421].

One of those cases is the phenomenon of "failed back surgery syndrome" or FBSS, which was defined by the International Association for the Study of Pain as "*Lumbar (cervical) spinal pain of unknown origin either persisting despite surgical intervention or appearing after surgical intervention for spinal pain originally in the same topographical location*" [422].

Patients with FBSS have had chronic back pain, with or without referred or radicular symptoms, and with at least one surgical intervention in the past which has failed to treat the pain. With conservative estimates, its prevalence could be up to 40% [423].

In 2005, Rasmussen reported implementation of nonsurgical clinics through multidisciplinary approach in Denmark was able to reduce annual rates of lumbar disk surgery for "sciatica with or without low back pain" to half and the rate of elective, first-time disk surgeries decreased by two-thirds in just 4 years [424].

Even for complex FBBS, which we mentioned above, based on the recent consensus on optimizing management and outcomes of FBBS by a European group, multidisciplinary approach, instead of repeated surgery, is strongly recommended [425].

Physical Therapy Treatment During Interdisciplinary Rehabilitation

Fear of movement, aka high kinesiophobia, has been shown to have a strong association with disability and pain intensity in people with chronic musculoskeletal [426, 427].

When considering fear of movement/kinesiophobia, or addressing fear-avoidance beliefs, it is important to note that exercise and multidisciplinary care have moderate levels of evidence for reducing fear.

Other conservative treatments that are common rehabilitation and may help with pain management such as manual therapy, electrotherapy or taping can be done in pain rehabilitation treatments have low levels of evidence to reduce fear of movement.

Physical therapists within interdisciplinary treatment settings may include exercise-based treatments such as cardiovascular and aerobic training, strength or resistance training, aquatic rehabilitation, alternative movement therapies such as yoga, dance, tai chi, or qi jong. These movement-based interventions listed have shown low-to-moderate treatment effect sizes when compared to placebo, education, or non-movement therapies for chronic musculoskeletal pain, including low back pain [428].

There is emerging evidence on the amount of dosing of exercise intensity, including HIIT exercise, for analgesic benefits that are both short- and long term for people suffering from chronic pain [429–431].

Physical therapists can provide expert guidance for patients to assist with dosing the proper amount of movement and exercise to help those with chronic pain, in addition to offer strategies for flare-up management, which can help decrease a patient's need for opiate pain medication after MSK injuries [432].

Occupational Therapy During Interdisciplinary Rehabilitation

Occupational therapy (OT) brings a specific and unique focus on function to an interdisciplinary pain management team. Occupational therapists are skilled in assessing multiple domains of functionality including activities of daily living (ADLs), instrumental activities of daily living (IADLs), functional mobility, sleep, sexual function, leisure engagement, work performance, and social participation. Many factors contribute to clients' abilities to engage in these daily routines, and objective measurements of physical, cognitive, and psychosocial functioning are considered building blocks for engagement in occupation. Occupational therapists take a holistic approach and consider how environmental, social, physiological, and personal factors influence the lived experience of pain. This information is utilized in collaboration with clients to develop unique self-management strategies with the ultimate goal of optimizing function and participation.

Occupational therapists not only utilize the biopsychosocial model of pain but also occupation-specific frameworks such as the person-environment-occupation performance (PEO) model or the model of human occupation (MOHO) [433].

These practice models provide a framework through which to conceptualize the complex relationship between pain and daily activities with consideration for complex internal and external factors shaping engagement.

The OT evaluation is guided by the OT Practice Framework and focuses on the intersection between pain, daily life, and quality of life. Specific factors such as activity patterns and engagement, routines and habits, important roles, environmental features, personal factors, and client goals are all explored. The occupational therapist also explores the patient's experience of pain including severity, quality,

Table 26.2 Occupational therapy assessments for chronic pain

Category	Assessment
Occupation-based assessments	Canadian Occupational Performance Measure (COPM) Disabilities of the arm shoulder and hand (DASH) Fear of daily activities questionnaire (FDAQ) Tampa Scale of Kinesiophobia (TSK) Chronic pain acceptance questionnaire (CPAQ) RAND-SF 36 The Role Checklist Version 3
Client-factors assessments	McGill Pain Questionnaire Leeds Assessment of Neuropathic Symptoms & Signs (S-LANSS) Central sensitization inventory Brief pain inventory Cognitive assessments Adult & Adolescent Sensory Profile (AASP) Diagnosis-specific assessments
Performance pattern assessments	Pain self-efficacy questionnaire Pain catastrophizing scale Patient activation measure Sleep hygiene index
Environmental assessments	Comprehensive Assessment and Solutions Process for Aging Residents (CASPAR)

location, aggravating factors, and relieving factors in order to tailor recommendations to the patient's needs. Table 26.2 summarizes commonly used evidence-based assessments.

Occupational Therapy Interventions

Occupational therapy practitioners not only plays a key role in the evaluation of function and daily routines but is an important player in the ongoing management and treatment of chronic pain. OT interventions emphasize the therapeutic use of occupations to target multiple domains, including promotion of healthy daily routines and graded engagement in valued activities.

Evidence-based interventions included patient and family education targeting pain neuroscience, self-management strategies, activity pacing, environmental and task modifications, and caregiver training with trusted family and friends [433–435].

Unfortunately, occupational therapists are less likely to be included in pain management teams than other allied health professions with wide variability from country to country [436].

The International Association for the Study of Pain (IASP) outlines recommendations for OTs role in the management of pain. They highlight the importance of establishing client-centered goals based on shared decision making and the importance of facilitating active coping, self-efficacy, and independence [437].

OT treatment strategies target patient education, self-management of symptoms, graded engagement in client-selected goals, and—if needed—prescription of compensatory strategies and adaptive equipment to optimize independence. A systematic review of OT's role in chronic pain management outlined the most common treatment strategies including enabling occupational engagement (38.5%), performance (28.8%), vocational rehabilitation (21.2%), promoting functional independence (9.6%), and addressing occupational balance (7.7%) [438].

These findings emphasize OT's focus on function as well as the diversity of strategies utilized.

Given ongoing calls for multidisciplinary care and the primacy of nonpharmacologic strategies for treating chronic pain, it is likely that the role of rehabilitation in chronic pain management will continue to grow and develop. Emerging technologies including virtual reality and wearables for activity monitoring as well as increased opportunities for telehealth services and remote monitoring offer synergistic opportunities for increased access to services and real-time feedback. There are many avenues for future research including optimal dosage of therapy as well as how best to target rehabilitative care within the chronic pain population [439].

Psychosocial Treatment During Interdisciplinary Rehabilitation

Interdisciplinary treatment is a gold standard for musculoskeletal pain. Regarding psychosocial treatment, over the past three decades, several evidence-based psychological treatments have been developed for pain. To date, cognitive behavioral therapy (CBT) is considered the first line of treatment. Acceptance and commitment therapy (ACT), mindfulness-based stress reduction (MBSR), hypnotherapy, and emotional awareness and expression therapy (EAET) have also been shown to be effective. Biofeedback, neurofeedback, and motivational interviewing are also offered as a standalone or adjunctive treatment for musculoskeletal pain. Offering these psychological treatments in parallel with other treatment modalities will be a multidisciplinary treatment approach. Interdisciplinary treatment will require coordinated efforts among clinicians from different disciplines. For example, CBT includes self-management strategies led by a psychologist, pain neuroscience education led by a physician, and activity planning led by a physical therapist. In interdisciplinary treatment, clinicians with different disciplines will work collaboratively in helping patients to manage their pain so that patients will naturally learn that they will not only need medical treatments but also psychosocial treatments.

Psychosocial Treatment

CBT is an evidence-based treatment for chronic musculoskeletal pain [440–442].

Typical CBT for chronic pain includes education about pain management and active pain coping skills [443–445].

The CBT education covers CBT model of pain, pain cycle, biopsychosocial approach, difference between acute and chronic pain, and stress responses. The active pain coping skills include a SMART goal, relaxation (e.g., breathing relaxation, progressive muscle relaxation, and imagery relaxation), activity pacing, cognitive restructuring, pleasant activity, sleep hygiene, communication skills, and a plan for pain flare-ups [443–455].

CBT can be delivered in an individual or group format. CBT class usually consists of 4–12 sessions and each CBT session takes 1 or 2 hours in length. Meta-analyses indicate that CBT has a small-to-moderate effect sizes in reducing pain intensity ($d = -0.37$), physical function($d = -0.40$), depression ($d = -0.44 \sim -0.48$), and anxiety ($d = -0.30$) in patients with musculoskeletal pain [359–361, 446].

When CBT is offered with an exercise program, outcomes show a trend for slightly better pain reduction ($d = -0.20 \sim -0.56$) and disability ($d = -0.14 \sim -0.77$) compared to when either treatment is offered alone [449, 450].

Operant behavioral therapy can be incorporated into CBT or offered as a single therapy to reduce pain behaviors and increase healthy behaviors [451].

Operant behavioral therapy aims to increase function, but does not aim to decrease pain [243].

In dealing with chronic pain, some patients may be lying down in bed all day and do nothing. Then, patients may receive extra attention from their caregivers. Subsequently, the behavior of lying to manage pain may be reinforced. On the other hand, other patients and their caregivers may focus on accomplishing activity goals such as daily walks or small household chores. As their caregivers show appreciation for the patient's effort of doing some activity and have time to do some activity together, the patient's behavior of engaging in activity may be reinforced [243].

CBT for insomnia (CBTi) is frequently offered because insomnia is common among patients with musculoskeletal pain [452, 453].

CBTi improves insomnia ($d = -0.99$) as well as pain ($d = -0.39$), disability ($d = -0.60$), and depression ($d = -0.58$) [454].

The CBTi's treatment components are neuroscience education about sleep and cognitive behavioral components. Behavioral treatment includes sleep diary, stimulus control, sleep restriction, and sleep hygiene. Cognitive treatment includes constructive worry and cognitive restructuring [455].

CBTi has been incorporated into CBT for pain [456] and physical therapy for pain rehabilitation [457].

ACT is an emerging pain psychology treatment and widely adopted by pain psychologists [356, 371] and physical therapists [443, 458–460].

The treatment outcomes between ACT and CBT for musculoskeletal pain have been similar in improving pain ($d = -0.37$), depression ($d = -0.32$), and anxiety ($d = -0.40$) [443].

Yet, ACT and CBT are different. While CBT teaches self-management tools and effective coping strategies to improve pain self-efficacy and pain control, ACT helps people to let go of control strategies, accept pain, improve psychological flexibility, use mindfulness techniques, and engage in value-based activities [458, 461, 462].

ACT helps patients think about the effectiveness of using problem-solving strategy, and workability of goals, find their own values, set an activity goal that aligns with their values, and rebuild a healthier routine to live a meaningful life with chronic pain. ACT usually consists of 4–10 sessions [458, 463, 464].

MBSR is another evidence-based treatment for musculoskeletal pain [465, 466] and mindfulness techniques have been incorporated into CBT, [467]ACT, [468] and physical therapy [469, 470].

MBSR aims to increase awareness, attend to the present moment, observe unpleasant thoughts, feelings, and sensations without judgment, and not attempt to change them [471].

MBSR treatment components are patient education, meditation practice, and yoga postures [472, 473].

A total of 8–10 sessions are offered weekly and each session is typically 2.5 hours. Participants are expected to practice guided mindfulness meditation or yoga posture daily for 45 minutes at home [473].

The effect of MBSR on pain (d = 0.43–0.86) is similar to that of CBT or ACT [474].

MBSR also improves physical function (d = 0.33), depression (d = 0.66), and anxiety (d = 0.72) [474].

Hypnotherapy has been developed and applied to acute, surgical/procedural, and chronic pain management [475–478].

The application of hypnotherapy to pain management has a long history. The first case of hypnotherapy for surgical pain was documented in the mid-1800s [479, 480].

Since then, its application has been extended to multiple medical conditions such as acute burn pain [481, 482], musculoskeletal pain [483, 484], and headache [480, 485].

During the therapy, a therapist induces a hypnotic trance ("altered state of consciousness"), makes various suggestions (e.g., dissociate with pain, imagine pain free, reduce pain, and engage in activity), and instructs patients to wake up from the hypnotic state [480].

Patients take a recorded hypnosis session and listen to the record for self-hypnosis practice at home. A total of four or five sessions are offered for hypnotherapy and each session takes 60 minutes [477, 486].

Meta-analysis reveals that the effect of hypnotherapy on pain is large for patients with fibromyalgia ($d = -1.17$) [484] and moderate for patients with musculoskeletal or neuropathic pain ($g = -0.37{\sim}{-0.47}$).

More recently, emotional awareness and expression therapy (*EAET*) has been developed and its effect on pain intensity has been observed to be similar to or better than CBT in treating patients with chronic musculoskeletal pain [487, 488].

EAET components are (a) neuroscience education about the relationship among pain, life traumas, and emotion, (b) processing life traumas and conflicts, (c) learning adaptive ways of expressing emotions, (d) practicing emotion expression and mindfulness meditation, (e) facing and re-engaging avoided emotional-laden situations, and (f) learning communication skills to express emotions in actual relationship [489].

Treatment duration ranges from one to eight sessions and it can be offered in individual or group formats.

Biofeedback, Neurofeedback, and Motivational Interviewing (MI) are used as a standalone or adjunctive treatment. Biofeedback and neurofeedback aim to improve self-control [490–493].

Patients observe changes in their physiological signals as they learn and use various regulation techniques. As receiving the feedback of physiological and neuronal signal responses to regulatory techniques, patients will learn effective regulatory techniques for stress responses in heart rate, heart rate variability (HRV), respiration rate, skin conductance, surface electromyography (EMG), and electroencephalography (EEG) [491].

EMG [494–496] and HRV are the two primary modules for musculoskeletal pain.

EMG will start with the collection of the 5-min baseline EMG values. Then, the goal is to reduce 5–90% of the baseline muscle tension. Auditory feedback is given when the goal is reached. Home activity is the daily practice of tension perception and tension-reduction exercise with a biofeedback apparatus [495].

During the EMG biofeedback session, patients are encouraged to develop their own strategies for tension management without receiving instruction from a therapist. EMG treatment typically requires 6–12 sessions [496].

EMG biofeedback is also used as an adjunctive treatment for physical therapy [497].

EMG biofeedback improves pain intensity ($g = 0.62$), muscle tension ($g = 0.44$), and disability ($g = 0.49$) to a small-to-moderate degree in patients with chronic back pain [495, 498, 499].

HRV changes in time intervals between heartbeats in synchronizing with breathing (faster heartbeats in inhalation and slower heartbeats in exhalation), which reflects autonomic nervous system function [500].

Lower synchronization or coherence indicates dysfunctional ANS, which may contribute to chronic pain and decline of physical function in patients with fibromyalgia [500].

HRV module aims to induce a vagal response as patients slow down respiration rates to 4–6 breaths/minute [501].

This slow breathing rate induces longer intervals between heartbeats and improves HRV coherence [501].

HRV treatment varies in the length of one session (15–60 minutes) and total number of sessions (3–10 sessions) [500].

More study is needed to understand the effectiveness of the HRV module for musculoskeletal pain, but it is hypothesized that routine practice of HRV sessions can lower pain and improve stress resilience [500–502].

EEG neurofeedback is an alternative option for fibromyalgia. Compared to EMG biofeedback, high-quality evidence has been lacking to support the effectiveness of neurofeedback in treating fibromyalgia [503, 504] but its application to pain management are promising and remains to be investigated.

So far, studies report that neurofeedback to increase sensorimotor rhythm (SRM) and decrease theta (4–7 Hz) are associated with pain reduction. It is also found that increased alpha (8–12 Hz) together with decreased beta (15–30 Hz) and/or decreased theta is associated with pain reduction [505].

SRM is oscillations in the 12–15 Hz range and this is a spindle-like pattern over the sensory-motor cortex. The number of sessions ranges from 3 to 145 and more sessions are associated with better pain reduction [505].

While *MI* is primarily an adjunctive treatment and clinical technique, MI is a critical component in pain care. The interdisciplinary treatment and biopsychosocial model of pain care are recommended for musculoskeletal pain, but not all patients are open and ready for it. MI will help patients find their own motivation to make behavioral changes [506].

According to the transtheoretical model, there are six stages in intentional human behavior change: Precontemplation, contemplation, preparation, action, maintenance, and relapse [506].

People do not notice any problem in precontemplation stage (e.g., "opioid medication is the only effective option for my pain"). In the contemplation stage, people acknowledge a problem (e.g., opioid medication provides limited benefit for my pain), but also feel ambivalence about making a change (e.g., multidisciplinary treatment). In the preparation stage, people start seeking medical advice and information about "what to do" and "how to start." Then, people in the action stage are trying different approaches, and undergoing trials and errors. As for finding new effective pain management strategies, people will continue using the strategies (maintenance stage) but may also return to old or different maladaptive strategies (relapse stage). Subsequently, clinicians should use MI at each encounter to assess where the patient is in the stage of change. MI has been shown to be effective in increasing adherence to prescribed chronic pain treatment [507] and faster opioid tapering after total hip or knee arthroplasty [508].

Compared to PT only, MI combined with PT is significantly better in improving pain intensity, mobility, pain self-efficacy, and anxiety symptoms in older adults with chronic pain [509].

Social Support Intervention

Support groups are excellent resources for social intervention. Patients can exchange information about pain management among the group members and attend online or offline meetings to provide emotional and social support. Types of social support groups include unstructured support groups, peer-led self-management programs, peer coaching, online community, and professional-led groups [510].

Based on the self-determination theory, peer group intervention works in promoting autonomy, relatedness, and competence [510].

People can also easily make a social media-based support group.

Religion and spirituality have been acknowledged as a way of coping with pain [511–513].

While research has been inconsistent in supporting the pain relief effect of religion and spirituality [511, 514] a more recent brain imaging study has revealed that praying reduces pain intensity by 11%, pain unpleasantness by 26%, and neural activity in the parietofrontal network [515].

These reductions are mediated by expectation, not by the opioidergic system [515].

Additionally, religious, spiritual, and volunteer activities are associated with better overall health and well-being in patients with chronic pain [516–519].

When possible, clinicians can validate patients' plans and efforts to engage in religious and volunteer activities for better health and quality of life.

Telehealth Option for Interdisciplinary Treatments

Since the onset of COVID-19 pandemic, telehealth option for pain care has been rapidly introduced and widely accepted by patients and clinicians [520].

Telehealth (also known as telemedicine) is defined as the use of an electronic communication tool to exchange medical information to improve a patient's health [521].

Electronic communication tools are telephone, smartphone apps [522], internet [520], and videoconference-based platforms [523].

Some treatment formats are self-guided (e.g., applications and recorded video sessions) [524–527] and others are interactive, therapist-guided formats (online, live video sessions) [528, 529].

Empirical data indicate that telehealth provides rapid access to interdisciplinary consultation for pain [530] and patient satisfaction is high for video consultation [531].

Further, web-based pain education, CBT, and ACT have been demonstrated to have a small effect on pain reduction ($d = -0.17{\sim}{-0.26}$) [524, 532, 533].

Early evidence indicate that telehealth-based multidisciplinary treatments are a promising tool to improve the health of patients with chronic widespread pain [534], low back pain [535], and musculoskeletal pain [523, 536–538].

Although there has been limited evidence to support the effectiveness of telehealth interventions compared to that of traditional, in-person interventions, telehealth is one way of addressing barriers to access interdisciplinary or multidisciplinary pain care [539, 540]. Research efforts should be put into improving the effectiveness of telehealth treatments.

Long-Term Care Plan

Interdisciplinary or multidisciplinary treatments are known to provide greater pain reduction, improved physical function, better mood, return to work, and reduced healthcare utilization [541–543].

However, the long-term benefits of interdisciplinary pain care are relatively unknown. A study has observed that patients report on average the same or better levels of pain, physical function, and negative mood at 10 or more years later compared to the levels shortly after the multidisciplinary treatments [544].

The pain stage of change questionnaire has been developed to assess the readiness to use a self-management strategy [545].

In reaching the action and maintenance stage, patients use more relaxation and exercise/stretch and they believe in having greater control over pain, less pain-related disability, and less fear avoidance [546].

However, according to the transtheoretical model of behavior change, individuals will have a period of relapse (i.e., returning to maladaptive and passive pain coping strategy) even after reaching the maintenance stage [547].

Subsequently, assessment should be continued even after patients have completed the interdisciplinary treatment programs. Over time, some patients may benefit from a brief motivational interview to remind them of effective pain management strategies that the patient already has learned and used. Others may benefit from attending maintenance or booster sessions after interdisciplinary treatments. Besides medical treatments, a chronic pain support group, [548, 549], health diary [550], or smart-device-based apps [551, 552] are excellent long-term care options to self-monitor daily health status and utilize active pain coping skills regularly.

Special Circumstances

Specialized interdisciplinary pain management programs may require additional disciplines to adequately serve their population. Table 26.3 reflects the additional team members that are considered desirable to offer certain specified services.

Additionally, Gatchel's group [553] has shown that early application of interdisciplinary pain management is cost-effective in high-risk patients with acute low back pain. These conclusions follow the natural application of these proven services to yet expanding populations of patients disabled by pain. Applying the interdisciplinary evaluation and treatment approach earlier in the course of a pain syndrome has the potential to dramatically increase the cost-effectiveness of interdisciplinary pain management and help reduce patient exposure to potentially harmful treatments. Every health system in the country needs to develop the capacity to provide their patients access to interdisciplinary evaluation and treatment for pain to prevent the consequences of chronic pain including the risk of long-term opioid therapy and poor quality of life.

Table 26.3 Specialty programs and needed personnel and resources

Specialized program	Core and additional disciplines required	Other needed resources
Standard pain clinic	Pain medicine physician Pain managenment psychologist Pain management physical therapist Pain management nurse	Dedicated space for all disciplines in one common clinic Group therapy room Case management Outcome database manager Psychiatry Addictionology Physical medicine and rehabilitation Occupational therapy Medical director Program director
Spine	Orthopedic spine surgery Neurological surgery	Comprehensive perioperative program, including internal medicine, regional and acute pain management, physical therapy
Musculoskeletal	Rheumatology Physical medicine and rehabilitation Orthopedic surgery	Comprehensive perioperative program including internal medicine, regional and acute pain management, physical therapy
Veterans hospital	Psychiatry with PTSD program	
Children's hospital	Pediatric pain physician Pediatric psychologist Pediatric physical therapist	Pediatric psychiatry Family therapy
Public hospital	Social work	
Inpatient/catastrophic pain program	Nursing pain management Regional and acute pain physician Pain medicine physician	Pharmacy Aquatics
Headache	Neurology	Infusion clinic
Cancer pain	Palliative care	Clergy, spiritual care
Wokers' compensation	Occupational therapy Vocational counselor and rehabilitation	Spanish speaking psychologist Translators for other providers
Commission for the Accreditation of Rehabilitation Facilities certified pain program (CARF)	See CARF guidelines	High level Admintrative support
Low back pain (nonoperative)	Acupuncture Tai Chi Yoga Low-level laser	
Opioid reduction program	Addictionology	Comprehensive addiction program
Interventional pain clinic	Interventional pain physician	Neurological surgeon Interventional radiologist
Abdominal pain clinic	Gastroenterologist	

Final Considerations

Interdisciplinary pain management programs are very safe and moderately effective treatments for many patients with a wide variety of chronic musculoskeletal pain syndromes. CDC, VA/DoD, and HHS guidelines for pain and opioid management endorse interdisciplinary pain management [554–556]. However, in 2012, Schatmann estimated that only one program existed for every 670,000 people in the United States [557]. With estimates that 20% of the US population experiences chronic back, hip knee, or foot pain, a woeful mismatch exists between available treatment capacity and existing need. Individual physician leadership and institutional support are needed to overcome barriers to establishing and maintaining these programs to serve the growing need.

References

1. Raja SN, et al. The revised International Association for the study of pain definition of pain: concepts, challenges, and compromises. Pain. 2020;161(9):1976–82.
2. Peacock S, Patel S. Cultural influences on pain. Rev Pain. 2008;1(2):6–9.
3. Benzon H. Essentials of pain medicine. 4th ed; 2018.
4. Laslett M, et al. Diagnosis of sacroiliac joint pain: validity of individual provocation tests and composites of tests. Man Ther. 2005;10(3):207–18.
5. Jensen MP, Karoly P, Braver S. The measurement of clinical pain intensity: a comparison of six methods. Pain. 1986;27(1):117–26.
6. Askew RL, et al. Evidence from diverse clinical populations supported clinical validity of PROMIS pain interference and pain behavior. J Clin Epidemiol. 2016;73:103–11.
7. Cheng J, Rosenquist RW. Fundamentals of pain medicine, 2017.
8. Fairbank JC, et al. The Oswestry low back pain disability questionnaire. Physiotherapy. 1980;66(8):271–3.
9. Cohen SP, Vase L, Hooten WM. Chronic pain: an update on burden, best practices, and new advances. Lancet. 2021;397(10289):2082–97.
10. Cohen SP, Mao J. Neuropathic pain: mechanisms and their clinical implications. BMJ. 2014;348:f7656.
11. (IASP), I.A.f.t.S.o.P., IASP terminology. Available online: https://www.iasp-pain.org/terminology?navItemNumber=576#Centralsensitization.
12. Fitzcharles MA, et al. Nociplastic pain: towards an understanding of prevalent pain conditions. Lancet. 2021;397(10289):2098–110.
13. Staats P, Wallace M. Pain medicine and management just the facts. New York: McGraw-Hill Education; 2015.
14. Lynch ME, Craig KD, Peng PW. Clinical pain management a practical guide. 2nd ed; 2022.
15. Mosher ZA, Sawyer JR, Kelly DM. MRI safety with orthopedic implants. Orthop Clin North Am. 2018;49(4):455–63.
16. Starling A, et al. Sensitivity of MRI of the spine compared with CT myelography in orthostatic headache with CSF leak. Neurology. 2013;81(20):1789–92.
17. American Association of Electrodiagnostic, M. and Y.T. So. Guidelines in electrodiagnostic medicine. Practice parameter for needle electromyographic evaluation of patients with suspected cervical radiculopathy. Muscle Nerve Suppl. 1999;8:S209–21.
18. Bhadola S, Daniello K. When to refer patients with pain for EMG. Pract Neurology. https://practicalneurology.com/articles/2018-sept/when-to-refer-patients-with-pain-for-emg/pdf, 2018.

19. Waldman SD. Pain review, 2016.
20. Donald F, Ward MM. Evaluative laboratory testing practices of United States rheumatologists. Arthritis Rheum. 1998;41(4):725–9.
21. West S, Kolfenbach J. Rheumatology secrets, 2019.
22. Straube S, et al. Vitamin D and chronic pain. Pain. 2009;141(1–2):10–3.
23. Deer TR, et al. A systematic literature review of peripheral nerve stimulation therapies for the treatment of pain. Pain Med. 2020;21(8):1590–603.
24. U.S. Department of Health and Human Services. Pain management best practices Inter-Agency Task Force Report: UPdates, Gaps, INconsistencies, and Recommendations, 2019. Retrieved from https://www.hhs.gov/sites/default/files/pmtf-final-report-2019-05-23.pdf.
25. Kamper SJ, Apeldoorn AT, Chiarotto A, Smeets RJEM, Ostelo RWJG, Guzman J, et al. Multidisciplinary biopsychosocial rehabilitation for chronic low back pain: Cochrane systematic review and meta-analysis. BMJ. 2015;350:h444. https://doi.org/10.1136/bmj.h444.
26. Rivano-Fischer MR, Schults ML, Stalnacke BM, Ekholm J, Persson EB, Lofgren M. Variability in patient characteristics and service provision of interdisciplinary pain rehabilitation: a study using the Swedish national quality registry for pain rehabilitation. J Rehabil Med. 2020;52(11):jrm00128. https://doi.org/10.2340/16501977-2765.
27. Treede R-D, Rief W, Barke A, et al. Chronic pain as a symptom or a disease: the IASP classification of chronic pain for the International Classification of Diseases (ICD-11). Pain. 2019;160(1):19–27.
28. Melzack R, Wall PD. Pain mechanisms: a new theory: a gate control system modulates sensory input from the skin before it evokes pain perception and response. Science. 1965;150(3699):971–9.
29. Engel GL. The need for a new medical model: a challenge for biomedicine. Science. 1977;196(4286):129–36.
30. McNee P, Shambrook J, Harris EC, et al. Predictors of long-term pain and disability in patients with low back pain investigated by magnetic resonance imaging: a longitudinal study. BMC Musculoskelet Disord. 2011;12(1):1–12.
31. Shambrook J, McNee P, Harris EC, et al. Clinical presentation of low back pain and association with risk factors according to findings on magnetic resonance imaging. Pain. 2011;152(7):1659–65.
32. Berg L, Hellum C, Gjertsen Ø, et al. Do more MRI findings imply worse disability or more intense low back pain? A cross-sectional study of candidates for lumbar disc prosthesis. Skeletal Radiol. 2013;42(11):1593–602.
33. Steffens D, Hancock M, Maher C, Williams C, Jensen TS, Latimer J. Does magnetic resonance imaging predict future low back pain? A systematic review. Eur J Pain. 2014;18(6):755–65.
34. Suri P, Boyko EJ, Goldberg J, Forsberg CW, Jarvik JG. Longitudinal associations between incident lumbar spine MRI findings and chronic low back pain or radicular symptoms: retrospective analysis of data from the longitudinal assessment of imaging and disability of the back (LAIDBACK). BMC Musculoskelet Disord. 2014;15(1):1–10.
35. Weber C, Giannadakis C, Rao V, et al. Is there an association between radiological severity of lumbar spinal stenosis and disability, pain, or surgical outcome?: a multicenter observational study. Spine. 2016;41(2):E78–83.
36. Moseley JB, O'malley K, Petersen NJ, et al. A controlled trial of arthroscopic surgery for osteoarthritis of the knee. N Engl J Med. 2002;347(2):81–8.
37. Enck P, Bingel U, Schedlowski M, Rief W. The placebo response in medicine: minimize, maximize or personalize? Nat Rev Drug Discov. 2013;12(3):191–204.
38. Holmes R, Tiwari A, Kennedy J. Mechanisms of the placebo effect in pain and psychiatric disorders. Pharmacogenomics J. 2016;16(6):491–500.
39. Levine J, Gordon N, Fields H. The mechanism of placebo analgesia. Lancet. 1978;312(8091):654–7.
40. Zubieta JK, Stohler CS. Neurobiological mechanisms of placebo responses. Ann N Y Acad Sci. 2009;1156(1):198–210.

41. Abhishek A, Doherty M. Mechanisms of the placebo response in pain in osteoarthritis. Osteoarthr Cartil. 2013;21(9):1229–35.
42. Engel GL. The clinical application of the biopsychosocial model, vol. 6. Oxford University Press; 1981. p. 101–24.
43. Turk DC, Fillingim RB, Ohrbach R, Patel KV. Assessment of psychosocial and functional impact of chronic pain. J Pain. 2016;17(9):T21–49.
44. Baria AM, Pangarkar S, Abrams G, Miaskowski C. Adaption of the biopsychosocial model of chronic noncancer pain in veterans. Pain Med. 2019;20(1):14–27.
45. Miaskowski C, Blyth F, Nicosia F, et al. A biopsychosocial model of chronic pain for older adults. Pain Med. 2020;21(9):1793–805.
46. Bevers K, Watts L, Kishino ND, Gatchel RJ. The biopsychosocial model of the assessment, prevention, and treatment of chronic pain. US Neurol. 2016;12(2):98–104.
47. Kassam A, Patten SB. Major depression, fibromyalgia and labour force participation: a population-based cross-sectional study. BMC Musculoskelet Disord. 2006;7(1):1–5.
48. Dworkin RH, Gitlin MJ. Clinical aspects of depression in chronic pain patients. Clin J Pain. 1991;7(2):79–94.
49. Patten SB, Williams JV, Wang J. Mental disorders in a population sample with musculoskeletal disorders. BMC Musculoskelet Disord. 2006;7(1):1–10.
50. Hasin DS, Sarvet AL, Meyers JL, et al. Epidemiology of adult DSM-5 major depressive disorder and its specifiers in the United States. JAMA Psychiatry. 2018;75(4):336–46.
51. Patten SB, Williams JV, Lavorato DH, Wang JL, McDonald K, Bulloch AG. Descriptive epidemiology of major depressive disorder in Canada in 2012. Can J Psychiatry. 2015;60(1):23–30.
52. Glombiewski JA, Hartwich-Tersek J, Rief W. Depression in chronic back pain patients: prediction of pain intensity and pain disability in cognitive-behavioral treatment. Psychosomatics. 2010;51(2):130–6.
53. Talaei-Khoei M, Fischerauer SF, Jha R, Ring D, Chen N, Vranceanu A-M. Bidirectional mediation of depression and pain intensity on their associations with upper extremity physical function. J Behav Med. 2018;41(3):309–17.
54. Kroenke K, Wu J, Bair MJ, Krebs EE, Damush TM, Tu W. Reciprocal relationship between pain and depression: a 12-month longitudinal analysis in primary care. J Pain. 2011;12(9):964–73.
55. Hung C-I, Liu C-Y, Fu T-S. Depression: an important factor associated with disability among patients with chronic low back pain. Int J Psychiatry Med. 2015;49(3):187–98.
56. Campbell P, Hope K, Dunn KM. The pain, depression, disability pathway in those with low back pain: a moderation analysis of health locus of control. J Pain Res. 2017;10:2331.
57. Alschuler KN, Theisen-Goodvich ME, Haig AJ, Geisser ME. A comparison of the relationship between depression, perceived disability, and physical performance in persons with chronic pain. Eur J Pain. 2008;12(6):757–64.
58. Börsbo B, Peolsson M, Gerdle B. The complex interplay between pain intensity, depression, anxiety and catastrophising with respect to quality of life and disability. Disabil Rehabil. 2009;31(19):1605–13.
59. Ramírez-Maestre C, Reyes-Pérez Á, Esteve R, López-Martínez AE, Bernardes S, Jensen MP. Opioid pain medication prescription for chronic pain in primary care centers: the roles of pain acceptance, pain intensity, depressive symptoms, pain catastrophizing, sex, and age. Int J Environ Res Public Health. 2020;17(17):6428.
60. Halbert B, Davis R, Wee CC. Disproportionate longer-term opioid use among US adults with mood disorders. Pain. 2016;157(11):2452.
61. Goesling J, Henry MJ, Moser SE, et al. Symptoms of depression are associated with opioid use regardless of pain severity and physical functioning among treatment-seeking patients with chronic pain. J Pain. 2015;16(9):844–51.
62. Bair MJ, Wu J, Damush TM, Sutherland JM, Kroenke K. Association of depression and anxiety alone and in combination with chronic musculoskeletal pain in primary care patients. Psychosom Med. 2008;70(8):890.

63. Tesio V, Di Tella M, Ghiggia A, et al. Alexithymia and depression affect quality of life in patients with chronic pain: a study on 205 patients with fibromyalgia. Front Psychol. 2018;9:442.
64. Slyer J, Scott S, Sheldon B, Hancu M, Bridger C, Pilitsis JG. Less pain relief, more depression, and female sex correlate with spinal cord stimulation explants. Neuromodulation Technol Neural Interface. 2020;23(5):673–9.
65. Cohen SP, Doshi TL, Kurihara C, et al. Multicenter study evaluating factors associated with treatment outcome for low back pain injections. Region Anesth Pain Med. 2022;47(2):89–99.
66. Merrill RK, Zebala LP, Peters C, Qureshi SA, McAnany SJ. Impact of depression on patient-reported outcome measures after lumbar spine decompression. Spine. 2018;43(6):434–9.
67. Lau BC, Scribani M, Wittstein J. Patients with depression and anxiety symptoms from adjustment disorder related to their shoulder may be ideal patients for arthroscopic rotator cuff repair. J Shoulder Elb Surg. 2020;29(7):S80–6.
68. Fishbain DA. The association of chronic pain and suicide. Semin Clin Neuropsychiatry. 1999;4:221–7.
69. Tang NK, Crane C. Suicidality in chronic pain: a review of the prevalence, risk factors and psychological links. Psychol Med. 2006;36(5):575–86.
70. Edwards RR, Smith MT, Kudel I, Haythornthwaite J. Pain-related catastrophizing as a risk factor for suicidal ideation in chronic pain. Pain. 2006;126(1–3):272–9.
71. Jimenez-Rodríguez I, Garcia-Leiva JM, Jimenez-Rodriguez BM, Condés-Moreno E, Rico-Villademoros F, Calandre EP. Suicidal ideation and the risk of suicide in patients with fibromyalgia: a comparison with non-pain controls and patients suffering from low-back pain. Neuropsychiatr Dis Treat. 2014;10:625.
72. Racine M. Chronic pain and suicide risk: a comprehensive review. Prog Neuro-Psychopharmacol Biol Psychiatry. 2018;87:269–80.
73. Grocott B, Sommer JL, El-Gabalawy R. Usual presence and intensity of pain are differentially associated with suicidality across chronic pain conditions: a population-based study. J Psychosom Res. 2021;148:110557.
74. Ashrafioun L, Kane C, Bishop TM, Britton PC, Pigeon WR. The association of pain intensity and suicide attempts among patients initiating pain specialty services. J Pain. 2019;20(7):852–9.
75. Kanzler KE, Bryan CJ, McGeary DD, Morrow CE. Suicidal ideation and perceived burdensomeness in patients with chronic pain. Pain Pract. 2012;12(8):602–9.
76. Shim E-J, Song YW, Park S-H, Lee K-M, Go DJ, Hahm B-J. Examining the relationship between pain catastrophizing and suicide risk in patients with rheumatic disease: the mediating role of depression, perceived social support, and perceived burdensomeness. Int J Behav Med. 2017;24(4):501–12.
77. Hassett AL, Aquino JK, Ilgen MA. The risk of suicide mortality in chronic pain patients. Curr Pain Headache Rep. 2014;18(8):1–7.
78. Owen-Smith AA, Ahmedani BK, Peterson E, et al. The mediating effect of sleep disturbance on the relationship between nonmalignant chronic pain and suicide death. Pain Pract. 2019;19(4):382–9.
79. Arnow BA, Blasey CM, Lee J, et al. Relationships among depression, chronic pain, chronic disabling pain, and medical costs. Psychiatr Serv. 2009;60(3):344–50.
80. First MB, Williams JB, Karg RS, Spitzer RL. User's guide for the SCID-5-CV structured clinical interview for DSM-5® disorders: clinical version. American Psychiatric Publishing, Inc.; 2016.
81. Sheehan DV, Lecrubier Y, Sheehan KH, et al. The Mini-International Neuropsychiatric Interview (MINI): the development and validation of a structured diagnostic psychiatric interview for DSM-IV and ICD-10. J Clin Psychiatry. 1998;59(20):22–33.
82. Kessler RC, Calabrese J, Farley P, et al. Composite International Diagnostic Interview screening scales for DSM-IV anxiety and mood disorders. Psychol Med. 2013;43(8):1625–37.

83. Kroenke K, Spitzer RL, Williams JB. The PHQ-9: validity of a brief depression severity measure. J Gen Intern Med. 2001;16(9):606–13.
84. Löwe B, Spitzer RL, Gräfe K, et al. Comparative validity of three screening questionnaires for DSM-IV depressive disorders and physicians' diagnoses. J Affect Disord. 2004;78(2):131–40.
85. Kroenke K, Spitzer RL, Williams JB. The patient health questionnaire-2: validity of a two-item depression screener. Med Care. 2003;41:1284–1292.
86. Radloff LS. The CES-D scale: a self-report depression scale for research in the general population. Appl Psychol Meas. 1977;1(3):385–401.
87. Zich JM, Attkisson CC, Greenfield TK. Screening for depression in primary care clinics: the CES-D and the BDI. Int J Psychiatr Med. 1990;20(3):259–77.
88. Zhang W, O'Brien N, Forrest JI, et al. Validating a shortened depression scale (10 item CES-D) among HIV-positive people in British Columbia, Canada. PLoS One. 2012;7(7):e40793.
89. Zigmond AS, Snaith RP. The hospital anxiety and depression scale. Acta Psychiatr Scand. 1983;67(6):361–70.
90. Bjelland I, Dahl AA, Haug TT, Neckelmann D. The validity of the Hospital Anxiety and Depression Scale: an updated literature review. J Psychosom Res. 2002;52(2):69–77.
91. Lovibond S, Lovibond P. Manual for the depression anxiety stress scales. 2nd ed. Sydney: Psychology Foundation; 1995. Google Scholar. pp. 4–42.
92. Bech P, Bille J, Møller SB, Hellström LC, Østergaard SD. Psychometric validation of the Hopkins Symptom Checklist (SCL-90) subscales for depression, anxiety, and interpersonal sensitivity. J Affect Disord. 2014;160:98–103.
93. Derogatis LR, Unger R. Symptom checklist-90-revised. In: The Corsini encyclopedia of psychology; 2010. p. 1–2.
94. Arnau RC, Meagher MW, Norris MP, Bramson R. Psychometric evaluation of the Beck Depression Inventory-II with primary care medical patients. Health Psychol. 2001;20(2):112.
95. Beck AT, Steer RA, Brown G. Beck depression inventory–II. Psychological assessment. APA PsycTests; 1996.
96. Pilkonis PA, Yu L, Dodds NE, Johnston KL, Maihoefer CC, Lawrence SM. Validation of the depression item bank from the Patient-Reported Outcomes Measurement Information System (PROMIS®) in a three-month observational study. J Psychiatr Res. 2014;56:112–9.
97. Beck AT, Brown GK, Steer RA. Psychometric characteristics of the Scale for Suicide Ideation with psychiatric outpatients. Behav Res Ther. 1997;35(11):1039–46.
98. De Beurs DP, Fokkema M, O'Connor RC. Optimizing the assessment of suicidal behavior: the application of curtailment techniques. J Affect Disord. 2016;196:218–24.
99. Posner K, Brent D, Lucas C, et al. Columbia-suicide severity rating scale (C-SSRS). New York: Columbia University Medical Center; 2008. p. 10.
100. Posner K, Brown GK, Stanley B, et al. The Columbia–Suicide Severity Rating Scale: initial validity and internal consistency findings from three multisite studies with adolescents and adults. Am J Psychiatry. 2011;168(12):1266–77.
101. Alphs L, Fu D-J, Williamson D, et al. Suicide ideation and behavior assessment tool (SIBAT): evaluation of intra-and inter-rater reliability, validity, and mapping to Columbia Classification Algorithm of Suicide Assessment. Psychiatry Res. 2020;294:113495.
102. Asmundson GJ, Katz J. Understanding the co-occurrence of anxiety disorders and chronic pain: state-of-the-art. Depress Anxiety. 2009;26(10):888–901.
103. Knaster P, Karlsson H, Estlander A-M, Kalso E. Psychiatric disorders as assessed with SCID in chronic pain patients: the anxiety disorders precede the onset of pain. Gen Hosp Psychiatry. 2012;34(1):46–52.
104. McWilliams LA, Cox BJ, Enns MW. Mood and anxiety disorders associated with chronic pain: an examination in a nationally representative sample. Pain. 2003;106(1–2):127–33.
105. McWilliams LA, Goodwin RD, Cox BJ. Depression and anxiety associated with three pain conditions: results from a nationally representative sample. Pain. 2004;111(1–2):77–83.

106. Littleton S, Cameron ID, Poustie SJ, et al. The association of compensation on longer term health status for people with musculoskeletal injuries following road traffic crashes: emergency department inception cohort study. Injury. 2011;42(9):927–33.
107. Bekeris J, Wilson LA, Fiasconaro M, et al. New onset depression and anxiety after spinal fusion surgery: incidence and risk factors. Spine. 2020;45(16):1161–9.
108. Alkassabi O, Voogt L, Andrews P, Alhowimel A, Nijs J, Alsobayel H. Risk factors to persistent pain following musculoskeletal injuries: a systematic literature review. Int J Environ Res Public Health. 2022;19(15):9318.
109. McGeary D, Moore M, Vriend CA, Peterson AL, Gatchel RJ. The evaluation and treatment of comorbid pain and PTSD in a military setting: an overview. J Clin Psychol Med Settings. 2011;18(2):155–63.
110. Muscatelli S, Spurr H, O'Hara NN, O'Hara LM, Sprague SA, Slobogean GP. Prevalence of depression and posttraumatic stress disorder after acute orthopaedic trauma: a systematic review and meta-analysis. J Orthop Trauma. 2017;31(1):47–55.
111. Asmundson GJ, Norton GR, Allerdings MD. Fear and avoidance in dysfunctional chronic back pain patients. Pain. 1997;69(3):231–6.
112. Lucchetti G, Oliveira AB, Mercante JPP, Peres MFP. Anxiety and fear-avoidance in musculoskeletal pain. Curr Pain Headache Rep. 2012;16(5):399–406.
113. Vlaeyen JW, Linton SJ. Fear-avoidance and its consequences in chronic musculoskeletal pain: a state of the art. Pain. 2000;85(3):317–32.
114. Dixon JJ, Monchaux CD, Sandler J. Patterns of anxiety: the phobias. Br J Med Psychol. 1957;30(1):34–40.
115. Shepard JF. Affective phenomena-experimental. Psychol Bull. 1916;13(5):202.
116. Spitzer RL, Kroenke K, Williams JB, Löwe B. A brief measure for assessing generalized anxiety disorder: the GAD-7. Arch Intern Med. 2006;166(10):1092–7.
117. Byrd-Bredbenner C, Eck K, Quick V. GAD-7, GAD-2, and GAD-mini: psychometric properties and norms of university students in the United States. Gen Hosp Psychiatry. 2021;69:61–6.
118. Kroenke K, Spitzer RL, Williams JB, Monahan PO, Löwe B. Anxiety disorders in primary care: prevalence, impairment, comorbidity, and detection. Ann Intern Med. 2007;146(5):317–25.
119. Spielberger CD, Sydeman SJ, Owen AE, Marsh BJ. Measuring anxiety and anger with the State-Trait Anxiety Inventory (STAI) and the State-Trait Anger Expression Inventory (STAXI). Lawrence Erlbaum Associates Publishers; 1999.
120. Beck AT, Steer RA. Manual for the Beck anxiety inventory. San Antonio: Psychological Corporation; 1990.
121. Pilkonis PA, Choi SW, Reise SP, et al. Item banks for measuring emotional distress from the Patient-Reported Outcomes Measurement Information System (PROMIS®): depression, anxiety, and anger. Assessment. 2011;18(3):263–83.
122. Schalet BD, Pilkonis PA, Yu L, et al. Clinical validity of PROMIS depression, anxiety, and anger across diverse clinical samples. J Clin Epidemiol. 2016;73:119–27.
123. McCracken LM, Zayfert C, Gross RT. The Pain Anxiety Symptoms Scale: development and validation of a scale to measure fear of pain. Pain. 1992;50(1):67–73.
124. Roelofs J, McCracken L, Peters ML, Crombez G, van Breukelen G, Vlaeyen JW. Psychometric evaluation of the Pain Anxiety Symptoms Scale (PASS) in chronic pain patients. J Behav Med. 2004;27(2):167–83.
125. McNeil DW, Rainwater AJ. Development of the fear of pain questionnaire-III. J Behav Med. 1998;21(4):389–410.
126. McNeil DW, Kennedy SG, Randall CL, et al. Fear of pain questionnaire-9: brief assessment of pain-related fear and anxiety. Eur J Pain. 2018;22(1):39–48.
127. Lundberg MK, Styf J, Carlsson SG. A psychometric evaluation of the Tampa Scale for Kinesiophobia—from a physiotherapeutic perspective. Physiother Theory Pract. 2004;20(2):121–33.
128. Tkachuk GA, Harris CA. Psychometric properties of the Tampa Scale for Kinesiophobia-11 (TSK-11). J Pain. 2012;13(10):970–7.

129. Edition F. Diagnostic and statistical manual of mental disorders. Am Psychiatr Assoc. 2013;21(21):591–643.
130. Barjandi G, Kosek E, Hedenberg-Magnusson B, Velly AM, Ernberg M. Comorbid conditions in temporomandibular disorders myalgia and myofascial pain compared to fibromyalgia. J Clin Med. 2021;10(14):3138.
131. Creed F. The relationship between somatic symptoms, health anxiety, and outcome in medical out-patients. Psychiatr Clin N Am. 2011;34(3):545–64.
132. Hartzell MM, Choi Y, Neblett R, Williams M, Mayer TG, Gatchel RJ. Somatization as a predictor of outcomes following functional restoration of chronic disabling occupational musculoskeletal pain disorder patients. J Appl Biobehav Res. 2013;18(2):59–81.
133. Tsui P, Deptula A, Yuan DY. Conversion disorder, functional neurological symptom disorder, and chronic pain: comorbidity, assessment, and treatment. Curr Pain Headache Rep. 2017;21(6):1–10.
134. Epstein SA, Maurer CW, LaFaver K, Ameli R, Sinclair S, Hallett M. Insights into chronic functional movement disorders: the value of qualitative psychiatric interviews. Psychosomatics. 2016;57(6):566–75.
135. Ettinger AB, Devinsky O, Weisbrot DM, Ramakrishna RK, Goyal A. A comprehensive profile of clinical, psychiatric, and psychosocial characteristics of patients with psychogenic nonepileptic seizures. Epilepsia. 1999;40(9):1292–8.
136. Kocalevent R-D, Hinz A, Brähler E. Standardization of a screening instrument (PHQ-15) for somatization syndromes in the general population. BMC Psychiatry. 2013;13(1):1–8.
137. Bernstein IH, Jaremko ME, Hinkley BS. On the utility of the SCL-90-R with low-back pain patients. Spine. 1994;19(1):42–8.
138. Pennebaker JW. Pennebaker inventory of Limbic Languidness. APA PsycTests; 1982.
139. Fink P, Ewald H, Jensen J, et al. Screening for somatization and hypochondriasis in primary care and neurological in-patients: a seven-item scale for hypochondriasis and somatization. J Psychosom Res. 1999;46(3):261–73.
140. Salkovskis PM, Rimes KA, Warwick H, Clark D. The Health Anxiety Inventory: development and validation of scales for the measurement of health anxiety and hypochondriasis. Psychol Med. 2002;32(5):843–53.
141. Hedman E, Ljótsson B, Andersson E, et al. Psychometric properties of Internet-administered measures of health anxiety: an investigation of the Health Anxiety Inventory, the Illness Attitude Scales, and the Whiteley Index. J Anxiety Disord. 2015;31:32–7.
142. Fishbain DA, Goldberg M, Meagher BR, Steele R, Rosomoff H. Male and female chronic pain patients categorized by DSM-III psychiatric diagnostic criteria. Pain. 1986;26(2):181–97.
143. Attademo L, Bernardini F. Prevalence of personality disorders in patients with fibromyalgia: a brief review. Prim Health Care Res Dev. 2018;19(5):523–8.
144. Dersh J, Gatchel RJ, Mayer T, Polatin P, Temple OR. Prevalence of psychiatric disorders in patients with chronic disabling occupational spinal disorders. Spine. 2006;31(10):1156–62.
145. Conrad R, Schilling G, Bausch C, et al. Temperament and character personality profiles and personality disorders in chronic pain patients. Pain. 2007;133(1–3):197–209. Kalira V, Treisman GJ, Clark MR. Borderline personality disorder and chronic pain: a practical approach to evaluation and treatment. Curr Pain Headache Rep. 2013;17(8):1–8.
146. Saper JR, Lake AE III. Borderline personality disorder and the chronic headache patient: review and management recommendations. Headache J Head Face Pain. 2002;42(7):663–74.
147. Dubovsky AN, Kiefer MM. Borderline personality disorder in the primary care setting. Med Clin. 2014;98(5):1049–64.
148. Doering S. Borderline personality disorder in patients with medical illness: a review of assessment, prevalence, and treatment options. Psychosom Med. 2019;81(7):584–94.
149. Johnson BN, Lumley MA, Cheavens JS, McKernan LC. Exploring the links among borderline personality disorder symptoms, trauma, and pain in patients with chronic pain disorders. J Psychosom Res. 2020;135:110164.
150. Ekselius L, von Knorring L, Enskog J, Ordeberg G. Effect of personality disorders on treatment outcome of surgery for low back pain. J Musculoskel Pain. 1996;4(3):87–96.

151. Linder J, Carlos Poston IIWS, Haddock KC, Foreyt PJ, Ericsson M. Does personality or psychopathology predict disability in chronic pain patients? Disabil Rehabil. 2000;22(6):281–7.
152. Sansone RA, Sinclair JD, Wiederman MW. Disability and borderline personality disorder in chronic pain patients. Pain Res Manag. 2010;15(6):369–70.
153. Reynolds CJ, Tragesser SL. Borderline personality disorder features are associated with concurrent pain-related disability in a chronic pain sample. Pain Med. 2019;20(2):233–45.
154. Butcher JN. International adaptations of the MMPI-2: Research and clinical applications. University of Minnesota Press; 1996.
155. Morey L. Personality Assessment Inventory (PAI) Odessa, Fla. Personality Assessment Resources (PAR), 1991.
156. Zanarini MC, Vujanovic AA, Parachini EA, Boulanger JL, Frankenburg FR, Hennen J. A screening measure for BPD: the McLean screening instrument for borderline personality disorder (MSI-BPD). J Personal Disord. 2003;17(6):568–73.
157. Poreh AM, Rawlings D, Claridge G, Freeman JL, Faulkner C, Shelton C. The BPQ: a scale for the assessment of borderline personality based on DSM-IV criteria. J Personal Disord. 2006;20(3):247–60.
158. Bohus M, Kleindienst N, Limberger MF, et al. The short version of the Borderline Symptom List (BSL-23): development and initial data on psychometric properties. Psychopathology. 2009;42(1):32–9.
159. Bohus M, Limberger MF, Frank U, Chapman AL, Kühler T, Stieglitz R-D. Psychometric properties of the borderline symptom list (BSL). Psychopathology. 2007;40(2):126–32.
160. Zanarini MC. Zanarini Rating Scale for Borderline Personality Disorder (ZAN-BPD): a continuous measure of DSM-IV borderline psychopathology. J Personal Disord. 2003;17(3):233.
161. Sadri SK, McEvoy PM, Pinto A, Anderson RA, Egan SJ. A psychometric examination of the Pathological Obsessive Compulsive Personality Scale (POPS): Initial study in an undergraduate sample. J Pers Assess. 2018;101:284.
162. Pinto A, Liebowitz MR, Foa EB, Simpson HB. Obsessive compulsive personality disorder as a predictor of exposure and ritual prevention outcome for obsessive compulsive disorder. Behav Res Ther. 2011;49(8):453–8.
163. Woody SR, Steketee G, Chambless DL. The usefulness of the obsessive compulsive scale of the Symptom Checklist-90-Revised. Behav Res Ther. 1995;33(5):607–11.
164. Söderfjell S, Molander B, Johansson H, Barnekow-Bergkvist M, Nilsson LG. Musculoskeletal pain complaints and performance on cognitive tasks over the adult life span. Scand J Psychol. 2006;47(5):349–59.
165. Ojeda B, Dueñas M, Salazar A, Mico JA, Torres LM, Failde I. Factors influencing cognitive impairment in neuropathic and musculoskeletal pain and fibromyalgia. Pain Med. 2018;19(3):499–510.
166. Kratz AL, Whibley D, Kim S, Sliwinski M, Clauw D, Williams DA. Fibrofog in daily life: an examination of ambulatory subjective and objective cognitive function in fibromyalgia. Arthritis Care Res. 2020;72(12):1669–77.
167. Lawlor PG. The panorama of opioid-related cognitive dysfunction in patients with cancer: a critical literature appraisal. Cancer. 2002;94(6):1836–53.
168. Moriarty O, McGuire BE, Finn DP. The effect of pain on cognitive function: a review of clinical and preclinical research. Prog Neurobiol. 2011;93(3):385–404.
169. Dick BD, Verrier MJ, Harker KT, Rashiq S. Disruption of cognitive function in fibromyalgia syndrome. Pain. 2008;139(3):610–6.
170. Lee D, Pendleton N, Tajar A, et al. Chronic widespread pain is associated with slower cognitive processing speed in middle-aged and older European men. Pain. 2010;151(1):30–6.
171. Fougnie D. The relationship between attention and working memory. New Res Short-Term Memor. 2008;1:45.
172. Jang SE, Bradshaw YS, Carr DB. Comparison of the impacts of under-treated pain and opioid pain medication on cognitive impairment. Cureus. 2022;14(2):e22037.

173. Reyes del Paso GA, Pulgar A, Duschek S, Garrido S. Cognitive impairment in fibromyalgia syndrome: the impact of cardiovascular regulation, pain, emotional disorders and medication. Eur J Pain. 2012;16(3):421–9.
174. Galvez-Sánchez CM, Reyes del Paso GA, Duschek S. Cognitive impairments in fibromyalgia syndrome: associations with positive and negative affect, alexithymia, pain catastrophizing and self-esteem. Front Psychol. 2018;9:377.
175. Ersek M, Cherrier MM, Overman SS, Irving GA. The cognitive effects of opioids. Pain Manag Nurs. 2004;5(2):75–93.
176. Golombok S, Moodley P, Lader M. Cognitive impairment in long-term benzodiazepine users. Psychol Med. 1988;18(2):365–74.
177. Schiltenwolf M, Akbar M, Hug A, et al. Evidence of specific cognitive deficits in patients with chronic low back pain under long-term substitution treatment of opioids. Pain Physician. 2014;17(1):9.
178. Soyka M, Limmer C, Lehnert R, et al. A comparison of cognitive function in patients under maintenance treatment with heroin, methadone, or buprenorphine and healthy controls: an open pilot study. Am J Drug Alcohol Abuse. 2011;37(6):497–508.
179. Nugent SM, Morasco BJ, O'Neil ME, et al. The effects of cannabis among adults with chronic pain and an overview of general harms: a systematic review. Ann Intern Med. 2017;167(5):319–31.
180. Wildes M, Bigand TL, Layton ME, Wilson M. Cannabis use and cognition in adults prescribed opioids for persistent pain. Pain Manag Nurs. 2020;21(1):94–9.
181. McCracken LM, Iverson GL. Predicting complaints of impaired cognitive functioning in patients with chronic pain. J Pain Symptom Manag. 2001;21(5):392–6.
182. Baker KS, Gibson S, Georgiou-Karistianis N, Roth RM, Giummarra MJ. Everyday executive functioning in chronic pain: specific deficits in working memory and emotion control, predicted by mood, medications, and pain interference. Clin J Pain. 2016;32(8):673–80.
183. Morone NE, Abebe KZ, Morrow LA, Weiner DK. Pain and decreased cognitive function negatively impact physical functioning in older adults with knee osteoarthritis. Pain Med. 2014;15(9):1481–7.
184. Van Der Leeuw G, Eggermont LH, Shi L, et al. Pain and cognitive function among older adults living in the community. J Gerontol Ser A Biomed Sci Med Sci. 2016;71(3):398–405.
185. Hirase T, Okubo Y, Delbaere K, Menant JC, Lord SR, Sturnieks DL. Predictors of development and persistence of musculoskeletal pain in community-dwelling older people: a two-year longitudinal study. Geriatr Gerontol Int. 2021;21(6):519–24.
186. Whitlock EL, Diaz-Ramirez LG, Glymour MM, Boscardin WJ, Covinsky KE, Smith AK. Association between persistent pain and memory decline and dementia in a longitudinal cohort of elders. JAMA Intern Med. 2017;177(8):1146–53.
187. Kao P-H, Fong-Lin J, Chung-Han H, et al. Chronic pain increases the risk of dementia: a nationwide population-based cohort study. Pain Physician. 2021;24(6):E849.
188. Wang K, Liu H. Association between widespread pain and dementia, Alzheimer's disease and stroke: a cohort study from the Framingham Heart Study. Region Anesth Pain Med. 2021;46(10):879–85.
189. Yoon BY, Lee J-H, Shin SY. Discrepancy between subjective and objective measures of cognitive impairment in patients with rheumatoid arthritis. Rheumatol Int. 2017;37(10):1635–41.
190. Gelonch O, Garolera M, Valls J, Rosselló L, Pifarré J. Cognitive complaints in women with fibromyalgia: are they due to depression or to objective cognitive dysfunction? J Clin Exp Neuropsychol. 2017;39(10):1013–25.
191. Pidal-Miranda M, González-Villar AJ, Carrillo-de-la-Peña MT, Andrade E, Rodríguez-Salgado D. Broad cognitive complaints but subtle objective working memory impairment in fibromyalgia patients. PeerJ. 2018;6:e5907.
192. Amariglio RE, Donohue MC, Marshall GA, et al. Tracking early decline in cognitive function in older individuals at risk for Alzheimer disease dementia: the Alzheimer's Disease Cooperative Study Cognitive Function Instrument. JAMA Neurol. 2015;72(4):446–54.

193. Munro CE, Buckley R, Vannini P, et al. Longitudinal trajectories of participant-and study partner-rated cognitive decline, in relation to Alzheimer's disease biomarkers and mood symptoms. Front Aging Neurosci. 2021;13:13.
194. Rodríguez-Andreu J, Ibáñez-Bosch R, Portero-Vázquez A, Masramon X, Rejas J, Gálvez R. Cognitive impairment in patients with fibromyalgia syndrome as assessed by the mini-mental state examination. BMC Musculoskelet Disord. 2009;10(1):1–5.
195. Cardoso J, Apagueno B, Lysne P, et al. Pain and the montreal cognitive assessment (MoCA) in aging. Pain Med. 2021;22(8):1776–83.
196. Hanmer J, Jensen RE, Rothrock N. A reporting checklist for HealthMeasures' patient-reported outcomes: ASCQ-Me, Neuro-QoL, NIH Toolbox, and PROMIS. J Patient-Rep Outcomes. 2020;4(1):1–7.
197. Weintraub S, Dikmen SS, Heaton RK, et al. Cognition assessment using the NIH Toolbox. Neurology. 2013;80(11 Supplement 3):S54–S64.
198. Peres MF, Lucchetti G. Coping strategies in chronic pain. Curr Pain Headache Rep. 2010;14(5):331–8.
199. Barry LC, Kerns RD, Guo Z, Duong BD, Iannone LP, Carrington RM. Identification of strategies used to cope with chronic pain in older persons receiving primary care from a Veterans Affairs Medical Center. J Am Geriatr Soc. 2004;52(6):950–6.
200. Reid M, Barry L, Kerns R, Duong B, Concato J. Coping strategies and their associations with levels of disability or pain, among older veterans receiving primary care. J Clin Epidemiol. 2002;55(6):629.
201. Keogh E, Denford S. Sex differences in perceptions of pain coping strategy usage. Eur J Pain. 2009;13(6):629–34.
202. Baastrup S, Schultz R, Brødsgaard I, et al. A comparison of coping strategies in patients with fibromyalgia, chronic neuropathic pain, and pain-free controls. Scand J Psychol. 2016;57(6):516–22.
203. Evers AW, Kraaimaat FW, Geenen R, Jacobs JW, Bijlsma JW. Pain coping and social support as predictors of long-term functional disability and pain in early rheumatoid arthritis. Behav Res Ther. 2003;41(11):1295–310.
204. López-Martínez AE, Esteve-Zarazaga R, Ramírez-Maestre C. Perceived social support and coping responses are independent variables explaining pain adjustment among chronic pain patients. J Pain. 2008;9(4):373–9.
205. Karsdorp PA, Vlaeyen JW. Active avoidance but not activity pacing is associated with disability in fibromyalgia. Pain. 2009;147(1–3):29–35.
206. Carroll LJ, Ferrari R, Cassidy JD, Côté P. Coping and recovery in whiplash-associated disorders: early use of passive coping strategies is associated with slower recovery of neck pain and pain-related disability. Clin J Pain. 2014;30(1):1–8.
207. Benyon K, Muller S, Hill S, Mallen C. Coping strategies as predictors of pain and disability in older people in primary care: a longitudinal study. BMC Fam Pract. 2013;14(1):1–7.
208. Sullivan MJ, Bishop SR, Pivik J. The pain catastrophizing scale: development and validation. Psychol Assess. 1995;7(4):524.
209. Sullivan MJ, Stanish W, Waite H, Sullivan M, Tripp DA. Catastrophizing, pain, and disability in patients with soft-tissue injuries. Pain. 1998;77(3):253–60.
210. Somers TJ, Keefe FJ, Pells JJ, et al. Pain catastrophizing and pain-related fear in osteoarthritis patients: relationships to pain and disability. J Pain Symptom Manag. 2009;37(5):863–72.
211. Severeijns R, Vlaeyen JW, van den Hout MA, Picavet HSJ. Pain catastrophizing is associated with health indices in musculoskeletal pain: a cross-sectional study in the Dutch community. Health Psychol. 2004;23(1):49.
212. Martinez-Calderon J, Jensen MP, Morales-Asencio JM, Luque-Suarez A. Pain catastrophizing and function in individuals with chronic musculoskeletal pain. Clin J Pain. 2019;35(3):279–93.
213. Coronado RA, George SZ, Devin CJ, Wegener ST, Archer KR. Pain sensitivity and pain catastrophizing are associated with persistent pain and disability after lumbar spine surgery. Arch Phys Med Rehabil. 2015;96(10):1763–70.

214. Besen E, Gaines B, Linton SJ, Shaw WS. The role of pain catastrophizing as a mediator in the work disability process following acute low back pain. J Appl Biobehav Res. 2017;22(1):e12085.
215. Brown GK, Nicassio PM. Development of a questionnaire for the assessment of active and passive coping strategies in chronic pain patients. Pain. 1987;31(1):53–64.
216. Hadjistavropoulos HD, MacLeod FK, Asmundson GJ. Validation of the chronic pain coping inventory. Pain. 1999;80(3):471–81.
217. Snow-Turek AL, Norris MP, Tan G. Active and passive coping strategies in chronic pain patients. Pain. 1996;64(3):455–62.
218. Tan G, Jensen MP, Robinson-Whelen S, Thornby JI, Monga TN. Coping with chronic pain: a comparison of two measures. Pain. 2001;90(1–2):127–33.
219. Meredith P, Strong J, Feeney JA. Adult attachment, anxiety, and pain self-efficacy as predictors of pain intensity and disability. Pain. 2006;123(1–2):146–54.
220. Asghari A, Nicholas MK. Pain self-efficacy beliefs and pain behaviour. A prospective study. Pain. 2001;94(1):85–100.
221. Costa LCM, Maher CG, McAuley JH, Hancock MJ, Smeets RJ. Self-efficacy is more important than fear of movement in mediating the relationship between pain and disability in chronic low back pain. Eur J Pain. 2011;15(2):213–9.
222. Skinner EA, Edge K, Altman J, Sherwood H. Searching for the structure of coping: a review and critique of category systems for classifying ways of coping. Psychol Bull. 2003;129(2):216. Esteve R, Ramírez-Maestre C, López-Martínez AE. Adjustment to chronic pain: the role of pain acceptance, coping strategies, and pain-related cognitions. Ann Behav Med. 2007;33(2):179–188
223. McCracken LM, Eccleston C. Coping or acceptance: what to do about chronic pain? Pain. 2003;105(1–2):197–204.
224. Wright MA, Wren AA, Somers TJ, et al. Pain acceptance, hope, and optimism: relationships to pain and adjustment in patients with chronic musculoskeletal pain. J Pain. 2011;12(11):1155–62.
225. Chen S, You B, Jackson T. Facets of mindfulness as predictors of emotional distress among Chinese adults with chronic musculoskeletal pain. Mindfulness. 2021;12(3):775–83.
226. McCracken LM, Thompson M. Components of mindfulness in patients with chronic pain. J Psychopathol Behav Assess. 2009;31(2):75–82.
227. Schütze R, Rees C, Preece M, Schütze M. Low mindfulness predicts pain catastrophizing in a fear-avoidance model of chronic pain. Pain. 2010;148(1):120–7.
228. Tuna E, Gençöz T. Pain perception, distress tolerance and self-compassion in Turkish young adults with and without a history of non-suicidal self-injury. Curr Psychol. 2021;40(8):4143–55.
229. Wegener ST, Castillo RC, Haythornthwaite J, MacKenzie EJ, Bosse MJ, Group LS. Psychological distress mediates the effect of pain on function. Pain. 2011;152(6):1349–57.
230. Utrillas-Compaired A, la Torre-Escuredo D, Basilio J, Tebar-Martínez AJ, Barco A-D. Does preoperative psychologic distress influence pain, function, and quality of life after TKA? Clin Orthop Relat Res. 2014;472(8):2457–65.
231. Van Damme S, Crombez G, Eccleston C. Coping with pain: a motivational perspective. Pain. 2008;139(1):1–4.
232. Vowles KE, McCracken LM, McLeod C, Eccleston C. The Chronic Pain Acceptance Questionnaire: confirmatory factor analysis and identification of patient subgroups. Pain. 2008;140(2):284–91.
233. Fish RA, McGuire B, Hogan M, Morrison TG, Stewart I. Validation of the Chronic Pain Acceptance Questionnaire (CPAQ) in an Internet sample and development and preliminary validation of the CPAQ-8. Pain. 2010;149(3):435–43.
234. Truchon M, Côté D. Predictive validity of the Chronic Pain Coping Inventory in subacute low back pain. Pain. 2005;116(3):205–12.

235. Romano JM, Jensen MP, Turner JA. The chronic pain coping inventory-42: reliability and validity. Pain. 2003;104(1–2):65–73.
236. Rosenstiel AK, Keefe FJ. The use of coping strategies in chronic low back pain patients: relationship to patient characteristics and current adjustment. Pain. 1983;17(1):33–44.
237. Huguet A, Miró J, Nieto R. The factor structure and factorial invariance of the Pain-Coping Questionnaire across age: evidence from community-based samples of children and adults. Eur J Pain. 2009;13(8):879–89.
238. Wicksell RK, Lekander M, Sorjonen K, Olsson GL. The Psychological Inflexibility in Pain Scale (PIPS)–statistical properties and model fit of an instrument to assess change processes in pain related disability. Eur J Pain. 2010;14(7):771. e1–771. e14.
239. Jensen MP, Turner JA, Romano JM, Lawler BK. Relationship of pain-specific beliefs to chronic pain adjustment. Pain. 1994;57(3):301–9.
240. Lefebvre J, Jensen M, Waters S, Molton I, Keefe F, Caldwell D. The development and assessment of the Worry About Pain Questionnaire. Eur J Pain. 2017;21(7):1154–64.
241. Slepian PM, Ankawi B, Himawan LK, France CR. Development and initial validation of the pain resilience scale. J Pain. 2016;17(4):462–72.
242. Flor H, Knost B, Birbaumer N. The role of operant conditioning in chronic pain: an experimental investigation. Pain. 2002;95(1–2):111–8.
243. Gatzounis R, Schrooten MG, Crombez G, Vlaeyen JW. Operant learning theory in pain and chronic pain rehabilitation. Curr Pain Headache Rep. 2012;16(2):117–26.
244. Turk DC. Cognitive-behavioral approach to the treatment of chronic pain patients. Region Anesth Pain Med. 2003;28(6):573–9.
245. Zarcone JR, Crosland K, Fisher WW, Worsdell AS, Herman K. A brief method for conducting a negative-reinforcement assessment. Res Dev Disabil. 1999;20(2):107–24.
246. Zale EL, Ditre JW. Pain-related fear, disability, and the fear-avoidance model of chronic pain. Curr Opin Psychol. 2015;5:24–30.
247. Meulders A. From fear of movement-related pain and avoidance to chronic pain disability: a state-of-the-art review. Curr Opin Behav Sci. 2019;26:130–6.
248. Vlaeyen JW, Kole-Snijders AM, Rotteveel AM, Ruesink R, Heuts PH. The role of fear of movement/(re) injury in pain disability. J Occup Rehabil. 1995;5(4):235–52.
249. Becker S, Kleinböhl D, Hölzl R. Awareness is awareness is awareness? Decomposing different aspects of awareness and their role in operant learning of pain sensitivity. Conscious Cogn. 2012;21(3):1073–84.
250. Hölzl R, Kleinböhl D, Huse E. Implicit operant learning of pain sensitization. Pain. 2005;115(1–2):12–20.
251. Barke A, Preis MA, Schmidt-Samoa C, Baudewig J, Kröner-Herwig B, Dechent P. Neural correlates differ in high and low fear-avoidant chronic low back pain patients when imagining back-straining movements. J Pain. 2016;17(8):930–43.
252. Revicki DA, Chen W-H, Harnam N, et al. Development and psychometric analysis of the PROMIS pain behavior item bank. Pain. 2009;146(1–2):158–69.
253. Cimmino MA, Ferrone C, Cutolo M. Epidemiology of chronic musculoskeletal pain. Best Pract Res Clin Rheumatol. 2011;25(2):173–83.
254. Stefansdottir R, Gudmundsdottir S. Sedentary behavior and musculoskeletal pain: a five-year longitudinal Icelandic study. Public Health. 2017;149(suppl C):71–3.
255. da Costa L, Lemes IR, Tebar WR, et al. Sedentary behavior is associated with musculoskeletal pain in adolescents: a cross sectional study. Braz J Phys Ther. 2022;26(5):100452.
256. Mahdavi SB, Riahi R, Vahdatpour B, Kelishadi R. Association between sedentary behavior and low back pain; A systematic review and meta-analysis. Health Promo Perspect. 2021;11(4):393.
257. Holth HS, Werpen HKB, Zwart J-A, Hagen K. Physical inactivity is associated with chronic musculoskeletal complaints 11 years later: results from the Nord-Trøndelag Health Study. BMC Musculoskelet Disord. 2008;9(1):1–7.
258. Heikkala E, Oura P, Korpela T, Karppinen J, Paananen M. Chronotypes and disabling musculoskeletal pain: a Finnish birth cohort study. Eur J Pain. 2022;26(5):1069–78.

259. Heikkala E, Paananen M, Merikanto I, Karppinen J, Oura P. Eveningness intensifies the association between musculoskeletal pain and health-related quality of life: a Northern Finland Birth Cohort Study 1966. Pain. 2022;163(11):2154–61.
260. Kantermann T, Theadom A, Roenneberg T, Cropley M. Fibromyalgia syndrome and chronotype: late chronotypes are more affected. J Biol Rhythm. 2012;27(2):176–9.
261. Smith MT, Haythornthwaite JA. How do sleep disturbance and chronic pain inter-relate? Insights from the longitudinal and cognitive-behavioral clinical trials literature. Sleep Med Rev. 2004;8(2):119–32.
262. Arnison T, Schrooten MG, Hesser H, Jansson-Fröjmark M, Persson J. Longitudinal, bidirectional relationships of insomnia symptoms and musculoskeletal pain across adolescence: the mediating role of mood. Pain. 2022;163(2):287–98.
263. Koffel E, Kroenke K, Bair MJ, Leverty D, Polusny MA, Krebs EE. The bidirectional relationship between sleep complaints and pain: analysis of data from a randomized trial. Health Psychol. 2016;35(1):41.
264. Tang NK, McBeth J, Jordan KP, Blagojevic-Bucknall M, Croft P, Wilkie R. Impact of musculoskeletal pain on insomnia onset: a prospective cohort study. Rheumatology. 2015;54(2):248–56.
265. Aili K, Åström-Paulsson S, Stoetzer U, Svartengren M, Hillert L. Reliability of actigraphy and subjective sleep measurements in adults: the design of sleep assessments. J Clin Sleep Med. 2017;13(1):39–47.
266. Case MA, Burwick HA, Volpp KG, Patel MS. Accuracy of smartphone applications and wearable devices for tracking physical activity data. JAMA. 2015;313(6):625–6.
267. Kushida CA, Chang A, Gadkary C, Guilleminault C, Carrillo O, Dement WC. Comparison of actigraphic, polysomnographic, and subjective assessment of sleep parameters in sleep-disordered patients. Sleep Med. 2001;2(5):389–96.
268. De Chazal P, Fox N, O'hare E, et al. Sleep/wake measurement using a non-contact biomotion sensor. J Sleep Res. 2011;20(2):356–66.
269. Yi R, Enayati M, Keller JM, Popescu M, Skubic M. Non-invasive in-home sleep stage classification using a ballistocardiography bed sensor. IEEE; 2019. p. 1–4.
270. Schalet BD, Hays RD, Jensen SE, Beaumont JL, Fries JF, Cella D. Validity of PROMIS physical function measured in diverse clinical samples. J Clin Epidemiol. 2016;73:112–8.
271. Hung M, Hon SD, Franklin JD, et al. Psychometric properties of the PROMIS physical function item bank in patients with spinal disorders. Spine. 2014;39(2):158–63.
272. Carvalho FA, Morelhão PK, Franco MR, et al. Reliability and validity of two multidimensional self-reported physical activity questionnaires in people with chronic low back pain. Musculoskel Sci Pract. 2017;27:65–70.
273. Baecke JA, Burema J, Frijters JE. A short questionnaire for the measurement of habitual physical activity in epidemiological studies. Am J Clin Nutr. 1982;36(5):936–42.
274. Ono R, Hirata S, Yamada M, Nishiyama T, Kurosaka M, Tamura Y. Reliability and validity of the Baecke physical activity questionnaire in adult women with hip disorders. BMC Musculoskelet Disord. 2007;8(1):1–6.
275. Craig CL, Marshall AL, Sjöström M, et al. International physical activity questionnaire: 12-country reliability and validity. Med Sci Sports Exerc. 2003;35(8):1381–95.
276. Elma Ö, Yilmaz ST, Deliens T, et al. Chronic musculoskeletal pain and nutrition: where are we and where are we heading? PM R. 2020;12(12):1268–78.
277. Elma Ö, Yilmaz ST, Deliens T, et al. Do nutritional factors interact with chronic musculoskeletal pain? a systematic review. J Clin Med. 2020;9(3):702.
278. Towery P, Guffey JS, Doerflein C, Stroup K, Saucedo S, Taylor J. Chronic musculoskeletal pain and function improve with a plant-based diet. Complement Ther Med. 2018;40:64–9.
279. Holton KF, Kirkland AE, Baron M, et al. The low glutamate diet effectively improves pain and other symptoms of Gulf War illness. Nutrients. 2020;12(9):2593.
280. Torres SJ, Nowson CA. Relationship between stress, eating behavior, and obesity. Nutrition. 2007;23(11–12):887–94.

281. Elran Barak R, Shuval K, Li Q, et al. Emotional eating in adults: the role of sociodemographics, lifestyle behaviors, and self-regulation—findings from a US National Study. Int J Environ Res Public Health. 2021;18(4):1744.
282. Amy EA, Kozak AT. "The more pain I have, the more I want to eat": obesity in the context of chronic pain. Obesity. 2012;20(10):2027–34.
283. Meleger AL, Froude CK, Walker J III. Nutrition and eating behavior in patients with chronic pain receiving long-term opioid therapy. PM R. 2014;6(1):7–12. e1
284. Van Strien T, Frijters JE, Bergers GP, Defares PB. The Dutch Eating Behavior Questionnaire (DEBQ) for assessment of restrained, emotional, and external eating behavior. Int J Eat Disord. 1986;5(2):295–315.
285. Nolan LJ, Halperin LB, Geliebter A. Emotional Appetite Questionnaire. Construct validity and relationship with BMI. Appetite. 2010;54(2):314–9.
286. Arnow B, Kenardy J, Agras WS. The Emotional Eating Scale: the development of a measure to assess coping with negative affect by eating. Int J Eat Disord. 1995;18(1):79–90.
287. Karlsson J, Persson L-O, Sjöström L, Sullivan M. Psychometric properties and factor structure of the Three-Factor Eating Questionnaire (TFEQ) in obese men and women. Results from the Swedish Obese Subjects (SOS) study. Int J Obes. 2000;24(12):1715–25.
288. Cappelleri J, Bushmakin A, Gerber R, et al. Psychometric analysis of the Three-Factor Eating Questionnaire-R21: results from a large diverse sample of obese and non-obese participants. Int J Obes. 2009;33(6):611–20.
289. Masheb RM, Douglas ME, Kutz AM, Marsh AG, Driscoll M. Pain and emotional eating: further investigation of the Yale Emotional Overeating Questionnaire in weight loss seeking patients. J Behav Med. 2020;43(3):479–86.
290. Di Maso M, Boffetta P, Negri E, La Vecchia C, Bravi F. Caffeinated coffee consumption and health outcomes in the US population: a dose–response meta-analysis and estimation of disease cases and deaths avoided. Adv Nutr. 2021;12(4):1160–76.
291. Carter GS, Hamdan H. Insomnia and caffeine. In: Comorbid Sleep and Psychiatric Disorders. Springer; 2019. p. 247–52.
292. Statland BE, Demas TJ. Serum caffeine half-lives: healthy subjects vs. patients having alcoholic hepatic disease. Am J Clin Pathol. 1980;73(3):390–3.
293. Benowitz NL. Clinical pharmacology of caffeine. Annu Rev Med. 1990;41(1):277–88.
294. Knutti R, Rothweiler H, Schlatter C. The effect of pregnancy on the pharmacokinetics of caffeine. In: New Toxicology for Old. Springer; 1982. p. 187–92.
295. Abuse S. Mental Health Services Administration. Key substance use and mental health indicators in the United States: results from the 2020 National Survey on Drug Use and Health (HHS Publication No. PEP21-07-01-003, NSDUH Series H-56). Rockville: Center for Behavioral Health Statistics and Quality; 2021. Substance Abuse and Mental Health Services Administration Retrieved from https://www.samhsa.gov/data. 2022.
296. Humeniuk R, Henry-Edwards S, Ali R, Poznyak V, Monteiro MG, Organization WH. The Alcohol, Smoking and Substance Involvement Screening Test (ASSIST): manual for use in primary care. World Health Organization; 2010.
297. McNeely J, Wu L-T, Subramaniam G, et al. Performance of the tobacco, alcohol, prescription medication, and other substance use (TAPS) tool for substance use screening in primary care patients. Ann Intern Med. 2016;165(10):690–9.
298. Levy SJ, Williams JF, Ryan SA, et al. Substance use screening, brief intervention, and referral to treatment. Pediatrics. 2016;138(1):e20161211.
299. Hammock K, Velasquez MM, Alwan H, von Sternberg K. Alcohol screening, brief intervention, and referral to treatment (SBIRT) for girls and women. Alcohol Res. 2020;40(2):07.
300. Butler SF, Budman SH, Fanciullo GJ, Jamison RN. Cross validation of the Current Opioid Misuse Measure (COMM) to monitor chronic pain patients on opioid therapy. Clin J Pain. 2010;26(9):770.

301. Dowling LS, Gatchel RJ, Adams LL, Stowell AW, Bernstein D. An evaluation of the predictive validity of the Pain Medication Questionnaire with a heterogeneous group of patients with chronic pain. J Opioid Manag. 2007;3(5):257–66.
302. Pilkonis PA, Yu L, Dodds NE, et al. An item bank for abuse of prescription pain medication from the patient-reported outcomes measurement information system (PROMIS®). Pain Med. 2017;18(8):1516–27.
303. You DS, Hah JM, Collins S, et al. Evaluation of the preliminary validity of misuse of prescription pain medication items from the Patient-Reported Outcomes Measurement Information System (PROMIS)®. Pain Med. 2019;20(10):1925–33.
304. Cheatle MD, Compton PA, Dhingra L, Wasser TE, O'Brien CP. Development of the revised opioid risk tool to predict opioid use disorder in patients with chronic nonmalignant pain. J Pain. 2019;20(7):842–51.
305. Olivieri P, Solitar B, Dubois M. Childhood risk factors for developing fibromyalgia. Open Access Rheumatol Res Rev. 2012;4:109.
306. Jones GT, Silman AJ, Power C, Macfarlane GJ. Are common symptoms in childhood associated with chronic widespread body pain in adulthood?: Results from the 1958 british birth cohort study. Arthritis Rheum. 2007;56(5):1669–75.
307. Generaal E, Vogelzangs N, Macfarlane GJ, et al. Biological stress systems, adverse life events and the onset of chronic multisite musculoskeletal pain: a 6-year cohort study. Ann Rheum Dis. 2016;75(5):847–54.
308. Miranda H, Punnett L, Gore RJ, Team PR. Musculoskeletal pain and reported workplace assault: a prospective study of clinical staff in nursing homes. Hum Factors. 2014;56(1):215–27.
309. Miranda H, Punnett L, Gore R, Boyer J. Violence at the workplace increases the risk of musculoskeletal pain among nursing home workers. Occup Environ Med. 2011;68(1):52–7.
310. Rezaee M, Ghasemi M. Prevalence of low back pain among nurses: predisposing factors and role of work place violence. Trauma Mon. 2014;19(4):e17926.
311. Poleshuck EL, Bair MJ, Kroenke K, et al. Psychosocial stress and anxiety in musculoskeletal pain patients with and without depression. Gen Hosp Psychiatry. 2009;31(2):116–22.
312. Craner JR, Lake ES, Barr AC, Kirby KE, O'Neill M. Childhood adversity among adults with chronic pain: prevalence and association with pain-related outcomes. Clin J Pain. 2022;38(9):551–61.
313. Nicol AL, Sieberg CB, Clauw DJ, Hassett AL, Moser SE, Brummett CM. The association between a history of lifetime traumatic events and pain severity, physical function, and affective distress in patients with chronic pain. J Pain. 2016;17(12):1334–48.
314. Van Houdenhove B, Neerinckx E, Onghena P, Vingerhoets A, Lysens R, Vertommen H. Daily hassles reported by chronic fatigue syndrome and fibromyalgia patients in tertiary care: a controlled quantitative and qualitative study. Psychother Psychosom. 2002;71(4):207–13.
315. Lobo CP, Pfalzgraf AR, Giannetti V, Kanyongo G. Impact of invalidation and trust in physicians on health outcomes in fibromyalgia patients. Prim Care Compan CNS Disorders. 2014;16(5):10.4088/PCC.14m01664.
316. Farin E, Gramm L, Schmidt E. The patient–physician relationship in patients with chronic low back pain as a predictor of outcomes after rehabilitation. J Behav Med. 2013;36(3):246–58.
317. Racine N, Killam T, Madigan S. Trauma-informed care as a universal precaution: beyond the adverse childhood experiences questionnaire. JAMA Pediatr. 2020;174(1):5–6.
318. Koetting C. Trauma-informed care: helping patients with a painful past. J Christ Nurs. 2016;33(4):206–13.
319. Ranjbar N, Erb M. Adverse childhood experiences and trauma-informed care in rehabilitation clinical practice. Arch Rehabil Res Clin Transl. 2019;1(1–2):100003.
320. Weickgenant AL, Slater MA, Patterson TL, Atkinson JH, Grant I, Garfin SR. Coping activities in chronic low back pain: relationship with depression. Pain. 1993;53(1):95–103.
321. Che X, Cash R, Ng SK, Fitzgerald P, Fitzgibbon BM. A systematic review of the processes underlying the main and the buffering effect of social support on the experience of pain. Clin J Pain. 2018;34(11):1061–76.

322. Prang K-H, Berecki-Gisolf J, Newnam S. Recovery from musculoskeletal injury: the role of social support following a transport accident. Health Qual Life Outcomes. 2015;13(1):1–17.
323. Suso-Ribera C, Sullivan MJ, Suso-Vergara S. Pain intensity is not always associated with poorer health status: exploring the moderating role of spouse personality. Pain Res Manag. 2018;2018:7927656.
324. Felitti VJ, Anda RF, Nordenberg D, et al. Relationship of childhood abuse and household dysfunction to many of the leading causes of death in adults: the Adverse Childhood Experiences (ACE) Study. Am J Prev Med. 1998;14(4):245–58.
325. Bernstein DP, Stein JA, Newcomb MD, et al. Development and validation of a brief screening version of the Childhood Trauma Questionnaire. Child Abuse Negl. 2003;27(2):169–90.
326. Aldwin CM. The Elders Life Stress Inventory (ELSI): research and clinical applications. In: Keller PA, Heyman SR, editors. Innovations in clinical practice: a source book, vol. 10. Professional Resource Press/Professional Resource Exchange; 1991. p. 355–64.
327. Cohen S, Kamarck T, Mermelstein R. Perceived stress scale. Measuring stress: a guide for health and social scientists. 1994;10(2):1–2.
328. Roohafza H, Ramezani M, Sadeghi M, Shahnam M, Zolfagari B, Sarafzadegan N. Development and validation of the stressful life event questionnaire. Int J Public Health. 2011;56(4):441–8.
329. Brantley PJ, Waggoner CD, Jones GN, Rappaport NB. A daily stress inventory: development, reliability, and validity. J Behav Med. 1987;10(1):61–73.
330. Holm JE, Holroyd KA. The daily hassles scale (revised): does it measure stress or symptoms? Behav Assess. 1992;14:465.
331. Kubany ES, Leisen MB, Kaplan AS, et al. Development and preliminary validation of a brief broad-spectrum measure of trauma exposure: the Traumatic Life Events Questionnaire. Psychol Assess. 2000;12(2):210.
332. Smith TO, Dainty JR, Williamson E, Martin KR. Association between musculoskeletal pain with social isolation and loneliness: analysis of the English Longitudinal Study of Ageing. Br J Pain. 2019;13(2):82–90.
333. Karayannis NV, Baumann I, Sturgeon JA, Melloh M, Mackey SC. The impact of social isolation on pain interference: a longitudinal study. Ann Behav Med. 2019;53(1):65–74.
334. Solé E, Racine M, Tomé-Pires C, Galán S, Jensen MP, Miró J. Social factors, disability, and depressive symptoms in adults with chronic pain. Clin J Pain. 2020;36(5):371–8.
335. Nicolson PJ, Williamson E, Morris A, et al. Musculoskeletal pain and loneliness, social support and social engagement among older adults: analysis of the Oxford Pain, Activity and Lifestyle cohort. Musculoskeletal Care. 2021;19(3):269–77.
336. Hahn EA, DeVellis RF, Bode RK, et al. Measuring social health in the patient-reported outcomes measurement information system (PROMIS): item bank development and testing. Qual Life Res. 2010;19(7):1035–44.
337. Nicholson NR Jr, Feinn R, Casey E, Dixon J. Psychometric evaluation of the social isolation scale in older adults. The Gerontologist. 2020;60(7):e491–501.
338. Chiu C-Y, Motl RW, Ditchman N. Validation of the Social Provisions Scale in people with multiple sclerosis. Rehabil Psychol. 2016;61(3):297.
339. Cutrona CE, Russell DW. The provisions of social relationships and adaptation to stress. Adv Person Relat. 1987;1(1):37–67.
340. Lee RM, Robbins SB. Measuring belongingness: the social connectedness and the social assurance scales. J Couns Psychol. 1995;42(2):232.
341. Russell DW. UCLA Loneliness Scale (Version 3): reliability, validity, and factor structure. J Pers Assess. 1996;66(1):20–40.
342. Ebesutani C, Drescher CF, Reise SP, et al. The loneliness questionnaire–short version: an evaluation of reverse-worded and non-reverse-worded items via item response theory. J Pers Assess. 2012;94(4):427–37.
343. Organization WH. The World health report 2001: mental health: new understanding, new hope, 2001.

344. De Ruddere L, Craig KD. Understanding stigma and chronic pain: a-state-of-the-art review. Pain. 2016;157(8):1607–10.
345. Samulowitz A, Gremyr I, Eriksson E, Hensing G. "Brave men" and "emotional women": a theory-guided literature review on gender bias in health care and gendered norms towards patients with chronic pain. Pain Res Manag. 2018;2018:6358624.
346. Kool MB, van Middendorp H, Lumley MA, Bijlsma JW, Geenen R. Social support and invalidation by others contribute uniquely to the understanding of physical and mental health of patients with rheumatic diseases. J Health Psychol. 2013;18(1):86–95.
347. Penn TM, Overstreet DS, Aroke EN, et al. Perceived injustice helps explain the association between chronic pain stigma and movement-evoked pain in adults with nonspecific chronic low back pain. Pain Med. 2020;21(11):3161–71.
348. Waugh OC, Byrne DG, Nicholas MK. Internalized stigma in people living with chronic pain. J Pain. 2014;15(5):550. e1–550. e10.
349. Steele CM. A threat in the air: how stereotypes shape intellectual identity and performance. Am Psychol. 1997;52(6):613.
350. Coyle J. Exploring the meaning of 'dissatisfaction'with health care: the importance of 'personal identity threat'. Sociol Health Illn. 1999;21(1):95–123.
351. Knapp S, Marziliano A, Moyer A. Identity threat and stigma in cancer patients. Health Psychol Open. 2014;1(1):2055102914552281.
352. McGonagle AK, Barnes-Farrell JL. Chronic illness in the workplace: stigma, identity threat and strain. Stress Health. 2014;30(4):310–21.
353. Vaala SE, Bleakley A, Hennessy M, Jordan AB. Weight stigmatization moderates the effects of sugar-sweetened beverage-related PSAs among US parents. Media Psychol. 2016;19(4):534–60.
354. Mensinger JL, Tylka TL, Calamari ME. Mechanisms underlying weight status and healthcare avoidance in women: a study of weight stigma, body-related shame and guilt, and healthcare stress. Body Image. 2018;25:139–47.
355. Bernardes SF, Lima ML. Being less of a man or less of a woman: perceptions of chronic pain patients' gender identities. Eur J Pain. 2010;14(2):194–9.
356. Marriott C, Thompson AR. Managing threats to femininity: personal and interpersonal experience of living with vulval pain. Psychol Health. 2008;23(2):243–58.
357. Gullacksen A-C, Lidbeck J. The life adjustment process in chronic pain: psychosocial assessment and clinical implications. Pain Res Manag. 2004;9(3):145–53.
358. Kowal J, Wilson KG, McWilliams LA, Péloquin K, Duong D. Self-perceived burden in chronic pain: relevance, prevalence, and predictors. Pain. 2012;153(8):1735–41.
359. Wilson KG, Kowal J, Henderson PR, McWilliams LA, Péloquin K. Chronic pain and the interpersonal theory of suicide. Rehabil Psychol. 2013;58(1):111.
360. Wilson KG, Kowal J, Caird SM, Castillo D, McWilliams LA, Heenan A. Self-perceived burden, perceived burdensomeness, and suicidal ideation in patients with chronic pain. Canad J Pain. 2017;1(1):127–36.
361. Kirtley OJ, Rodham K, Crane C. Understanding suicidal ideation and behaviour in individuals with chronic pain: a review of the role of novel transdiagnostic psychological factors. Lancet Psychiatry. 2020;7(3):282–90.
362. Cousineau N, McDowell I, Hotz S, Hébert P. Measuring chronic patients' feelings of being a burden to their caregivers: development and preliminary validation of a scale. Med Care. 2003;41:110–118.
363. Hood CM, Gennuso KP, Swain GR, Catlin BB. County health rankings: relationships between determinant factors and health outcomes. Am J Prev Med. 2016;50(2):129–35.
364. Rethorn ZD, Cook C, Reneker JC. Social determinants of health: if you aren't measuring them, you aren't seeing the big picture. J Orthop Sports Phys Ther. 2019;49(12):872–4.
365. Karran EL, Grant AR, Moseley GL. Low back pain and the social determinants of health: a systematic review and narrative synthesis. Pain. 2020;161(11):2476–93.
366. Guillemin F, Carruthers E, Li LC. Determinants of MSK health and disability–social determinants of inequities in MSK health. Best Pract Res Clin Rheumatol. 2014;28(3):411–33.

367. Wandner LD, Fenton BT, Goulet JL, et al. Treatment of a large Cohort of veterans experiencing musculoskeletal disorders with spinal cord stimulation in the veterans health administration: veteran characteristics and outcomes. J Pain Res. 2020;13:1687.
368. Campwala Z, Datta P, DiMarzio M, Sukul V, Feustel PJ, Pilitsis JG. Spinal cord stimulation to treat low back pain in patients with and without previous spine surgery. Neuromodulation Technol Neural Interface. 2021;24(8):1363–9.
369. Petta D, D'Amora U, D'Arrigo D, et al. Musculoskeletal tissues-on-a-chip: role of natural polymers in reproducing tissue-specific microenvironments. Biofabrication. 2022;14:4.
370. Ajalik RE, Alenchery RG, Cognetti JS, et al. Human organ-on-a-chip microphysiological systems to model musculoskeletal pathologies and accelerate therapeutic discovery. Front Bioeng Biotechnol. 2022;10:846230.
371. Bruns D, Disorbio JM. Assessment of biopsychosocial risk factors for medical treatment: a collaborative approach. J Clin Psychol Med Settings. 2009;16(2):127–47.
372. Beltrutti D, Lamberto A, Barolat G, et al. The psychological assessment of candidates for spinal cord stimulation for chronic pain management. Pain Pract. 2004;4(3):204–21.
373. Atkinson L, Sundaraj S, Brooker C, et al. Recommendations for patient selection in spinal cord stimulation. J Clin Neurosci. 2011;18(10):1295–302.
374. Mammis A. Spinal cord stimulation: principles and practice. Nova Biomedical; 2016.
375. Campbell CM, Jamison RN, Edwards RR. Psychological screening/phenotyping as predictors for spinal cord stimulation. Curr Pain Headache Rep. 2013;17(1):1–8.
376. De La Cruz P, Fama C, Roth S, et al. Predictors of spinal cord stimulation success. Neuromodulation Technol Neural Interface. 2015;18(7):599–602.
377. Marola O, Cherala R, Prusik J, et al. BMI as a predictor of spinal cord stimulation success in chronic pain patients. Neuromodulation Technol Neural Interface. 2017;20(3):269–73.
378. Celestin J, Edwards RR, Jamison RN. Pretreatment psychosocial variables as predictors of outcomes following lumbar surgery and spinal cord stimulation: a systematic review and literature synthesis. Pain Med. 2009;10(4):639–53.
379. Odonkor C, Kwak R, Ting K, Hao D, Collins B, Shihab A. Fantastic four: age, spinal cord stimulator waveform, pain localization and history of spine surgery influence the odds of successful spinal cord stimulator trial. Pain Physician. 2020;23(1):E19.
380. Strauss I, Taha K, Krishna V, Hodaie M. Younger age predicts greater effectiveness of spinal cord stimulation for chronic pain. Acta Neurochir. 2016;158(5):999–1003.
381. Sparkes E, Duarte RV, Mann S, Lawrence TR, Raphael JH. Analysis of psychological characteristics impacting spinal cord stimulation treatment outcomes: a prospective assessment. Pain Physician. 2015;18(3):E369.
382. Paroli M, Bernini O, De Carolis G, et al. Are Multidimensional pain inventory coping strategy profiles associated with long-term spinal cord stimulation effectiveness? Pain Med. 2018;19(5):1023–32.
383. Stanos S. Topical analgesics. Phys Med Rehabil Clin N Am. 2020;31(2):233–44.
384. Waxman SG, et al. Sodium channels and pain. Proc Natl Acad Sci USA. 1999;96(14):7635–9.
385. Stanos SP, Galluzzi KE. Topical therapies in the management of chronic pain. Postgrad Med. 2013;125(4 Suppl 1):25–33.
386. Gasparini D, Ljubicic R, Mrsic-Pelcic J. Capsaicin - potential solution for chronic pain treatment. Psychiatr Danub. 2020;32(Suppl 4):420–8.
387. Derry S, et al. Topical capsaicin (high concentration) for chronic neuropathic pain in adults. Cochrane Database Syst Rev. 2017;1:CD007393.
388. Finnerup NB, et al. Pharmacotherapy for neuropathic pain in adults: a systematic review and meta-analysis. Lancet Neurol. 2015;14(2):162–73.
389. Derry S, et al. Topical NSAIDs for acute musculoskeletal pain in adults. Cochrane Database Syst Rev. 2015;6:CD007402.
390. Haroutiunian S, Drennan DA, Lipman AG. Topical NSAID therapy for musculoskeletal pain. Pain Med. 2010;11(4):535–49.
391. Bonezzi C, et al. Capsaicin 8% dermal patch in clinical practice: an expert opinion. Expert Opin Pharmacother. 2020;21(11):1377–87.

392. Arora V, Campbell JN, Chung MK. Fight fire with fire: neurobiology of capsaicin-induced analgesia for chronic pain. Pharmacol Ther. 2021;220:107743.
393. Bravo L, et al. Monoamines as drug targets in chronic pain: focusing on neuropathic pain. Front Neurosci. 2019;13:1268.
394. Nelson JC. Tricyclic and tetracyclic drugs. In: Schatzberg AF, Nemeroff CB, editors. The American Psychiatric Association publishing textbook of psychopharmacology. 5th ed. Arlington: American Psychiatric Association Publishing; 2017. p. 305.
395. Saarto T, Wiffen PJ. Antidepressants for neuropathic pain. Cochrane Database Syst Rev. 2007;4:CD005454.
396. Cruccu G, Di Stefano G, Truini A. Trigeminal neuralgia. N Engl J Med. 2020;383(8):754–62.
397. Zakrzewska JM, Linskey ME. Trigeminal neuralgia. BMJ. 2014;348:g474.
398. Moshe SL. Mechanisms of action of anticonvulsant agents. Neurology. 2000;55(5 Suppl 1):S32–40; discussion S54-8.
399. Dickenson AH, Matthews EA, Suzuki R. Neurobiology of neuropathic pain: mode of action of anticonvulsants. Eur J Pain. 2002;6 Suppl A:51–60.
400. Sidhu HS, Sadhotra A. Current status of the new antiepileptic drugs in chronic pain. Front Pharmacol. 2016;7:276. Dobecki DA, Schocket SM, Wallace MS. Update on pharmacotherapy guidelines for the treatment of neuropathic pain. Curr Pain Headache Rep. 2006;10(3):185–90.
401. Hirsch LJ, et al. Cross-sensitivity of skin rashes with antiepileptic drug use. Neurology. 2008;71(19):1527–34.
402. Sobotka JL, Alexander B, Cook BL. A review of carbamazepine's hematologic reactions and monitoring recommendations. DICP. 1990;24(12):1214–9.
403. Stoner SC, et al. Historical review of carbamazepine for the treatment of bipolar disorder. Pharmacotherapy. 2007;27(1):68–88.
404. Mannheimer B, et al. The effect of carbamazepine on warfarin anticoagulation: a register-based nationwide cohort study involving the Swedish population. J Thromb Haemost. 2016;14(4):765–71.
405. Yagi T, et al. Impact of concomitant antacid administration on gabapentin plasma exposure and oral bioavailability in healthy adult subjects. Drug Metab Pharmacokinet. 2012;27(2):248–54.
406. Hauser W, Schug S, Furlan AD. The opioid epidemic and national guidelines for opioid therapy for chronic noncancer pain: a perspective from different continents. Pain Rep. 2017;2(3):e599.
407. Antoniou T, et al. "Like being put on an ice floe and shoved away": a qualitative study of the impacts of opioid-related policy changes on people who take opioids. Int J Drug Policy. 2019;66:15–22.
408. Gomes T, et al. The burden of opioid-related mortality in the United States. JAMA Netw Open. 2018;1(2):e180217.
409. Dowell D, Haegerich TM, Chou R. CDC guideline for prescribing opioids for chronic pain — United States, 2016. MMWR Recomm Rep. 2016;65(1):1–49.
410. Adams K, Guerra M. Unintended consequences of United States chronic pain guidelines. Int J Clin Pharm. 2021;43(2):313–7.
411. CDC, CDC advises against misapplication of the guideline for prescribing opioids for chronic pain, 2019.
412. Reinecke H, et al. Analgesic efficacy of opioids in chronic pain: recent meta-analyses. Br J Pharmacol. 2015;172(2):324–33.
413. Krebs EE, et al. Effect of opioid vs nonopioid medications on pain-related function in patients with chronic back pain or hip or knee osteoarthritis pain: the SPACE randomized clinical trial. JAMA. 2018;319(9):872–82.
414. Chaparro LE, et al. Opioids compared with placebo or other treatments for chronic low back pain: an update of the Cochrane Review. Spine (Phila Pa 1976). 2014;39(7):556–63.
415. Vasudevan S. Multidisciplinary management of chronic pain. Cham: Springer; 2015.

416. Roth RS, Geisser ME, Williams DA. Interventional pain medicine: retreat from the biopsychosocial model of pain. Transl Behav Med. 2012;2(1):106–16.
417. Turk DC. Clinical effectiveness and cost-effectiveness of treatments for patients with chronic pain. Clin J Pain. 2002;18(6):355–65.
418. Breuer B, et al. U.S. board-certified pain physician practices: uniformity and census data of their locations. J Pain. 2007;8(3):244–50.
419. Schofferman J. Interventional pain medicine: financial success and ethical practice: an oxymoron? Pain Med. 2006;7(5):457–60.
420. Jonas WB, et al. Are invasive procedures effective for chronic pain? a systematic review. Pain Med. 2019;20(7):1281–93.
421. Skolasky RL, et al. The impact of reduction of pain after lumbar spine surgery: the relationship between changes in pain and physical function and disability. Spine (Phila Pa 1976). 2014;39(17):1426–32.
422. Baber Z, Erdek MA. Failed back surgery syndrome: current perspectives. J Pain Res. 2016;9:979–87.
423. Thomson S. Failed back surgery syndrome - definition, epidemiology and demographics. Br J Pain. 2013;7(1):56–9.
424. Rasmussen C, et al. Rates of lumbar disc surgery before and after implementation of multidisciplinary nonsurgical spine clinics. Spine (Phila Pa 1976). 2005;30(21):2469–73.
425. Rigoard P, et al. Optimizing the management and outcomes of failed back surgery syndrome: a consensus statement on definition and outlines for patient assessment. Pain Res Manag. 2019;2019:3126464.
426. Luque-Suarez A, Martinez-Calderon J, Falla D. Role of kinesiophobia on pain, disability and quality of life in people suffering from chronic musculoskeletal pain: a systematic review. Br J Sports Med. 2019;53:554.
427. Thomas JS, France CR. The relationship between pain-related fear and lumbar flexion during natural recovery from low back pain. Eur Spine J. 2008;17(1):97–103.
428. Prabhu C, Dadmi P. Effect of aquatic therapy v/s relaxation therapy in chronic low back pain. Int J Orthop Sci. 2019;5(1):279–84.
429. Booth J, Moseley GL, Schiltenwolf M, Cashin A, Davies M, Hübscher M. Exercise for chronic musculoskeletal pain: a biopsychosocial approach. Musculoskeletal Care. 2017;15:413. https://doi.org/10.1002/msc.1191.
430. Botta RM, Palermi S, Tarantino D. High-intensity interval training for chronic pain conditions: a narrative review. J Exerc Rehabil. 2022;18(1):10–9. https://doi.org/10.12965/jer.2142718.359. PMID: 35356137; PMCID: PMC8934613.
431. Polaski AM, Phelps AL, Kostek MC, Szucs KA, Kolber BJ. Exercise-induced hypoalgesia: a meta-analysis of exercise dosing for the treatment of chronic pain. PLoS One. 2019;14(1):e0210418. https://doi.org/10.1371/journal.pone.0210418. PMID: 30625201; PMCID: PMC6326521.
432. Sun E, Moshfegh J, Rishel CA, Cook CE, Goode AP, George SZ. Association of early physical therapy with long-term opioid use among opioid-naive patients with musculoskeletal pain. JAMA Netw Open. 2018;1(8):e185909.
433. Reeves L, Sako M, Malloy J, Goldstein A, Bennett K. Role of occupational therapy in comprehensive integrative pain management. American Occupational Therapy Association; 2022. Retrieved from https://www.aota.org/practice/practice-essentials/quality/quality-resources/role-of-ot-pain-management.
434. Antcliff D, Keeley P, Campbell M, Woby S, Keenan A-M, McGowan L. Activity pacing: moving beyond taking breaks and slowing down. Qal Life Res. 2018;27(7):1933–5. Department of Health and Human Services (2019). Department of health and human services pain management best practices inter-agency task force report. https://www.hhs.gov/sites/default/files/pmtf-final-report-2019-05-23.pdf

435. Louw A, Diener I, Butler DS, Puentedura EJ. The effect of neuroscience education on pain, disability, anxiety and dress in chronic musculoskeletal pain. Arch Phys Med Rehabil. 2011;92(12):2041–56.
436. Fashler S, Cooper L, Oosenbrug E, Burns L, Razavi S, Goldberg L, Katz J. Systematic review of multidisciplinary chronic pain treatment facilities. Pain Res Manag. 2016;2016:1. https://doi.org/10.1155/2016/5960987.
437. IASP. IASP curriculum outline on pain for occupational therapy; 2021. Retrieved from https://www.iasp-pain.org/education/curricula/iasp-curriculum-outline-on-pain-for-occupational-therapy/.
438. Lagueux E, Depelteau A, Masse J. Occupational therapy's unique contribution to pain management: a scoping review. Pain Res Manag. 2018;2018:1. https://doi.org/10.1155/2018/5378451.
439. Reneman MF, Waterschoot FPC, Burgerhof JGM, Geertzen JHB, Schiphorst Preuper HR, Dijkstra PU. Dosage of pain rehabilitation programmes for patients with chronic musculoskeletal pain: a non-inferiority randomised controlled trial. Disabil Rehabil. 2020;42(6):814–21. https://doi.org/10.1080/09638288.2018.1510549. Epub 2018 Dec 18. PMID: 30563365.
440. Knoerl R, Lavoie Smith EM, Weisberg J. Chronic pain and cognitive behavioral therapy: an integrative review. West J Nurs Res. 2016;38(5):596–628.
441. Castro M, Daltro C, Kraychete DC, Lopes J. The cognitive behavioral therapy causes an improvement in quality of life in patients with chronic musculoskeletal pain. Arq Neuropsiquiatr. 2012;70:864–8.
442. Leon L, Jover JA, Candelas G, et al. Effectiveness of an early cognitive–behavioral treatment in patients with work disability due to musculoskeletal disorders. Arthritis Care Res. 2009;61(7):996–1003.
443. Wetherell JL, Afari N, Rutledge T, et al. A randomized, controlled trial of acceptance and commitment therapy and cognitive-behavioral therapy for chronic pain. Pain. 2011;152(9):2098–107.
444. Murphy JL, Cordova MJ, Dedert EA. Cognitive behavioral therapy for chronic pain in veterans: evidence for clinical effectiveness in a model program. Psychol Serv. 2022;19(1):95.
445. Bennett R, Nelson D. Cognitive behavioral therapy for fibromyalgia. Nat Clin Pract Rheumatol. 2006;2(8):416–24.
446. Cheng JOS, Cheng S-T. Effectiveness of physical and cognitive-behavioural intervention programmes for chronic musculoskeletal pain in adults: a systematic review and meta-analysis of randomised controlled trials. PLoS One. 2019;14(10):e0223367.
447. Shen B, Li Y, Du X, et al. Effects of cognitive behavioral therapy for patients with rheumatoid arthritis: a systematic review and meta-analysis. Psychol Health Med. 2020;25(10):1179–91.
448. Khoo E-L, Small R, Cheng W, et al. Comparative evaluation of group-based mindfulness-based stress reduction and cognitive behavioural therapy for the treatment and management of chronic pain: a systematic review and network meta-analysis. Evid Based Ment Health. 2019;22(1):26–35.
449. Fleckenstein J, Flössel P, Engel T, et al. Individualized exercise in chronic non-specific low back pain: a systematic review with meta-analysis on the effects of exercise alone or in combination with psychological interventions on pain and disability. J Pain. 2022;23(11):1856.
450. Casey M-B, Smart KM, Segurado R, Doody C. Multidisciplinary-based Rehabilitation (MBR) compared with active physical interventions for pain and disability in adults with chronic pain: a systematic review and meta-analysis. Clin J Pain. 2020;36(11):874–86.
451. Thieme K, Turk D. Cognitive-behavioral and operant-behavioral therapy for people with fibromyalgia. Reumatismo. 2012;64(4):275–85.
452. Selvanathan J, Pham C, Nagappa M, et al. Cognitive behavioral therapy for insomnia in patients with chronic pain–a systematic review and meta-analysis of randomized controlled trials. Sleep Med Rev. 2021;60:101460.
453. Asih S, Neblett R, Mayer TG, Brede E, Gatchel RJ. Insomnia in a chronic musculoskeletal pain with disability population is independent of pain and depression. Spine J. 2014;14(9):2000–7.

454. Enomoto K, Adachi T, Fujino H, Kugo M, Tatsumi S, Sasaki J. Comparison of the effectiveness of cognitive behavioral therapy for insomnia, cognitive behavioral therapy for pain, and hybrid cognitive behavioral therapy for insomnia and pain in individuals with comorbid insomnia and chronic pain: a systematic review and network meta-analysis. Sleep Med Rev. 2022;66:101693.
455. Edinger JD, Carney CE. Overcoming insomnia: a cognitive-behavioral therapy approach, therapist guide. Oxford University Press; 2014.
456. Tang NK. CBT-I protocol for insomnia co-morbid with chronic pain. In: Cognitive-behavioural therapy for insomnia (CBT-I) across the life span: guidelines and clinical protocols for health professionals; 2022. p. 169–79.
457. Van Looveren E, Meeus M, Cagnie B, et al. Combining cognitive behavioral therapy for insomnia and chronic spinal pain within physical therapy: a practical guide for the implementation of an integrated approach. Phys Ther. 2022;102(8):pzac075.
458. McCracken LM, Gutiérrez-Martínez O. Processes of change in psychological flexibility in an interdisciplinary group-based treatment for chronic pain based on Acceptance and Commitment Therapy. Behav Res Ther. 2011;49(4):267–74.
459. Godfrey E, Wileman V, Holmes MG, et al. Physical therapy informed by acceptance and commitment therapy (PACT) versus usual care physical therapy for adults with chronic low back pain: a randomized controlled trial. J Pain. 2020;21(1–2):71–81.
460. Coronado RA, Brintz CE, McKernan LC, et al. Psychologically informed physical therapy for musculoskeletal pain: current approaches, implications, and future directions from recent randomized trials. Pain Rep. 2020;5(5):e847.
461. Hughes LS, Clark J, Colclough JA, Dale E, McMillan D. Acceptance and commitment therapy (ACT) for chronic pain. Clin J Pain. 2017;33(6):552–68.
462. Wicksell RK, Olsson GL, Hayes SC. Mediators of change in acceptance and commitment therapy for pediatric chronic pain. Pain. 2011;152(12):2792–801.
463. Dahl J, Wilson KG, Nilsson A. Acceptance and commitment therapy and the treatment of persons at risk for long-term disability resulting from stress and pain symptoms: a preliminary randomized trial. Behav Ther. 2004;35(4):785–801.
464. Wicksell RK, Melin L, Lekander M, Olsson GL. Evaluating the effectiveness of exposure and acceptance strategies to improve functioning and quality of life in longstanding pediatric pain–a randomized controlled trial. Pain. 2009;141(3):248–57.
465. Andrés-Rodríguez L, Borràs X, Feliu-Soler A, et al. Immune-inflammatory pathways and clinical changes in fibromyalgia patients treated with Mindfulness-Based Stress Reduction (MBSR): a randomized, controlled clinical trial. Brain Behav Immun. 2019;80:109–19.
466. Cherkin DC, Sherman KJ, Balderson BH, et al. Effect of mindfulness-based stress reduction vs cognitive behavioral therapy or usual care on back pain and functional limitations in adults with chronic low back pain: a randomized clinical trial. JAMA. 2016;315(12):1240–9.
467. Marchand WR. Mindfulness-based stress reduction, mindfulness-based cognitive therapy, and Zen meditation for depression, anxiety, pain, and psychological distress. J Psychiatr Pract. 2012;18(4):233–52.
468. Veehof MM, Oskam M-J, Schreurs KM, Bohlmeijer ET. Acceptance-based interventions for the treatment of chronic pain: a systematic review and meta-analysis. Pain. 2011;152(3):533–42.
469. Jay K, Brandt M, Jakobsen MD, et al. Ten weeks of physical-cognitive-mindfulness training reduces fear-avoidance beliefs about work-related activity: randomized controlled trial. Medicine. 2016;95(34):e3945.
470. Tatta J, Willgens AM, Palombaro KM. Mindfulness and acceptance–based interventions in physical therapist practice: the time is now. Phys Ther. 2022;102(3):pzab293.
471. Irving JA, Dobkin PL, Park J. Cultivating mindfulness in health care professionals: a review of empirical studies of mindfulness-based stress reduction (MBSR). Complement Ther Clin Pract. 2009;15(2):61–6.
472. Kabat-Zinn J. Mindfulness-based interventions in context: past, present, and future, vol. 10. American Psychological Association; 2003. p. 144.

473. Grossman P, Niemann L, Schmidt S, Walach H. Mindfulness-based stress reduction and health benefits: a meta-analysis. J Psychosom Res. 2004;57(1):35–43.
474. Rosenzweig S, Greeson JM, Reibel DK, Green JS, Jasser SA, Beasley D. Mindfulness-based stress reduction for chronic pain conditions: variation in treatment outcomes and role of home meditation practice. J Psychosom Res. 2010;68(1):29–36.
475. Elkins G, Johnson A, Fisher W. Cognitive hypnotherapy for pain management. Am J Clin Hypn. 2012;54(4):294–310.
476. Geagea D, Tyack Z, Kimble R, Eriksson L, Polito V, Griffin B. Hypnotherapy for procedural pain and distress in children: a scoping review protocol. Pain Med. 2021;22(12):2818–26.
477. Elkins G, Jensen MP, Patterson DR. Hypnotherapy for the management of chronic pain. Int J Clin Exp Hypnos. 2007;55(3):275–87.
478. Császár N, Scholkmann F, Bókkon I. Implications on hypnotherapy: neuroplasticity, epigenetics and pain. Neurosci Biobehav Rev. 2021;131:755–64.
479. Edmonston WE. Hypnosis and social suggestibility. Behav Brain Sci. 1986;9(3):470–1.
480. Elkins GR. Handbook of medical and psychological hypnosis: foundations, applications, and professional issues. Springer Publishing Company; 2016.
481. Geagea D, Griffin B, Kimble R, Polito V, Terhune DB, Tyack Z. Hypnotherapy for procedural pain, itch, and state anxiety in children with acute burns: a feasibility and acceptability study protocol. Pilot Feasib Stud. 2022;8(1):1–18.
482. Patterson DR, Questad KA, Boltwood MD. Hypnotherapy as a treatment for pain in patients with burns: research and clinical considerations. J Burn Care Rehabil. 1987;8(4):263–8.
483. Langlois P, Perrochon A, David R, et al. Hypnosis to manage musculoskeletal and neuropathic chronic pain: a systematic review and meta-analysis. Neurosci Biobehav Rev. 2022;135:104591.
484. Bernardy K, Füber N, Klose P, Häuser W. Efficacy of hypnosis/guided imagery in fibromyalgia syndrome-a systematic review and meta-analysis of controlled trials. BMC Musculoskelet Disord. 2011;12(1):1–11.
485. Flynn N. Systematic review of the effectiveness of hypnosis for the management of headache. Int J Clin Exp Hypn. 2018;66(4):343–52.
486. Jensen MP. Hypnosis for chronic pain management: a new hope. Pain. 2009;146(3):235–7.
487. Yarns BC, Lumley MA, Cassidy JT, et al. Emotional awareness and expression therapy achieves greater pain reduction than cognitive behavioral therapy in older adults with chronic musculoskeletal pain: a preliminary randomized comparison trial. Pain Med. 2020;21(11):2811–22.
488. Lumley MA, Schubiner H, Lockhart NA, et al. Emotional awareness and expression therapy, cognitive-behavioral therapy, and education for fibromyalgia: a cluster-randomized controlled trial. Pain. 2017;158(12):2354.
489. Lumley MA, Schubiner H. Emotional awareness and expression therapy for chronic pain: rationale, principles and techniques, evidence, and critical review. Curr Rheumatol Rep. 2019;21(7):1–8.
490. Mackay AM, Buckingham R, Schwartz RS, Hodgkinson S, Beran RG, Cordato DJ. The effect of biofeedback as a psychological intervention in multiple sclerosis: a randomized controlled study. Int J MS Care. 2015;17(3):101–8.
491. Frank DL, Khorshid L, Kiffer JF, Moravec CS, McKee MG. Biofeedback in medicine: who, when, why and how? Ment Health Fam Med. 2010;7(2):85.
492. Marzbani H, Marateb HR, Mansourian M. Neurofeedback: a comprehensive review on system design, methodology and clinical applications. Basic Clin Neurosci. 2016;7(2):143.
493. Sitaram R, Ros T, Stoeckel L, et al. Closed-loop brain training: the science of neurofeedback. Nat Rev Neurosci. 2017;18(2):86–100.
494. Angoules AG, Balakatounis KC, Panagiotopoulou KA, Mavrogenis AF, Mitsiokapa EA, Papagelopoulos PJ. Effectiveness of electromyographic biofeedback in the treatment of musculoskeletal pain. Orthopedics. 2011;31(10):e980–4.

495. Flor H, Birbaumer N. Comparison of the efficacy of electromyographic biofeedback, cognitive-behavioral therapy, and conservative medical interventions in the treatment of chronic musculoskeletal pain. J Consult Clin Psychol. 1993;61(4):653.
496. Gatchel RJ, Robinson RC, Pulliam C, Maddrey AM. Biofeedback with pain patients: evidence for its effectiveness, vol. 1. Elsevier; 2003. p. 55–66.
497. Neblett R, Gatchel RJ, Mayer TG. A clinical guide to surface-EMG-assisted stretching as an adjunct to chronic musculoskeletal pain rehabilitation. Appl Psychophysiol Biofeedback. 2003;28(2):147–60.
498. Newton-John TR, Spence SH, Schotte D. Cognitive-behavioural therapy versus EMG biofeedback in the treatment of chronic low back pain. Behav Res Ther. 1995;33(6):691–7.
499. Sielski R, Rief W, Glombiewski JA. Efficacy of biofeedback in chronic back pain: a meta-analysis. Int J Behav Med. 2017;24(1):25–41.
500. Reneau M. Heart rate variability biofeedback to treat fibromyalgia: an integrative literature review. Pain Manag Nurs. 2020;21(3):225–32.
501. McCraty R, Shaffer F. Heart rate variability: new perspectives on physiological mechanisms, assessment of self-regulatory capacity, and health risk. Global Adv Health Med. 2015;4(1):46–61.
502. Cohen H, Neumann L, Shore M, Amir M, Cassuto Y, Buskila D. Autonomic dysfunction in patients with fibromyalgia: application of power spectral analysis of heart rate variability, vol. 29. Elsevier; 2000. p. 217–27.
503. Santoro M, Cronan T. A systematic review of neurofeedback as a treatment for fibromyalgia syndrome symptoms. J Musculoskel Pain. 2014;22(3):286–300.
504. Glombiewski JA, Bernardy K, Häuser W. Efficacy of EMG-and EEG-biofeedback in fibromyalgia syndrome: a meta-analysis and a systematic review of randomized controlled trials. Evid Based Complement Alternat Med. 2013;2013:962741.
505. Patel K, Sutherland H, Henshaw J, et al. Effects of neurofeedback in the management of chronic pain: a systematic review and meta-analysis of clinical trials. Eur J Pain. 2020;24(8):1440–57.
506. Miller WR, Rollnick S. Motivational interviewing: helping people change. Guilford Press; 2012.
507. Alperstein D, Sharpe L. The efficacy of motivational interviewing in adults with chronic pain: a meta-analysis and systematic review. J Pain. 2016;17(4):393–403.
508. Hah JM, Trafton JA, Narasimhan B, et al. Efficacy of motivational-interviewing and guided opioid tapering support for patients undergoing orthopedic surgery (MI-Opioid Taper): a prospective, assessor-blind, randomized controlled pilot trial. EClinicalMedicine. 2020;28:100596.
509. Tse MM, Vong SK, Tang SK. Motivational interviewing and exercise programme for community-dwelling older persons with chronic pain: a randomised controlled study. J Clin Nurs. 2013;22(13–14):1843–56.
510. Stenberg N, Gillison F, Rodham K. How do peer support interventions for the self-management of chronic pain, support basic psychological needs? a systematic review and framework synthesis using self-determination theory. Patient Educ Couns. 2022;105(11):3225.
511. Rippentrop AE, Altmaier EM, Chen JJ, Found EM, Keffala VJ. The relationship between religion/spirituality and physical health, mental health, and pain in a chronic pain population. Pain. 2005;116(3):311–21.
512. Wachholtz AB, Pearce MJ, Koenig H. Exploring the relationship between spirituality, coping, and pain. J Behav Med. 2007;30(4):311–8.
513. Dedeli O, Kaptan G. Spirituality and religion in pain and pain management. Health Psychol Res. 2013;1(3):e29.
514. Rippentrop AE. A review of the role of religion and spirituality in chronic pain populations. Rehabil Psychol. 2005;50(3):278.
515. Elmholdt E-M, Skewes J, Dietz M, et al. Reduced pain sensation and reduced BOLD signal in parietofrontal networks during religious prayer. Front Hum Neurosci. 2017;11:337.

516. Mueller PS, Plevak DJ, Rummans TA. Religious involvement, spirituality, and medicine: implications for clinical practice, vol. 76. Elsevier; 2001. p. 1225–35.
517. Arnstein P, Vidal M, Wells-Federman C, Morgan B, Caudill M. From chronic pain patient to peer: benefits and risks of volunteering. Pain Manag Nurs. 2002;3(3):94–103.
518. Salt E, Crofford LJ, Segerstrom S. The mediating and moderating effect of volunteering on pain and depression, life purpose, well-being, and physical activity. Pain Manag Nurs. 2017;18(4):243–9.
519. Ferreira-Valente A, Sharma S, Torres S, et al. Does religiosity/spirituality play a role in function, pain-related beliefs, and coping in patients with chronic pain? a systematic review. J Relig Health. 2022;61(3):2331–85.
520. Tauben DJ, Langford DJ, Sturgeon JA, et al. Optimizing telehealth pain care after COVID-19. Pain. 2020;161(11):2437.
521. Tuckson RV, Edmunds M, Hodgkins ML. Telehealth. N Engl J Med. 2017;377(16):1585–92.
522. Turolla A, Rossettini G, Viceconti A, Palese A, Geri T. Musculoskeletal physical therapy during the COVID-19 pandemic: is telerehabilitation the answer? Phys Ther. 2020;100(8):1260–4.
523. Fernandes LG, Devan H, Fioratti I, Kamper SJ, Williams CM, Saragiotto BT. At my own pace, space, and place: a systematic review of qualitative studies of enablers and barriers to telehealth interventions for people with chronic pain. Pain. 2022;163(2):e165–81.
524. de Oliveira LL, Saragiotto BT, Costa LOP, Nogueira LC, Meziat-Filho N, Reis FJ. Self-guided web-based pain education for people with musculoskeletal pain: a systematic review and meta-analysis. Phys Ther. 2021;101(10):pzab167.
525. Calner T, Nordin C, Eriksson MK, Nyberg L, Gard G, Michaelson P. Effects of a self-guided, web-based activity programme for patients with persistent musculoskeletal pain in primary healthcare: a randomized controlled trial. Eur J Pain. 2017;21(6):1110–20.
526. Ziadni MS, You DS, Keane R, et al. "My Surgical Success": feasibility and impact of a single-session digital behavioral pain medicine intervention on pain intensity, pain catastrophizing, and time to opioid cessation after orthopedic trauma surgery—a randomized trial. Anesth Analg. 2022;135(2):394.
527. Evedal DC, Wang C, Oberleitner L, Schwartz S, Williams AM. Effects of an individually tailored web-based chronic pain management program on pain severity, psychological health, and functioning. J Med Internet Res. 2013;15(9):e2296.
528. Ziadni MS, Gonzalez-Castro L, Anderson S, Krishnamurthy P, Darnall BD. Efficacy of a single-session "empowered relief" zoom-delivered group intervention for chronic pain: randomized controlled trial conducted during the COVID-19 pandemic. J Med Internet Res. 2021;23(9):e29672.
529. Fritz JM, Minick KI, Brennan GP, et al. Outcomes of telehealth physical therapy provided using real-time, videoconferencing for patients with chronic low back pain: a longitudinal observational study. Arch Phys Med Rehabil. 2022;103(10):1924–34.
530. Theodore BR, Whittington J, Towle C, et al. Transaction cost analysis of in-clinic versus telehealth consultations for chronic pain: preliminary evidence for rapid and affordable access to interdisciplinary collaborative consultation. Pain Med. 2015;16(6):1045–56.
531. Hohenschurz-Schmidt D, Scott W, Park C, Christopoulos G, Vogel S, Draper-Rodi J. Remote management of musculoskeletal pain: a pragmatic approach to the implementation of video and phone consultations in musculoskeletal practice. Pain Rep. 2020;5(6):e878.
532. Trindade IA, Guiomar R, Carvalho SA, et al. Efficacy of online-based acceptance and commitment therapy for chronic pain: a systematic review and meta-analysis. J Pain. 2021;22(11):1328–42.
533. Cuenca-Martínez F, López-Bueno L, Suso-Martí L, et al. Implementation of online behavior modification techniques in the management of chronic musculoskeletal pain: a systematic review and meta-analysis. J Clin Med. 2022;11(7):1806.
534. McBeth J, Prescott G, Scotland G, et al. Cognitive behavior therapy, exercise, or both for treating chronic widespread pain. Arch Intern Med. 2012;172(1):48–57.

535. Raiszadeh K, Tapicer J, Taitano L, Wu J, Shahidi B. In-clinic versus web-based multidisciplinary exercise-based rehabilitation for treatment of low back pain: prospective clinical trial in an integrated practice unit model. J Med Internet Res. 2021;23(3):e22548.
536. Kravitz RL, Schmid CH, Marois M, et al. Effect of Mobile device–supported single-patient multi-crossover trials on treatment of chronic musculoskeletal pain: a randomized clinical trial. JAMA Intern Med. 2018;178(10):1368–77.
537. Platts-Mills TF, Hollowell AG, Burke GF, et al. Randomized controlled pilot study of an educational video plus telecare for the early outpatient management of musculoskeletal pain among older emergency department patients. Trials. 2018;19(1):1–9.
538. Barton C, Ezzat A, Merolli M, et al. "It's second best": a mixed-methods evaluation of the experiences and attitudes of people with musculoskeletal pain towards physiotherapist delivered telehealth during the COVID-19 pandemic. Musculoskel Sci Pract. 2022;58:102500.
539. Rod K. Finding ways to lift barriers to care for chronic pain patients: outcomes of using internet-based self-management activities to reduce pain and improve quality of life. Pain Res Manag. 2016;2016:8714785.
540. Cottrell MA, Hill AJ, O'Leary SP, Raymer ME, Russell TG. Patients are willing to use telehealth for the multidisciplinary management of chronic musculoskeletal conditions: a cross-sectional survey. J Telemed Telecare. 2018;24(7):445–52.
541. Flor H, Fydrich T, Turk DC. Efficacy of multidisciplinary pain treatment centers: a meta-analytic review. Pain. 1992;49(2):221–30.
542. Kamper SJ, Apeldoorn AT, Chiarotto A, et al. Multidisciplinary biopsychosocial rehabilitation for chronic low back pain: Cochrane systematic review and meta-analysis. BMJ. 2015;350:h444.
543. Volker G, van Vree F, Wolterbeek R, et al. Long-term outcomes of multidisciplinary rehabilitation for chronic musculoskeletal pain. Musculoskeletal Care. 2017;15(1):59–68.
544. Patrick LE, Altmaier EM, Found EM. Long-term outcomes in multidisciplinary treatment of chronic low back pain: results of a 13-year follow-up. Spine. 2004;29(8):850–5.
545. Kerns RD, Rosenberg R, Jamison RN, Caudill MA, Haythornthwaite J. Readiness to adopt a self-management approach to chronic pain: the Pain Stages of Change Questionnaire (PSOCQ). Pain. 1997;72(1–2):227–34.
546. Jensen MP, Nielson WR, Romano JM, Hill ML, Turner JA. Further evaluation of the pain stages of change questionnaire: is the transtheoretical model of change useful for patients with chronic pain? Pain. 2000;86(3):255–64.
547. Prochaska JO, Prochaska JM, Transtheoretical model. Lifestyle medicine. CRC Press; 2019. p. 219–28.
548. Finlay KA, Peacock S, Elander J. Developing successful social support: an interpretative phenomenological analysis of mechanisms and processes in a chronic pain support group. Psychol Health. 2018;33(7):846–71.
549. Finlay KA, Elander J. Reflecting the transition from pain management services to chronic pain support group attendance: an interpretative phenomenological analysis. Br J Health Psychol. 2016;21(3):660–76.
550. Jacob E, Stinson J, Duran J, et al. Usability testing of a Smartphone for accessing a web-based e-diary for self-monitoring of pain and symptoms in sickle cell disease. J Pediatr Hematol Oncol. 2012;34(5):326.
551. Rosser BA, Eccleston C. Smartphone applications for pain management. J Telemed Telecare. 2011;17(6):308–12.
552. Lou J, Pourkazemi F, Mackenzie L. Exploring the experiences of individuals living with persistent pain using a visual art diary. Br J Occup Ther. 2022;85:03080226221079239.
553. Rogerson MD, Gatchel RJ, Bierner SM. A cost utility analysis of interdisciplinary early intervention versus treatment as usual for high-risk acute low back pain patients. Pain Pract. 2010;10(5):382–95. https://doi.org/10.1111/j.1533-2500.2009.00344.x. PMID: 20384967.

554. Dowell D, Ragan KR, Jones CM, Baldwin GT, Chou R. CDC clinical practice guideline for prescribing opioids for pain — United States, 2022. MMWR Recomm Rep. 2022;71(No. RR-3):1–95. https://doi.org/10.15585/mmwr.rr7103a1.
555. U.S. Department of Health and Human Services. Pain Management Best Practices Inter-Agency Task Force Report: updates, Gaps, Inconsistencies, and Recommendations. Retrieved from U. S. Department of Health and Human Services website; 2019. https://www.hhs.gov/ash/advisory-committees/pain/reports/index.htm
556. VA/DoD Clinical Practice Guideline. Use of opioids in the Management of Chronic Pain Work Group. Washington, DC: U.S. Government Printing Office; 2022.
557. Schatman ME. Interdisciplinary chronic pain management: international perspectives. Pain Clin Updates. 2012;XX(7):1.

Who Benefits from Opioids? A Best Practices Approach

27

Carl Edward Noe, Standiford Helm, and Gabor Racz

Why Have Opioids Fallen Out of Favor?

With the awareness of the risks associated with opioid use, physicians have moved away from prescribing opioids. The switch away from opioids leaves unanswered the question of whether there is any role for using opioids in treating chronic pain, and, if so, what is that role? This chapter seeks to stimulate debate on that question.

Historical Perspective

A one paragraph letter to the editor of the New England Journal of Medicine in 1980 suggested that addiction was rare in patients treated with narcotics [1]. Based on the thought that opioids were safe and pain was undertreated, access to opioids was viewed as a fundamental right. An example is the passage in 1990 of the Pain Patient's Bill of Rights by the California Legislature [2]. This legislation codified a pain patient's right to have opioids and a physician's ability to prescribe "a dosage deemed medically necessary to relieve the pain."

With this advocacy, prescription opioid prescribing increased dramatically. With that increase came new, contravening, insights. In 2002, Mao introduced the

C. E. Noe (✉)
The University of Texas Southwestern Med, Dallas, TX, USA

S. Helm
Department of Anesthesia and Perioperative Medicine, University of California Irvine, Irvine, CA, USA
e-mail: drhelm@thehelmcenter.com

G. Racz
Department of Anesthesiology, Texas Tech University Health Sciences Center, Lubbock, TX, USA

C. E. Noe (ed.), *Musculoskeletal Pain*,
https://doi.org/10.1007/978-3-031-86057-7_27

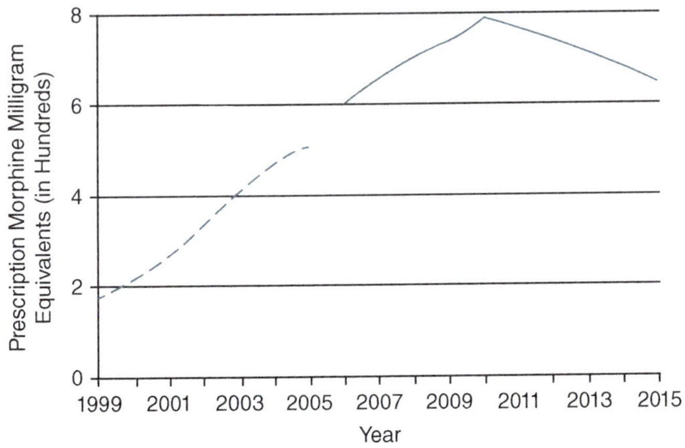

Fig. 27.1 Per capita prescription opioid sales 1999–2015 [5]

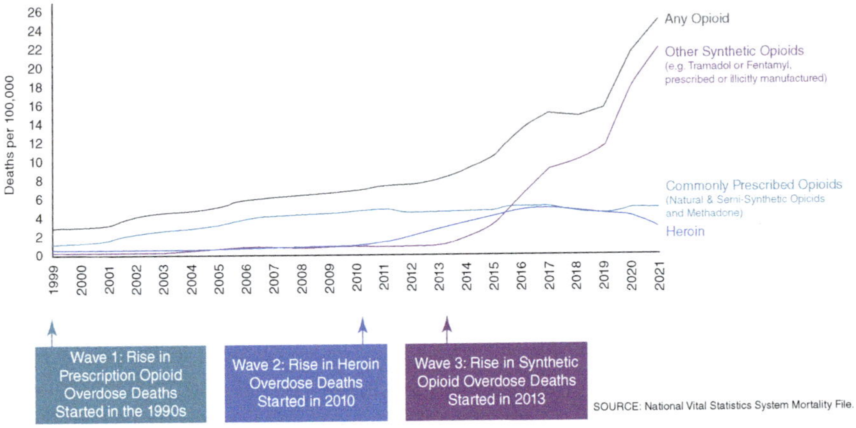

Fig. 27.2 Three waves of opioid overdose deaths 1999–2019 [6]

concept of opioid-induced hyperalgesia [3]. By the end of the first decade of this century, it was clear that opioids had side effects and unforeseen risks and that prescription opioid use was leading to a surge in overdose deaths [4]. Regulatory oversight, primarily by licensing boards, led to a decrease in opioid prescribing in the United States (Fig. 27.1) [5].

Despite the reduction in prescribed opioids, the increased use of illicit opioids has led to a continuing increase in drug-related deaths. These opioid deaths have come in waves, as shown in Fig. 27.2 [6]. The first wave was prescription opioids; the second, heroin; and the third, synthetic opioids, particularly fentanyl [7]. The major source of fentanyl is from overseas, particularly from China, despite prohibitions [8].

Given the difficulty in stopping illicit opioids, the ongoing increase in opioid deaths has led to ongoing scrutiny by licensing authorities and the drug enforcement administration (DEA) of physicians prescribing opioids.

Shifting the Paradigm

Huber et al. suggested in 2016 that the focus should be shifted from "who is not a candidate for chronic opioid therapy" to "who would benefit from opioids" [9]. Despite the widespread early belief that opioids were underused, high-quality evidence that the long-term effectiveness of opioids did not emerge [10]. The screening questionnaires, such as Pain Medication Questionnaire (PMQ), Opioid Risk Tool (ORT), Current Opioid Misuse Measure (COMM), and Screening and Opioid Assessment for Patients with Pain (SOAPP), emphasized opioid dangers and were focused on excluding patients rather than identifying patients who would benefit from therapy [11].

Two problems arise with the use of screening tools attempting to define who is not a candidate for opioid therapy. First, it is not clear that they accurately identify these patients. Second, and more importantly, simply because a patient is felt to be at low-risk for opioid misuse, respiratory depression, and side effects does not mean that the patient would benefit from opioids.

The aim of this chapter is to review the evolving understanding of patient selection considerations for chronic opioid therapy. This is particularly relevant for patients with chronic musculoskeletal pain.

Evidence of Efficacy: Present or Not?

Opioids appear to provide only small improvement in pain and function compared to placebo. Non-opioid medications, and non-pharmacological approaches, may be as, or more, effective than opioids to treat chronic pain [12]. Jones et al. found that acute low-back-pain patients provided opioids had worse pain, possibly because of opioid-induced hyperalgesia, and more side effects than the placebo group [13]. Conversely, Busse et al. performed a meta-analysis showing small pain and functional benefits from opioids [12]. Guidelines and position papers, such as those prepared by the centers for disease control and prevention (CDC) and the American Academy of Neurology, have recommended that at morphine equivalent doses (MED) of approximately 80 mg/day, consultation with a pain management specialist be considered [14, 15].

Enriched enrollment studies are a form of randomized controlled trials in which patients who have been documented to respond to opioids are enrolled into the trial. The advantage of enriched enrollment studies is that they allow smaller sizes, although they may underestimate adverse effects [16]. Meske et al. performed a meta-analysis of opioids in noncancer pain, using the FDA's requirement of three months follow-up to approve an opioid for chronic pain [17], finding that opioids were efficacious. This finding suggests that there is a subgroup of patients in whom opioid use may be appropriate, although the question of long-term use of opioids remains open. It is unclear how to identify this subgroup.

One difficulty with extrapolating the results of opioid studies to clinical practice is the exclusion of diagnoses such as abdominal pain, dental pain, ischemic pain, and migraine pain, all of which are indications for opioid therapy, from these studies.

Another study design occasionally used to evaluate opioids, particularly formulations designed to minimize risk deterrence, are drug likability studies. These studies are generally performed using enrollees known to be attracted to the side effects of opioids, such as mood modulation. Drug likability studies have been criticized because of the difficulty of getting reliable, consistent information from this patient population [18].

Guidelines

The CDC is the most widely recognized source of guidelines for using opioids for chronic pain. The 2022 version is focused on adult patients with pain, excluding sickle cell disease, cancer pain, palliative care, and end-of-life care [19, 20]. Unlike the 2016 version, the 2022 version extends beyond primary care providers to include surgeons, dentists, and emergency department physicians. The CDC guidelines' recommendations provide an excellent foundation for opioid prescribing and are summarized in Table 27.1.

The American College of Physicians has similarly developed guidelines for the treatment of acute low back pain, with the recommendation that opioids not be used initially, with the first recommended treatment being topical non steroidal antiinflammatory drug (NSAIDs) [21].

Table 27.1 Summary of the 2022 CDC guidelines recommendations

1. Non-opioid therapies should be considered first for acute pain, with opioids considered only if benefits outweigh risks.
2. Non-opioid therapies are preferred for subacute and chronic pain; opioids should only be initiated if expected benefits outweigh risks.
3. Immediate-release opioids should be prescribed over extended-release and long acting opioids when starting opioid therapy.
4. The lowest effective dosage of opioids should be prescribed, and caution should be exercised when considering dosage increases.
5. Clinicians should carefully evaluate the benefits and risks of opioid therapy and work closely with patients to optimize other therapies if benefits do not outweigh risks.
6. Clinicians should prescribe no greater quantity of opioids than needed for the expected duration of pain.
7. Benefits and risks of opioid therapy should be evaluated with patients within 1–4 weeks of starting opioid therapy or dosage escalation.
8. Clinicians should evaluate the risk for opioid-related harms and discuss risk mitigation strategies with patients.
9. Prescription drug monitoring program (PDMP) data should be used to assess the patient's history of controlled substance prescriptions.
10. Consideration should be given to toxicology testing when prescribing opioids for subacute or chronic pain.
11. Caution should be exercised when prescribing opioid pain medication and benzodiazepines concurrently.
12. Treatment with evidence-based medications should be offered or arranged for patients with opioid use disorder.

Multidisciplinary functional restoration programs appear to be one of the most effective ways to treat chronic pain [22, 23], although cost and availability limit their usefulness.

Neuropathic pain, including from diabetes, herpes zoster, fibromyalgia, cancer or cancer therapy, or HIV, is generally felt to be unresponsive to opioid therapy [24]. Generally, non-opioid therapy is recommended for these conditions. Exercise and psychological techniques such as cognitive behavioral and mindfulness therapy have also been shown to be helpful [25, 26].

Acute Pain: When Should Opioids Be Stopped?

Even though guidelines are recommended against using opioids as a first-line drug for acute pain, they are widely used in that setting. Because of concerns that the use of opioids in the acute setting can lead to chronic use, various barriers have been implemented to minimize the occurrence of the acute to chronic opioid use transition. Many states have implemented restrictions, such as a seven-day supply limit without refills for the initial prescription.

Patients who report persistent pain after the expected healing period of an acute episode, perhaps because of neuropathic pain or complications such as an infection or hematoma, should be treated with non-opioid analgesics or non-pharmacological techniques as a base of analgesic therapy before opioids are added on top of that for breakthrough pain if required.

A special case are patients who are on chronic opioid therapy prior to surgery. Some have advocated tapering opioids prior to surgery to prevent escalating doses after surgery. Nguyen, Sing, and Bozic, for example, found that those patients who were on chronic opioid therapy prior to total joint replacement and who were able to wean their opioid dose by at least 50% prior to surgery did better functionally 6–12 months after surgery than those who did not wean [27].

Generally, opioids should be stopped within 90 days of surgery or trauma unless the opioids were being provided prior to surgery for an unrelated reason. Burn patients or those with major spinal surgery, such as scoliosis repair, may require a longer time to taper. Tapering opioid preoperatively allows the use of usual opioid doses that are effective for postoperative pain rather than dangerously high doses.

Sickle cell disease represents a special situation. In addition to the short-term use of opioids for acute crises, a substantial number of patients are on chronic opioid therapy. One reason for the 2022 CDC's guidelines excluding sickle cell patients from those guidelines is the finding that the decreased provision of opioids to those patients after the 2016 guidelines led to their requiring increased pain-related hospitalizations [28].

Treatment of cancer-related pain is generally felt, like sickle cell disease, to be less restricted than treatment of noncancer-related pain. Despite less rigorous scrutiny by regulatory authorities, cancer patients are at risk of being under or over prescribed because of fragmentation of care [29]. Patients who develop cancer therapy-induced neuropathy are particularly at risk as continued opioid use may hinder their transition to their pre-cancer activities [29].

Diversion of opioids after a cancer patient's death is a significant risk. Planning for disposal prior to death can minimize this problem.

Chronic Pain

Chronic pain, defined variously as pain lasting more than three or six months or beyond the expected healing time, represents specific problems. Given the absence of evidence for long-term efficacy, there is not a consensus that opioids need to be prescribed long term. Further, patients on long-term opioids are also at long-term risk for the side effects of opioids. Any clinician, however, who has had to deal with the consequences of a patient committing suicide because of inadequate pain control will argue that there is some subset of patients for whom the long-term use of opioids is an appropriate component of the treatment plan.

When Should Opioids Be Trialed?

Beyond the confines of postoperative pain, cancer pain, sickle cell disease, palliative care, or end-of-life care, no specific chronic pain condition exists that mandates the use of opioids. The use of opioids therefore would rest on the contraindication or failure of other options. Contraindications would include the inability to use NSAIDs or acetaminophen, such as gastrointestinal bleeding risk, renal insufficiency, recent myocardial infarction or high-risk coronary disease, or hepatic issues. The inability to tolerate or the failure of non-opioid medications, such as the various serotonin or norepinephrine reuptake inhibitors, or the gabapentinoid preparations, often used for neuropathic pain, provide a basis for considering opioid therapy, although the evidence is not strong. Finally, conservative treatments, such as physical or chiropractic therapy, acupuncture, self-directed exercise, cognitive behavioral or mindfulness therapies, along with dietary support as indicated, should be considered prior to initiation of opioid therapy.

Several patient considerations should be taken into account when considering opioids. Younger patients, with an active limbic system, are more likely to misuse opioids. Older patients, with senescence influencing metabolism, balance, the various bodily systems, are at greater risk for side effects and drug interactions [30–32]. Women are prescribed opioids more frequently than men, often in combination with a sedative-hypnotic drug, putting them at risk for overdose and dependence [33]. Patients with dual pain and psychiatric diagnoses can use the language of pain to describe their psychological pain. The perceived beneficial effects on psychological pain can lead to the continued use of opioids despite limited benefit for physical pain [34, 35].

Risk Stratification

Risk stratification has become an accepted tool when considering whether to initiate or maintain opioids. As discussed above, the goal of risk stratification is to determine who is not a candidate for opioids rather than who is a candidate.

Broadly taken, risk stratification includes both physical and psychological/use disorder risks, including the presence or risk of use disorders, risk of diversion, sedation, respiratory depression, or overdose, cognitive dysfunction, nausea, constipation, pruritus, hormonal and sexual dysfunction, or fall risk. Many tools have been developed for risk assessment, one of which, Risk Index for Overdose or Serious Opioid-Induced Respiratory Depression (RIOSORD) is shown in Fig. 27.3 [36].

Risk Index for Overdose or Serious Opioid-Induced Respiratory Depression (RIOSORD)

Description	Y/N	Score
In the past 6 months, has the patient had a health care visit (outpatient, inpatient, or ED) involving:		
Opioid dependence?		15
Chronic hepatitis or cirrhosis?		9
Bipolar disorder or schizophrenia?		7
Chronic pulmonary disease? (e.g., emphysema, chronic bronchitis, asthma, pneumoconiosis, asbestosis)		5
Chronic kidney disease with clinically significant renal impairment?		5
Active traumatic injury, excluding burns? (e.g., fracture, dislocation, contusion, laceration, wound)		4
Sleep apnea?		3
Does the patient consume:		
An extended-release or long-acting (ER/LA) formulation of any prescription opioid or opioid with long and/or variable half-life? (e.g.,OxyContin, Oramorph-SR, methadone, fentanyl patch, levorphanol)		9
Methadone? (Methadone is a long-acting opioid, so also write Y for "ER/LA formulation")		9
Oxycodone? (If it has an ER/LA formulation [e.g., OxyContin], also write Y for "ER/LA formulation")		3
A prescription antidepressant? (e.g., fluoxetine, citalopram, venlafaxine, amitriptyline)		7
A prescription benzodiazepine? (e.g., diazepam, alprazolam)		4
Is the patient's current maximum prescribed opioid dose:		
>100 mg morphine equivalents per day?		16
50-100 mg morphine equivalents per day?		9
20-50 mg morphine equivalents per day?		5
In the past 6 months, has the patient:		
Had 1 or more ED visits?		11
Been hospitalized for 1 or more days?		8
Total Score		**115**

Opioid Induced Respiratory Depression (OIRD) Probability based on Calculated Risk Index

Risk index score	OIRD probability (%)
0-24	3
25-32	14
33-37	23
38-42	37
43-46	51
47-49	55
50-54	60
55-59	79
60-66	75
≥67	86

Adapted from: Zedler B, Xie L, Wang L et al. Development of a Risk Index for Serious Prescription Opioid-Induced Respiratory Depression or Overdose in Veterans' Health Administration Patients. Pain Medicine. Jun 2015. 16;1566-1579

Fig. 27.3 Risk index for overdose or serious opioid-induced respiratory depression (RIOSORD) [36]

Monitoring

Monitoring falls into two broad categories, monitoring of efficacy and monitoring of risks. This process has been summarized as the "Four A's," analgesia, activities of daily living, adverse events, and aberrant behavior [37]. Given the subjectivity of reports of analgesia, maintenance or improvement in function should be the primary end point. Palliative care patients are an exception since their function is expected to decline with or without opioid therapy. Signs of acute intoxication, such as overt sedation, pupillary constriction, or decreased oxygen saturation, are rarely seen in chronic pain patients, if only because most patients who are abusing drugs are not able to present to the office acutely intoxicated. It is important that prescribing physicians are informed of emergency encounters for overdose.

Naloxone should be offered to patients. Some states, such as California, have legislatively required the offering of naloxone to patients with an MED of 90 or more, taking both opioids at any dose and benzodiazepines, or certain high-risk patients.

Consistent with the CDC guidelines, documentation should include a detailed history and physical examination providing the rationale for the use of opioids, along with the treatment plan, informed consent/pain agreement, periodic review to confirm that the use of opioids is successful, and appropriate referrals. Generally, pain management specialists are held to a higher standard than primary care physicians in terms of complying with guidelines. Primary care physicians often lack awareness of all the nuances of documenting their care of patients on chronic opioids, exposing them to regulatory risk. Most opioids, however, are prescribed by primary care physicians [38].

Figure 27.4 provides a summary of steps to take with new patients requiring long-term opioids.

Legacy Patients

Legacy patients are patients who have been on long-term, generally high dose opioids, often started by another physician at a time when higher doses were accepted. Legacy patients are often resistant to trialing lower doses, claiming that they are functioning well on their current dose. Many physicians feel obliged to continue opioid medications for such patients, similar to managing other chronic diseases like hypertension or diabetes.

Patients switch practices for many reasons, including changes in insurance or location. If possible, a conversation with or a review of records of the previous providers should be done. The need for chronic opioid therapy needs to be confirmed, rather than simply rubber stamping previous treatments [39].

These patients need to be closely evaluated prior to electing to maintain their prior opioid doses, as the risk of opioid substance use disorder (SUD) increases with duration of treatment and markedly as the dose increases [40]. Figure 27.5 shows the relationship between dose and relative risk of having substance use disorder. A patient on >120 MED has a relative risk of SUD 122 times higher than the reference

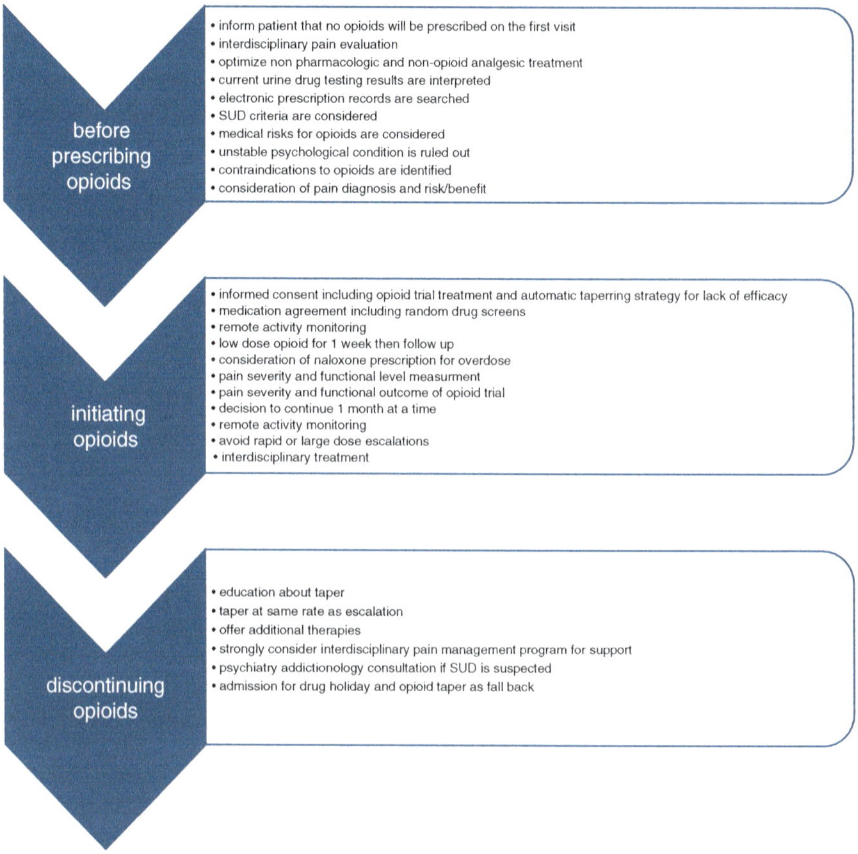

Fig. 27.4 Management of new patient on long-term opioids

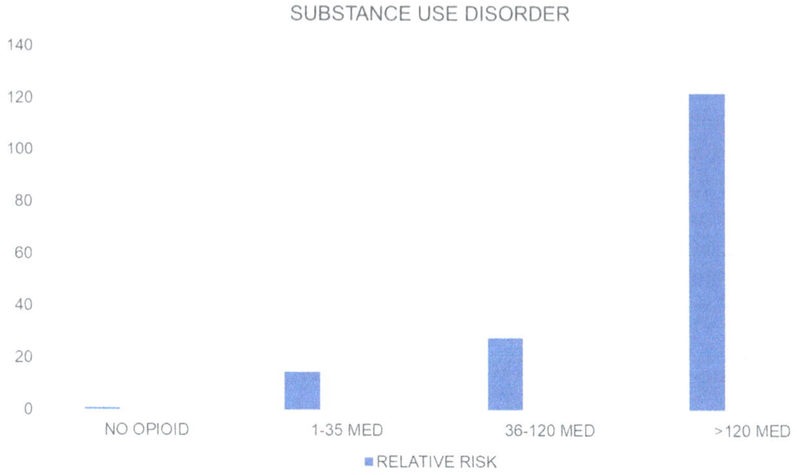

Fig. 27.5 Increasing risk of substance use disorder with increasing daily morphine dose equivalents

group. Patients should be evaluated for SUD, as defined by the DSM-5 [41]. These patients should at least have a consultation with a pain management physician, or, if possible, managed by one, because the use of higher opioid doses has drawn regulatory scrutiny. Primary care physicians who have maintained high doses because of the inability to transfer care and the patient's unwillingness to move have found themselves facing sanctions.

At the same time, Dowell, Haegerich, and Chou have clearly highlighted the risks of overaggressive and inappropriate weaning [42]. While the number of opioids prescribed is ultimately at the discretion of the physician who is writing the prescription, nonconsensual tapering of legacy patients has been criticized [43]. Part of the art of pain medicine is knowing how to work with patients.

Legacy patients pose a special challenge to the practitioners, as there is no one or simple way to easily reduce the risk of opioid prescribing to either the patient or the practitioner [44].

How to Approach Opioid Tapering

Guidelines recommend trials of opioid tapering for patients on chronic opioid therapy, even when the patient is stable on current doses. While tapering is often resisted by patients, Veterans Affairs studies show that dose reduction is not associated with changes in pain severity, even when the dose reduction was done against the patient's wishes [45, 46]. Research and clinical experience also show that patients will claim that their pain was better controlled on the previous, higher, doses, while review of the medical records does not support that claim [47].

Due to opioid-induced hyperalgesia, pain may actually be reduced on lower doses.

Patients need to be listened to and respected during tapering trials, although not necessarily fully deferred to. Support services such as group therapy with education, individual support, and skills-based learning have been successful in reducing opioid dosing [48]. Further, non-opioid pharmacological and non-pharmacological therapies can also be helpful, as documented by the Pain Management Best Practices Inter-Agency Task Force [49].

Sullivan et al. documented long-term opioid reduction using an interdisciplinary approach to support patients during the taper [50].

Our experience with opioid reduction in patients treated in our interdisciplinary pain program has been favorable. The percentage of patients taking opioids daily preprogram was 56% and 30% after the program. Two years later, the percentage decreased further to 20%, and at 5 years, 8.9%. The average dose index decreased from 1.9 to 1 after the program, then 0.67 at 2 years, and 0.19 at 5 years.

Office-Based Medication Assisted Treatment

Patients who have been provided opioids for apparent medical indications who either do not have relief of the pain complaints or who develop signs of substance use disorder can successfully be tapered and treated in an office-based setting, whether pain management or primary care. Buprenorphine, an opioid partial agonist antagonist, is effective both at preventing withdrawal symptoms and providing pain relief [51–56]. The Substance Abuse and Mental Health Services Administration's (SMHSA) 2023 removal of the DATA waiver (X-waiver) allows any practitioner with a DEA registration number to treat opioid use disorder. However, the online training program for buprenorphine prescribing is recommended to avoid precipitating withdrawal. Also, CDC guidelines recommend a comprehensive addiction program for patients with substance use disorder. While the capacity of these programs is not adequate to meet the demand, and the cost is prohibitive, simply replacing one drug for another is unlikely to address the underlying psychosocial issues that many patients have.

The use of methadone to treat opioid use disorder is limited to certified opioid treatment programs (OTP). Outside of OTPs, physicians can use methadone to treat pain, being aware of the specific risk factors associated with that drug, but not use disorder. Methadone has highly variable oral bioavailability and long half-life that has led to overdoses when doses are escalated too rapidly.

The DEA has also developed rules for the telemedicine prescribing of buprenorphine for substance use disorder, so that an initial 30-day supply can be provided to a patient without an in-person examination. Given the narrow window that patients suffering from SUD often provide to get treatment, this ability to provide medication quickly is important. Further, patients who have had an in-person examination by a referring doctor can receive buprenorphine from the consultant using telemedicine [57].

When Should Opioids Not Be Used for Chronic Pain?

There is no diagnosis which mandates the use of opioids. Many of the diagnoses which are felt to provide a medical rationale for the chronic use of opioids have not been shown to respond well to opioids. Examples of such diagnoses include low back pain, chronic lumbar radiculopathy, chronic abdominal pain, primary headaches including migraines, dental pain, and fibromyalgia [58–64].

Patients with psychiatric disorders, including untreated Axis I disorders, such as bipolar disorders or schizophrenia, or Axis II personality disorders, need to be approached cautiously, as it can be difficult to distinguish between the use of opioids to treat physical versus psychological pain [65]. Patients with depression are more likely to transition to long-term opioid use than patients without depression, again highlighting the question as to whether physical or psychological issues are being treated [66].

It should go without saying that patients with somatic symptom disorder or functional neurological disorders would not be expected to benefit from opioids.

A history of SUD is not an absolute contraindication for chronic opioid use. However, if opioids are used in this setting, low doses and vigilant monitoring are recommended.

Patient Satisfaction

Successful pain management requires trust between the provider and the patient. Anecdotally, some patients whose self-perception is that they have successfully dealt with their chronic pain issues stated that a major factor in their success is that their providers believed in them. At the same time, a survey of patient satisfaction across all specialties at a major teaching hospital found that the pain management physicians and clinics received the lowest satisfaction rating, a result felt to be related to the issues the patients were facing [67]. One has to accept that these issues are inherent in a pain practice and the cross-specialty satisfaction scores need to be understood in context.

Patients Whose Actions Disrupt the Doctor–Patient Relationship

Occasionally, patients will demonstrate behavior which documents that they are not candidates for opioid therapy. Examples include repeated loss of medication, repeated inappropriate urine drug screens, doctor shopping, or overdoses. These situations are easily handled by simply explaining to the patient that their actions prevent you, the provider, from continuing to prescribe more opioids. There is no need to discharge the patient from the practice in this setting, the doctor–patient relationship can continue, should the patient desire, absent opioids.

Rarely, however, patients can become abusive or threatening. These situations can lead to termination of the doctor–patient relationship. Prior to following the process proscribed by the State, while the licensee is in the process of terminating the relationship, several steps should be considered:

1. *Establish Clear Boundaries*: These include a pain management agreement, follow-up requirements, and the implementation of monitoring protocols.
2. *Document Incidents*: The provider and the office staff should carefully document any incidents or abusive behaviors. This document is particularly useful if the patient later files a complaint against you with the medical board. Documentation should be factual, objective and include the specific dates, times, and details of each incident.
3. *Communication*: Attempt to address the perceived issues with the patient through open and honest communication. Express concerns about their behavior and emphasize the importance of a respectful and cooperative doctor–patient relationship.
4. *Offer support and Resources*: For patients struggling with SUD or behavioral issues offer resources and support services, such as addiction counseling, mental health treatment, or support groups.

5. *Consider Consultation with Specialists*: Referral to an addictionologist or psychiatrist may be indicated.
6. *Termination of the Doctor–Patient relationship*: Termination may be necessary. Follow the local guidelines. Your medical association or malpractice carrier can help with the details of what is required. Generally, written notice is required, along with information as to how to obtain further care, and maintenance of medication, generally for 30 days.

Items to Consider When Considering Prescribing

Table 27.2 provides an inclusionary checklist for the acute use of opioids.

Table 27.3 provides an inclusionary checklist for initiating longer term opioid therapy.

Table 27.4 provides an inclusionary checklist for continuing longer term opioid therapy.

These checklists are proposed as a guide but do not replace informed consent, pain management agreements, or documentation of patient assessment and ongoing management.

Table 27.2 Inclusionary checklist for acute pain opioid treatment

1. The patient has cancer pain, palliative care pain, end-of-life shortness of breath, or the patient needs opioid for breakthrough pain after trauma or surgery or painful medical condition.
2. Non-pharmacological and non-opioid treatment have been optimized.
3. The patient risk factors have been evaluated and are acceptable.
4. The patient has a diagnosis likely to respond to opioid.
5. The patient responds well to initial doses of opioid.

Table 27.3 Inclusionary checklist for initiating longer term opioid treatment on an existing patient

1. The patient has a clear, unmistakable diagnosis known to be painful and likely to respond to an opioid such as postherpetic neuralgia.
2. The patient has poor pain control despite tedious trials of other evidence-based therapies.
3. The patient responds well to a trial of opioid.
4. The patient has good respiratory and airway function.
5. The patient has good psychosocial function.
6. Regulatory requirements are met- informed consent, medication agreement, drug screen, naloxone prescription, etc.
7. The patient is able to follow up frequently.
8. The patient is reliable and able to secure their medications and manage medications independently.
9. The patient is willing to engage actively in interdisciplinary pain management and alternatives to opioids as indicated.
10. Prescribing opioids for the patients' diagnosis is defensible in the event of an adverse outcome.

Table 27.4 Additional inclusionary checklist before continuing longer term opioid treatment on a new patient or existing patient

1. Patient informed that the first visit is for evaluation only, and no medication will be prescribed, and additional evaluations may be required before an opinion about opioid treatment is made.
2. Medical records including drug screen results are complete and consistent with continuing opioid treatment.
3. Discussion with previous prescriber before evaluation visit is consistent with continuing opioid treatment.
4. Interdisciplinary screening or evaluation is completed.
5. Consultation with an addictionologist if indicated.
6. Patient has a track record of responsible medication use.
7. Family members and other physicians are unanimously supportive of opioid therapy.
8. Psychosocial function has remained good on opioid treatment.
9. Physical activity is not worsened by opioid use (physical activity may worsen from disease progression and aging).
10. Opioids produce significant analgesia and no unsafe side effects.

Marijuana and Opioids

While many States have legalized the non-medicinal use of marijuana, physicians holding DEA registrations should remember that marijuana is still classified as Schedule I under Federal Law. Individual physicians have taken varying stands regarding providing opioids to patients using marijuana. Currently, there is no consensus to help physicians decide whether to prescribe opioids only if patients abstain from marijuana, or if patients get a license to use marijuana for medical reasons, or if patients use marijuana solely recreationally.

The evidence for the medical use of marijuana is limited. Finnerup et al. found some benefit for HIV neuropathy and central pain from cannabinoids [68]. A recent review of the literature by Ang et al. found some benefit for neuropathic pain, fibromyalgia, and geriatric pain, but the evidence does not currently support the use of cannabinoids as a first-line treatment [69]. Another recent review found that cannabidiol (CBD) for pain may be ineffective and potentially harmful [70].

Acetaminophen works via the endogenous cannabinoid systems and is a safer option for incorporating this mechanism into an analgesic package.

It is important to remember that mood-altering, sedative, or anxiolytic drugs, such as alcohol, diphenhydramine, or marijuana, may lower pain scores without providing therapeutic analgesic effects or functional improvement.

Cannabis use disorder, with the increased potency of cannabis, is prevalent and may be a contraindication for opioid use.

The use of multiple sedation drugs is generally avoided in pain management. In that marijuana is a sedating drug, its use with opioids, with or without the other drugs commonly used in pain management, should be approached with caution. Safer options for co-analgesics include the standard choices, such as NSAIDs, acetaminophen, selective reuptake inhibitors, or gabapentinoids.

Opioids and Non-pain Diagnoses

Opioids have been used for several non-pain diagnoses, including restless leg syndrome, chronic idiopathic diarrhea, and chronic cough [71–73]. The restless leg study was done with an oxycodone/naloxone proprietary formulation, suggesting its limited applicability [71]. Chronic diarrhea and cough are not complaints generally treated by pain management physicians. The general conclusion is that pain management physicians should limit themselves to using opioids for pain diagnoses.

Should Opioid Prescribing Be Done by One Physician or a Team?

The evolution of opioid prescribing regulations in Texas, particularly with the passage of the Intractable Pain Treatment Act in 1989, played a significant role in shaping the landscape of pain management and the opioid epidemic in the United States. Before this act, physicians were restricted in prescribing opioids to individuals deemed "habitual users" or those the physician "should have known" were habitual users, highlighting the importance of understanding patients' histories and potential risks before prescribing opioids.

The Intractable Pain Treatment Act, by allowing physicians to prescribe opioids for pain management without fear of disciplinary action, inadvertently contributed to the rise of the opioid epidemic by facilitating more liberal opioid prescribing practices. This legislative change, followed by similar actions in other states, catalyzed the widespread use of opioids for pain management and contributed to the normalization of opioids as a primary treatment modality for chronic pain.

Currently, the prescribing physician assumes any risk of regulatory action when prescribing opioids. Given the complexities of treating pain, including the difficulties of treating a patient with both pain and psychological disorders, including substance use disorder, some have advocated for an interdisciplinary approach to chronic pain management. The exact structure of such a chronic approach, as compared to the time-limited functional restoration program, is unclear, but would include medical, psychological, likely group sessions, and functional, likely supervision of home exercise programs, components.

Certification of interdisciplinary pain management teams by state medical boards could provide a framework for safe opioid prescribing practices, while ensuring that patients receive comprehensive care that prioritizes their well-being. Such initiatives could potentially lead to better outcomes for patients with chronic pain, while mitigating the risks associated with opioid misuse and addiction.

Conclusions

This chapter examines the questions as to which patients are candidates for chronic opioid therapy. The short answer is that no one is mandated to need opioids, yet there are patients who do live more fulfilling lives, given whatever functional limitations they may have, if they are provided opioids. These patients will have already been provided access to non-opioid and non-pharmacological therapies. Generally, success is achieved at low MEDs of opioids. Buprenorphine, with its agonist/partial antagonist properties, is an excellent option, but not the only choice for long-term therapy. While tolerance can occur, dose escalation over years does not necessarily occur; patients may stay on stable doses ad infinitum.

Shared decision-making between physicians and patients is important, but the physician's decision may be paramount in situations of substance use disorder or the potential for self-harm.

Evaluation, both before and after providing opioids, is an absolute requirement. The CDC guidelines, including their exclusion of sickle cell disease, cancer-related pain, palliative care, and end-of-life care, provide a good outline of this evaluation.

Prescribing opioids long term is treacherous since it may be argued that prescribing opioids is ineffective or even placebo. In the event of a complication, well-intentioned physicians are subject to extremely harsh treatment from the medicolegal and regulatory arenas. Avoiding the appearance of conflicts of interest by not investing in opioid preparation or manufacturing companies is helpful in the event of a legal action.

The medicolegal cases that are won by the prescribing physicians are done so with evidence. Documenting evidence of improvement with opioid treatment and good intentions of the prescribing physician are essential.

References

1. Porter J, Jick H. Addiction rare in patients treated with narcotics. NEJM. 1980;302(2):123. https://doi.org/10.1056/nejm198001103020221.
2. Pain Patient's Bill of Rights, Cal Health & Saf Code § 124961 (1990). http://www.leginfo.ca.gov/pub/11-12/bill/asm/ab_0501-0550/ab_507_cfa_20110623_143905_sen_comm.html
3. Mao J. Opioid-induced abnormal pain sensitivity: implications in clinical opioid therapy. Pain. 2002;100(3):213–7.
4. Dunn KM, Saunders KW, Rutter CM, et al. Opioid prescriptions for chronic pain and overdose: a cohort study. Ann Intern Med. 2010;152(2):85–92.
5. Dowell D, Noonan RK, Houry D. Underlying factors in drug overdose deaths. JAMA. 2017;318:2295. https://doi.org/10.1001/jama.2017.15971. [October 11, 2017].
6. Understanding the Opioid Overdose Epidemic. April 5, 2024. CDC. Retrieved from https://www.cdc.gov/overdose-prevention/about/understanding-the-opioid-overdose-epidemic.html
7. Manchikanti L, Singh VM, Staats PS, et al. Fourth wave of opioid (illicit drug) overdose deaths and diminishing access to prescription opioids and interventional techniques: cause and effect. Pain Physician. 2022;25(2):97–124.
8. Feng E. 'We Are Shipping To The U.S.': Inside China's Online Synthetic Drug Networks: NPR; 2020. Available from: https://www.npr.org/2020/11/17/916890880/we-are-shipping-to-the-u-s-china-s-fentanyl-sellers-find-new-routes-to-drug-user. Accessed 6/26/24 2024.

9. Huber E, Robinson RC, Noe CE, Van Ness O. Who benefits from chronic opioid therapy? Rethinking the question of opioid misuse risk. Healthcare (MDPI). 2016;4:29.
10. Chou R, Turner JA, Devine EB, et al. The effectiveness and risks of long-term opioid therapy for chronic pain: a systematic review for a National Institutes of Health Pathways to Prevention Workshop. Ann Intern Med. 2015;162(4):276–86.
11. Holmes CP, Gatchel RJ, Adams LL, et al. An opioid screening instrument: long-term evaluation of the utility of the pain medication questionnaire. Pain Pract. 2006;6(2):74–88.
12. Busse JW, Wang L, Kamaleldin M, et al. Opioids for chronic noncancer pain: a systematic review and meta-analysis. JAMA. 2018;320(23):2448–60.
13. Jones CM, Day RO, Koes BW, et al. Opioid analgesia for acute low back pain and neck pain (the OPAL trial): a randomised placebo-controlled trial. Lancet. 2023;402(10398):304–12.
14. Franklin GM. Opioids for chronic noncancer pain: a position paper of the American Academy of Neurology. Neurology. 2014;83(14):1277–84.
15. Dowell D, Haegerich TM, Chou R. CDC guideline for prescribing opioids for chronic pain —United States. 2016. Morbidity and Mortality Weekly Reports Retrieved from https://www.cdc.gov/mmwr/volumes/65/rr/pdfs/rr6501e1.pdf
16. Furlan AD, Chaparro LE, Irvin E, Mailis-Gagnon A. A comparison between enriched and nonenriched enrollment randomized withdrawal trials of opioids for chronic noncancer pain. Pain Res Manag. 2011;16:337–51.
17. Meske DS, Lawal OD, Elder H, Langberg V, Paillard F, Katz N. Efficacy of opioids versus placebo in chronic pain: a systematic review and meta-analysis of enriched enrollment randomized withdrawal trials. J Pain Res. 2018;Volume 11:923–34.
18. Setnik B, Roland CL, Pixton G, Webster L. Measurement of drug liking in abuse potential studies: a comparison of unipolar and bipolar visual analog scales. J Clin Pharmacol. 2017;57(2):266–74.
19. Dowell D, Ragan KR, Jones CM, Baldwin GT, Chou R. CDC clinical practice guideline for prescribing opioids for pain—United States, 2022. MMWR Recomm Rep 2022;71(No. RR-3):1–95. https://doi.org/10.15585/mmwr.rr7103a1.
20. Dowell DMD, Ragan KR, Jones CM, Baldwin GT, Chou R. Prescribing opioids for pain — the new CDC clinical practice guideline. NEJM. 2022;387:2011. https://doi.org/10.1056/NEJMp2211040.
21. Qaseem A, McLean RM, O'Gurek D, Batur P, Lin K, Kansagara DL. Nonpharmacologic and pharmacologic management of acute pain from non–low back, musculoskeletal injuries in adults: a clinical guideline from the American College of Physicians and American Academy of Family Physicians. Ann Intern Med. 2020;173(9):739–48. https://doi.org/10.7326/M19-3602. [Epub Date 2020 Aug 18]. Erratum in: Ann Intern Med 2023 Apr;176(4):584. PMID: 32805126
22. Davergne T, Bailly F, Foltz V, Lambert A, Fautrel B, Gossec L. Effectiveness of a short functional restoration program for patients with chronic low back pain: a cohort study of 193 patients. Joint Bone Spine. 2020;87(6):640–6.
23. Ward R, Rauch SA, Axon RN, Saenger MS. Evaluation of a non-pharmacological interdisciplinary pain rehabilitation and functional restoration program for chronic pain in veterans. Health Serv Res. 2023;58(2):365–74.
24. Sandbrink F, Murphy JL, Johansson M, et al. The use of opioids in the management of chronic pain: synopsis of the 2022 updated US Department of Veterans Affairs and US Department of Defense clinical practice guideline. Ann Int Med. 2023;176(3):388–97.
25. Leitzelar BN, Koltyn KF. Exercise and neuropathic pain: a general overview of preclinical and clinical research. Sports Med. 2021;7:1–16. https://doi.org/10.1186/s40798-021-00307-9.
26. Zhang Y-H, Hu H-Y, Xiong Y-C, et al. Exercise for neuropathic pain: a systematic review and expert consensus. Front Med. 2021;8:756940. https://doi.org/10.3389/fmed.2021.756940.
27. Nguyen L-CL, Sing DC, Bozic KJ. Preoperative reduction of opioid use before total joint arthroplasty. J Arthroplast. 2016;31(9):282–7. https://doi.org/10.1016/j.arth.2016.01.068. [Epub 2016 Mar 17]

28. Kang HA, Wang B, Barner JC, et al. Opioid prescribing and outcomes in patients with sickle cell disease post–2016 CDC guideline. JAMA Int Med. 2024;184(5):510–8. https://doi.org/10.1001/jamainternmed.2023.8538.
29. Bulls HW, Hamm M, Wasilewski J, Olejniczak D, Bell SG, Liebschutz JM. "To prescribe or not to prescribe, that is the question": perspectives on opioid prescribing for chronic, cancer-related pain from clinicians who treat pain in survivorship. Cancer. 2024;130:3034. https://doi.org/10.1002/cncr.35299.
30. Schepis TS, McCabe SE. Trends in older adult nonmedical prescription drug use prevalence: results from the 2002–2003 and 2012–2013 National Survey on Drug Use and Health. Addict Behav. 2016;60:219–22.
31. Lipari RN, Hedden SL, Hughes A. Substance use and mental health estimates from the 2013 National Survey on Drug Use and Health: overview of findings. Rockville. 2016.
32. Rose AJ, McBain R, Schuler MS, et al. Effect of age on opioid prescribing, overdose, and mortality in Massachusetts, 2011 to 2015. J Am Geriatr Soc. 2019;67(1):128–32. https://doi.org/10.1111/jgs.15659. [Epub 2018 Nov 24]
33. Campbell CI, Weisner C, LeResche L, et al. Age and gender trends in long-term opioid analgesic use for noncancer pain. Am J Public Health. 2010;100(12):2541–7. https://doi.org/10.2105/AJPH.2009.180646. [Epub Date: September 20, 2011]
34. Sullivan MD, Howe CQ. Opioid therapy for chronic pain in the United States: promises and perils. Pain. 2013;(154):S94–S100. https://doi.org/10.1016/j.pain.2013.09.009. [Epub 2013 Sep 11]
35. Leung J, Santo T Jr, Colledge-Frisby S, et al. Mood and anxiety symptoms in persons taking prescription opioids: a systematic review with meta-analyses of longitudinal studies. Pain Med. 2022;23(8):1442–56. https://doi.org/10.1093/pm/pnac029.
36. Zedler BK, Saunders WB, Joyce AR, Vick CC, Murrelle EL. Validation of a screening risk index for serious prescription opioid-induced respiratory depression or overdose in a US commercial health plan claims database. Pain Med. 2018;19(1):68–78. https://doi.org/10.1093/pm/pnx009.
37. Passik SD, Kirsh KL, Whitcomb L, et al. A new tool to assess and document pain outcomes in chronic pain patients receiving opioid therapy. Clin Ther. 2004;26(4):552–61.
38. Chen JH, Humphreys K, Shah NH, Lembke A. Distribution of opioids by different types of Medicare prescribers. JAMA Int Med. 2016;176(2):259–61.
39. Callinan CE, Neuman MD, Lacy KE, Gabison C, Ashburn MA. The initiation of chronic opioids: a survey of chronic pain patients. J Pain. 2017;18(4):360–5. https://doi.org/10.1016/j.jpain.2016.11.001. [Epub 2016 Dec 3]
40. Bohnert AS, Valenstein M, Bair MJ, Ganoczy D, McCarthy JF, Ilgen MA. Association between opioid prescribing patterns and opioid overdose-related deaths. JAMA. 2011;305:1315–21.
41. American Psychiatric Association. Diagnostic and statistical manual of mental disorders (5th ed). 2013. https://doi.org/10.1176/appi.books.9780890425596.
42. Dowell D, Haegerich TM, Chou R. No shortcuts to safer opioid prescribing. NEJM. 2019;380:2285. https://doi.org/10.1056/NEJMp1904190. [Published online first 4/24/19]
43. Darnall BD, Juurlink D, Kerns RD, et al. International stakeholder community of pain experts and leaders call for an urgent action on forced opioid tapering. Pain Med. 2019;20(3):429–33. https://doi.org/10.1093/pm/pny228PMC6657573.
44. Eccleston C, Fisher E, Thomas KH, et al. Interventions for the reduction of prescribed opioid use in chronic non-cancer pain. Cochrane Database Syst Rev. 2017;11 https://doi.org/10.1002/14651858.CD010323.pub3.
45. McPherson S, Smith CL, Dobscha SK, et al. Changes in pain intensity after discontinuation of long-term opioid therapy for chronic noncancer pain. Pain. 2018;159(10):2097–104. https://doi.org/10.1097/j.pain.0000000000001315.
46. Frank JW, Carey E, Nolan C, Hale A, Nugent S, Krebs EE. Association between opioid dose reduction against patients' wishes and change in pain severity. J Gen Intern Med. 2020;(35):910–7. https://doi.org/10.1007/s11606-020-06294-z. [Epub 2020 Nov 3]

47. Goesling J, Moser SE, Lin LA, Hassett AL, Wasserman RA, Brummett CM. Discrepancies between perceived benefit of opioids and self-reported patient outcomes. Pain Med. 2018;19(2):297–306. https://doi.org/10.1093/pm/pnw263.
48. Sandhu HK, Booth K, Furlan AD, et al. Reducing opioid use for chronic pain with a group-based intervention: a randomized clinical trial. JAMA. 2023;329(20):1745–56. https://doi.org/10.1001/jama.2023.6454. [Epub Date 2023 May 23]
49. Singh V. Pain management best practices inter-agency task force: pain management: best practices. 2019. Washington, D.C. Retrieved from https://www.hhs.gov/sites/default/files/pain-mgmt-best-practices-draft-final-report-05062019.pdf
50. Sullivan MD, Turner JA, DiLodovico C, D'Appollonio A, Stephens K, Chan Y-F. Prescription opioid taper support for outpatients with chronic pain: a randomized controlled trial. J Pain. 2017;18(3):308–18. https://doi.org/10.1016/j.jpain.2016.11.003. [Epub 2016 Nov 28]
51. Powell VD, Rosenberg JM, Yaganti A, et al. Evaluation of buprenorphine rotation in patients receiving long-term opioids for chronic pain: a systematic review. JAMA Netw Open. 2021;4(9):e2124152. https://doi.org/10.1001/jamanetworkopen.2021.24152.
52. Thakrar AP, Jablonski L, Ratner J, Rastegar DA. Micro-dosing intravenous buprenorphine to rapidly transition from full opioid agonists. J Addict Med. 2022;16(1):122–4. https://doi.org/10.1097/ADM.0000000000000838.
53. Randhawa PA, Brar R, Nolan S. Buprenorphine–naloxone "microdosing": an alternative induction approach for the treatment of opioid use disorder in the wake of North America's increasingly potent illicit drug market. CMAJ. 2020;192(3):E73. https://doi.org/10.1503/cmaj.74018.
54. Raheemullah A, Benhamou O-M, Kuo J, Lembke A. Buprenorphine microdosing cross tapers: a time for change. Int J Environ Res Public Health. 2022;19(24):16436. https://doi.org/10.3390/ijerph192416436.
55. Dahan A, Yassen A, Bijl H, et al. Comparison of the respiratory effects of intravenous buprenorphine and fentanyl in humans and rats. Br J Anaesth. 2005;94(6):825–34. [Epub 2005 Apr 15]
56. Koppert W, Ihmsen H, Körber N, et al. Different profiles of buprenorphine-induced analgesia and antihyperalgesia in a human pain model. Pain. 2005;118(1–2):15–22.
57. Expansion of induction of buprenorphine via telemedicine encounter. National Archives. (3/1/2023). Retrieved from https://www.federalregister.gov/documents/2023/03/01/2023-04217/expansion-of-induction-of-buprenorphine-via-telemedicine-encounter
58. Khoromi S, Cui L, Nackers L, Max MB. Morphine, nortriptyline and their combination vs. placebo in patients with chronic lumbar root pain. Pain. 2007;130(1–2):66–75. https://doi.org/10.1016/j.pain.2006.10.029. [Epub 2006 Dec 19]
59. Goldenberg DL, Clauw DJ, Palmer RE, Clair AG. Opioid use in fibromyalgia: a cautionary tale. Mayo Clin Proc. 2016;91(5):640–8. https://doi.org/10.1016/j.mayocp.2016.02.002. [Epub 2016 Mar 11]
60. Drossman DA, Morris CB, Edwards H, et al. Diagnosis, characterization, and 3-month outcome after detoxification of 39 patients with narcotic bowel syndrome. Am J Gastroenterol. 2012;107(9):1426–40. https://doi.org/10.1038/ajg.2012.142. [Epub 2012 Jun 19]
61. Langer-Gould AM, Anderson WE, Armstrong MJ, et al. The American Academy of Neurology's top five choosing wisely recommendations. Neurology. 2013;81(11):1004–11. https://doi.org/10.1212/WNL.0b013e31828aab14. [Epub 2013 Feb 20]
62. Casucci G, Cevoli S. Controversies in migraine treatment: opioids should be avoided. Neurol Sci. 2013;34:125–8. https://doi.org/10.1007/s10072-013-1395-8.
63. Mikosz CA, Zhang K, Haegerich T, et al. Indication-specific opioid prescribing for US patients with Medicaid or private insurance, 2017. JAMA Netw Open. 2020;3(5):e204514. https://doi.org/10.1001/jamanetworkopen.2020.4514.
64. Pasricha SV, Tadrous M, Khuu W, et al. Clinical indications associated with opioid initiation for pain management in Ontario, Canada: a population-based cohort study. Pain. 2018;159(8):1562–8. https://doi.org/10.1097/j.pain.0000000000001242.
65. Sullivan MD, Edlund MJ, Zhang L, Unützer J, Wells KB. Association between mental health disorders, problem drug use, and regular prescription opioid use. Arch Intern Med. 2006;166(19):2087–93. https://doi.org/10.1001/archinte.166.19.2087.

66. Sullivan MD. Depression effects on long-term prescription opioid use, abuse, and addiction. Clin J Pain. 2018;34(9):878–84. https://doi.org/10.1097/AJP.0000000000000603.
67. Stephens AR, Presson AP, Chen D, Tyser AR, Kazmers NH. Inter-specialty variation of the Press Ganey outpatient medical practice survey. Medicine. 2021;100(12):e25211. https://doi.org/10.1097/MD.0000000000025211.
68. Finnerup NB, Attal N, Haroutounian S, et al. Pharmacotherapy for neuropathic pain in adults: a systematic review and meta-analysis. Lancet Neurol. 2015;14(2):162–73.
69. Ang SP, Sidharthan S, Lai W, et al. Cannabinoids as a potential alternative to opioids in the management of various pain subtypes: benefits, limitations, and risks. Pain Ther. 2023;12(2):355–75.
70. Moore A, Straube S, Fisher E, Eccleston C. Cannabidiol (CBD) products for pain: ineffective, expensive, and with potential harms. J Pain. 2024;25(4):833–42. https://doi.org/10.1016/j.jpain.2023.10.009. [Epub 2023 Oct 18]
71. de Oliveira CO, Carvalho LB, Carlos K, et al. Opioids for restless legs syndrome. Cochrane Database Syst Rev. 2016;2016:6. https://doi.org/10.1002/14651858.CD006941.pub2.
72. Graven-Nielsen CS, Knoph CS, Okdahl T, et al. Opioids in the treatment of chronic idiopathic diarrhea in humans—a systematic review and treatment guideline. J Clin Med. 2023;12(7):2488. https://doi.org/10.3390/jcm12072488.
73. Belvisi M, Geppetti P. Cough• 7: current and future drugs for the treatment of chronic cough. Thorax. 2004;59(5):438–40.

Index

C. E. Noe (ed.), *Musculoskeletal Pain*,
https://doi.org/10.1007/978-3-031-86057-7

P

GPSR Compliance

The European Union's (EU) General Product Safety Regulation (GPSR) is a set of rules that requires consumer products to be safe and our obligations to ensure this.

If you have any concerns about our products, you can contact us on ProductSafety@springernature.com

In case Publisher is established outside the EU, the EU authorized representative is:

Springer Nature Customer Service Center GmbH
Europaplatz 3
69115 Heidelberg, Germany

Batch number: 10126020

Printed by Printforce, the Netherlands